Innovations in BEHAVIOURAL HEALTH ARCHITECTURE

Innovations in Behavioural Health Architecture is the most comprehensive book written on this topic in more than 40 years. It examines the ways in which healthcare architecture can contribute, as a highly valued informational and reference source, to the provision of psychiatric and addictive disorder treatment in communities around the world. It provides an overview of the need for a new generation of progressively planned and designed treatment centres – both inpatient and outpatient care environments – and the advantages, challenges, and opportunities associated with meeting the burgeoning need for treatment settings of this type. Additional chapters address the specifics of geriatric psychiatry and its architectural ramifications in light of the rapid aging of societies globally and provide a comprehensive compendium of planning and design considerations for these places in both inpatient and outpatient care contexts. Finally, the book presents an expansive and fully illustrated set of international case studies that express state-of-the-art advancements in architecture for behavioural healthcare.

Stephen Verderber is an award-winning scholar, researcher, and registered architect (US) whose core specialty is architecture, design therapeutics, and health. He is Professor at the John H. Daniels Faculty of Architecture, Landscape and Design and at the Dalla Lana School of Public Health, at the University of Toronto, Canada. He holds a doctorate in architecture from the University of Michigan, is cofounder of R-2ARCH, and is widely published. His books include *Healthcare Architecture in an Era of Radical Transformation* (2000), *Compassion in Architecture: Evidence-Based Design for Health* (2005), *Innovations in Hospice Architecture* (2005), *Innovations in Hospital Architecture* (2010), *Sprawling Cities and Our Endangered Public Health* (2012), and *Innovations in Transportable Healthcare Architecture* (2016).

Innovations in BEHAVIOURAL HEALTH ARCHITECTURE

Stephen Verderber

Routledge
Taylor & Francis Group
LONDON AND NEW YORK

First published 2018
by Routledge
2 Park Square, Milton Park, Abingdon, Oxon OX14 4RN

and by Routledge
711 Third Avenue, New York, NY 10017

Routledge is an imprint of the Taylor & Francis Group, an informa business

British Library Cataloguing-in-Publication Data
A catalogue record for this book is available from the British Library

Library of Congress Cataloging-in-Publication Data
Names: Verderber, Stephen, author.
Title: Innovations in behavioural health architecture / Stephen Verderber.
Description: Milton Park, Abingdon ; New York, NY : Routledge, 2018. |
Includes bibliographical references and index.
Identifiers: LCCN 2017038226 | ISBN 9780415789646 (hbk : alk. paper) |
ISBN 9781315213866 (ebk)
Subjects: LCSH: Hospital architecture. | Health facilities—Design and
construction. | Architecture—Health aspects.
Classification: LCC RA967 .V4735 2018 | DDC 725/.51—dc23
LC record available at https://lccn.loc.gov/2017038226

ISBN: 978-0-415-78964-6 (hbk)
ISBN: 978-1-315-21386-6 (ebk)

Typeset in Avenir LT Std
by Apex CoVantage, LLC

Printed and bound in India by Replika Press Pvt. Ltd.

For my amazing children, Elyssa Leigh Verderber and Alexander Verderber.

Contents

Illustration credits

FRONT COVER PHOTO

Centre for the Mentally Handicapped in Alcolea, Cordoba, Spain. Taller de Arquitectura/Rico+Roa, Cordoba, Spain. Photo: D. Fernando Alda.

PREFACE AND ACKNOWLEDGMENTS

Figures P.1 and P.2: Courtesy of the Historic New Orleans Collection. Photos: Source Unknown. xv

BACK COVER PHOTOS

Kingfisher Court, Radlett, Hertfordshire, Greater London, UK: P+HS Architects, Leeds, UK. Photo: David Churchill.

Vermont Psychiatric Care Hospital, Berlin, Vermont, USA: architecture+, Troy, New York, USA/Black River Design, Montpelier, Vermont, USA.

Helsingor Psychiatric Hospital and Clinic, Helsingor, Denmark: JDS/BIG, Copenhagen, Denmark.

Linn Dara Child and Adolescent Centre at Cherry Hill Hospital, Dublin, Ireland: Reddy Architecture + Urbanism, London, UK. Photo: Ros Kavanagh.

CHAPTER 2

2.1	Photo: Source unknown.	17
2.2–2.5	Photo: Oscar Menzer.	21–22
2.6	Drawing: Mengjii Cheng.	23
2.7a–c	Photo: Earl Saundres.	24
2.8	Photo: Source unknown.	25
2.9	Drawing: Mengjie Cheng.	25
2.10–2.11	Photos: Source unknown.	26
2.12	Photo: Orlando R. Cabanban.	26
2.13	Drawing: Skidmore, Owings, and Merrill.	27
2.14	Photo: Orlando R. Cabanban.	27
2.15	Drawing: Hougen, Good & Pfaller Associates.	28
2.16	Drawing: Shih-En (Grace) Chang.	30
2.17a–j	Illustration: Stephen Verderber/Gabriel Valdivieso.	31
2.18–2.20	Photos: Source unknown.	32–33
2.21a-c to 2.22	Drawings/Photo: Courtesy Richard Meier Architects.	33

CHAPTER 6

Preface and acknowledgments

When she boarded the streetcar that fall afternoon in Toronto, we all sensed something was amiss. She suddenly pushed a woman aside and scolded her to sit down. The offended woman protested, and then the real offender became abusive, cursing loudly. She then spat on the seated woman, again and again as the profanities continued. Was it an alcoholic seizure? A passenger called out toward the driver at the front of the streetcar for help. We sat frozen. It was packed. I was near the rear of the car as the scene unfolded. Could the operator see or hear what was happening? Another passenger grasped the cursing woman as she started to convulse. Another called for help. A small crowd gathered around her. Eventually the streetcar stopped. Then the ambulance arrived. Afterward, she told the paramedics she had no recollection of what just happened. As they asked her questions, she categorically denied having a drinking problem or ever even having sought treatment. She became indignant once again, refusing to get into the ambulance and repeatedly yelling, 'I *do not* have a drinking problem!' It appeared as if she was in fact quite humiliated by all of this, although she steadfastly refused to admit her need for help.

I am repeatedly stunned by how much social stigma persists toward persons suffering from a mental illness or addiction disorder. It's as if these persons are terminally flawed or inferior in some way. In most cases, self-destruction is not their intent, nor is it their intent to destroy the lives of all those close to them. The gnarly connotations of social stigma make it difficult for many to admit they could benefit from treatment. Tragically, access to treatment is denied to millions each day. Many end up on the streets. Homelessness is a chronic challenge for modern society. In San Francisco, a haven for the homeless in the United States, mental health specialists now routinely shadow the city's police officers while on duty because there are so many homeless on the streets its social service infrastructure is on the verge of total collapse. Isn't it ironic that in a city so wealthy and dependent on tourism, this last-ditch effort occurs in the face of widespread taxpayer indifference?

In Venezuela, the nation's psychiatric hospitals by 2017 ran nearly completely out of medications to treat its increasingly hopeless, forgotten population of addicted and mentally ill persons. The government attributed the absence of funding for these services to the recent collapse in global oil prices. Disenfranchised, the affected individuals are first removed from mainstream society and then left to rot in remote, forsaken psychiatric hospitals. In Nigeria, professional psychiatric care is virtually inaccessible for any person with psychosis. Fewer than 200 psychiatrists work in a country of 168 million, and since Nigerian culture treats psychosis as a supernatural affliction, psychiatrists are rarely seen first, if ever. As a result, supernatural spiritualists provide frontline mental health diagnoses and treatment. But even they are becoming overwhelmed by ever-expanding need, especially in light of the fact that the 'cure' administered by rural Nigerian folk-faith healers is often far worse than the initial illness itself.

Nearly one in five children in the United States each year suffer from a psychiatric disorder, and a current national shortage of medical specialists and inpatient facilities means many individuals will remain improperly, if completely, untreated (Shefali Luthra, 'How Gaps in Mental Health Care Play Out in Emergency Rooms', *National Public Radio*, 17 October 2016). Research presented at the 2016 annual meeting of the American College of Emergency Physicians provided some further insight into how frequently patients with mental health issues wind up in their nearest hospital emergency department (ED). This usually occurs because earlier opportunities to intervene were either misdiagnosed or left untreated, and pediatricians and child psychologists believe children to be among the hardest hit of all. The US *National Hospital Ambulatory Medical Care Survey*, which ranked health visits to all hospital EDs between 2001 and 2011, found that 6% of all ED patients of all ages had a preexisting psychiatric condition. More than 20% were admitted to hospital as inpatients for observation, compared with just 13% of all other persons coming to the ED. And about 11% of these mental health admittances required transfer to another hospital, compared to just 1.4% of those with a physical ailment.

A national shortage of inpatient beds for psychiatric patients is a big part of the problem in the United States. The American Academy of Child and Adolescent Psychiatry estimates that only 8,300 such specialists exist for as many as 15 million young persons in need, annually. Often, these persons end up in a pediatric or family practice clinic where neither the staff nor the facility is able to provide the needed support. Bed-availability tracking technology, for its part, also often fails in this quest to close the treatment gap. In Canada, 60% of those who suffer from a mental or addiction disorder do not seek out help for fear of being stigmatized in their community, according to the Mental Health Commission of Canada. In Toronto, a city that prides itself on having a relatively well-educated population and a formidable social safety net, 5,000 homeless persons on average sleep on the streets nightly. Many continue to hide their mental health issues from their workplace, family, and friends. Greater public advocacy and awareness is needed to help address this dilemma. And what of the hundreds of thousands of dispossessed migrants streaming into Europe from Africa and the Middle East? Do their growing, unmet mental health needs not constitute a major crisis? Working-class neighborhoods in the northern section of Paris filled up in 2016 with thousands of refugees, persons barely eking out an existence amid densely packed enclaves of pup tents hurriedly set up along sidewalks, under bridges, and in rail stations. These *ad hoc* 'wildcat encampments' thrust to the public forefront the severe and growing inadequacies of existing social services.

My first real exposure to the built environment needs of the mentally ill and persons with addiction disorders was in New Orleans. The venerable DePaul Hospital, an institution located next to Audubon Park in the uptown section of that city, had commissioned our firm, R-2ARCH, to develop a campus master plan for them; it focused on identifying repurposing options for its existing buildings and make recommendations for the design of a new residential pavilion. This work began with a postoccupancy assessment of its historic 11-acre campus and all its buildings. The Catholic Sisters of St. Vincent DePaul provided care for the mentally ill in New Orleans dating from 1841, at Charity Hospital in downtown New Orleans. In 1863 the sisters established the first dedicated psychiatric ward in the city in that hospital. In 1876 they opened this freestanding asylum uptown (Figures P.1 and P.2). Side wings were added later to the main building and outbuildings were constructed in the intervening decades, although sadly, the original 1876 building was demolished after sustaining wind damage in Hurricane Betsy in 1965. Until the mid-20th century, the protected grounds of this asylum included a small farm and modest structures housing occupational workshops for patients. The same type of high wall that surrounded virtually every asylum surrounded this asylum (and still does, partially). After a due-diligence assessment of the campus, we proposed a multiphased redevelopment plan, a plan later to receive national recognition in a *Progressive Architecture* award (1991). I had been taken aback by its lockdown units, similar to those in the iconic 1976 film *One Flew Over the Cuckoo's Nest*, and especially because DePaul was by then a for-profit institution, owned and operated by Hospital Corporation of American (HCA), one of nearly 40 psychiatric facilities it owned across the United States at the time.

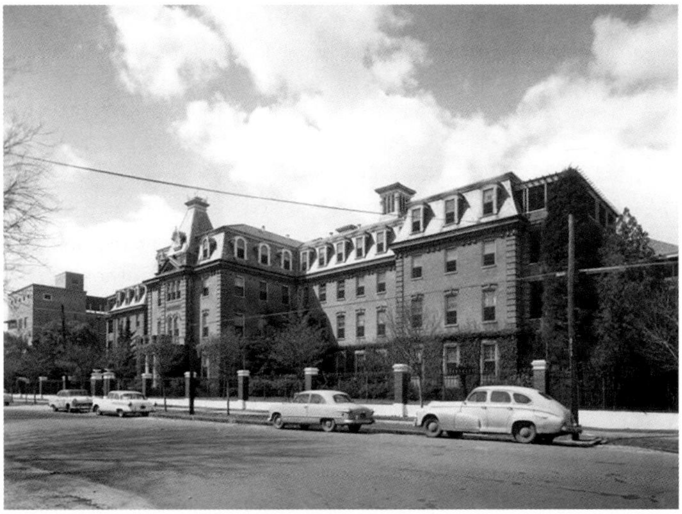

P.1 DePaul Hospital, New Orleans, circa 1955.

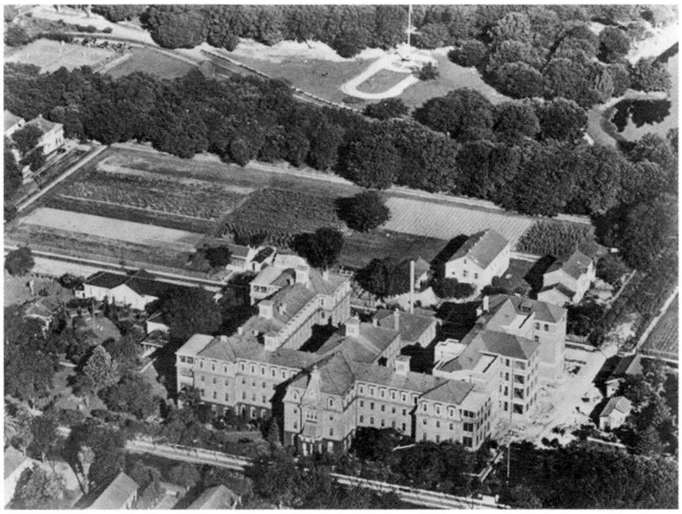

P.2 DePaul Hospital, New Orleans, circa 1885.

My second upfront exposure to individuals with mental health disorders would be different because it was so personal. It occurred in the aftermath of Hurricane Katrina in 2005. It was no secret that in the years preceding the disaster, New Orleans suffered from a severe shortage of inpatient psychiatric beds and very few neighborhood mental health clinics. Prior to Katrina, the city's mental health support network was already in tatters; then things got much worse. Tens of thousands faced long-term displacement after 80% of the city flooded and as people attempted to return to the hardest hit neighborhoods, the sheer stress of it all simply overwhelmed them. The poorest were hit disproportionally hard, as is always the case in the aftermath of disaster. The mental health needs of displaced and dispossessed persons (1,863 died, in all) were acute. Many with a prior, diagnosed mental illness experienced total emotional breakdown because it was simply too much bear. Others wandered about in an aimless daze, up and down the devastated streets of their old neighborhoods as if now on some different, unrecognizable planet. An article published some five years later, titled 'The Impact of Hurricane Katrina on the Mental and Physical Health of Low-Income Parents in New Orleans' (American Journal of Orthopsychiatry 2010, 80(2):237–247), recounted the struggles of returnees' attempts to cope with Katrina's aftermath. A disaster knows no geographic, socioeconomic, racial, or mental health boundaries and the cumulative stress took its toll on thousands of families, including my own.

The idea for this book evolved from these life experiences, in client-architect relationships, and in working with those who have counseled my then-14-year-old daughter in the years since 2005. I am grateful to so many on both a personal and professional level, and this list of persons who helped in some way is definitely long, in terms of architectural support and encouragement for this project, this includes Frank Pitt and Barbara Miszkiel, who participated in graduate design studio 'laboratory experiments' I directed in 2015 and 2016 at the University of Toronto. Numerous specialists have been a source of guidance and inspiration, including the firms and individuals who contributed their work in the form of case studies.

That said, this book would have been impossible without the support and encouragement of family, friends, colleagues, and the inspiring, fearless work of Christopher Alexander and Jane Jacobs. I am grateful for the support provided by my team of graduate research assistants at the University of Toronto. Timothy Boll served as lead research assistant from 2013 to 2017 and worked diligently to shape the various chapters. I am thankful for the valuable assistance provided by Ramsey Leung, Esther Cheng, Yishan Yue, and

Jordan Livings for help in developing specific sections including the review of recently built projects globally, historical precursors, recent evidence-based research on the subject, and the history of the Centre for Addiction and Mental Health in Toronto. Thanks also to research assistants Gabriel Valdivieso, Mengjie Cheng, Shih-En (Grace) Chang, Kian Hosseinnia, Josh Sinet, and Josie Harrison for helping to bring the project across the finish line. I am grateful for the support of the John H. Daniels Faculty of Architecture, Landscape and Design, and its Dean, Richard Sommer, at the University of Toronto; as well as the Dalla Lana School of Public Health, and its former Dean, Howard Hu; and to Adelstein Brown, director of the Institute for Health Policy, Management and Evaluation at the University of Toronto (currently Interim Dean at the Dalla Lana School of Public Health). Thanks also to Shirley Chan, grants and sponsored research specialist at the Daniels Faculty at the University of Toronto.

As large numbers of people begin the process of migrating further inland in the *great retreat* from threatened coastal regions in the 21st century, existing healthcare support networks will be hard-pressed to adroitly respond to the social and psychological needs of the displaced. Forced dislocation is something I have experienced firsthand, and what the future portends will likely dwarf what has been experienced thus far. Despite the false promises of government, and the shrill chorus of climate change deniers and their vested financial interests, the reality is that global societies are dangerously unprepared to cope with the consequences of the environmental, economic, and sociopolitical upheaval likely ahead. The magnitude of this upheaval will be intensified since nearly 80% of the world's population lives in a coastal region. The United Nations reports the world's overall population in 2016 was 7.3 billion, a number expected to balloon to 9.7 billion by 2050, with medically underserved communities in the poorest countries and poorest cities most acutely vulnerable.

This is the fourth book in the series *Innovations in Architecture and Health* published by Routledge in the United Kingdom. The previous three titles I authored were *Innovations in Hospice Architecture* (2005), with Ben J. Refuerzo as second author; *Innovations in Hospital Architecture* (2010); and *Innovations in Transportable Healthcare Architecture* (2016). This series has focused on typologically based inquiries into current issues in the planning and design of the built environment for human and environmental health, and as such has provided a rare opportunity. For this I am most grateful to Routledge for its continuing support of these publications for the international community. Special thanks to my editors, Caroline Mallinder (Book 1) and Fran Ford and Grace Harrison (Books 2–4). May this fourth installment serve you well.

TORONTO,
NOVEMBER 2017

PART 1

Background

Introduction

CHAPTER 1

Dramatic events are transforming the global mental health landscape. In developing regions, where four fifths of the world's population reside, noncommunicable diseases (NCDs) are supplanting traditional diseases as leading causes of disability and premature death. By the year 2020, NCDs are expected to account for 7 out of every 10 deaths in developing regions, due in large part to an aging global population, combined with declining birth rates. The rate of change combined with the absolute numbers impacted will pose serious challenges to healthcare systems, requiring difficult decisions. Worse, many governments lack basic health status population data, so necessary in effective policy making.[1] Recent reports in the *Lancet* and the *Lancet Psychiatry* have underscored the gravity of this situation, concluding the growing burden of untreated mental disorders in the world's two most populous countries, China and India alone, cannot be adequately addressed without fundamental changes to their internal healthcare systems.[2] In these two countries, less than 10% of those who suffer from a mental disorder ever receive treatment, and the burden of disability is higher in these places than in all Western nations combined. These two countries, accounting for one third of the world's entire population, are in the midst of major economic transformations, and will need to invest significantly more than the less than 1% they currently devote to mental health care services.

China is especially ill prepared for the coming tsunami of need as its population ages. Its central government started a program in 2004 that, to date, has trained 10,000 psychiatrists and built hundreds of outpatient community mental health centers, representing an unprecedented national investment in psychiatric care.[3] In addition, folk medicine is an integral if unorthodox component of the healthcare system in numerous countries: this includes the work of traditional faith healers, herbalists, and spiritualists who have practiced their traditions for centuries. In China, many doctors receive some exposure to the traditional healing arts (i.e., herbal treatments, acupuncture, and qigong). In India, similarly, many physicians incorporate yoga and Ayurveda traditions in their practices, and medical doctors and folk healers are just now beginning to collaborate in some places. In Nigeria, folk tribal healers are becoming ever-slightly willing to treat conventional diagnoses such as depression and anxiety, although not schizophrenia or bipolar disorder, both traditionally considered demonic afflictions.[4]

The rate of occurrence of depression, alcohol dependency, and schizophrenia tend to be underestimated by researchers who take account of only a nation's death rate and not the occurrence of mental disability. The reasons for this bias are many, but one reason has been an overarching focus on infectious disease; this has accounted for historically blasé attitudes toward the study of mental health in many parts of the world.[5] While psychiatric illnesses are responsible for little more than 1% of all deaths worldwide, annually, they account for nearly 11% of the total global disease burden. Adults under the age of 70 in sub-Saharan Africa now face a higher probability of death from an NCD than adults of the same age in highly developed societies.[6] How are various disease burdens comparatively measured? Research in the past two decades has identified a set of metrics for documenting health outcomes associated with disease and disability. This research has yielded a metric widely known as the *Disability-Adjusted Life Year* (DALY) index. The DALY index documents the total years of life lost due to premature death as a fraction of the total years lived with a disability. One DALY is therefore the equivalent of one lost year of a healthy life. A premature death is defined as one that occurs before the age a dying person could have been expected to live if she or he were a member of a standardized population with a life expectancy at birth equivalent to that of the world's longest-surviving population (Japan).[7]

The unseen burdens of psychiatric illness are both timeless and omnipresent, and epidemiological research on the quantification of the disease burden index has until recently been rather undependable. Of the 10 leading causes of disability worldwide in 1990 – as measured in years lived with a disability – 5 were psychiatric conditions: unipolar depression, alcohol and substance abuse, bipolar affective disorders (manic depression), schizophrenia, and obsessive compulsive disorders. Unipolar depression alone is responsible for more than 1 in every 10 years of life lived with a disability worldwide. Altogether, psychiatric and neurological conditions account for 28% of all years of living with a disease, compared with only 1.4% of all deaths globally. Alcohol abuse is a leading cause of male disability in advanced developed societies and fifth highest in less-developed societies.[8] That said, mental illness and other NCDs are rapidly emerging as dominant causes of ill health worldwide and this trend shows no signs of diminishing.[9] In 2010, mental and substance abuse disorders accounted for 183.9 million aggregate DALYs, translating into 7.4% of all DALYs worldwide. Overall, these disorders are the fifth leading disease category of all global DALYs, with such disorders having increased by 37.6% in a 20-year period between 1990 and 2010.[10] What is the function of the physical environment and the effects of human mistreatment of planet Earth in predicting the occurrence of mental illness and substance addiction?

Urbanization

The world's population as of 2015 was 7.3 billion, a number expected to rise to 8.5 billion by the year 2030. By 2050, 66% of the world's population is expected to live in urbanized regions.[11] Globalization, combined with advancements made possible by telecommunication networks, long-distance air travel, and the Internet, is fueling accelerated rates of urbanization. Rural-to-urban migratory shifts are happening with increasing frequency as people relocate to cities in unprecedented numbers. By comparison, in the mid-1970s, less than 40% of the world's population lived in cities.[12] Back in 1950, 41 of the world's 100 largest cities were in less-developed countries. By 1995 this statistic had risen to 64 cities and keeps arcing ever upward.[13] Rapid urbanization warrants examining the complex interrelationships between the experience of living in increasingly dense cities and the status of their residents' mental health and well-being. Admission rates to psychiatric institutions are often significantly higher in urban areas compared to rural areas. In one nationwide study in the Netherlands, hospital admission rates were twice as high in the most highly urbanized municipalities compared to the least urbanized municipalities in the country.[14] In another study, of 4.4 million persons living in Sweden, a similar rural-versus-urban pattern was found to exist with higher incidences of psychosis occurring in the latter contexts.[15] This pattern was consistent across all major psychiatric disorders and across study groups of children and adolescents, the aged, men and women, married couples, and among unmarried individuals.[16]

Systematic research on the incidence of mental illness among urban residents dates from the 1950s, stemming from findings showing first-time hospitalization rates for schizophrenics were higher in the densest inner urban neighborhoods of Chicago, with comparable admission rates gradually decreasing outward toward the urban periphery.[17] It was concluded population density *per se*, combined with an inadequate social and physical infrastructural support network, is associated with a higher level of mental illness, irrespective of ethnicity, race, or income level.[18] From the 1970s to the present, the work of psychiatric researchers has focused on further understanding this interrelationship. Urbanization in many less-developed countries has been linked to increasing occurrences of depression and anxiety disorders, and particularly among low-income women.[19] Not until 1991 did the World Health Organization (WHO) officially acknowledge this pending crisis, and only then did it act to define eight specific diseases believed to be deserving of particular attention and policy action, reflective of clearly discernable quality-of-life risk factors in urban environments.[20]

Often, these risk factors become magnified as the size of the city and its surrounding region intensifies, and length of residency in such places has been linked with higher probabilities for developing psychosis within one's lifetime.[21] In a recent meta-analysis of numerous research studies, the occurrence of schizophrenia in dense cities was found to increase by as much as 72%. It is now estimated that urbanization accounts for nearly 30% of all reported cases of schizophrenia in all Western countries.[22] Effective social support infrastructures, for their part, are a necessary ingredient in order to help in early detection. By contrast, a socially fragmented urban community – that is, one with high social and income inequality; pervasive crime; and poor, ineffective neighborhood-level social supports – is in general associated with higher rates of psychosis. The concept of urban *social capital* has become widely known in the past 15 years in terms of how it can help explain these outcomes, for better and worse. Urban areas with relatively high levels of intrinsic, or built-in, social capital tend to report lower rates of mental illness and substance addiction, and this has been attributed to a higher overall social cohesiveness quotient as defined by their existing physical, environmental, and sociocultural infrastructures.[23]

While specific definitions of social capital are many, the sociologist Robert Putnam postulates it is definable by five key characteristics, centered on the presence of (1) viable community social networks; (2) active civic engagement and participation; (3) a shared collective sense of civic identity and of belonging to something larger and more important than oneself, solidarity, and social equality; (4) reciprocity and effective, normative communication channels to achieve mutual cooperation, a shared sense of purpose, and a sense of obligation to help others in need, with the confidence this will be reciprocated if and when needed; and (5) a general presence of trust in the community and throughout its constituent social networks.[24] The social capital construct has been extended more recently to include the impact of urbanization on individuals' mental health status, with higher social capital associated with lower rates of mental illness and addictive disorders. Restated, cities with more in-place 'bridging' social capital infrastructure will more naturally produce and sustain the types of social safety nets necessary to buffer the psychological impacts of adverse life events.[25]

These urban communities are also better positioned to more successfully acquire and hold on to educational, health, and housing resources linked to improved mental health outcomes. Kwame McKenzie views urban social capital as relatively easy to destroy, but tediously slow to build back up, once lost. This is because it takes so much time to reestablish trust and to rebuild social structures that previously fostered positive life outcomes, before having been disrupted. He views rapid, unplanned urban sprawl as undermining the development of social cohesiveness because it destroys innumerable cognitive and structural horizontal bonds, and predictably, this results in a greater propensity for mental illness because the needed social buttresses and buffers erode and in time become completely dysfunctional. Cities with a characteristically low level of social capital tend to be associated with a characteristically high level of mistrust and the need to look out for oneself, above all else. This inadvertently results in a toxicogenic psychological environment of high stress compounded by low mutual social support. This manifests in disconnection from one's neighbors, the people one works with, one's spouse and children, and even prior friendships from long ago.[26]

The United Nations (UN) contends that strong, effective government at all levels is the necessary foundation for building positive urban social capital in the world's burgeoning cities.[27] A recent UN report concluded that good governance must be a genuinely participatory proposition, a process drawing into the manifold of concern the best interests of all stakeholders in a given society, and especially the interests of the historically marginalized and economically disadvantaged. It views the prerequisites for this urban condition consist of transparency, responsiveness, consensus orientation, and mutual accountability. A prior WHO report on this same subject (2003) concluded the fundamental premise of urban planning and development at all levels must be to promote and implement policies and built initiatives that serve the best interests of everyone because a city and its surrounding region is both a human and an environmental ecosystem, and because of this, positive social supports are needed on multiple levels, including physical, social, economic, and psychological. To this end, the most recent WHO guide to planning for urban communities has listed among its key health objectives the establishment of policies to encourage and promote social cohesiveness, premised on the assumption that mass urbanization itself is often traumatic, with significant human health consequences.[28]

Climate change

Global climate change is a reality, and will increasingly contribute to mental illnesses in human populations.[29] For thousands of years, civilization flourished within specific geographic-climatic ranges, ranges that remained relatively unchanged across the millennia.[30] As climate science advances, our species must brace for dramatic population dislocations, with the greatest challenges coming from a lack of food and drinkable water – food and water insecurity – vector-borne diseases, and weather-induced disruptions, including the deleterious impacts of significantly higher temperature levels. Comparatively little attention, however, is devoted currently to the myriad ways in which climate change is likely to impact our mental health and well-being.[31] It is predicted to have an adverse, widespread impact regardless.[32] This is because adverse mental health outcomes are beginning to be experienced in many places in the form of psychological trauma due to posttraumatic stress disorder (PTSD) and related disorders associated with climate change.[33] Identified as an adverse mental health outcome, PTSD is occurring more and more in the aftermath of natural, as well as human-induced, disasters.[34] Vulnerable populations, particularly in the poorest countries, are especially at risk psychologically, although the citizens of rich and poor regions alike will be significantly affected.[35]

In the United States, Hurricane Katrina in 2005 was one of the worst natural disasters in that nation's history.[36] Beyond the sheer physical devastation, this hurricane resulted in elevated levels of mental disorders among its survivors (discussed in some greater length in Chapter 3).[37] The region's healthcare network was ravaged, as only 1 of 11 hospitals was able to remain open.[38] The tedious pace of psychological recovery in post-Katrina New Orleans and across the Mississippi Gulf Coast demonstrated why additional, much improved mental health support resources would be needed in the aftermath of future major disasters.[39] It is the poorest who disproportionately bear the direct psychological brunt, including, as became apparent in Katrina, many thousands of low-income African-American single mothers.[40] Adverse mental health consequences can persist for years after the actual disaster event and remain most severe for those who sustained the greatest losses, including the aftereffects of permanent displacement (see Chapter 3).[41]

Impacted populations include those fleeing droughts and other natural disasters, marauders in South Sudan, drug gangs in Central America, and the activities of the Islamic State in the Middle East.[42] Economic malaise is also a contributor. In times of recession and high unemployment, the need for mental health support rises significantly.[43] More knowledge is needed on the relationship between economic adversities triggered by climate change and psychopathologies, including suicide, antisocialism, behavioural mood disorders, substance abuse, and depression.[44] The term *treatment gap* is being used more frequently to describe the difference between the need for treatment versus the actual availability of treatment services in a given locale. This gap persists in rural and urban contexts, impacting rich and poor alike. Research is delineating a fuller picture of the treatment gap's extensiveness related to the distribution of current mental health care resources throughout the world, the generation of more accurate statistics on rates of occurrence, and a more precise classification system.[45] That said, the WHO has recently identified several issues of priority:

Chronic lack of funding – The political will to invest in mental health is slowly growing but remains astonishingly low. Currently, only about 2% of the total healthcare budget is spent on mental health services in majority low- and middle-income countries, and this funding is mainly in the form of support for inpatient psychiatric care. Similarly, while global investment in mental health services did increase ever so slightly between 2007 and 2013, in both relative and absolute terms, reaching US$134 million annually (on average), as a proportion of overall support for health it still remained less than 1% of total healthcare expenditures.

A global dementia epidemic – Recent epidemiological incidence projections indicate the number of people living with dementia and Alzheimer's syndrome will continue to expand dramatically, particularly among the oldest-old population cohort (285) in countries already experiencing dramatic demographic changes. The enormous cost of this trend for healthcare systems is just one of myriad challenges to be faced in the 21st century. Family members are often ill prepared to provide care for these persons, and the lack of affordable residential alternatives is becoming a worrisome challenge in many countries.

Lack of reliable mental health statistics – On a country-by-country basis, many ministries of health agencies do not currently have sophisticated health informatics databases on mental illness occurrences within their jurisdiction. This unfortunate situation persists in over two thirds of all nations globally, with these jurisdictions neither able to document their own internal needs nor able to contribute reliable information to the global discourse on the extent of service coverage for even the most severe types of mental disorders that exist within their own geographic borders.

Continued stigmatization – Negative stereotypes toward people living with a mental or substance addiction abound and seem to continue relatively unchecked. These are compounded by a lack of 'objective' markers or diagnostic tests that, often, is interpreted as further evidence of these cases somehow not being 'real' or genuinely physical in a classical sense compared to types of physical ailments and diseases far more easily observable. Comorbidities also remain widely misunderstood in countries, resulting in further stigmatization of those afflicted, compounded by the reality that cultural barriers continue to thwart an individual from seeking out and obtaining proper diagnosis and treatment.

Lack of grassroots advocacy – Stronger patients' rights advocacy groups, such as those that spawned the social movement on the need to research the HIV/AIDS phenomenon in the early 1980s, are needed at this time. In the case of HIV/AIDS, this effort had a profound positive impact worldwide. Further successes in establishing greater societal awareness and the will to take subsequent political action with regards to mental health and substance addiction awareness will be dependent on mounting a comparable movement. The absence of this global movement unfortunately prevents the widespread attention and support it deserves.

Health workforce inadequacies – The human resource challenges remain immense with regard to providing effective diagnosis and care for individuals with mental health and substance addictions, including the aforementioned need to diagnose and treat individuals experiencing comorbidity where a mental health disorder is part of the equation. Social and financial investments are in need of pronounced expansion to provide educational opportunities to train more specialists in the fields of social work, medicine, nursing, psychiatry and related health disciplines. This will result in more effective interdisciplinary, team-based models of care.

Lack of access to appropriate care – Widespread substance abuse, such as the current heroin and opioid epidemics, and associated high death rates, are a cold reminder that these are conditions many unscrupulous for-profit healthcare organizations tend to view as 'profit-driven diseases'. In other words, they are diseases that invite all forms of fraud and deceptive practices on the part of so-called care providers. To counter this, clearly articulated regulatory policies are necessary to rein in brazen commercial interests, and to do so without undermining broader public health goals. The ongoing undersupply of dedicated psychiatric beds in 24/7 treatment centers and in community hospitals further contributes to this crisis.[46]

These challenges are persistent and continue to worsen, although, as trends, they are by no means intractable.[47] Interestingly (but not surprisingly) the reams of research reports produced that address these challenges generally conclude the same thing – underfunding is pervasive and additional funding is needed to confront the unmet need for psychiatric diagnosis and treatment.[48] In one such recent meta-analysis, 37 independent studies were cross-analyzed, all focusing on individuals with schizophrenia, diagnosed (yet untreated) nonaffective psychotic disorders, major depression, dysthymia, bipolar disorder, generalized anxiety disorder (GAD), panic disorder, obsessive compulsive disorder (OCD), and alcohol and related addictive disorders. The authors (again, unsurprisingly) concluded the treatment gap remains universally broad based and severe.[49] The WHO has issued dire prognostications for those regions to be most severely impacted by climate change and the probability for its direct intersection with increased rates of mental illnesses and substance addictions. These places include sub-Saharan Africa,[50] Uganda, East Africa,[51] Chile,[52] the United Kingdom (where a reported 1,711 inpatient psychiatric beds were lost in 24/7 institutions between 2011 and 2013 alone),[53] and in Canada.[54] Despite the need to close the treatment gap, critics of the National Health Service (NHS), in a wealthy nation such as the United Kingdom, paint its relative disregard for persons with mental illnesses as a form of 'structural social discrimination'.[55] This is all the more compounded by the impact of chronic fiscal underinvestment.[56] Other risk factors include the psychological impact of disemployment. Robotics and automated manufacturing is resulting in the loss of hundreds of thousands of stable, full-time jobs in many countries. In the United States alone in the past decade, more than 100,000 bank teller jobs have been lost due to automation. What are all these people to do? For many, with no job, and no income, despair sets in. It soon can become a downward spiral leading to depression, or worse. One asks, what do these global trends have to do with architecture and the design of therapeutic environments for persons in need of this type of healthcare?

On the therapeutic role of architecture and landscape

The previous discussion sets the context for a closer look at the relationship between landscape, architecture, mental health and addictive disorders. Connellan and colleagues at the University of South Australia recently published a review of the literature on this subject. There, a team of interdisciplinary researchers perused 165 articles and reports.[57] Diverse sources of information were reviewed and categorized, and key themes identified included the current debate on nursing station design, the importance of natural light in the therapeutic milieu, the role of security, privacy, special considerations for children and adolescents, forensic facilities, interior design, patient room configuration and amenity, therapeutic benefits of art and music, design for persons with dementia, nature and therapeutic gardens, postoccupancy evaluations of psychiatric treatment settings, and effective methods for eliciting the day-to-day occupant's participation in the facility design process.

Physical aggression and violence in psychiatric treatment settings is an undercurrent in this literature, although this has been a key theme for years in the professional and scientific healthcare literature.[58] The debate over the use of forced restraint and seclusion continues, as it is viewed as a time-tested method to control patients with anxiety and a proclivity for outward acts of physical aggression.[59] As social science–based research continues on this issue in an effort to pinpoint its antecedent causes, the role of the built environment comes into play. And in the arena of evidence-based healthcare design research, this has not gone unnoticed. In response, a 'tentative theory' for the design of psychiatric facilities was recently put forth by the environmental psychologist Roger Ulrich and colleagues in Sweden. This theory represents an attempt to drill down into a set of 10 evidence-based design variables, each one based on an assumption that when all 10 are physically present in a given psychiatric treatment setting, the result will be a reduced use of chemical and physical restraints.[60]

An alternative view put forth here (by this author), in this chapter, is premised on the assumption that perhaps the Ulrich et al. conceptualization is somewhat reductive, even premature, to put forth at this time until additional corroborating studies are carried out in other contexts. Despite this problem, Ulrich et al. argue that (only) these 10 design attributes, when simultaneously in evidence in a treatment facility, will result in the hypothesized outcome – as manifest in a reduction in the use of physical restraint methods.[61] The aim here is to describe this alternative theory and methodology to Ulrich et al. The goal is to advance knowledge on this subject in a way that *equally* and more broadly addresses the everyday experience of the mental health *caregiver*, as well as the reality of the *patient* experience.[62] For example, as for the critical role of the caregiver, one recent study found unit understaffing persists as a contributing factor in patients' violent outbursts, and yet this finding was not accounted for by Ulrich et al. Second, as for the role of the physical setting itself, environmental trigger factors such as excessive noise levels, poor lighting, lack of respite space, and the facility's site context and type (rural, suburban, or urban; low rise, midrise, high rise) have been correlated with nurses' decreased overall job performance and yet neither of these determinants were addressed by Ulrich et al.[63]

Taken further, additional investigative, evidence-based design research on this subject needs to address broader questions such as, 'What are the functions and ramifications of architecture and landscape architecture as therapeutic modalities in psychiatric and addictive disorders treatment?'[64] On this point, it is equally instructive to take a broad view from the outset of any research activity on this subject; it has been learned that certain architectural and landscape design 'lessons' can be borrowed from prior research on allied healthcare types, including from recent research conducted in hospice residential environments.[65] Numerous parallels exist between the palliative care milieu and mental health and substance abuse treatment milieu.[66] These parallels include the importance of personal autonomy, individuality, dignity, privacy, meaningful interpersonal interactions, security and safety, comfort, spiritual well-being, functional competency support mechanisms, staff amenities, and the ability to engage in a sustained level of engagement with nature.[67] Ulrich et al., unfortunately, do not specifically address these additional, yet possibly quite important, variables and their potentially significant ripple effects on patient and caregiver well-being.

Additionally, adverse outcomes in physical settings that need to be addressed in evidence-based research on this subject should be grounded in a broader definition of physical violence itself – patient-to-patient, patient-to-caregiver, and sometimes staff-to-patient acts of aggression. This relationship, as a 'triad of codependency', warrants being included in the manifold of investigative concern. The alternative framework described here for investigating this subject is structured into a series of sequential steps that build upon one another, with input/output causality (cause/effect). First, it is important to keep abreast of the current literature being published across numerous disciplines on this general topic. Next, a fuller portrait of the users of the physical setting needs to be identified, with regard to data gathered about or directly from the study's participants (the caregivers and patients), as well as certain archival personal background information, as this will provide a foundation for further investigating person-environment transactions, respondent satisfaction, and psychological health status in psychiatric treatment environments. This research strategy is illustrated in Figure 1.1.

The early stages in this protocol lead to the ascertainment of intermediary risk factors and outcome behaviours for the caregiver cohort, as well as the patient cohort. A datum line threads continuously from left to right, through a series of intermediary stages; the penultimate stage is where findings are summarized and translated into healthcare organizational policies and architectural and landscape planning and design considerations (Figure 1.1). The six intervals in this theory/method consist of (1) respondent characteristics, (2) respondents' lifestyle and background, (3) built environment characteristics, (4) additional respondent background information elicited in a second phase (as indicated in Figure 1.1), (5) the translation of these data into a useful format for application in professional policy-making and architectural contexts, and (6) the assessment of 'outcome' in terms of occupant health status and one's predilection to engage in an aggressive or violent act that in some way, to some degree, may have been set off by one or more antecedent attributes present in the built physical environment.

In this alternative investigative strategy, the treatment setting is, first, thoroughly documented for the purpose of studying the ways it might influence occupants' behaviour. Methodologically, this is accomplished by means of photography, videography, drawings, diagrams, and other methods, without compromising patient, visitor, or caregiver privacy or confidentiality. Once the physical setting (or settings if more than one facility is being investigated) has been systematically documented, a *behavioural mapping analysis* is conducted to identify occupants' patterns of movement within the facility and the immediate exterior site environs.[68] Correspondingly, the role of occupants' actual physical impact upon his or her physical setting – physical *traces* – are mapped, then compared and contrasted.[69] It then becomes feasible to comparatively examine a broad set of architectural and landscape design variables within the unit, and also in the broader context of the hospital or clinic.[70] For instance, the occupant's access to nature and landscape is documented and examined for its potential influence on outcome behaviour. If works of art are to be documented – how many, and what types? Where are they located? What themes are addressed? Are artworks on display in the inpatient treatment unit? Is there an ongoing program to rotate or add to the number of artworks in the treatment setting? Is artwork present in every patient room, throughout the facility, or only in social activity areas? Do patients or the direct caregiving staff have a say in the type of art on display?[71]

This information can be examined in relation to respondents' background data and incorporated in further statistical analyses where patient and facility attributes are studied to identify any causal (cause/effect) patterns.[72] In the mental health nursing literature, for example, it is widely accepted that in psychiatric units,

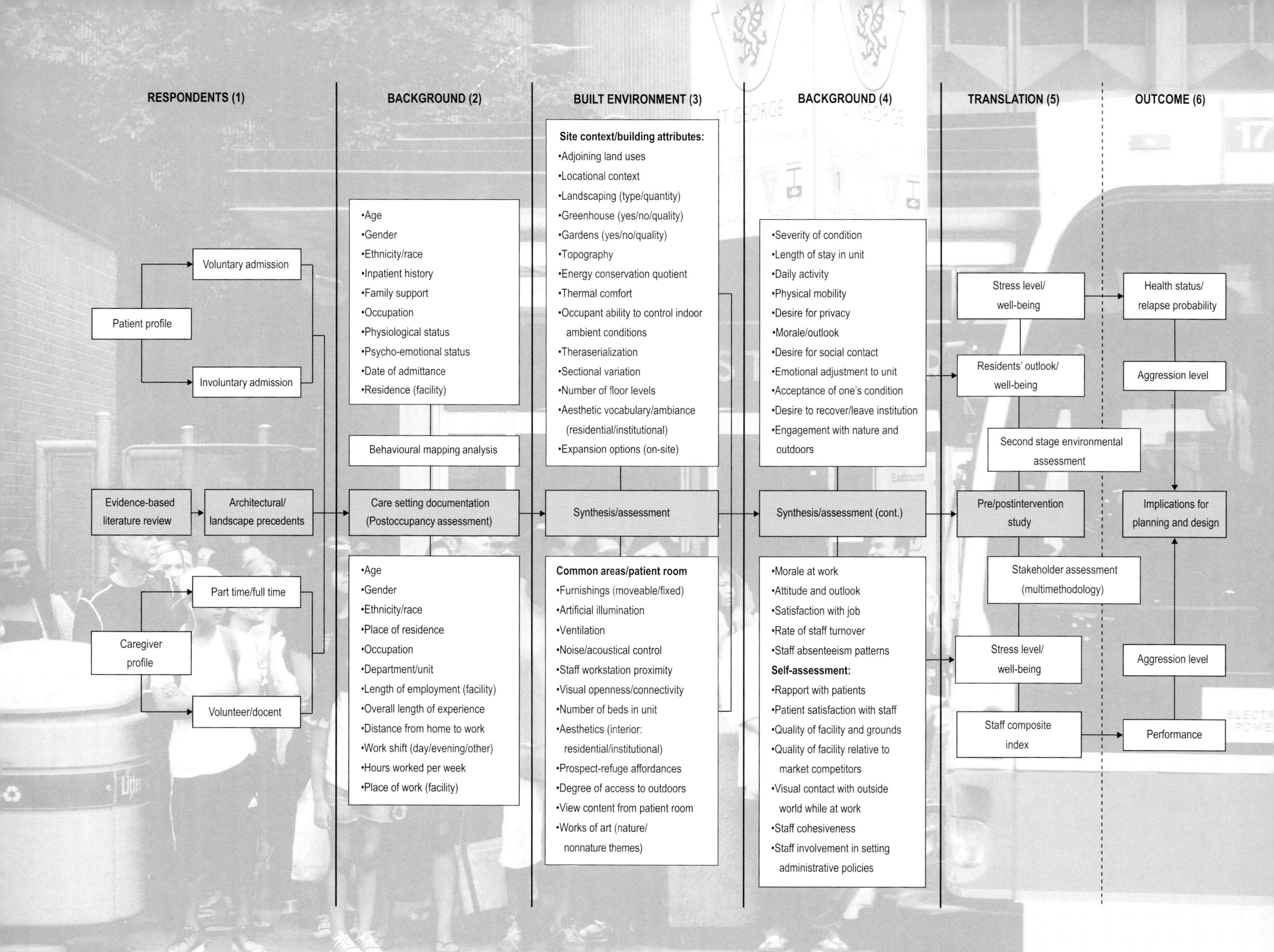

1.1 Relationship between behavioural health environments and occupant well-being

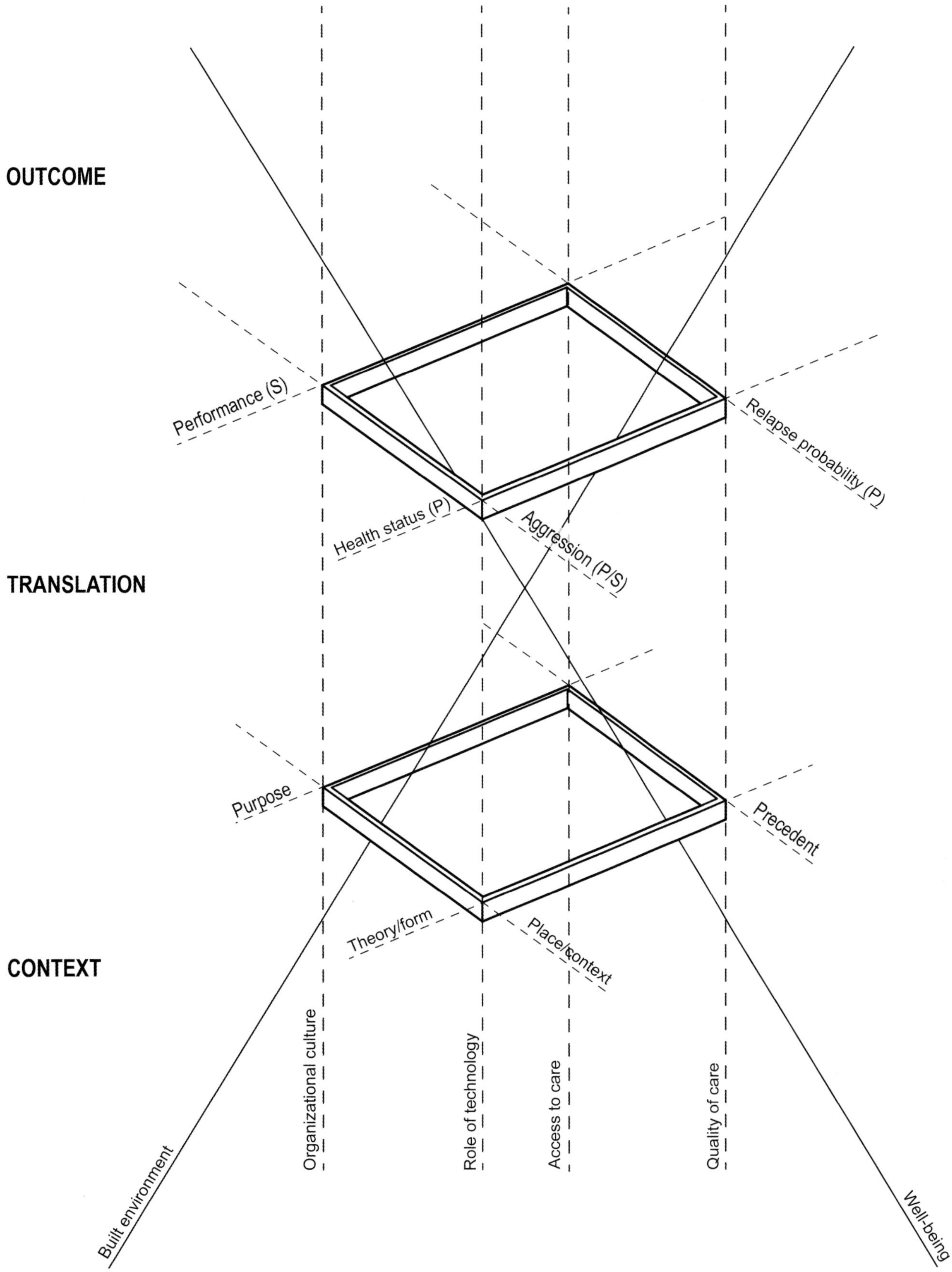

1.2 Relationship between contextual and translational determinants and behavioural outcomes.

inpatient aggression and conflict arises from a complex mix of factors, including the backgrounds of patients and the staff, together with potential influencing aspects of the physical environment.[73] In a major study of psychiatric hospitals in the Netherlands, the researchers noted how a large number of architectural considerations can factor into a reduction in the use of restraints and coercive measures relating to aggression, including the outcome of better patient-staff communication, higher staffing levels, better aggression management training, and improved risk-assessment training.[74]

In another review of the literature on environmental design research conducted in healthcare settings, Laursen, Danielson, and Rosenburg (2014) found stimulating sensory interventions including music, murals, plants, and natural daylight to have a positive effect on patients' self-reported anxiety and pain levels in the postoperative phase of their hospitalization.[75] In summary, the thrust of any alternate, more expansive research strategy such as that proposed here is solely to broaden the discourse. It is to allow for more resonant comparisons between the patient, his or her caregiver, and the role of the physical setting. This is but one approach, yet it represents an effort to more holistically approach the root causes of patient aggression and the use or nonuse of physical restraints in psychiatric settings. It is a holistic evidence-based research strategy encompassing the role of the broader institution and its organizational policies.

This investigative paradigm is composed of two *tiers* of inquiry related to the research context, the translation of information, and behavioural-psychological outcomes. In Tier 1, purpose, theory/form, place/context, and design precedents are of fundamental concern. In Tier 2, respondents' behavioural performance, health status, and outcomes are of principal focus. These two tiers are drawn together by means of an axis representing the continuous 24/7 role of the *built environment*, and a second diagonal axis representing the similar continuous role of *well-being* as it specifically relates to patient and staff assessment of the physical setting (Figure 1.2). The influence of organizational culture, the role of technology, access to care, and the quality of care provided is to be taken into account relative to the occurrence of patients' acts of aggression and physical violence.

The evidence-based research reported by Ulrich et al. in 2013 therefore remains underdeveloped, by comparison, making its generalizability very difficult. It remains unclear exactly *how* patient stress was defined and measured. The use of chemical and physical restraints with patients was presumably the sole outcome measured, yet this left many questions unanswered. Second, only patients were included in the study, not their caregivers. Third, a very limited set of design attributes (10) were included. Fourth, it was not possible to tell if any particular types of respondents are more predisposed to engage in these adverse behavioural outcomes. In other words, do younger patients need to be restrained more often than older patients? Despite the existence of their single study, Ulrich authored an op-ed piece in the *New York Times* in 2013 titled 'Designing for Calm'.[76] In it, he described his and his colleagues' research in Sweden in 2013.[77]

In reality, there does not yet exist enough evidence-based research on this subject to justify firm conclusions as to which specific aspects of the physical setting, and which specific person-environment transactions, are of most influence, and which features do (or do not) function as antecedent influences in triggering a given patient's act of aggression or violence. This is because so little environmental design research of any type has been conducted in residential psychiatric facilities built in the past decade (see Chapter 6).[78] Interestingly, the lead architect of the Östra Hospital, Stefan Lundin (where the 2013 Ulrich et al. study was conducted), has stated he had received no research information *a priori* pertaining to Ulrich's 10 design attributes. Instead, he based his preliminary information-seeking and design process phases on many interactions with the client/agency, with the direct caregivers at the future new hospital, and on his own intuitive judgment.[79] This all points to a persistent knowledge transference gap between evidence-based health facility research and architectural design, and how the attainment of design excellence continues to be a less-than-foolproof proposition. In contrast to relying on intuitive knowledge, the alternate investigative model presented here depends on a mixture of qualitative (intuitive/informal), as well as quantitative (scientific/formal), data collection methods and instruments. Qualitative methods include focused interviews, behavioural observation, and perusal of archival data on the history of the institution and related organizational information, together with knowledge of the current design and research literature. Quantitative methods and instruments include the documenting physical setting; performing surveys and statistical analyses; and measuring indoor ambient air quality, environment comfort, lighting levels, and so forth.

The challenge

Beyond issues concerning specific research methodologies, or investigative scope, the far harsher reality is that much of the world lacks adequate mental health care treatment environments. The *treatment gap* remains problematic even though the number of available psychiatric beds varies between countries on a per-capita basis.[80] In Australia, a new generation of inpatient and outpatient facilities is currently being built, and in the 2000–2015 period, many high-quality psychiatric hospitals and community clinics were built.[81] In South America, the unmet need for services varies greatly from country to country. A recent study in six South American nations linked the closure of inpatient beds in state-run psychiatric hospitals to an increase in prison populations. Prison populations rose proportionately to the number of psychiatric bed closures since 1990 in all six countries. Researchers used government data on the availability of psychiatric beds since 1990 in Argentina, Bolivia, Brazil, Chile, Paraguay, and Uruguay. On average, it was learned the prison populations in these countries had increased by about three persons for every one psychiatric hospital bed eliminated.[82] In many places, 'psychiatric prisons' range from crude tent hospitals surrounded by rough barbed-wire fencing, to 50-plus-year-old International Style hospitals, neglected for decades and lacking running water and proper sanitation.[83]

One would imagine the situation in the United States to be far better, but back in 1955 there were 558,239 state- and county-run psychiatric beds, or about 340 beds per 100,000 population. By 2015, there were less than 35,000 state- and county-run beds remaining, or only 11 beds per 100,000 population![84] The extensive inventory of shuttered public psychiatric hospitals in the United States between then and now has left local communities in a quandary regarding (or even whether) to repurpose them. Options range from total adaptive reuse, as in the case with H.H. Richardson's state hospital in Buffalo, New York (see Chapter 5), to the repurposed state asylum in Traverse City, Michigan. This campus was closed in 1989 and destined for demolition. Its 480 acres, which once included a fully functional dairy farm run by patients, is now a tourist attraction called the Village at Grand Traverse Commons.[85] In Vancouver, Canada, the historic Riverview Hospital was closed in 2015. When this custodial institution opened in 1913 it was 'The Hospital for the Mind', home to 340 inpatients (all male). By 1955 nearly 80 buildings had been built on the grounds in support of a peak patient census of 4,726, and 2,200 staff. The British Columbia Mental Health Act of 1965 precipitated its downsizing and the transfer of patients elsewhere, while the future of dozens of empty historic buildings there remains unresolved.[86]

The following chapters represent an attempt to breathe life into, and further examine, the issues raised here. In Chapter 2, a brief history of the relationship between mental health services and architecture is presented in the 50-year period from 1960 to 2010. In Chapter 3, the narratives of individuals representing special populations across diverse contexts are presented. Chapter 4 consists of the tale of how a venerable, urban mental health and substance addiction treatment center in Canada is reinventing itself in the 21st century, together with the presentation of an alternative plan for its phased, in-place redevelopment. In Chapter 5, a compendium of campus- and facility-planning design considerations is presented for use by architects, their client constituencies, landscape architects, interior designers, engineers, allied built-environment professionals, patients' rights advocacy groups, and a broad range of healthcare professionals; in Chapter 6, a compendium of 25 recently built case studies is presented – representing diverse philosophies and design strategies in the provision of high-quality architecture for health.

CHAPTER 2

Architecture for mental and behavioural health: a brief history (1960–2010)

In 1953, the American Psychiatric Association and the American Institute of Architects jointly launched the 'Architectural Study Project'. It was financed by grants from the US Public Health Service and the Division Fund of Chicago, and consisted of an international survey of 'mental hospital' design with the explicit goal of putting forth 'good design' precepts for application by architects and administrators. This work resulted in the 1959 book *Psychiatric Architecture: A Review of Contemporary Developments in the Architecture of Mental Hospitals, Schools for the Mentally Retarded and Related Facilities.*[1] The Kirkbride psychiatric hospital template, dating from the publication of his influential 1854 book, was a precursor to this study in a number of ways. By the early 1950s, Kirkbride asylums were still in use in many places, and it had taken architects nearly a century to become thoroughly disillusioned with them.[2] The Kirkbride model had provided the platform for 'moral treatment' of the insane, but by then these asylums and the newer buildings built around them had fallen into benign neglect, having been expanded between the world wars into 'human warehouses' characterized by unimaginatively harsh, indestructible materials. In time, these places became indistinguishable from the nearest prison.

A few facilities stood apart, architecturally, from the dated institutionalism of these warehouses, and the exemplars included the Chestnut Lodge in Maryland and the Austin Riggs Center in Massachusetts, both facilities built in the 1930s, with the latter praised for an innovative use of a hotel to house its inpatients.[3] Even the treatments inside them had fallen into disrepute. In the 1930s and 1940s the frontline 'physiological therapies' – electric shock and prefrontal lobotomy – had risen to prominence, and these 'scientific' procedures at first were performed in private hospitals although soon, they were mostly performed at Kirkbride and post-Kirkbride psychiatric hospitals. These methods predominated until the late 1950s and the advent of the early 'tranquilizing' drug-based therapies. In 1960, 95% of all hospitalized psychiatric patients in the United States (as in most countries) resided in these institutions, places built for one prime function – custodial care – with few exhibiting any genuinely 'contemporary' design strategies. In this regard, the 'Architectural Study Project' was unable to learn very much about innovative architectural design strategies from any existing American psychiatric hospitals, because most of these places by then stood out boldly for precisely what *not* to do.[4]

Up to 1960, state governments across the U.S. were under immense pressure to expand their inventories of aging facilities to meet the burgeoning need for psychiatric beds. After 1960, however, this trend would be reversed, dramatically due to a confluence of events. At about this time a groundbreaking book was published, focusing international attention on the plight of the patients in these forlorn warehouses for the disenfranchised and forgotten. This book, *Asylums: Essays on the Condition of the Social Situation of Mental Patients and Other Inmates*, was a collection of four essays by the sociologist Erving Goffman.[5] Based on his participant-observer fieldwork employed as a physical therapist's assistant under a US federal grant in the late 1950s, Goffman put forth the theory of the *total institution*. A total institution is a place where a great number of similarly situated people are cut off from the wider community for a considerable time, and together lead an inward-focused, cloistered existence within a formalized, totalitarian-like world.[6]

In his words,

> Every institution captures something of the time and interest of its members and provides a world for them . . . every institution has its encompassing tendencies. Their total character is symbolized by their barriers to social intercourse with the outside . . . this is often built right into the physical plant, such as their locked doors, high walls, barbed wire, cliffs, water, forests, and moors. These establishments I am calling *total institutions* . . . First, all aspects of life are conducted in the same place and under the same single authority. Second, all daily activity is carried on in the immediate company of a large batch of others, all of whom are treated alike and required to do the same thing together. Third, all phases of the day's activities are tightly scheduled . . . finally, the various enforced activities are brought together into a single rational plan purportedly designed to fulfill the official aims of the institution . . . supervised by personnel whose chief activity is surveillance.[7]

Goffman examined the deep discontinuities within large, managed patient cohorts and their comparatively small supervisory staffs. The former live 24/7 inside the institution whereas the latter operate on an 8-hour shift and have regular contact with the world outside. The two constituencies view one another with resentment, suspicion, and through generally hostile stereotypes, with the staff viewing the patient-inmate as 'bitter, secretive, and untrustworthy', while the patient-inmate saw the staff as 'condescending, highhanded, and mean'. He characterized staff as feeling superior and righteous. Patient-inmates, for their part, felt 'inferior, weak, blameworthy, and guilty'. Social mobility between these two social strata was restricted, with social distances considerable and always formally prescribed. Even verbal communications across this boundary line were terse.[8] Goffman referred to this process as role dispossession, premised on a series of abasements, degradations, humiliations, and profanations of self where the victim (patient) becomes systematically mortified at oneself at how one could possibly have arrived at such a low point and in such a physical place in life.[9] He concluded that effectively subjugating the patient-inmate was at least as important as any cure.[10]

At this same time, the iconoclastic French philosopher Michel Foucault had, interestingly, also acquired firsthand experience from working in a psychiatric hospital. Foucault took a different approach to the decoding of the phenomena he observed firsthand, diving deeply into the history of the incarceration of the insane in his influential 1961 book *Madness and Civilization: A History of Insanity in the Age of Reason*.[11] Foucault examined the evolving conceptualization of madness through the lens of Anglo-European culture, law, politics, philosophy, and medicine from the Middle Ages to the end of the 18th century, and critiqued, along the way, historical methodologies and the viability of the formal historical narrative itself. This work represented a pronounced shift in his work away from phenomenology toward structuralism; Foucault insisted that madness itself was not a natural, unchanging condition, but rather one entirely codependent with society's strictures. Ultimately, he saw madness as having been consigned to a purgatorial 'cultural space' with prescribed properties and ramifications wholly dependent upon the prevailing society's prescriptive class-based order.[12]

The death of the asylum and the rise of psychopharmaceuticals

Numerous International Style psychiatric hospitals were built in the 1946–1960 period in developed countries in the West and, to a lesser extent, in less-developed places. These institutions were guided nearly exclusively by the dictum *form follows function*, often to the exclusion, or sublimation, of humanist concerns. The narrative of *One Flew Over the Cuckoo's Nest* (1976 film), in its depiction of the postwar state-run psychiatric hospital, was centered on starkness, minimalism, and an inability for the patient to feel in control of one's personal space to any real degree. In psychiatric medical and in academic circles, meanwhile, their rather reductivist appearance and their operation, and even the International Style itself, were now viewed with growing skepticism. In declaring the custodial building type bankrupt morally, sociologically, and now architecturally, the moment was ripe for innovation. To progressively minded psychiatrists and their architects at the time, anything that resembled the oppressiveness of an asylum or its International Style counterpart successor institution was seen as antithetical to the rapidly evolving aims of mental rehabilitation. The architecture of the psychiatric hospital was in need of being recast into the role of either blindly furthering institutionalism or in pointing the way toward new alternatives – a new way forward (Figure 2.1). In the words of Dr. Charles Goshen,

> In many institutions, destructiveness is the only way patients find to express themselves; there seems to be a direct ratio between the amount of destructiveness in a hospital and the extent it restricts . . . since 1900 there has been a steady increase in the number of security features built into mental hospitals, as if both psychiatrists and architects took great pride in the ingenuity of their efforts to outwit patients' attempts to express themselves destructively! Yet hospital design . . . can obviate the atmosphere which fosters destructive patient expression. The mistakes of the past do indeed make for gloomy reading.[13]

In citing 17 glaring architectural mistakes of recent decades, Goshen called out the neoclassicism of the asylum as well as the unsuitability of the modernist dictum 'form follows function' for its failure to support the everyday complexities of what actually needs to occur in these places. He called for a complete reappraisal of dormitories, dining halls, spaces for personal hygiene, storage for personal possessions, living and activity spaces, working spaces, outdoor recreational spaces ('Architects consistently fail to allow for the use of outdoor facilities'), spaces for individual therapy, group therapy, and spaces for visitation. He called for a complete rethinking of the nurses' station, the open ward, and all counseling offices and administrative areas. In conclusion, he called for smaller-scale, one-level outpatient clinics of between 5,000–10,000 square feet in size; for specialized long-term retirement facilities versus warehousing the aged *en masse* in generic psychiatric institutions; for the improved prescreening of patients; and the need for greatly improved professional training of direct caregivers.[14]

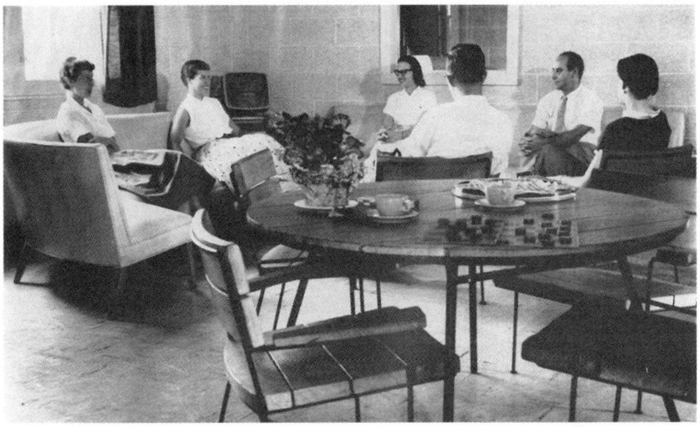

2.1 Group therapy room in an American psychiatric hospital, circa 1960.

Aside from architecture, this was the era of new, experimental psychiatric medications. For centuries, psychotropic plant-derived drugs had played an important role in religious practices, tribal rituals, and faith healing. Substances best known in this regard were opium, hashish, and hellebore, and the medicinal remedies practiced in India and throughout Southeast Asia.[15] René Spiegel writes that far earlier, around 400 BC, Hippocrates had elevated natural (i.e., physical) causes of mental illnesses to the forefront as expressions of an imbalance between the bodily fluids (humors), which are normally present in harmonious proportions and seasonal environmental conditions. The *humoral theory of Hippocrates*, among the most influential concepts in the history of psychology and psychiatry, was premised on four basic fluids corresponding to four temperaments, or character types, and in the case of pathological behaviour, to four types of mental disorders:

Humor	*Temperament: affectivity*	*Mental illness*
Blood	Sanguine: lively and weak	Mania, insanity
Phlegm	Phlegmatic: slow and weak	Calm insanity
Black bile	Melancholic: slow and strong	Melancholy
Choler	Choleric: lively and strong	Hysteria

In Rome in the second century, Galen of Pergamon adopted the humoral theory of Hippocrates, and this included his early classification of mental illnesses. Accordingly, his therapeutic recommendations centered on the tradition of the Hippocratic school: diet, vomiting, bloodletting, and soporifics. Later, during the Middle Ages, the darkest time in the history of psychiatry, the insane were thought to be possessed by the demonic spirits, and this resulted in witch burning and gruesome exorcisms of evil spirits. Suffice to say, medical science did not advance in medieval Christian Europe. Meanwhile, in the growing ranks of state-run asylums, the task of the prison (i.e., asylum) 'watcher' was to 'beat the hell' out of any 'possessed' wretched soul to rid him or her of evil predilections. In the Middle East, by contrast, physicians there had adopted the Hippocratic-Galenic tradition, and Arabic physicians furthered these humane teachings and applied practices; hospitals with separate departments for the mentally ill were available in Baghdad as early as AD 750 and in Cairo from AD 873.[16] By and large, medical models of mental illness, with the aim of detection and treatment (rehabilitation), were still far off.

The 19th century was a period of considerable innovation. In 1824, a treatise on psychopharmacology was authored by P.J. Schneider, a German. His book contained more than 600 pages of psychiatric therapy best practices in the early 19th century. Schneider's detailed analysis of the subject was well received and remained relevant for a century and more. It stands today as an important precursor to the modern practice of psychiatry. Few major advancements occurred until 1891, when Paul Ehrlich first observed the antimalarial effects of methylene blue, a phenothiazine derivative.[17] Later, the first phenothiazine medications were developed for their antihistaminergic possibilities. In 1951, in France, Laborit and Huguenard administered for the first time the aliphatic phenothiazine, *chlorpromazine*, to patients, and also examined its potential anesthetic affordances during surgery. However, some historians cite the dawn of modern psychopharmacology as J. Cada's discovery of the *antimanic* effect of lithium at the end of the 1940s. The impact of these medications would be profound, far beyond France; by 1953 many patients had experienced chlorpromazine-induced 'cures' and of particular significance was its effectiveness in treating schizophrenia and manic-depressive disorder.[18]

Other research teams extended this treatment approach in patients to exploit its antipsychotic benefits. The therapeutic efficacy of chlorpromazine, a soon-to-be widely used drug, would not be definitively established until the completion of a study by the US Veterans Administration Collaborative Study Group in the late 1950s.[19] Between 1954 and 1975, more than 15 antipsychotic drugs were introduced in the United States alone and about 40 throughout the world. Thereafter, a hiatus of sorts would occur in the development of new antipsychotics until the introduction of clozapine treatment in the United States in 1990, ushering in a new generation of antipsychotic drugs. These medications held promise in countering the adverse symptoms of schizophrenia.[20]

Spiegel writes,

> Thanks to chlorpromazine, the character of psychiatric clinics and of psychiatric care in general underwent a radical change. Lunatic asylums became peaceful hospitals; many patients who previously had to be admitted to hospital on account of the danger which they represented to their surroundings and to themselves could be discharged and partially rehabilitated. There was a marked reduction in the average stay in psychiatric hospitals . . . and the following years were to see a marked upswing in biologically oriented psychiatry.[21]

With the prior emphasis on psychoanalytic treatment now being called into question, purely biochemical approaches introduced in the 1960s would in time predominate.[22] Architecturally, the post-World War II medication revolution would profoundly influence what would (or, more accurately, would not) be built over the following 50 years as a parade of new psychopharmaceuticals were developed and mass marketed.[23] Correspondingly, beginning in 1960 the number of inpatient hospital beds would precipitously decline.[24] By 2000, four new types of 'alternative' antipsychotic drugs (clozapine, risperidone, olanzapine, and quetiapine) were widely available, and these eclipsed the earlier generation of drug-based therapies.[25] As this shift occurred, the vast majority of persons with mental and behavioural illnesses went from receiving treatment as inpatients in custodial institutions to being discharged, with many being treated as outpatients from then on.[26]

Deinstitutionalization: 1960–1980

The death of the asylum and, in time, its postwar modernist successors, mirrored the reappraisal of custodialism. This centered on the gross inadequacies of total institutionalism. For its part, the World Health Organization (WHO) argued the status quo needed to change.[27] Frequently cited problems included the ill-treatment of patients, geographic and professional isolation of the institutions and their staffs, poor reporting and accounting procedures, management failures in leadership and administration, chronic underfunding, ineffective staff training, and inadequate inspection and quality assurance measures. The bureaucratic response – *deinstitutionalization* – would be characterized by three component reactions: (1) the prevention of inappropriate mental hospital admissions by providing alternative treatment in nonresidential facility types; (2) the discharge of long-term institutionalized patients directly into the community (many without adequate preparation); and (3) the need to invent new types of community-based support systems because readmittance to custodial institutions was fast becoming a nonoption.

The asylum and its modernist counterpart had been where the lobotomy, electroshock therapy, and other medically based interventions flourished, all discredited by the late 1960s.[28] One physician, Walter J. Freeman, who died in 1972, presided over an estimated 3,500 lobotomies performed between 1936 and 1967. This gruesome procedure involved sawing two holes into a patient's skull and, with a device called a *leucotomy*, lopping off cells in the brain's frontal lobes. In one 12-day period, Freeman operated on 225 patients during a swing through West Virginia in the United States. Dr. Freeman insisted that many of his patients, persons previously suffering from depression, anxiety, and insomnia, showed positive results afterward. But in reality, most found no relief, ending up in far worse shape. By 1970, lobotomies were completely eclipsed by drugs such as Thorazine, followed by a host of mood-altering pharmaceuticals, including Prozac.[29]

In 1961, when Franco Basaglia arrived outside the grim walls of the Gorizia Asylum, on the Italian border with what was then Yugoslavia, it was to him a sight of horror, a warehouse where patients were frequently restrained for long periods and therapy was largely a matter of electroshock and insulin injections. The corridors stank and most patients were locked inside, for life. Dr. Basaglia, the new director, commenced to transform this institution from the inside out and his work would bring new freedoms to the patients and to the staff as well. Inspired by the writings of Primo Levi, R.D. Laing, Erving Goffman, Michael Foucault, and Frantz Fanon, he contributed significantly to the national and international deinstitutionalization movement. In 1978, in Italy, a law was passed, known as Law 180, or 'Basaglia's Law'. This landmark legislation resulted in the closure of the *entire* state-run Italian psychiatric hospital network by 1998.[30]

In the United Kingdom, the Royal Commission on the Law Relating to Mental Illness and Mental Deficiency, known as the Percy Commission, had established medically defined parameters of mental illness. Subsequently, the Mental Health Act of 1959 transferred mental health issues from the courts to physicians, and this enabled direct admissions to psychiatric institutions, unlike before. This law empowered both the medical profession and the patient, insofar as therapy was now viewed (once again) as a more viable alternative than the lobotomy, electroshock, or similar asylum-based 'medical' interventions. This remained the bedrock of UK law until 1983, and it influenced legislation in many other countries. In the eyes of many, the 1959 law rechanneled the mentally ill back to the community mainly as a way to reduce costs. Indeed, the UK Hospital Plan of 1962 would place further emphasis on deinstitutionalization, and a reconfiguration of National Health Service (NHS) resources commenced at this time.

In 1959, the WHO had published a book, *Psychiatric Services and Architecture*. Its authors, A. Baker, R. Llewelyn Davies, and P. Sivadon, put forward proposals for housing acute psychiatric inpatients in village-like communities in which clusters of buildings, each housing 14 patients, were grouped around a communal social activity center; this ensemble was to be analogous to a 'normative' community. This publication (and others, at the time) would influence psychiatric hospital facility planning and design for the next 30 years.[31] For psychiatric hospital architecture, a new way forward would now emphasize a distinctively informal arrangement of multiple residential-like pavilions in a campus setting, with no institution housing more than 280 beds total, and without deadly long corridors, intimidating large-scale buildings, or an unwelcoming aesthetic.[32]

As for existing psychiatric hospitals, the 1959 WHO publication disapproved of institutions larger than 1,000 beds, advocating no more than 300 beds on a given campus, and called for retrofitting initiatives as necessary for their 'modernization'. It called for family-stakeholder involvement, the incorporation of current psychosocial theories in campus planning and architectural design, and basically for a total rejection of the asylum and its harmful associated social stigmas.[33] With this call for new typologies, large asylums were now intensively subjected to a process of functional *deconstruction* – entailing the systematic decoupling of their various constituent parts, once highly centralized – to autonomous facility networks of small-scale local mental health clinics. This effort would slightly predate but generally parallel the movement to deconstruct the enormous acute care *megahospitals* that were built in many places in the 1970s and 1980s.[34] Dated, asylum-like psychiatric hospitals by the 1960s had become highly visible sociological targets, flashpoints – culminating in the summer of 1968. A reform movement would dovetail with the widespread defunding of state-run mental health facilities. The architectural winds of change at this time were succinctly captured in a feature article in the June 1965 issue of the *Architectural Review*:

> Traditionally in Britain and in most parts of the world patients in need of psychiatric treatment have been housed in very large groups of buildings designed primarily for custodial care. These are usually remote from the communities they serve and deliberately isolated from them by large grounds. It is becoming increasingly difficult to recruit staff for these institutions due not only to the obsolete equipment . . . and their generally depressing nature, but also because their very remoteness isolates staff . . . custodial care is now replaced by active therapy and the stay of patients has been greatly reduced in length. This physical remoteness from communities is now recognized as anti-therapeutic.[35]

If custodialism was now dead, would its replacement prove any better? The first report in the United States on this, called 'Planning, Programming and Design of the Community Mental Health Center', described in broad terms the types of care to be provided along with a pilot case study clinic, designed for an inner urban neighborhood in San Francisco. The Community Mental Health Center, or CHMC, was to be a new type, a place providing full diagnostic and rehabilitation services, vocational education, precare and aftercare services including foster home placement, home visitation by nurses, the training of mental health professionals, and a place to conduct field research.[36] A 1967 feature in Architectural Record declared each clinic is to serve a population of between 75,000 and 200,000 persons and in some instances be integrated into an existing healthcare campus setting:

> The community mental health professional has found that hospital beds can no longer be considered the single yardstick in planning facilities for the treatment of mental disability. The comprehensive range of community-based services has made it possible to emphasize early detection of symptoms . . . thus minimizing re-hospitalization . . . with many patients being treated without being admitted overnight.[37]

With the Vietnam War raging and the United States' military commitment expanding, massive social upheaval back home was the order of the day. A wave of social counterprotests swept across the country with student-led and worker-led demonstrations, with similar events occurring abroad. This would manifest in new alternative political parties, and well as in a period of popular counterculture literature, art, and music. The growing antiwar movement and the mood and spirit of the times led to a questioning of all social institutions, including the 'insane asylum' and the abject oppressiveness it symbolized. Its grassroots counterculture advocates saw the CMHC as a viable, peoples' alternative for dispensing mental health care much closer to where people actually live. Soon, CMHCs would be housed in converted storefronts, office buildings, former private residences, and in newly built freestanding facilities for the provision of outpatient care, partial hospitalization programs, and nontrauma emergency psychiatric care.

In the first 15 years of this federally funded program, 700 CMHCs opened in the United States, while the nation's custodial institutions were being closed or severely downsized. Every CMHC served a catchment area, although frequently, the local community chosen for a new CMHC often opposed it and this resulted in a new slogan, the term NIMBY (Not in my backyard!), used for the first time. This backlash was further exacerbated by a large new wave of mentally ill persons discharged from the old state-run psychiatric institutions, who now were homeless. These persons had few or no other options, with most simply lacking the basic life skills needed to succeed 'on the outside'. The new CMHCs, for their part, were ill equipped to accommodate this influx of individuals, with so many having been so long accustomed to custodial care. This dilemma was further compounded by a lack of affordable housing in cities, and premature discharging also burdened families unable to cope with this new order. Throughout the 1970s and 1980s, the limited availability of high-quality care options in communities throughout the United States resulted in a revolving-door syndrome of retreatment.

Psychiatry, psychology, and social work were themselves also now under fire for their collective inability to cope with the new wave of 'mainstreamed' patients.[38]

In Europe, following the social upheaval of May 1968, Italy, France, and Belgium, among other countries, also mandated large numbers of long-term institutionalized patients to be redirected to newly built neighborhood outpatient clinics. These mainstreaming policies, personified in Scandinavia's 'normalization' efforts (i.e., a new emphasis on residential-like local facilities), and in the United Kingdom (on newly built 'residential villages' for this same purpose). H. Goodman, chief architect of the British Ministry of Health, advocated at this time for a normative aesthetic of pitched roofs; contextualism; and residential-like interiors, materials, and furnishings. He viewed suicide as preventable through appropriate architectural design, combined with progressive treatment methods. However, critics saw all of this as purely reactionary, lacking in any substantive, evidence-based research. Second, it represented a knee-jerk repudiation of the scientific foundations of earlier 20th-century psychiatry. Meanwhile, experience out in the community was proving that 'institutional' behaviour did not only occur while in hospitalization insofar as this new generation of community-based clinics could also provoke patients' antisocial and aggressive behaviour.[39]

In 1960, the hospital board of the State of Arkansas (US) initiated a project that would garner architectural design awards. This institution housed and treated patients in a regional psychiatric hospital, serving as the hub of a network of affiliated outpatient CMHCs. This 400-bed residential campus, the Orval Eugene Faubus Intensive Treatment and Administrative Center, in Little Rock, designed by Wittenberg, Delony & Davidson (1962–1964), was the first of this new wave of 'normative' institutions to be built in the United States. It replaced the Arkansas State Hospital (asylum), a place by then wholly overcrowded and dilapidated. Its 1,775 beds were by then 400 beyond its licensed capacity, and of this total more than 1,000 beds had recently been condemned as 'unacceptable' by the American Psychiatric Association (APA). Three semidetached, dormitory-like residential treatment pavilions each housed 72 beds for women, and 72 beds for men, with other components housing two intensive care units, for a total of 450 beds (Figure 2.2 and Figure 2.3). The units were 'open' in the sense that only the campus perimeter exterior doors were locked at night. The architects used a series of survey questionnaires and focus groups to elicit feedback from staff and from community stakeholders; this information was supplemented with US Public Health Service published guidelines and those of the APA. In the architects' words,

> The building elements are organized by the device of a podium, an elevated square base bearing the structures and spaces that serve the adjacent living units. This podium is approximately 11.5 feet above the ground floor of the living units . . . one of the most striking features is an abundance of light, and their openness [Figure 2.4 and Figure 2.5]. There are no dead ends; every corridor ends with a window. Rooms and corridors have skylights . . . since it [the campus] covers a large expanse, we took pains to avoid spatial ambiguities that might add to patients' sense of confusion.

These measures also included pitched roofs and the creation of open landscaped space between the pavilions. The campus site plan indicated a strong emphasis on the by-now in-vogue 'residential village' concept (Figure 2.6 and Figure 2.7a–c).[40]

In building lower bed capacity, village-like campuses such as this, the die was cast. However, the construction of campuses with fewer beds overall would later spawn a large upswing in psychiatric admittances to acute care hospital emergency rooms. Eventually overwhelmed, urban hospitals would be forced to establish *ad hoc* psychiatric units. Soon, community-based nonpsychiatric general hospitals in the United States were admitting more psychiatric inpatients than the old state and county-run mental institutions

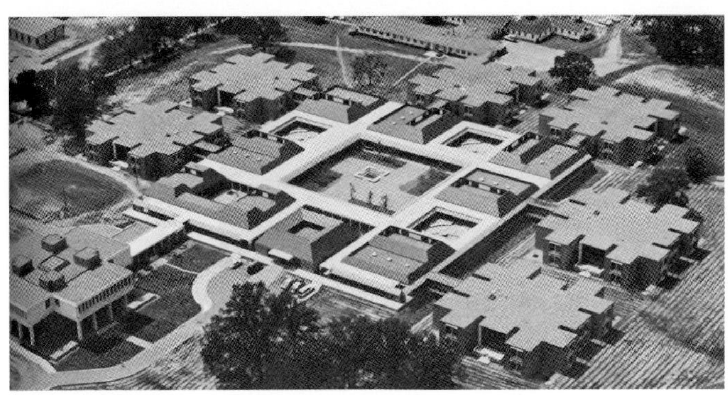

2.2 Faubus Intensive Treatment and Administrative Center, Little Rock, Arkansas (1962–1964).

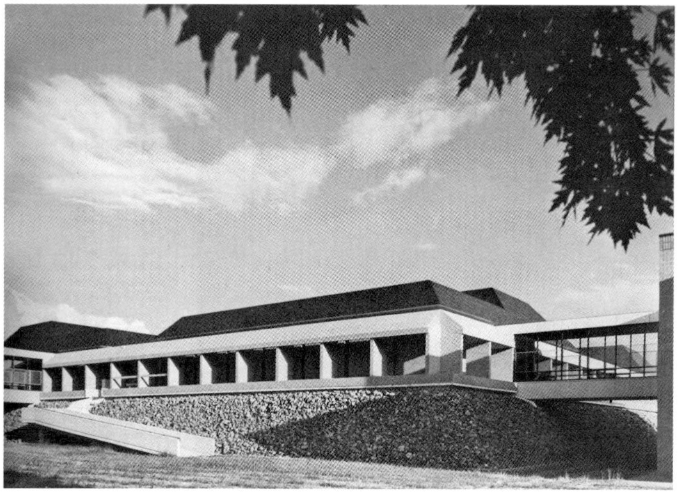

2.3 Residential pavilion at the Faubus Intensive Treatment and Administrative Center, Arkansas.

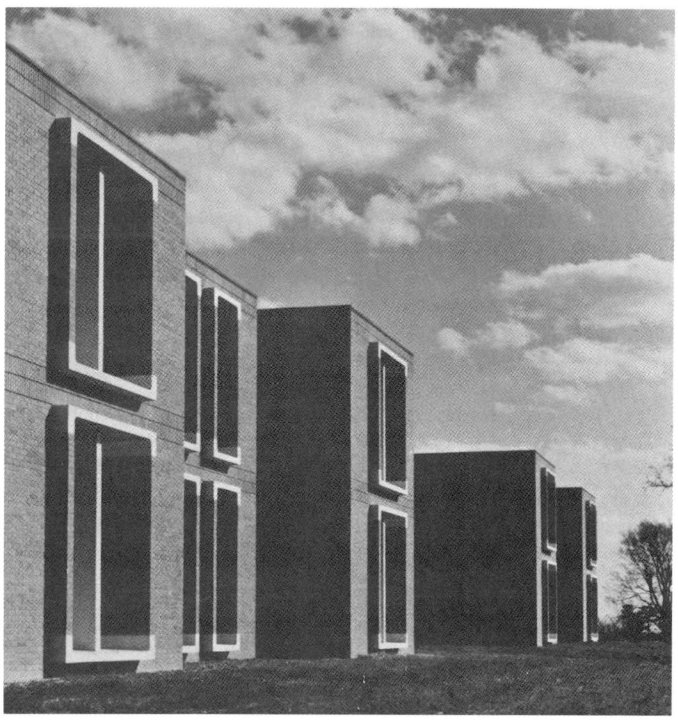

2.4 Fenestration pattern at the Faubus Intensive Treatment and Administrative Center, Arkansas.

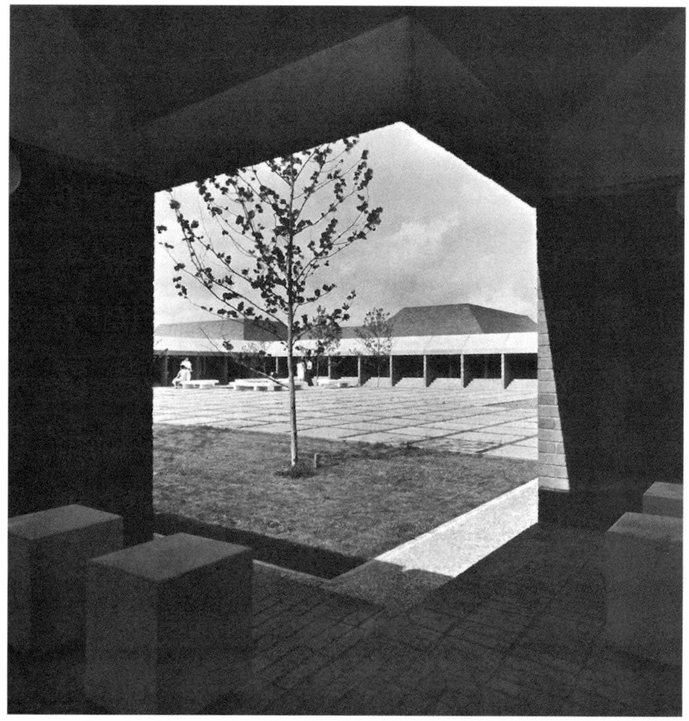

2.5 Central courtyard at the Faubus Intensive Treatment and Administrative Center, Arkansas.

had admitted *combined*.[41] At the Los Angeles County+USC Medical Center, overcrowding became acute on its psychiatric floor. By 1968, far more were being admitted nationwide but for far shorter stays (5.5 average days' length of stay, or ALOS) compared to the state- and county-run psychiatric hospitals, where the ALOS remained 21 days.[42] In Italy at this time, architectural design competitions were held on the theme of psychiatric hospitals as a way to generate new ideas about an old type and to break away from the status quo. The best of the submissions by Italian architectural firms were featured in an issue of *Lotus*, accompanied by an essay by Costantino Dardi.[43] In another such competition, finalists' entries were published in the magazine *Casabella*, including the work of a numerous rising young design firms in Europe.[44]

In the 1970s, the British debated the best method for downsizing their psychiatric hospitals – many of which by then were at least a century old. From the inception of the NHS in 1948 the community mental health center was to be an integral part of its mental health service network but by the late 1950s, as more new towns were built, this goal had fallen out of the equation. By the late 1960s interest reawakened to the point where new facilities were commissioned and in 1970 alone 69 new clinics opened in Britain.[45] In France, national facility design criteria were adopted, subdividing the nation into various discrete mental health districts. The strategy was to construct miniature mental 'health villages' not dissimilar from elsewhere in Europe and the United States at the time.[46] In the United States, as the CMHC network expanded, the most conspicuous, unintended consequence was a rise in the number of *their own* patients being referred to the nearest acute care community hospital although the original aim of the CMHC was, ironically, to *decrease* the patient demand for far costlier hospitalization.[47]

In Japan, a number of similarly designed inpatient psychiatric hospitals were built at this time, especially in rural districts, including the Kita Hospital (1965–1967) in Yamanashi Prefecture,

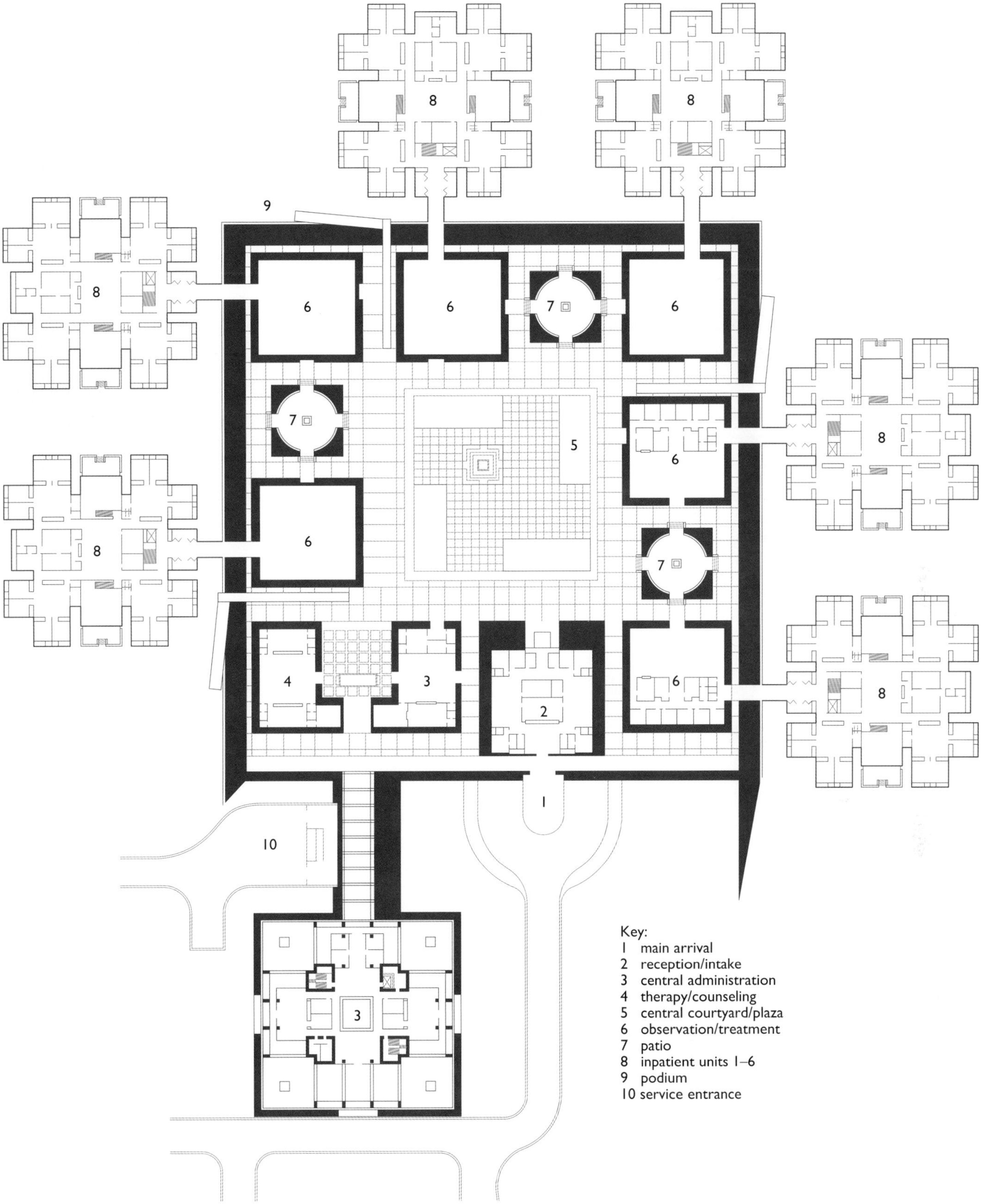
8
8
9
8
6
6
7
6
7
5
6
8
8
6
6
7
8
4
3
6
2
1
10
3
Key:
1 main arrival
2 reception/intake
3 central administration
4 therapy/counseling
5 central courtyard/plaza
6 observation/treatment
7 patio
8 inpatient units 1–6
9 podium
10 service entrance

2.6 Combined site and floor plan, Faubus Intensive Treatment and Administrative Center, Little Rock, Arkansas. Six pavilions were linked to support services housed within an 'internal zone' of structures surrounding a central courtyard.

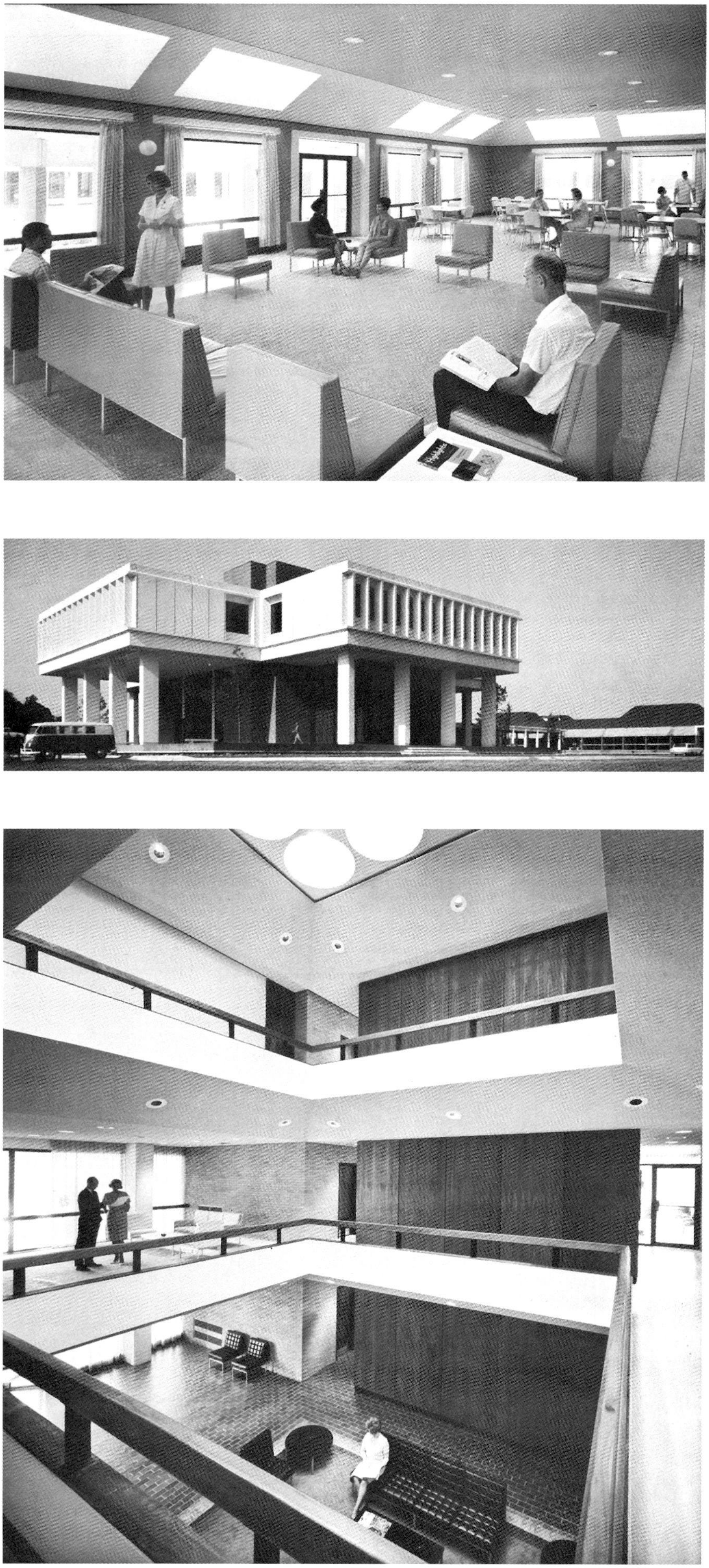

2.7a–c Faubus Intensive Treatment and Administrative Center: Residential unit's dayroom (top), exterior view of the administration building (middle), and the enclosed atrium (bottom).

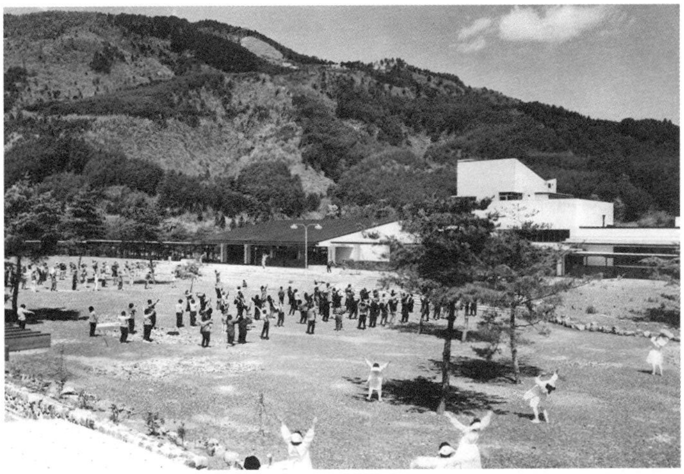

2.8 Central courtyard at the Kita Hospital, Yamanashi Prefecture, Japan (1965–1967), with nearby mountains.

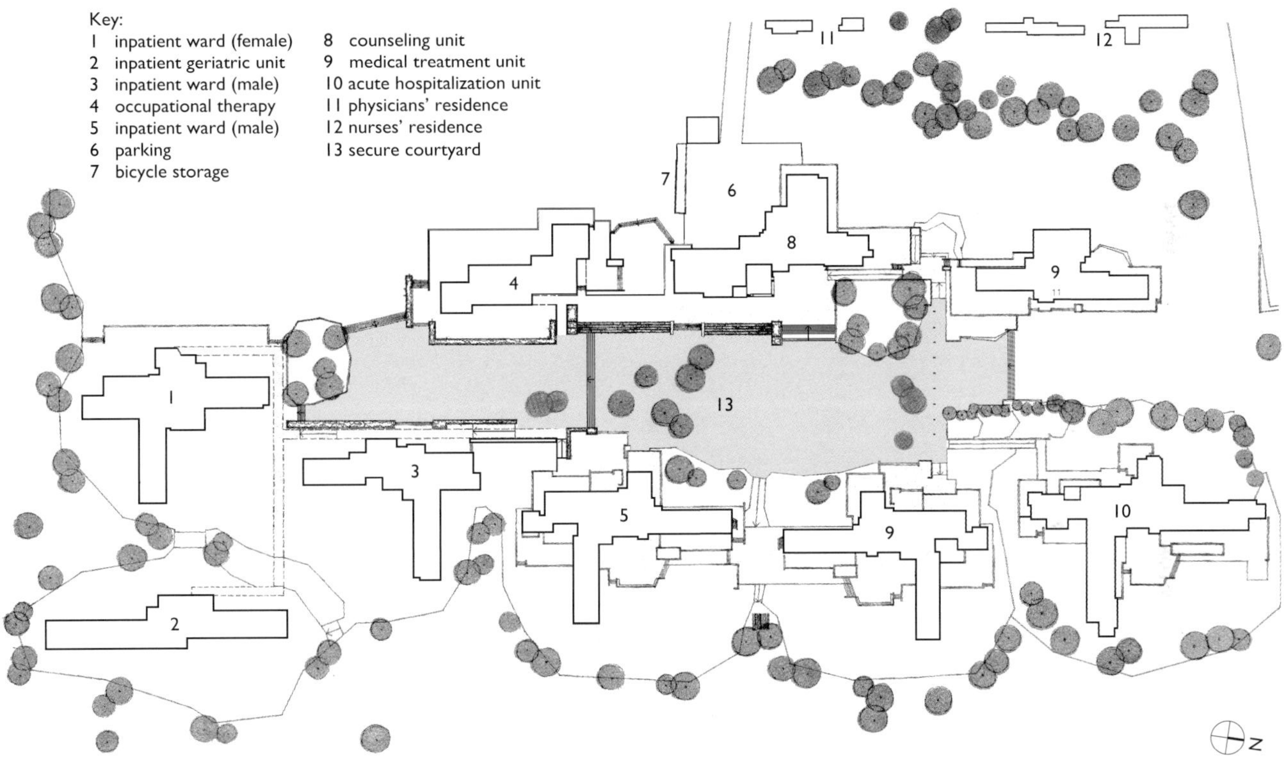

2.9 Site plan, Kita Hospital, Japan, indicating the deployment of residential pavilions and additional campus buildings.

designed by the Yoshitake Laboratory at the University of Tokyo. This idyllic campus was master planned as a series of interlocking residential pavilions connected to corresponding exterior landscaped plazas. A temperate local climate allowed for an unusual degree of transparency between indoor and outdoor spaces, and engagement with landscape was integral in treatment (Figure 2.8 and Figure 2.9). This campus's 'daily-life therapy building', not unlike the other pavilions, all two to four levels in height, was lifted above the ground plane, thereby providing sheltered space below for year-round uses (Figure 2.10 and Figure 2.11).[48]

In the United States, some architects took on the challenge to design something genuinely different. This was the case with the Winnebago Children's Health Clinic, built in Neillsville, Wisconsin (1971–1972), and designed by Skidmore, Owings, and Merrill. This

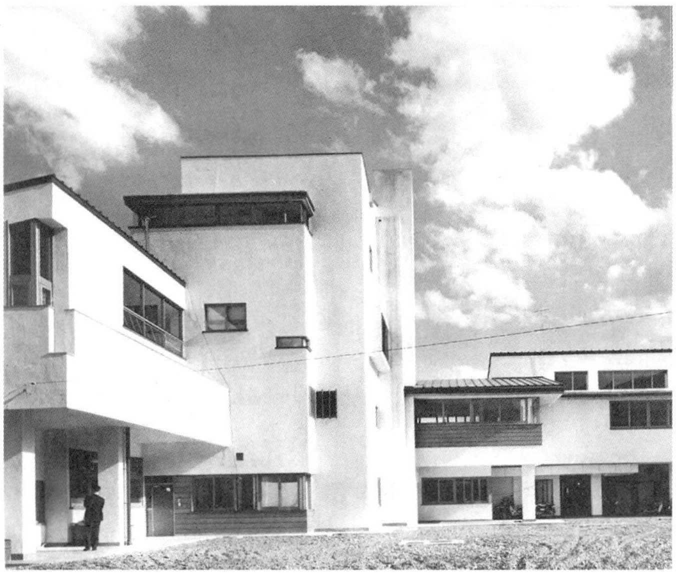

2.10 The administration building at Kita Hospital, depicting the influence of the International Style in psychiatric hospital architecture in post-World War II Japan.

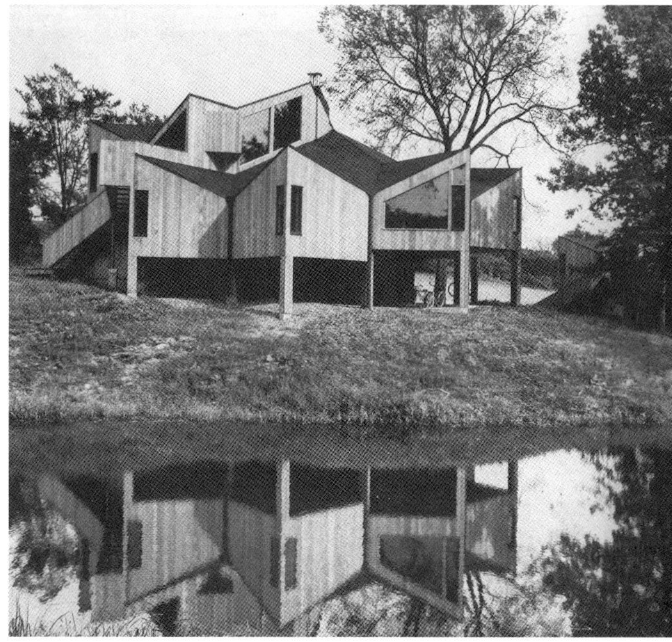

2.12 The angular, modularized forms of the Winnebago Children's Health Clinic, Neillsville, Wisconsin (1971–1972), by Skidmore, Owings, and Merrill.

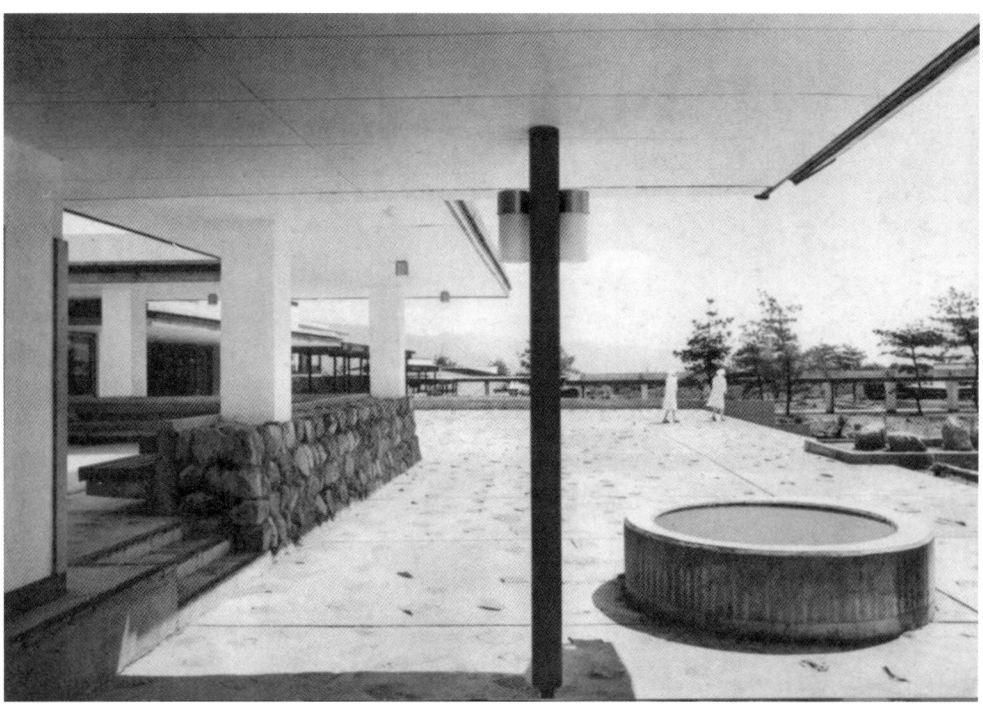

2.11 Sheltered outdoor activity space at Kita Hospital in Japan.

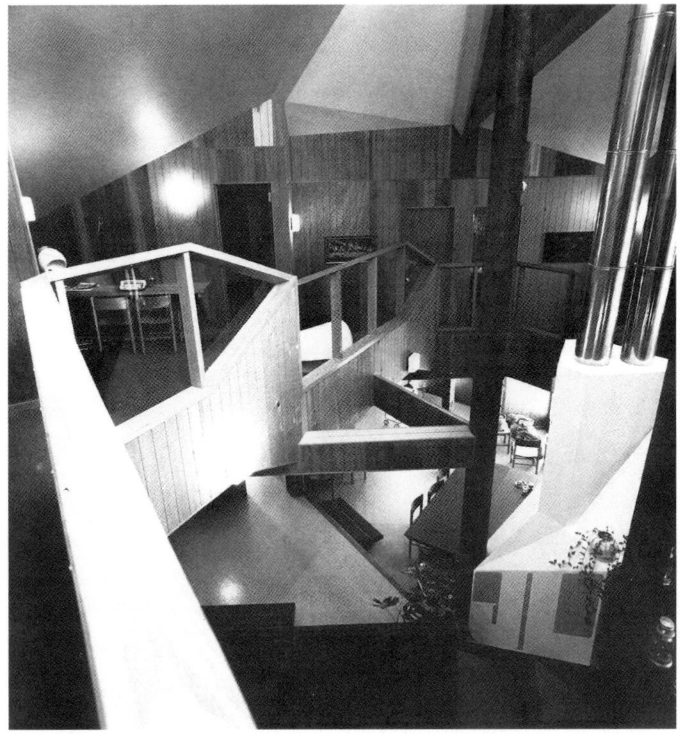

2.14 Interior volumes and circulation collided and intersected in the Winnebago Children's Health Clinic.

10-bed inpatient residential facility was developed for children and adolescents, and its floor plan resembled a flower in various stages of bloom. Its striking appearance was matched by an angular floor plan, corresponding to the zigzag exterior (Figure 2.12). Its exterior wood sheathing expressed a quasi-rustic vernacular, and this aesthetic was carried into the interior, and throughout, in plan (Figure 2.13a–c and Figure 2.14). The main level was lifted up above the ground to allow for sheltered exterior space below.[49] In Israel, the Geha Psychiatric Hospital, in Tel Aviv (1971–1973), by Arieh Sharon of Sharon & Associates, was built as a 170-bed facility, designed in accord with then-prevailing architectural trends in Europe and in North America. The campus was essentially a grid, in plan (as were most psychiatric hospital campuses built during the period), with a support/arrival core at the center composed of an administration building and an adjacent therapy/activity structure. Patients were housed in four surrounding residential pavilions, connected to the central support core by means of an outdoor 'racetrack' loop-circulation element. This two-level structure was built of cast-in-place concrete, expressing the in-vogue brutalism of the period. Its rather severe, vertical, ribbon-like fenestration featured deep-set windows in response to the intense sunlight in the region.[50]

The Norwood Mental Health Center, in Marshfield, Wisconsin (1972–1974), by Hougen, Good, Pfaller & Associates, was designed

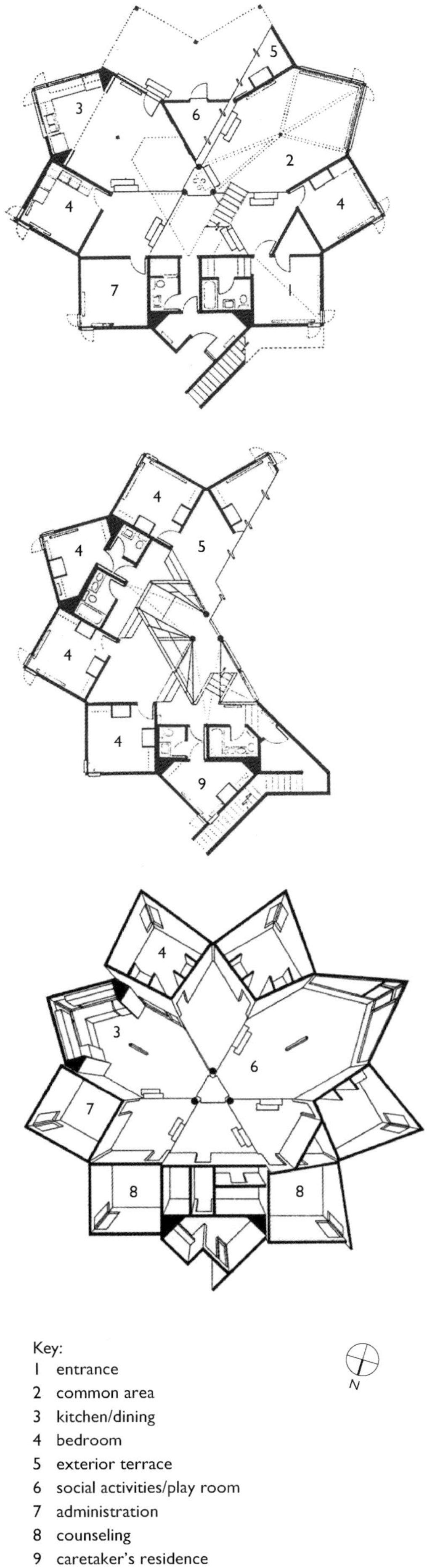

2.13a–c Winnebago Children's Health Clinic expressed, in plan, an origami-like series of intersecting, unfolding volumes.

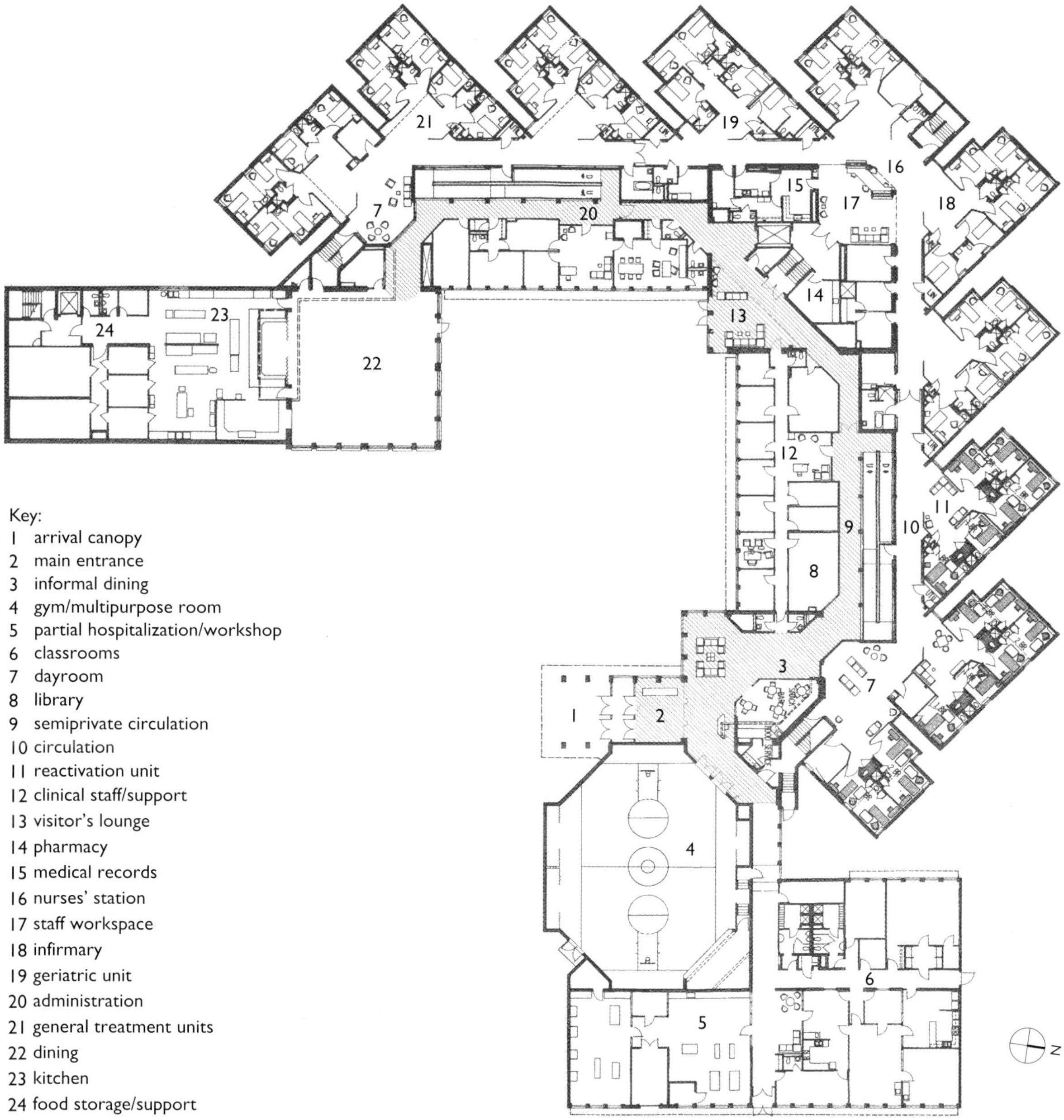

2.15 The L-configured plan of the one-level Norwood Mental Health Center, Marshfield, Wisconsin (1972–1974), by Hougen, Good, Pfaller & Associates. The clustering of patient rooms began in earnest in the 1970s in order to reduce staff walking distances.

as a replacement facility for the nearby, antiquated Wood County Hospital. Wood County Hospital opened in 1911 as part of Wisconsin's then-unique system of county mental hospitals. In time, it descended into the typical dysfunctionality, becoming severely overcrowded. This two-level Kirkbride-inspired institution of 275 beds was replaced with a 100-bed facility housing 55 beds on each of two levels. The plan was an L configuration, with patients' bedrooms arrayed in a sawtooth pattern on the outboard side of the floor and with staff support and patient activity functions housed on the inboard side. Every patient room was private, although bathing and hygiene accommodations were generally not (Figure 2.15). After one year of operations, a postoccupancy evaluation was conducted at this new facility, by its architects; it was an assessment based on eight structured interviews with hospital staff and with key administrators. Subsequently, a detailed account of this performance assessment, including a floor plan and photographs, was published in the professional journal *Hospital and Community Psychiatry* in 1976.[51] At about this time, a new-wave 166-bed replacement psychiatric hospital opened in Topeka, Kansas, designed by Skidmore, Owings, and Merrill for the Menninger Foundation (1979–1981). The floor plan was, similarly, an L configuration, although here the patient rooms (24 beds per unit) were clustered along both sides of an undulating corridor, with social activity and staff support spaces located at the intersection of two principal wings.[52]

In Canada, the firm of Somerville, McMurrich & Oxley was commissioned by the Province of Ontario to develop a master plan and new campus buildings for what was then known as the Queen Street Mental Health Centre (now CAMH), in Toronto. This firm developed a phased plan to replace the provincial asylum that had opened in 1850, with a new complex of structures. Four residential pavilions were built, plus various support buildings (1972–1974); each pavilion housed 35 beds on multiple levels. The residential units were cruciform, in plan, with the staff support core at the center (Figure 2.16); each pavilion was connected to an enclosed shopping mall–inspired atrium 'community' structure. This redevelopment strategy symbolized an effort to strike a balance between dormitory-like buildings and administrative centrality (this facility is discussed in considerably greater length in Chapter 4). It was but one of many experiments to occur in the 1960s and 1970s, representing new strategies in campus planning and architectural design (Figure 2.17a–j). By 1975, deinstitutionalization, once hailed as so promising in the United States and elsewhere, had devolved into something entirely different from what was first envisioned:

> About 12 years ago, the concept of 'deinstitutionalization' was hailed as a grand vision for reforming the care of mentally impaired people, a welcome alternative to the wretched conditions found in many huge, overcrowded state mental hospitals. Since then, the vision has become a nightmare, and the very word 'deinstitutionalization' has been twisted into a cruel euphemism for dumping hundreds of thousands of sick, dazed people into an unprepared society. Reacting to the acknowledged failures of large state institutions, reformers of the early 1960s proposed treatment of the mentally impaired should take place in small, community-based mental health centers. In 1963, President Kennedy and Congress brought forth the Community Mental Health Act, but the exhilaration of the concept exceeded the commitment to its execution. Of the 2,500 community mental health centers authorized by Congress 12 years ago, only 443 have become fully operational . . . state governments, however, clung steadfastly to their plans for discharging patients from state (custodial) institutions. Medicare and Medicaid came into being (in 1965), and states – which were groaning under the financial burden . . . found they could shift the weight to federal programs . . . States took advantage (and) discharged their inpatients to nursing homes, board and care facilities and, worse, to the streets. On a national scale, this exodus is chilling. In 1955, the peak year, state mental hospitals served more than a million persons (as inpatients). By 1974, that patient population had fallen 61 percent, to less than one-quarter million. Inpatient admissions to state hospitals in that year fell to 374,554, while discharges climbed to 448,203.[53]

This author continued,

> Where do these patients go? The most disquieting report comes from Illinois, where accounts have surfaced of a 'psycho bus' that takes patients from Manteno State Hospital and simply deposits them on Chicago streets. According to one registered nurse: 'Many of the patients who are discharged off the bus are hallucinating; many have urinated on themselves, and some are so confused and disoriented they don't know how to find their way home . . . the police have picked up patients and brought them to a state hospital or clinic for safekeeping, and we receive them back the very next day . . . patients who have been placed in halfway houses also are frequently brought back to the state hospitals . . . a social worker will be told any number of patients have to be discharged by a certain date, even if there are none fit to be discharged.[54]

Meanwhile, the federal response remained lukewarm in relation to the growing severity of the crisis. The situation deteriorated in Illinois to the point where public protests were held by nursing caregivers in the face of severe state budget cuts in mental health care, including 1,700 staff layoffs statewide in a single fiscal year.[55] In Italy,

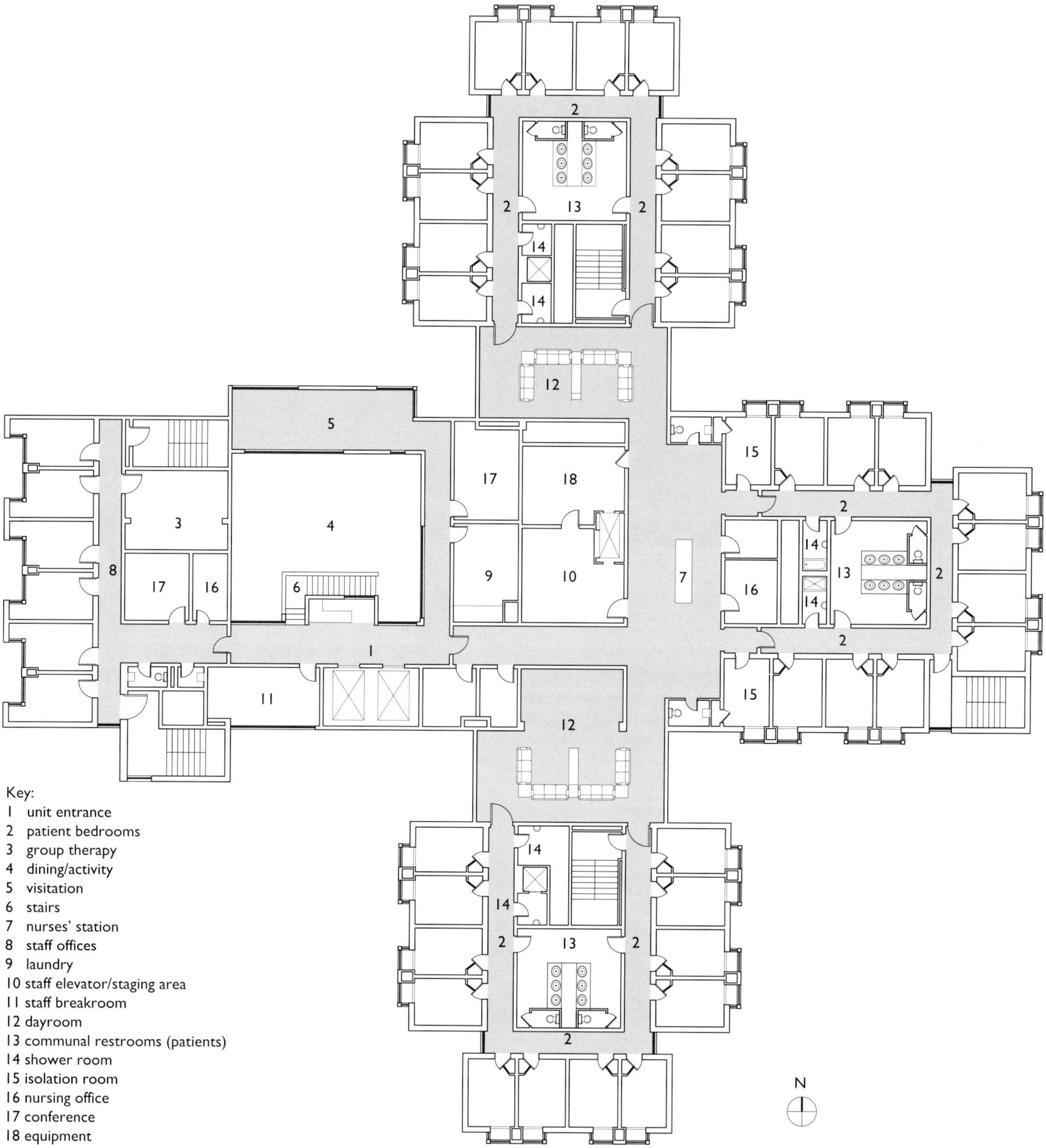

2.16 Cruciform plan, typical residential unit, Queen Street Mental Health Center (now the Center for Addiction and Mental Health), Toronto (1972–74), depicting multiple clusters of patient rooms and communal bath and shower rooms.

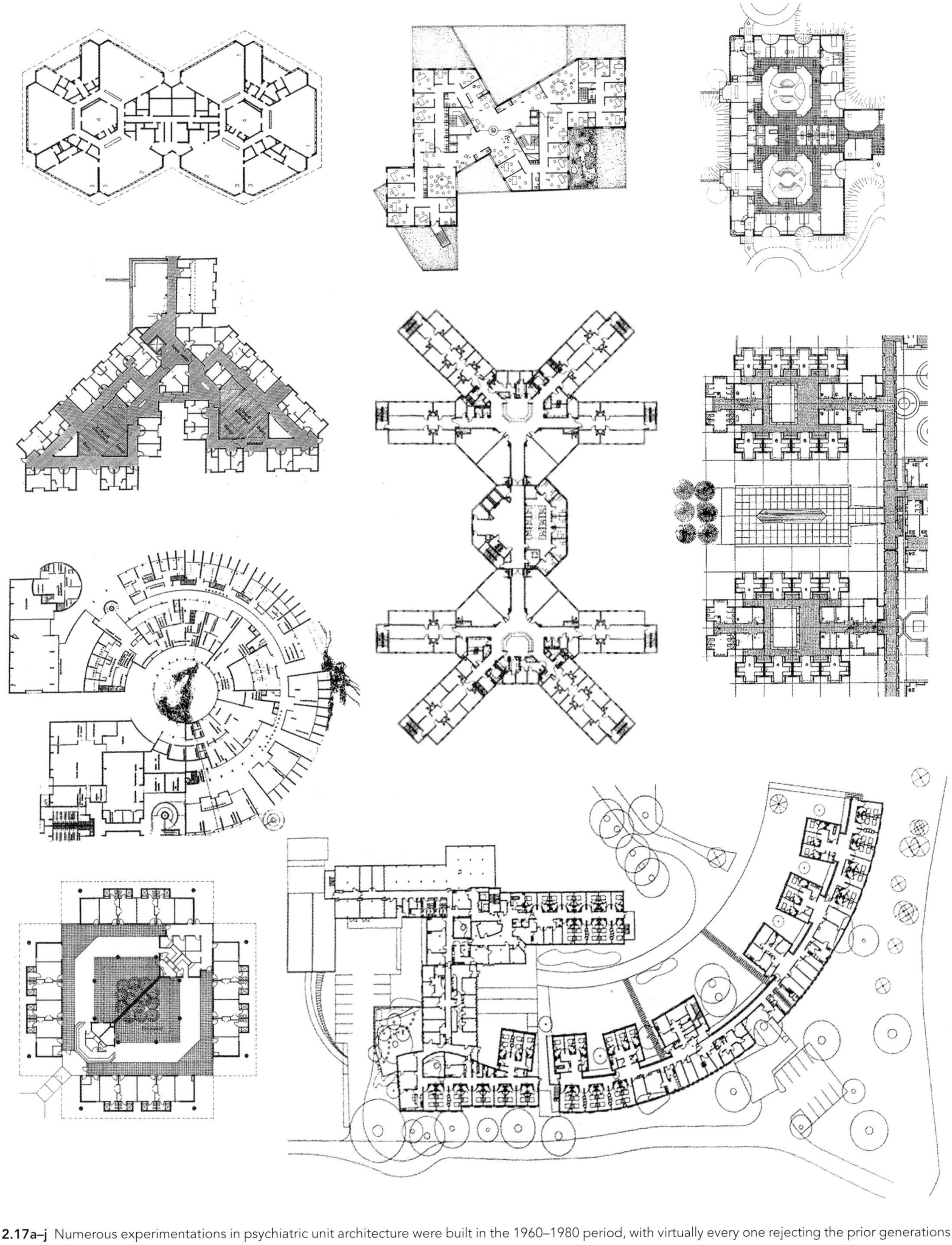

2.17a–j Numerous experimentations in psychiatric unit architecture were built in the 1960–1980 period, with virtually every one rejecting the prior generations of custodial asylums.

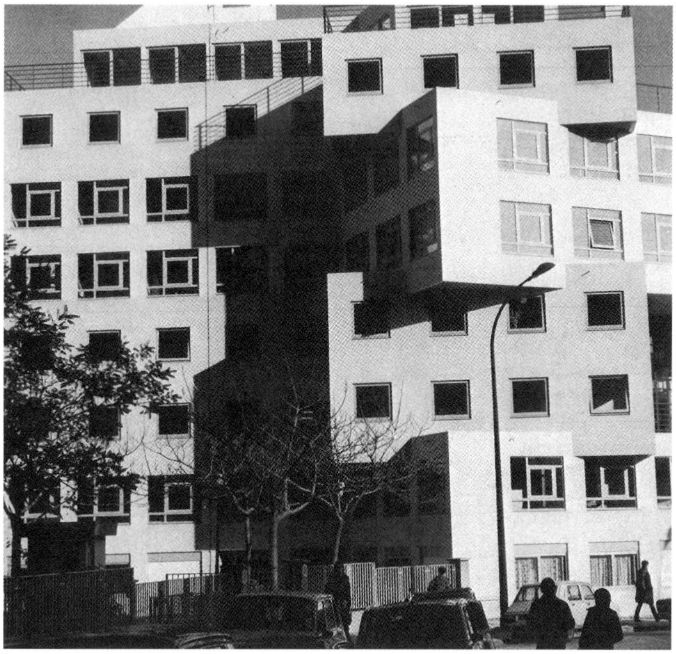

2.18 Exterior view, Centre de Santé Mentale, Paris (1978–1981).

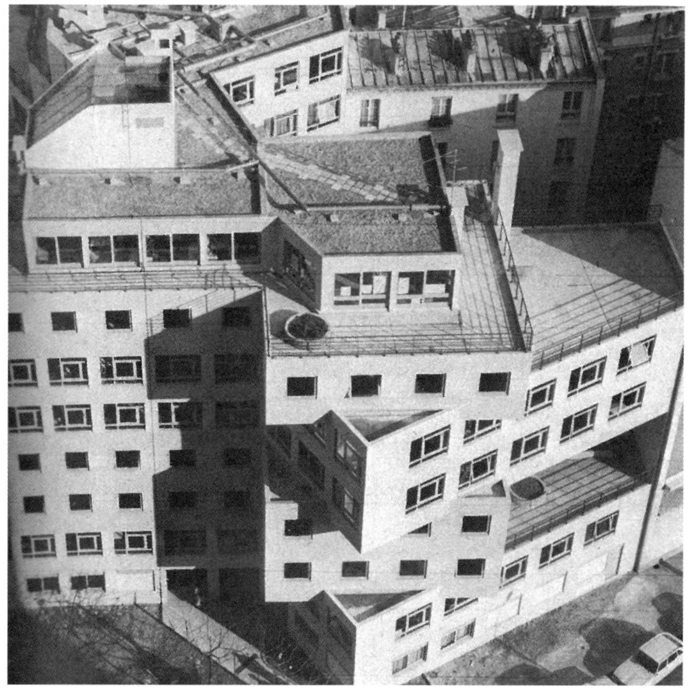

2.19 The clinic's angularity was a function of its rotated floor plates (in pairs).

the new wave of government-operated psychiatric hospitals built in the 1970s included the innovative, 225-bed Unità Ospedaliera Psichiatrica a Girifalco, in Catanzaro (1975–1978), by the firm of Michele Capobianco, Antonio Capobianco, and Daniele Zagaria. Here, on a rolling rural site, a series of highly articulated, compositionally varied administrative, therapy/treatment, and residential care pavilions were positioned in an informal campus arrangement, compared to the grid-driven symmetry of US counterpart psychiatric institutions. The structures were of cast-in-place concrete and steel-panel curtain wall construction, each one expressing its individual function. A central spine connected all structures, and this element undulated from one end of the campus to the other.[56]

1980–2000

In the United Kingdom and elsewhere, by 1980 the acute care hospital had nearly succumbed to an advancing wave of medical technologies to the point where renovations were often required, from opening day. Their technological apparatus had become highly complex, with new types of equipment and procedures introduced at such a rapid rate that premature hospital obsolescence was becoming a widespread concern. These hospitals were intensifying in scale, and gave rise to this author's coining of the term *megahospital* in 2000 to describe their enormous scale, overcomplexity, and inadvertent minimization of the role of the patient and patient's family. This term was applied at the time, and since, particularly to the massive interstitial hospitals built in wealthy advanced countries, principally in Europe and North America.[57] Architectural journals in many countries continued the practice of devoting an entire annual issue to the topic of healthcare architecture, including a special issue of the *Architectural Review*, in 1980. There, recent trends in community-based hospitals were described, including the Nucleus System recently launched by the NHS.[58]

In France, the Centre de Santé Mentale, built in an urban district in Paris by Nicole Sonolet, Maria Baran, Olek Kujawski, and Tristian Darros (1978–1981), was an exercise in taking a basic cube and then rotating the floor plates 45 degrees, creating an off-kilter composition. Was its various floor levels appearing somewhat unstable a wry reference to its occupants' unstable mental condition (Figure 2.18)? From above, rooftop open-air terraces were visible although only one such terrace was for actual use by patients (Figure 2.19). The windows were operable throughout, with their Mondrianesque frames, including in patients' rooms. Therapy/treatment and social activity rooms featured full-height windows (Figure 2.20).[59] In a similar vein, the 225-bed Centro Psichiatrico a Tirat Carmel, in Haifa, Israel, opened in 1981, designed by Elbanani Architects.[60] This residential treatment center carried forward the new, more normative approach to psychiatric care, in a series of pavilions connected to a central circulation spine. Less than a decade later, a second new facility, the Chaim Sheba Medical Center Psychiatric Hospital, would open in Tel-Hashomer, Israel.

The continued influence of high-style late modernism was in evidence in Richard Meier and Partners' Bronx Developmental Center (1978–1980), built in New York City.[61] This project featured Meier's well-known palette of ubiquitous white porcelain-baked exterior panels, a characteristic formal minimalism, and articulated massings (Figure 2.21a–c). Balconies and courtyards provided intermediary spaces for patients to interact with landscape and the outdoors. This freedom, compositionally, was possible

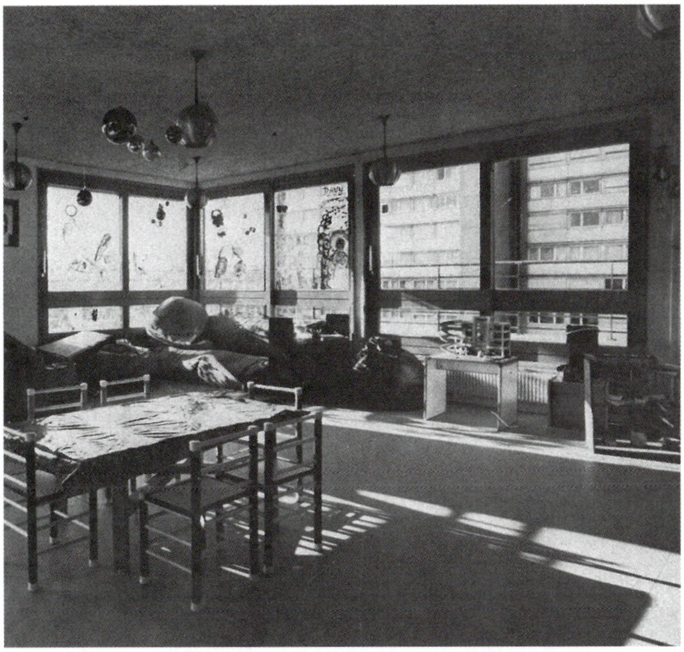

2.20 Recreational therapy room, Centre de Santé Mentale, Paris.

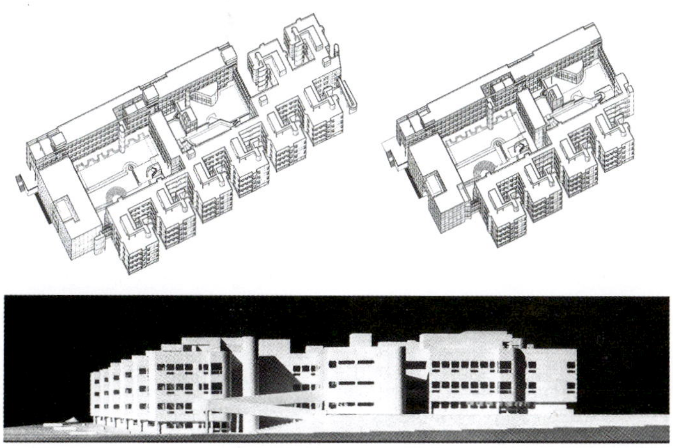

2.21a–c Bronx Developmental Center, New York (1978–1980), Richard Meier and Partners.

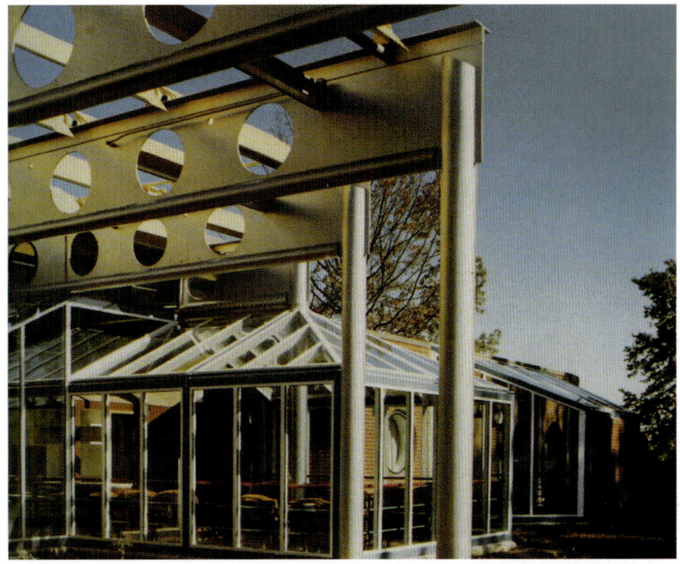

2.23 The high-tech expression of the Paul L. Barone Medical Building (a residential treatment facility), Nevada, Missouri (1980–1981), was (and remains) iconoclastic.

because this institution was significantly smaller in bed capacity compared to prior generations of state-run facilities (Figure 2.22). This project was also noteworthy for two reasons. First, it was one of the few hospitals of the period designed by an internationally established architect who had become known for commissions *other* than hospitals. Second, because it was designed by a renowned architect, this alone would prove influential in the subsequent work of specialized 'hospital architects' in the United States and elsewhere.[62]

The Paul L. Barone Medical Building (1980–1981) was built in Nevada, Missouri, designed by the firm Abend Singleton Associates. This 21-bed facility stood in stark contrast to the architectural status quo (Figure 2.23), insofar as then-popular language of high-tech expressionism was employed throughout, as inspired by the Pompidou Centre in Paris (1975–1977) by Richard Rogers and Renzo Piano. The aesthetic vocabulary of both of these buildings invoked the imagery of an industrial facility, a factory. The Barone Medical Building was built on the grounds of an old state asylum and starkly, even blithely, contrasted its adjacent neoclassical context (Figure 2.24a–b). Barone was a one-level structure, with soaring ceilings and expansive windows that allowed ample natural light to be drawn deep into the interior envelope. The residential unit was essentially triangular, in plan, with support functions clustered at the center of its triangulated *racetrack*. All patient rooms were private, with communal bath/hygiene rooms located at the end of the corridor. Therapy/treatment and administrative functions were housed in a connecting wing (Figure 2.25a–d).[63]

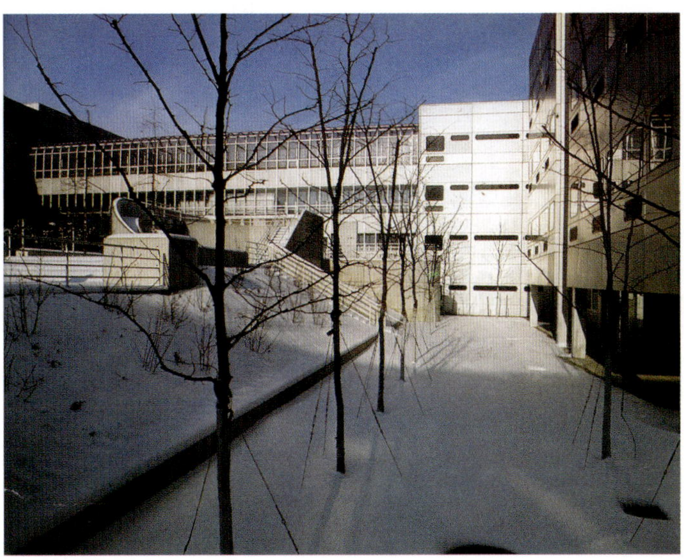

2.22 Main courtyard at the Bronx Developmental Center, which provides a protective enclosure for patients.

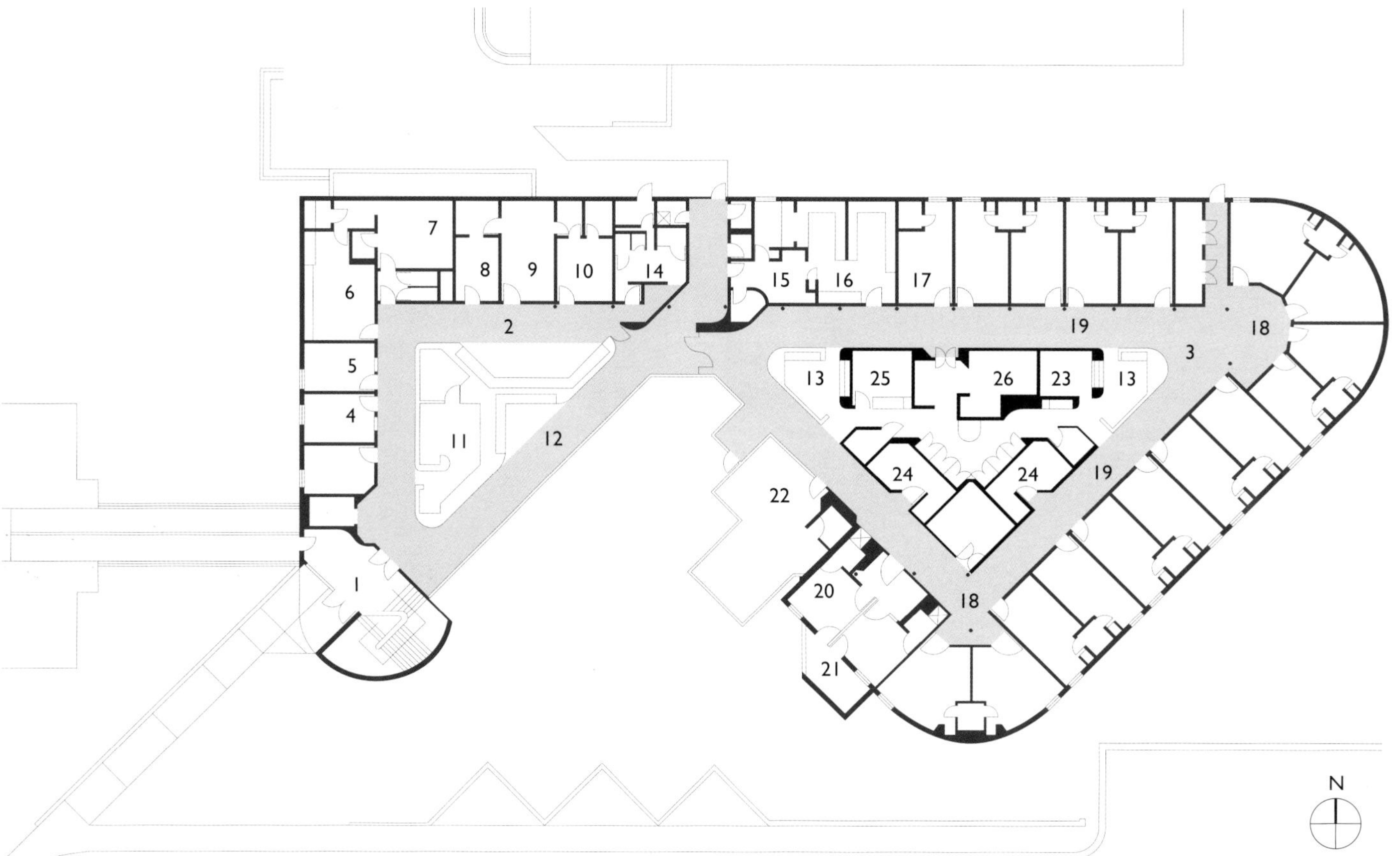

Key:

1 entrance	15 dispensary
2 therapy/treatment	16 pharmacy
3 residential unit	17 laboratory
4 clinical director	18 private bedrooms
5 administrator	19 semiprivate bedrooms
6 staff workroom	20 isolation
7 radiology	21 patio
8 assessment	22 solarium/dining
9 counseling	23 medications room
10 inhalation therapy	24 shower room
11 staff workroom	25 supervisor unit
12 waiting	26 clean/soiled utility
13 nurses' station	
14 restrooms	

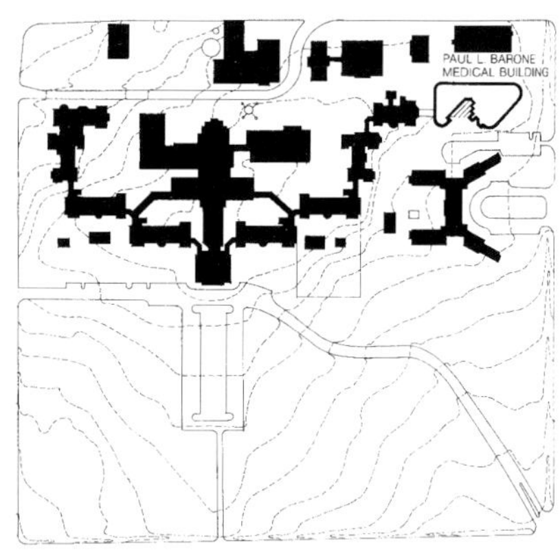

2.24a–b The Barone treatment center is dual triangular in plan, divided into an outpatient/administration zone and an inpatient unit, and the facility was built next to a 19th-century state-run asylum.

In the United States, for-profit chains soon built, or acquired, freestanding psychiatric hospitals, although the total number of beds remained insufficient in the face of the concurrent loss of many thousands of beds in the state-run hospitals.[64] Beyond this, these for-profit beds were disproportionally distributed, geographically. The recently enacted *diagnostic related group* (DRG) federal legislation in the United States was the first attempt in the post-World War II era in that country to rein in soaring governmental healthcare expenditures, though the introduction of a fixed, fee-for-service system; this resulted in an extensive classification system, or taxonomy, of treatment types then variously adjusted to account for regional differences in costs. Psychiatric treatment was exempted from the initial DRG legislation, and therefore not initially subject to any type of *capped* reimbursement system. The prospect of any fee-restricted pricing system for psychiatric hospitals was feared to inflict large financial losses for some providers and possibly windfall gains for others. This was the conclusion of a report by the National Association of Private Psychiatric

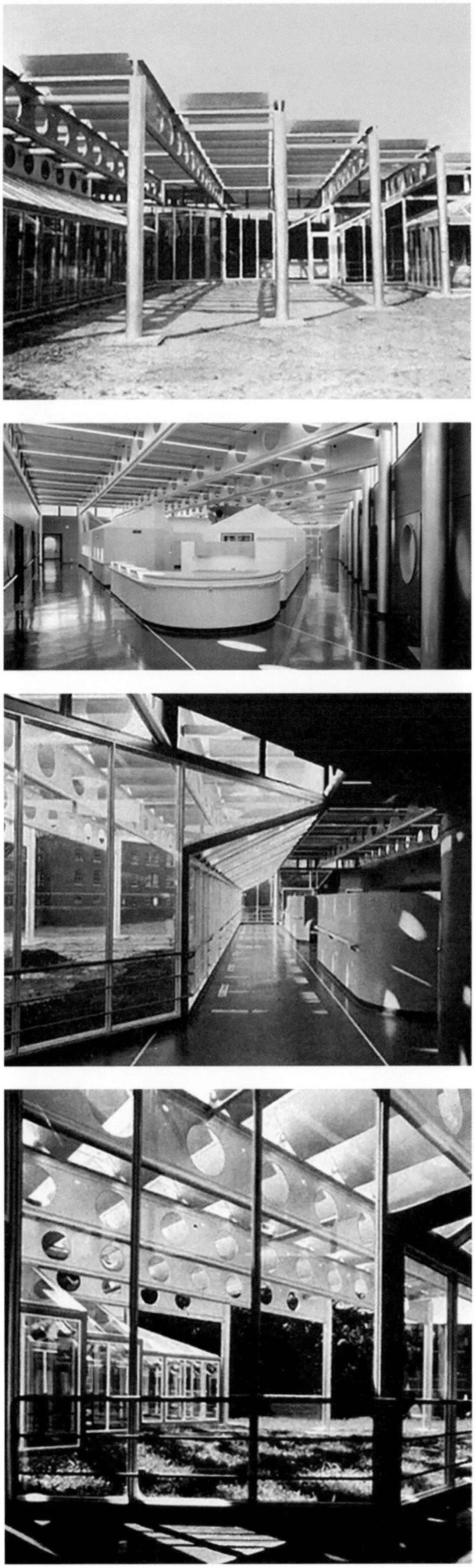

Hospitals. This trade group lobbied in 1985 (and won, for a time at least) for the privileged status of being able to charge on a fee-for-service basis (uncapped). This immediately fueled even more private investment in a growing and profitable industry just as the public sector was doing all it could to divest itself of its custodial care obligations – *privatization*. Privatization was therefore a direct response to the public-sector deinstitutionalization movement.[65] Concurrently, the for-profit psychiatric hospital industry began to engage in high-profile public media campaigns including costly print and television ads. Specific types of treatment – now including addictive disorder residential and outpatient treatments – were marketed for the first time to niche audiences, including teens, the aged, and middle-aged women.[66] Specialty programs, such as for eating disorders and obsessive compulsive disorder, also appeared in the for-profit healthcare marketplace at this time, as this was seen as yet another new means to fill otherwise empty hospital beds.[67] This expansionism continued throughout the 1980s, and appeared to have no end in sight.[68]

In architecture, postmodernism was the rage at this time. The Renfrew Center in Philadelphia (1983–1985), by Tony Atkins and Associates of Philadelphia, was a prominent example of the New Residentialism in for-profit healthcare architecture. This postmodern-inspired residential center was modeled on a 19th-century rural estate retreat (i.e., institutions built in the British countryside for the wealthier upper classes). Similar to these precursors, the Renfrew Center was situated amid a bucolic, pastoral campus. The 35-bed main facility and its immediate environs featured a strong axial orientation, with the main entrance at one end and a treatment and recreational therapy building forming a circulation spine, with narrow footprints that maximized natural light and ventilation transmission to the interiors. The 'Main Residence' was reminiscent of a country manor house, with its pitched roof, stucco façade, and portico, and this provided protection from the elements. The main living-dayroom and the patient rooms were well appointed, although the majority of patient rooms were semiprivate (two-beds) with four patients sharing a common bath/shower (situated between each pair of bedrooms). The Renfrew

2.25a–d The exterior and interior of the Barone facility in Missouri (1980–1981) expressed its structural frame and anatomical systems in a manner not unlike the Pompidou Centre in Paris, which opened in 1977.

Center symbolized an alternative, if elitist approach, including aesthetically, for its reprise of 19th-century neoclassical motifs and its romanticized landscape imagery, and for these reasons it was fêted by the architectural profession.[69]

These were indeed the halcyon days of postmodernism. Charles Jencks, writing a few years earlier (1977), argued a 'Post-Modern' building was one

> which speaks on at least two levels at once: to other architects and a concerned minority who care about specifically architectural meanings, and to the public at large, or the local inhabitants, who care about other issues, with comfort, traditional building, and a way of life . . . the architect can read the implicit metaphors and subtle meanings of the column drums, whereas the public can respond to the explicit metaphors . . . it is this discontinuity in taste cultures which creates both the 'theoretical base' and 'dual coding' of Post-Modernism . . . [these] buildings show a marked duality and a conscious schizophrenia.[70]

This new wave of postmodern, *New Residentialist* psychiatric and substance addiction treatment facilities in the United States was being recognized in the annual design awards program sponsored by the leading healthcare provider industry publication, *Modern Healthcare* magazine. These recognized buildings included the Kahi Mohala Psychiatric Hospital in Honolulu, Hawaii, by HKS of Dallas (1985); Kimberly Woods, in Columbus, Ohio, by Bohm-NBBJ of Columbus (1987); and the Laurel Ridge Psychiatric Hospital, in San Antonio, also by HKS, of Dallas (1989).[71] An evidence-based design initiative (codesigned by this author) was commissioned by Hospital Corporation of America (HCA) in 1991 with the aim of reinventing a 19th-century asylum campus in New Orleans (De Paul). It received a national award from *Progressive Architecture* magazine at the time.[72]

A postmodern 'village' concept was applied at the Yale Psychiatric Institute, in New Haven, Connecticut, by Frank O. Gehry and Associates (1987–1989). This campus, built in a high-crime neighborhood, housed 36 beds for adolescents in a 76,000-square-foot facility whose partí was composed of three main elements – a central administrative building flanked by two inpatient and therapy/treatment wings. These elements faced a central courtyard, open on one side to the city vis-à-vis a steel see-through fence. A postoccupancy assessment was conducted 4 years after its opening, and this yielded a number of deficiencies, including dysfunctional nurses' stations (they were perceived by nursing staff as too open, and lacking in physical protection), staff counseling offices too small for their intended use, and patients' belief the facility, overall, compromised one's sense of confidentiality and personal privacy.[73]

As deinstitutionalization was advancing on all fronts, governments in many jurisdictions realized that new 24/7 replacement facilities were needed, including specialized forensic facilities for housing at-risk patients deemed not guilty by the courts by reason of mental illness. One such facility, a 550-bed psychiatric care unit in Sugarland, Texas, designed by HOK of Dallas for the Texas Department of Criminal Justice, opened in 1995. This facility, aesthetically uninspired, to say the least, featured a stark, all-white exterior with few windows and a bare-bones aesthetic.[74]

At the opposite, nonpunitive end of this spectrum, in that same year, a wittily designed outpatient psychiatric center for children and adolescents opened in Leeuwarden, the Netherlands, designed by Sybolt Meindertsma and Eric Eijsbouts. It featured a playful site plan and human-scale (one-level) curvilinear buildings arrayed around an informal grouping of outdoor structures whose intent was to encourage a variety of recreational therapy activities.[75] In 1998, a similarly bold, alternative strategy was adopted in the design of the Pôle Psychiatric Hospital, in France, by Gaëlle Peneau (1996–1998). This one-level, 32-bed inpatient treatment center, the majority of which is a single curvilinear wing, in plan, featured semiprivate bedrooms on the outer side, with staff support and treatment functions on the inner side of a footprint spanning the length of its winding radius. Its exterior imagery was low slung and informal, with residential-like fenestration, an undulating roof line, and extended eaves.[76]

In Germany, the need similarly arose for new psychiatric hospitals, including the Karl-Bonhoeffer-Nervenklinik Forensic Hospital, built in Berlin (1984–1987), designed by Ganz E. Rolfes Architects. With postmodernism still raging, the architects elected to use exterior-face brick with banded accentuated courses, a strategy in vogue and specifically in the work of Caesar Pelli, James Sterling, Michael Graves, and other notable postmodern architects. This same masonry pattern was applied throughout the entire campus (Figure 2.26 and Figure 2.27a–j). In plan, the campus was orthogonal, dominated by a large high-security courtyard at the center of a superblock. This space was enclosed by formidable walls, an array of inpatient units, and miscellaneous supports (Figure 2.28a–b). The

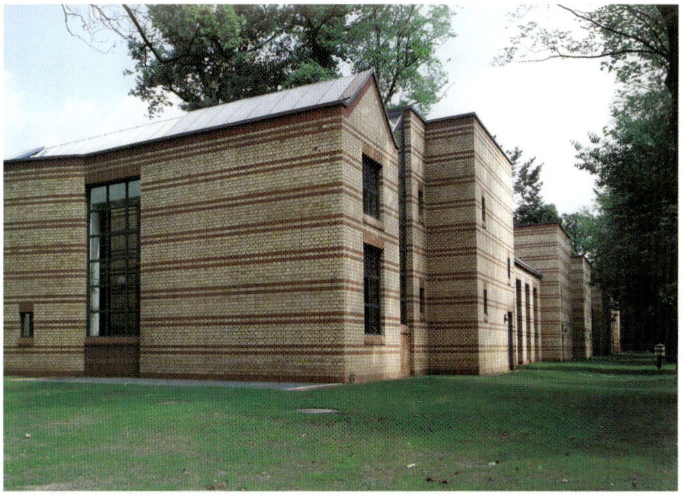

2.26 The high postmodern aesthetic of the Karl-Bonhoeffer-Nervenklinik, Berlin, Germany (1984–1987).

exterior courtyards between the two-level residential units allowed for 'passive activity' patient contact with the outdoors, whereas the large, high-secured courtyard allowed for active use, including athletic fields, walking paths, a small outdoor amphitheater, and the seclusion unit (Figure 2.29). The interior of the Spartan, semiprivate patient bedrooms featured built-in bunk beds and desks affixed to full-height window frames (Figure 2.30). One concern with this arrangement was that patients' personal visual privacy was compromised while sitting at the bedroom desk because he or she could be readily seen from the outside.[77]

As for comparable large-scale undertakings in North America, the Ontario Provincial Government embarked in the early 1990s on the construction of a 300-bed publicly run replacement psychiatric hospital, to be the first such comprehensive residential campus built in 20 years in Canada or the United States. This campus, originally known as the Whitby Psychiatric Hospital, would later be rechristened the Ontario Shores Centre for Mental Health Sciences. It was built in on the shores of Lake Ontario in Whitby, Ontario, approximately an hour's drive east of Toronto, in Canada. A design competition was held at a time when, in its large neighboring country to the south, the emphasis was on cost cutting when it came to inpatient psychiatric beds. As early as 1977, the Ministry of Health and Long-Term Care recognized that the 1917 Whitby hospital would require total replacement. This sprawling complex (36 buildings, 370 beds, 155 acres, 915,000 square feet) did not meet life safety codes and was costly to maintain due to new types of treatment. In 1989, the ministry prepared a master plan guide. The proposed project consolidated all buildings in an interconnected two-level superstructure of 500,000 square feet, allowing for flexibility to ensure future advancements in diagnosis and treatment can be readily accommodated. The new facility occupied 86 acres with a total construction budget of US$156 million of which US$89 million was for the actual facility.

The design competition attracted 17 teams responding to a Request for Information issued in September 1990. From these, six teams' schematic concepts were chosen for further development. Three finalists were then selected: Shore Tilbe Henschel Irwin Peters of Toronto with HKS of Dallas, Texas; Crang & Boake, Moffat Kinoshita Associates, of Toronto, with Cannon, of Grand Island, New York; and the Ziedler Roberts Partnership of Toronto. Each competitor team was allotted US$75,000 up front to cover project expenses. The design selection committee was composed of 12 members; the three finalist teams' submissions were each quite different.

The winning scheme, by Moffat Kinoshita Associates/Crang & Boake/Cannon Partnership, established a residential aesthetic with pitched roofs, familiar materials, ample natural light, and a sense of horizontal spaciousness maximizing the natural amenity of its shoreline site.[78] The partí was dominated by a series of pavilions connected to a single pedestrian 'street'. This circulation element (an example of *theraserialization*; see Chapters 4 and 5) functionally linked all spaces so that one need not venture outdoors in inclement weather, as the spacing of the pavilions allowed for courtyards to be interspersed between various residential and constituent support functions (Figure 2.31 and Figure 2.32). Therapeutic supports were housed to one side of this circulation spine, with residential units located on the opposing side. Many opportunities were provided for occupants to engage with the outdoors and lakefront site and special attention was devoted to campus landscape design.[79]

The courtyards were attuned to the therapeutic needs of patients, who were housed in 14 adjoining pavilions. Two outpatient units were provided as well, together with a partial hospitalization unit, and a 24/7 forensic unit. Residential units were oriented such that views outward were either to an adjoining courtyard or the shoreline beyond (Figure 2.33). Each residential unit featured a solarium and a day-activity room – adjacent to the unit nurses' station. These nurses' stations, initially designed without a glass separation, were later retrofitted to include shatterproof transparent glass, for protection. Most rooms' windows were operable, allowing for natural ventilation. A main cafeteria-dining area at the apex of two superordinate wings of the facility afforded direct views outward. The landscape architect, Vertechs Design, Inc., produced a low-maintenance scheme emphasizing trellises, pockets of seating, and plant species not unlike the backyard of a home in one of the nearby residential neighborhoods. During warmer months, social activities are held ranging from recreational

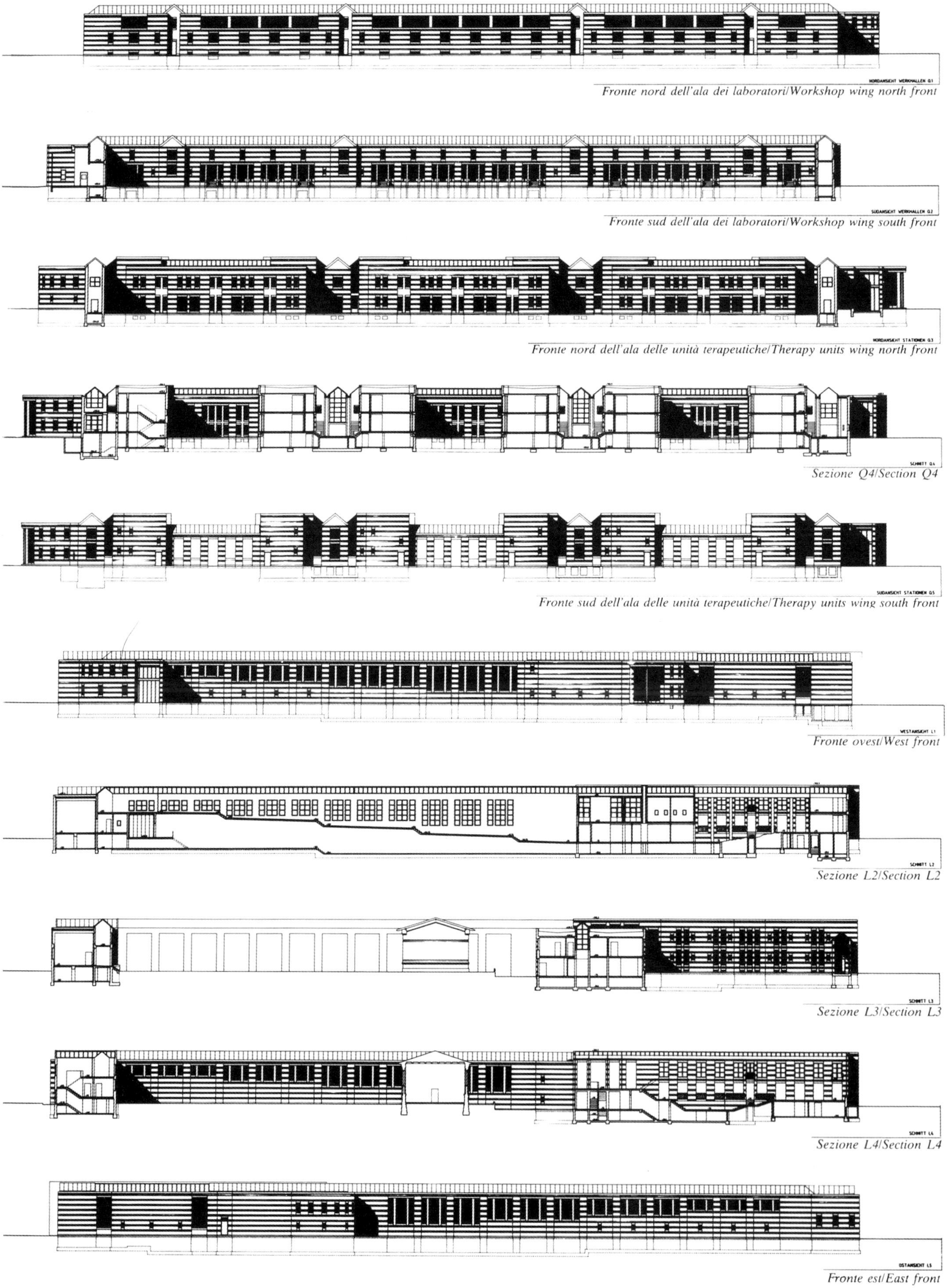

2.27a–j The exterior of this psychiatric hospital in Berlin was in banded, tinted-face brick, in an expression of postmodernism at its zenith.

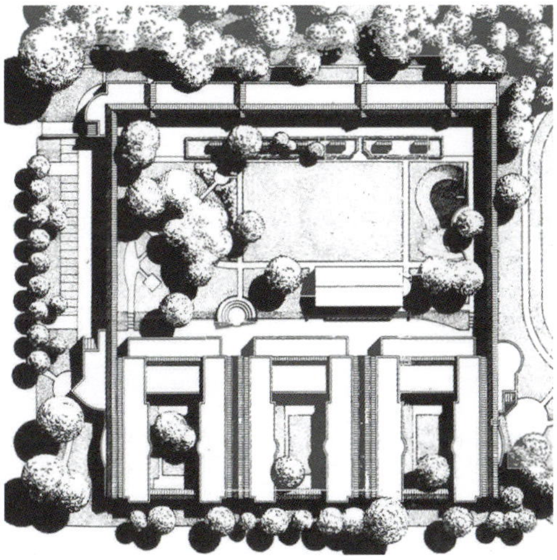

Key:
1 inpatient wards
2 workshops
3 main entry
4 service corridor
5 internal ring route
6 garden/courtyards
7 vegetable garden
8 therapeutic landscape
9 open-air theater
10 gymnasium
11 sports/recreation
12 pond
13 gardens
14 parking
15 staff/service entry

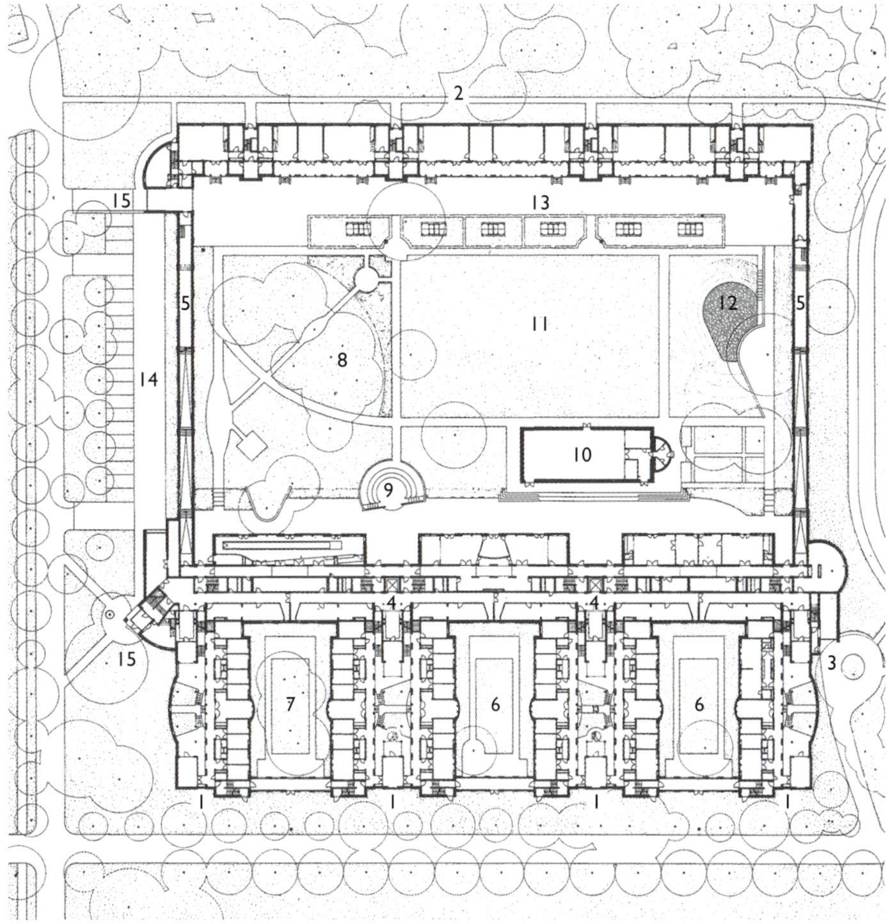

2.28a–b The six inpatient units at the Karl-Bonhoeffer-Nervenklinik psychiatric hospital were arrayed along of a central secure courtyard, connected to functions across the open space via a racetrack circulation system. The courtyard was subdivided into numerous passive- and active-use zones.

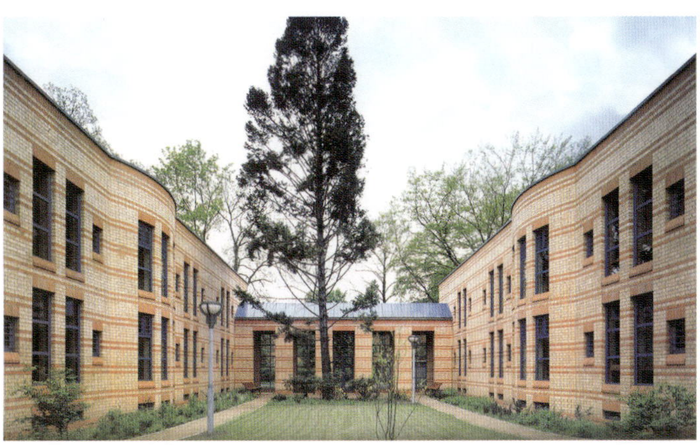

2.29 Exterior spaces at the Karl-Bonhoeffer-Nervenklinik psychiatric hospital were relatively Spartan in amenity and appearance.

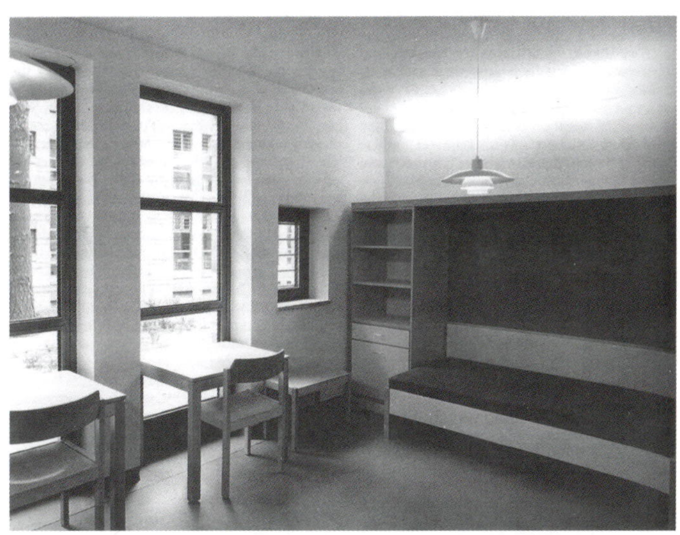

2.30 The patient rooms were semiprivate (two-bed) with dual windows, desks, beds, and storage.

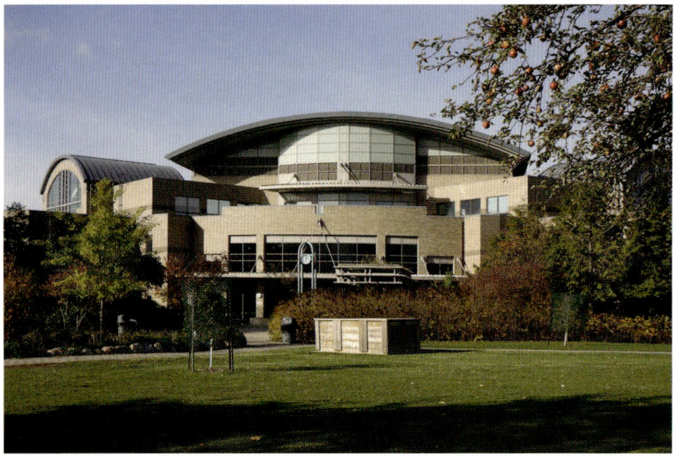

2.31 Ontario Shores Centre for Mental Health Sciences, Whitby, Ontario (1974–1976).

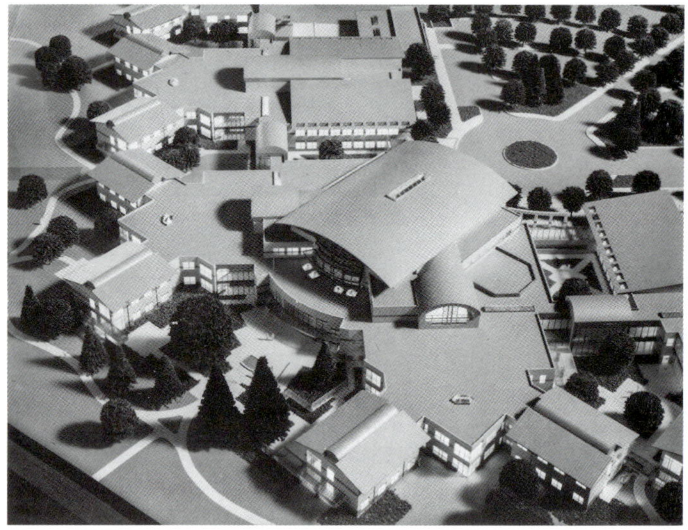

2.32 Architects' model, Ontario Shores, 1975.

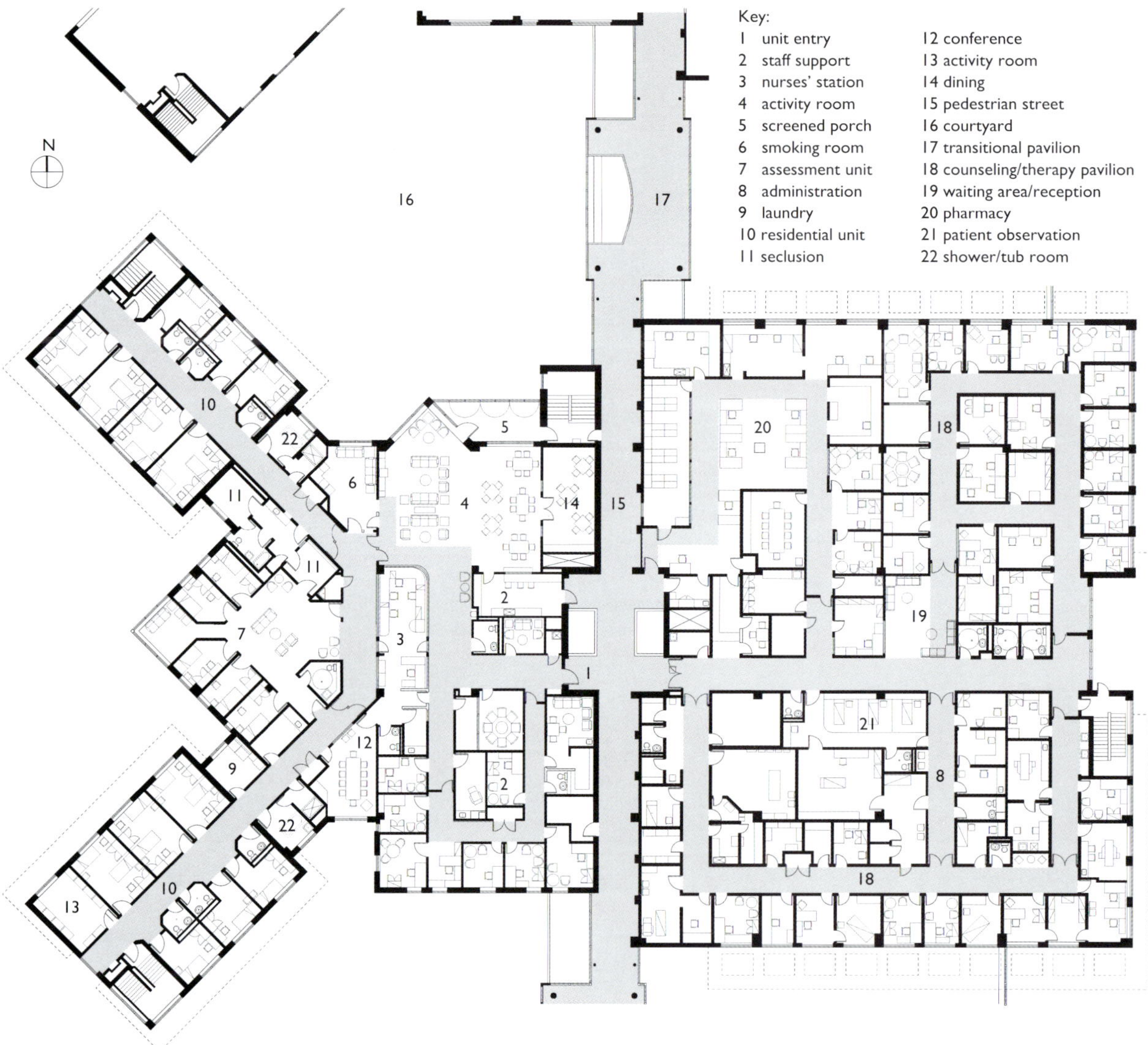

2.33 Residential pavilions were arrayed along a V-shaped 'street', with related supports housed directly across and in a main building at the campus center. Each unit's wing housed seven inpatient rooms (all private), communal toilets accessed via the corridor, and an assessment unit. The staff workstation (enclosed) was at the center of the unit.

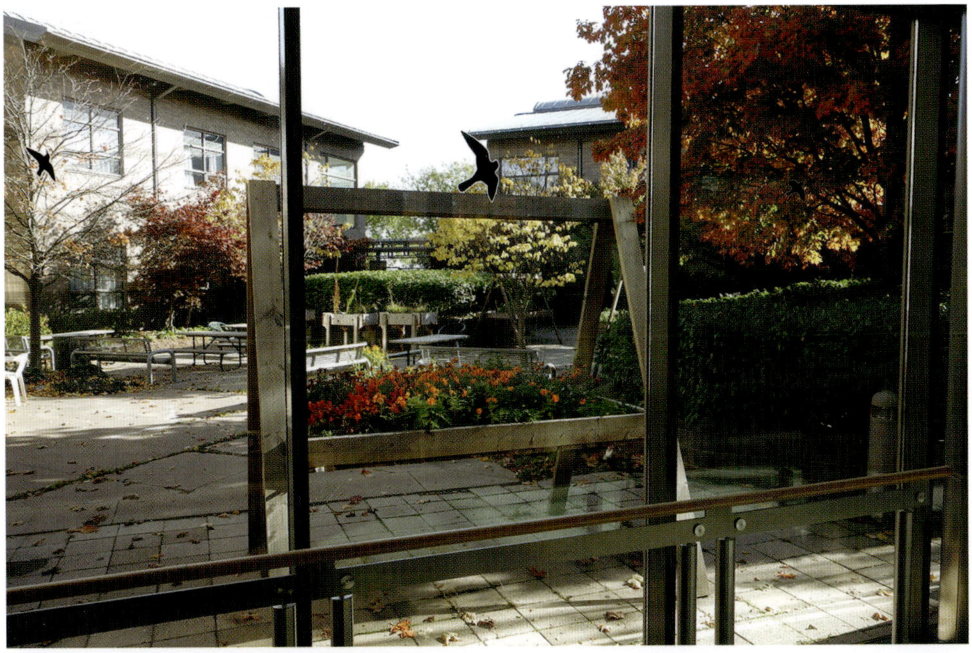

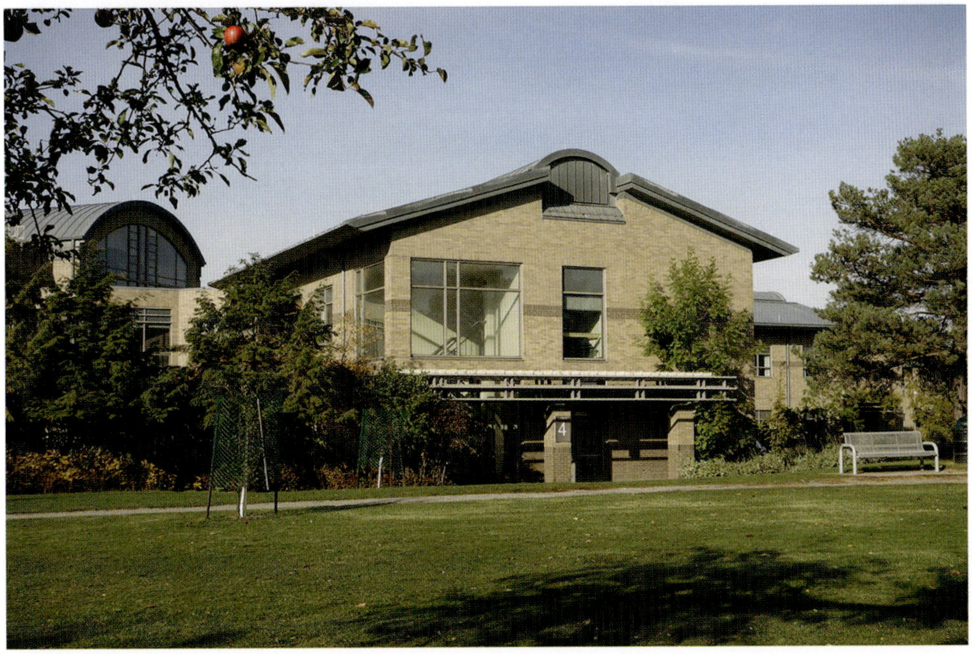

2.34a–b View of a courtyard from the main circulation street (top), and an exterior view of a residential unit at Ontario Shores (bottom).

therapy to sports and picnics. The trellised seating nodes provided shade and work well as settings for informal consultation. A see-through wrought-iron fence surrounded the courtyards. The main arrival atrium lobby houses an art gallery and the central administration. The forensic unit consists of two 20-bed units on the upper level, a forensic rehabilitation unit on the main level, and an exterior courtyard buffered from the rest of the campus. This campus also bordered the Lynde Marsh, a no-build wildlife habitat conservation area. Pedestrian/bike lanes traverse the campus, along with seating and places for respite. A significant portion of the grounds, and the interior 'street', are open to the general public, as are the shoreline and wildlife sanctuary areas.[80] This campus retains its aesthetic and functional integrity after serving its community for more than twenty years, at this writing (Figure 2.34a–b).

A counterpoint to Ontario Shores was the New York Psychiatric Institute, or NYPI (1996–1999), in New York City, by

Ellerbe Becket. This 312,000-square-foot, 58-bed treatment facility and research center was built on a dense urban site near the George Washington Bridge adjacent to the Hudson River, near the northern tip of Manhattan. First announced in 1992, this project was the focus of considerable NIMBY-ism on the part of its nearby irate residential neighbors. The narrow site, squeezed in between the heavily trafficked Henry Hudson Parkway and Riverside Drive, had previously been notorious for illicit drug dealing. The parti is curvilinear and continuously glazed on the river-facing side, establishing a unified (if quasi-corporate) image, and it is sheathed in laminated low-emitting (low-e) reflective glass with horizontal spandrel glass banding. Public access to the building is on three different levels and the structure provides parking for 100 vehicles one level below the street. Two pedestrian bridges (at the sixth level) provide umbilical links to the adjacent (and older) institute buildings situated directly across the roadway. An architectural journal account of the NYPI cited its positive impact on patients' behaviour insofar as fewer patient-restraint (lockdown) incidents occur now, as compared to the older building that formerly housed the institute. From above, this building is vessel-like, appearing not entirely unlike one of the nautical vessels passing by on the river.[81]

At this same time, the financial prospects of the for-profit psychiatric and addictive disorder healthcare industry in the United States began to dramatically shift course.[82] The federal government had by now clamped down on its previously uncapped reimbursement rates for psychiatric care and as a result many for-profit corporations found themselves with a losing hand – in one case, a hospital had a staff of 80 onboard, with only eight inpatients! Soon thereafter the federal government stepped in further, as it began to investigate and scrutinize the for-profit chains' questionable business practices, including widespread popular media reports of 'patient dumping' at nearby general hospital emergency departments.[83] With reimbursement models now firmly focused on outpatient treatment, patient dumping was becoming widespread (but by no means a new practice in the long, long history of psychiatric institutions).[84] Many countries by 2000 now found themselves in the *self-inflicted* predicament of having too many patients in need of 24/7 support, and with far too few hospital beds available to meet the growing need.[85] One desperate for-profit chain, HCA, even resorted to auctioning off its inventory of unwanted psychiatric hospitals at this time because they had become so unprofitable.[86]

In the United Kingdom, study after study continued to proclaim inpatient treatment was now vastly too expensive (deinstitutionalization) and a further emphasis on less costly outpatient treatment was of absolute necessity.[87]

A legacy of environmental design research

While this was happening in the public marketplace, a sizeable contingent of environmental design researchers was focused on studying the impact of the post-World War II psychiatric ward on occupants' well-being and satisfaction. This history of environmental design research is impressive in the 1960–2010 period. Unfortunately, space limitations do not allow a comprehensive appraisal of this work here; therefore, only certain landmark developments are cited (though this topic would warrant a complete chapter unto itself). The interested reader is encouraged to pursue these references further to learn of the specific studies and books published on this subject over the past half century. On the one hand, it is a distinguished body of work, while on the other, it was handicapped somewhat by inconsistency from the standpoint of data reliability, questionable methodology, and the at-times overgeneralization of results from a single, freestanding study (see Chapter 1 as to the persistence of this to this day). Moreover, most architects had difficulty in discerning useful 'takeaway' design insights for application in professional practice. Because the earliest studies and reports are now quite dated, in retrospect, these are not recounted in detail here in terms of their (if any) recommendations for design. The reader is encouraged, instead, to peruse the more recent examples cited in this section. Second, the field of psychiatry has itself continually evolved during this period, and finally, as mentioned, this summary is by no means intended to be seen as exhaustive.

1960s

In this decade, numerous publications and nongovernmental organization (NGO) reports appeared on the design and construction of psychiatric hospitals. Two major research trends in this decade are discernable. First, researchers' interest was centered at this time on the assumption that thousands of additional inpatient beds would be needed by the 1970s. The International Style was the prevailing architectural language, as was the 'form follows function' dictum, and the buildings built were, as to be expected, minimalist, with their campuses having been designed of rigid orthogonal grids. For example, in 1958, the article 'Architectural Research and the Construction of Mental Hospitals' was published, followed by the aforementioned WHO report 'Psychiatric Services and Architecture', a 1968 article 'Architectural Considerations in the Design of Places and Facilities for the Care and Treatment of the Mentally Ill', and the 1968 book by C.B. Moller, *Architectural Environment and Our Mental Health*.[88] In the early 1960s, research, as mentioned previously, began at the Topeka State Hospital (Kansas) on the efficacy of adapting a traditional open-ward unit to a more personalized, privacy-attuned treatment setting, and this work was published in an *AIA Journal* article and in a book.[89]

Another discernable trend was a new emphasis on creating empirically rigorous environmental assessment scales for evaluating the impact of the built setting of the inpatient ward/unit on inpatient well-being and health status. Rudolph Moos, who developed an instrument referred to as the Ward Atmosphere Scale, led the most prominent work on this. Moos's intent was for this assessment tool to be applicable in most psychiatric ward settings.[90] This thread of work culminated in his 1989 *The Ward Atmosphere Scale Manual*.[91] Researchers in Europe were keenly interested in this subject, and Moos's approach to creating prevalidated rating scales has endured over the years.[92] In addition, Kasmar et al. published multiple studies on outpatients' mood and their perceptions as a function of the psychiatric built environment; this included a review of the literature on this topic up to that point in time. In 1969, E.V. Zeller, a contemporary of Kasmar, published the book *Psychiatric Treatment Environment and Function*.[93]

1970s

The focus of environment-behaviour researchers during this decade on this subject remained firmly on the 'psych ward' and its impact on occupants' psychological and physical well-being. Patient ward layout, size, amenities, and aesthetic appearance remained primary foci. The decade began with a study reported by Ittelson, Proshansky, and Rivlin (1970) on patient bedroom size and its impact on social interactions. Rivlin and Wolfe (1972) published a descriptive narrative of a children's psychiatric hospitals' impact on the behaviour of its occupants. Holahan and Saegert (1973) reported the results of an investigation on the most suitable number of patients in an inpatient ward. Willer et al. (1974) addressed the socialization and well-being functions of therapy activities in an inpatient ward, and Wolfe (1975) reported on the function of room size, group size, and density factors on the well-being in a children's ward.[94] At the end of this decade, an essay was published in a leading psychiatry journal by Davis et al. on architectural design issues in psychiatric facilities (1979). David Canter and Sandra Canter's influential book, *Designing for Therapeutic Environments: A Review of Research* (1979), was published containing reviews of landmark recent environment-behaviour research on this subject.[95] An additional trend emerged during this decade: numerous postoccupancy assessments of psychiatric facilities were published, including Sivadon's previously mentioned research (1970), an article in the *AIA Journal* (1971), an essay by Osmond and Izumi and design guidelines (1971), and a method for evaluating an existing mental health facility and incorporating this information in facility renovation projects (1976).[96]

1980s and 1990s

Three broad trends in the environment-behaviour research emerged during these years. First, an increasing emphasis on research on specialized user constituencies, including further work on child and adolescent facilities (1984), the impact of various furniture arrangements in a forensic hospital (1985), further comparative work on patient versus staff perceptions of their facility (1991), a focus on personal safety with regards to specific types of patients (1991), and design factors in support of hospitalized schizophrenic patients (1992).[97] A second trend was a more pronounced focus on the adaptive use and renovation of existing mental health facilities, including the impact of new furnishings on patient and staff satisfaction. These studies included pre- and postrelocation investigations (1984), the subjective versus objective assessment of facilities (1984), and the role of interior design in the retrofitting of facilities (1986; 1992).[98] A third discernable trend in these years

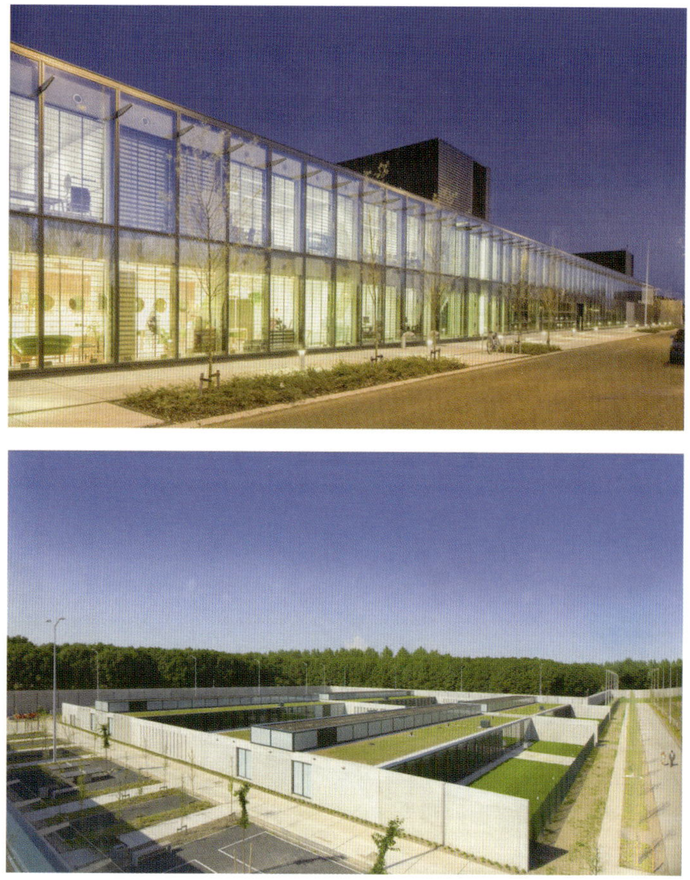

2.35a–b TBS Kliniek, Almere, the Netherlands (2005–2008). Exterior view (top) and view of secure outdoor activity space (bottom).

was an increasing dissatisfaction with institutionalism and health-care professionals' growing advocacy calls for a higher-quality built environment for psychiatric care. This advocacy focus included Meyer Spivak's book *Institutional Settings* (1984), and Kiesler and Sibulkin's *Mental Hospitalization: Myths and Facts About a National Crisis* (1987). A new generation of minimum architectural design guideline standards were published (1991 and 1993, respectively) aimed at improving overall aesthetics, functional design quality, and life safety-code compliance while less overtly advocating for the total obliteration of institutionalism.[99]

2000–2015

These years were characterized by an eclectic range of environmental design research on this subject, including work on the full emergence of specialized facilities for substance addiction treatment (2000); studies on assessing nurses' satisfaction with their unit's architectural design amenities (2002); the opening of the first Planetree inpatient psychiatric unit (2004); and the study of psychological impacts on patient and staff personnel after having relocated to new, purpose-built treatment facilities (2005; 2009).[100] A second discernable trend was a continued emphasis, particularly in Europe, on Moos's ward assessment scales and their various applications including in high-security forensic hospitals (2001; 2005; 2010), the comparative assessment of an open versus a closed inpatient residential ward (2002), and the interrelationship between depression and a ward's perceived atmosphere (2011).[101] Additional research investigations were reported on environmental interventions to reduce the use of seclusion as a treatment measure (2007) and on the role of visual art in reducing patient anxiety and agitation (2010).[102] Finally, in addition to the recent research conducted by Ulrich and colleagues in Sweden (see Chapter 1), essays were published on the need to reinvent the therapeutic milieu in the 21st century (2009), and the promise of *salutogenic* design precepts (2010 and 2012).[103] Would the international research community turn its attention to the sociocultural and political relevance, aesthetics, and functional performance of a new wave of treatment environments – not unlike the landmark research a generation earlier on Goffman and Foucault's total institutions of the 1950s and 1960s?

Architectural trends: 2000–2010

In the early years of this century, newly built, specialized, and architecturally noteworthy psychiatric and substance addiction treatment campuses and community clinics did not proliferate. Was this attributable to chronic underfunding, political ineptitude, or the continued stigma associated with mental health and addictive disorders? Space precludes a comprehensive survey here, although a subset of indicative examples is discussed, examples illustrating a prevailing pluralism from neo-modernism to postmodern historicism to unbridled expressiveness. In the Netherlands, Studio M10's TBS Kliniek (2005–2008), built in Almere, the Netherlands, was strongly influenced by the 20th-century European modernist aesthetic of minimalism established at the Bauhaus in the 1920s (Figure 2.35a–b). This two-level, 440-bed inpatient forensic psychiatric treatment center was configured, in plan, as virtually symmetrical, with multiple pairs of rectangular building elements connected at midsection by a bisecting circulation spine. Its open courts were situated between long, unbroken, repetitive blocks of patient rooms, with administrative, therapy/treatment, and recreational functions located along a central service 'street' spanning the length of the complex (Figure 2.36a–d). Relative transparency was achieved in the complex's public spaces, yet not in its Spartan,

Key:
A arrival/parking
B main building
C medium-security units
D maximum-security units

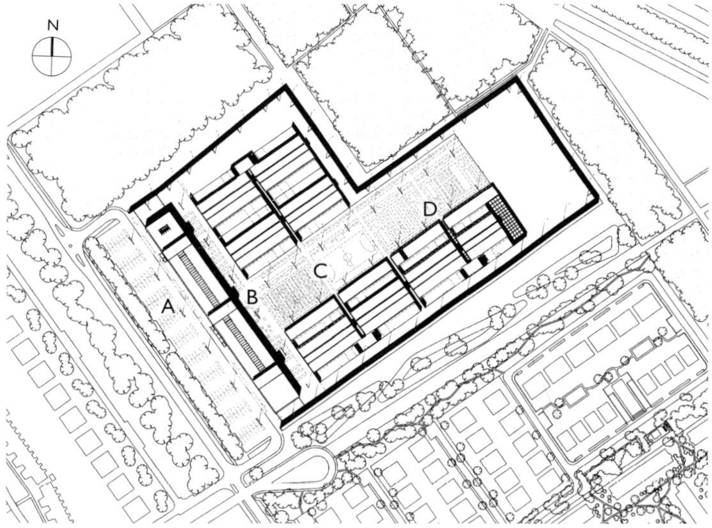

Site Plan

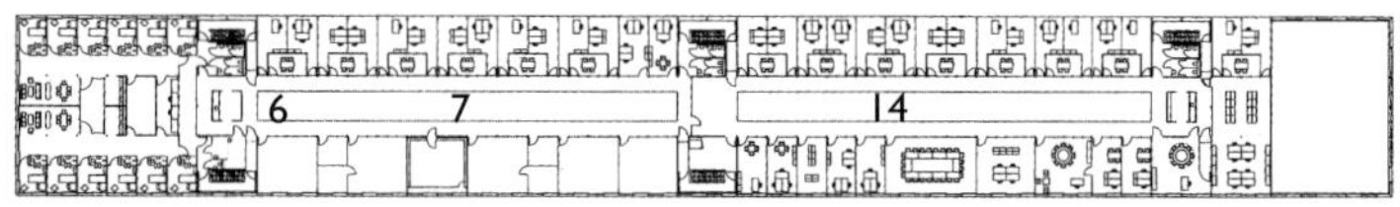

Second Floor Administration

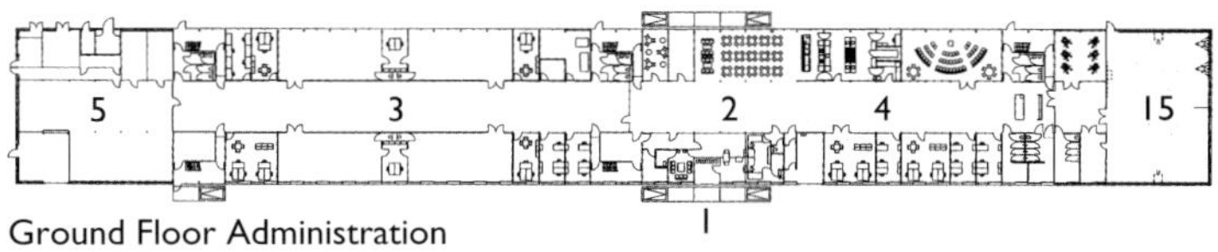

Ground Floor Administration

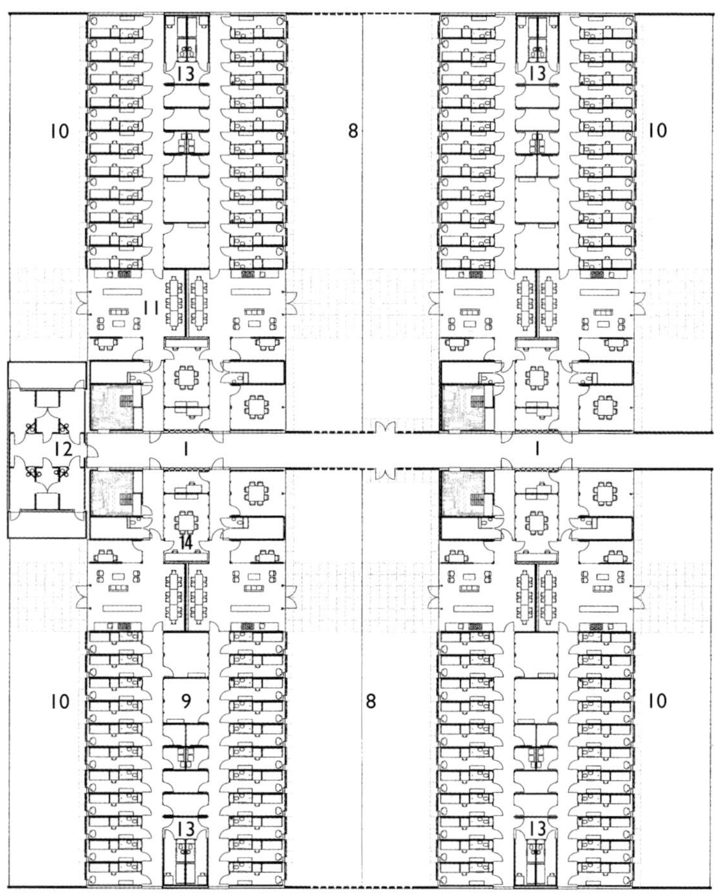

Ground Floor Inpatient Unit

Key:
1 entrance
2 reception
3 staff and training
4 recreational therapy
5 storeroom/facility management
6 rehabilitation unit
7 counseling
8 secure courtyard
9 game room
10 patient rooms
11 activity/dayroom
12 communal bath/showers
13 isolation
14 administration
15 gym

2.36a–d TBS Kliniek, campus plan (top), linear plan of administration building (middle), and inpatient housing 'blocks' (bottom).

dormitory-like living units. Its partí was reminiscent of a neo-Miesian orthogonality, not unlike the grids Mies used to master plan his Lafayette Gardens housing complex in Detroit and the Illinois Institute of Technology campus in Chicago in the 1950s.[104]

A strikingly different, postmodernist formal language was adopted in the case of the William Wake House (2008–2011), built in Northhamptonshire, United Kingdom, designed by ADAM Architecture. This comprehensive psychiatric hospital was the largest new (and also classically inspired) civic building built anywhere in Britain in more than 50 years. A dramatic, 70,000-square-foot facility, it was designed in consultation with healthcare planning experts Oxford Architects in the United Kingdom. It represented phase one of the Cliftonville site redevelopment, and in plan, was completely symmetrical, with a strong arrival and administration axis, and with its various inpatient residential units situated to the left and right, establishing a uniform rhythm throughout. A historicist, postmodern aesthetic was unabashedly expressed throughout the campus, with fenestration reminiscent of the 19th-century British asylums (Figure 2.37). The architectural vocabulary was contextually in keeping with the original hospital buildings on the grounds, the old asylum designed by George Wallet in 1835 (Figure 2.38). The principal programmatic components of the William Wake House resulted in a series of pavilions, with open-air courtyards featuring simplified classical detailing, in two tones of brick and a main public arrival entrance sequence with a rusticated circular window above a 'user's' (staff personnel) entrance and a glazed portico overlooking the nearby town, from its elevated vantage point.

In the architect's words, 'The building shows how modern classical design is not limited to private houses or historic settings but can provide high-quality public and institutional buildings.'[105] The overall effect of an unyielding formal symmetry and authoritative imagery was striking. This becomes particularly so when contrasted with more normative-appearing, ecologically attuned, residential-like alternatives (see Chapter 6). That said, it remained somewhat difficult to comprehend why a client agency would submit to this design strategy. If the treatment provided within was to be the most advanced, up to date, and progressive, it begged the question: Should not new architecture express the spirit of its times? This question, in point of fact, was equally pertinent, beyond whether the built outcome was inspired by Bauhaus historicism (Studio M10), a formal reprise of early 19th-century authoritarian British asylum architecture (Adam), or a rejection of both (Frank O. Gehry, to be discussed next).

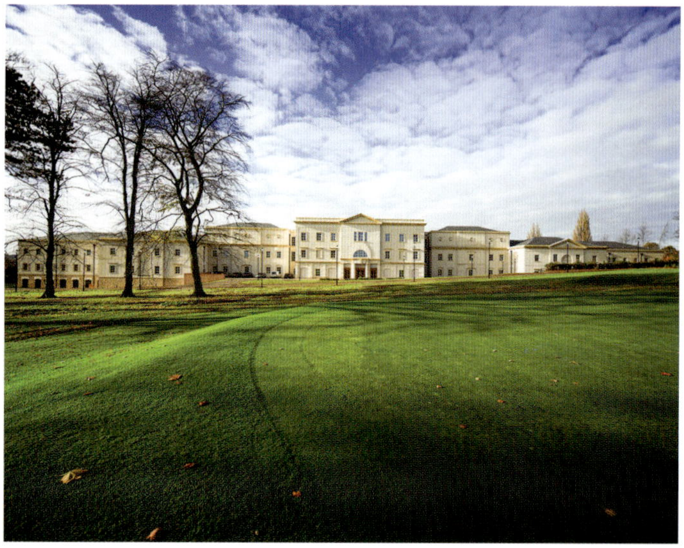

2.37 William Wake House, United Kingdom (2008–2011), front façade, shown set beyond an expanse of lawn.

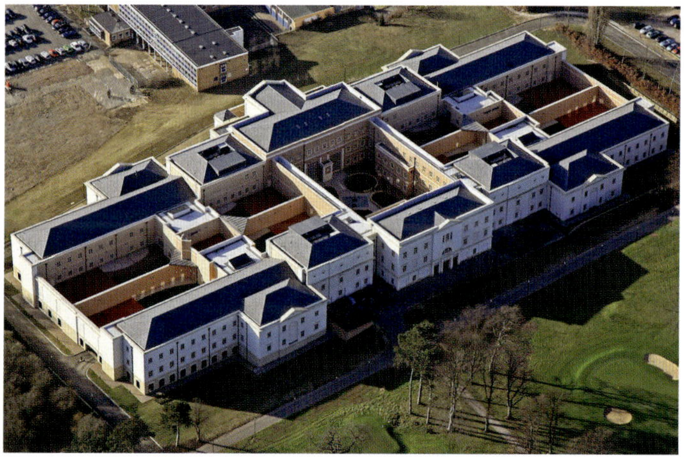

2.38 William Wake House, aerial view.

In the United States, the Cleveland Clinic Lou Ruvo Center for Brain Health, by Frank O. Gehry and Associates (2006–2010), now Gehry Associates, established a striking presence. It was sited at a prominent vehicular gateway to downtown Las Vegas (Figure 2.39). This center provided comprehensive diagnostic and outpatient treatment, including education, research, neuroimaging suites, a reference library, a Museum of the Mind, and a multipurpose center accommodating up to 450 persons. The research facilities were housed in a four-level building articulated as a series of offset rectangular volumes. In direct contrast to this backdrop, the public functions of the Ruvo Center complex, housed directly across an open-air circulation/arrival space, established an oppositional narrative of spontaneity, uncertainty, even randomness. Its public outreach functions were housed in

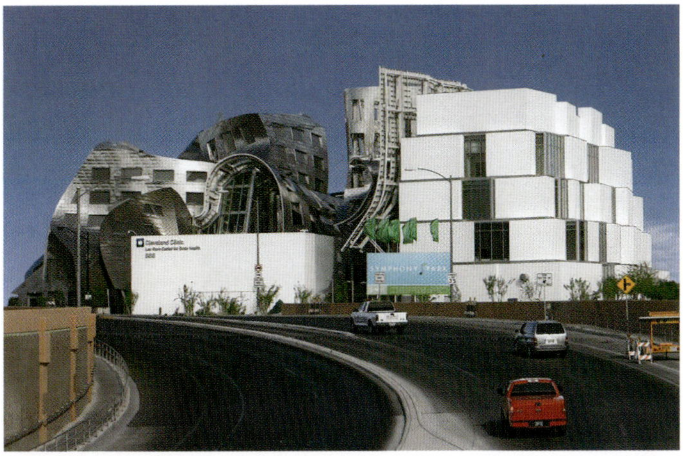

2.39 The aesthetic diversity of Frank Gehry's Cleveland Clinic Lou Ruvo Center for Brain Health, Las Vegas (2006–2010).

multiple interlocking, expressive shapes colliding at seemingly random angles as if about to all tumble to the ground in a heap. Interestingly, the dissociative identities of the two realms of the complex extended themes first examined in his Yale Psychiatric Institute years earlier. Here, Gehry rejected (overall) a more normative approach – while also rejecting the restraint of the TBS Kliniek – as he appears to have opted to examine the possibilities of anthropomorphically expressing the inner turmoil experienced by an individual wrestling with a severe mental disorder. At Ruvo in Las Vegas, he begins with a prosaic block 'background building' functioning as a 'normative' foil, and then proceeds to apply freeform experimentation to the liberated 'other self' of the center's more public realm. This yielded a sort of bifurcated split personality in physical architectural form. While ostensibly focused on community education, awareness, outreach programs, and outpatient treatment, it sought to transcend – to self-consciously push beyond – mainstream conventions of what behavioural health architecture should look (and feel) like.[106]

Summary

The consequences of the antihospitalization movement that originated in the early 1960s persist today, as its impact continues to be widespread.[107] Indeed, no one wishes for a return to custodialism, although some rather quixotic parallels did take place between 1960 and 2010. Then, in many countries, a disproportionately high number of psychiatric beds were housed in 24/7 warehouses for the mentally ill (with correspondingly few outpatient community-based mental health clinics). By 2010, *too few* inpatient beds were available in any type of 24/7 treatment center (albeit significantly more outpatient clinics existed than in 1960). Now, however, a shortage of *all types* of treatment options is the norm. Because of this it is arguable that by 2010 the situation represented a 'worst of both worlds' scenario. In rich and poor nations alike, a patchwork-quilt of services was shutting out tens of millions. And wealthy nations were by no means immune, with more than half of American adults with a mental illness or substance addiction never receiving proper, sustained treatment. Nationally, in the United States there were 43,318 public-sector psychiatric inpatient beds in 2010, compared with 50,509 a mere 5 years earlier, according to a widely cited report from the Treatment Advocacy Center. Corporate healthcare providers, for their part, continued to inadequately fill this treatment gap.[108] As a result, service networks continued to be distended, resulting in a growing number of medically underserved communities from a psychiatric and addiction disorders healthcare standpoint.[109] A tipping point had been reached, as community hospitals were at overcapacity, with mentally ill patients arriving at their local emergency department, with no other place to go.[110]

In the United States, the healthcare industry by 2010 was fully enmeshed and complicit in the mental health and substance addiction crisis.[111] This fact was used as a brickbat by critics of the system, for they cited this as the main reason why so many mass murders and other tragic events were occurring with increasing frequency. The situation had deteriorated into a combustible stew of inconsistencies, resulting in intensified social problems including homelessness and the incarceration of millions of mentally ill and chronically addicted persons who did not belong in jail. For example, the city of Chicago at this time elected to close down its network of outpatient mental health clinics due to budget cutbacks, while it provided no inpatient care alternatives except the Cook County Jail. This tragic turn of events was examined in the *Atlantic* in a feature titled 'America's Largest Mental Hospital Is a Jail.'[112] The record now showed that architects had ably lent their expertise to a generation of psychiatric hospitals and outpatient clinics in the 1960–2010 period. But a broken infrastructure begged virtually the same question for the architect as in 1960 – was it legitimate to claim that architectural innovation had been stymied during the previous 50-year period by ineffective, misguided clients, and had their architects been part of the problem, or the solution? Second, was the modernist psychiatric hospital to be declared dead as a type?

Special populations: children and adolescents, the aged, and the displaced

CHAPTER 3

Every day, we are bombarded with an unprecedented amount of information, and for a young person this can be overwhelming. In adolescence, generally defined as ages 10–19, a host of social, environmental, and cultural determinants compete for our limited attention spans. Childhood and adolescence is complicated enough as it is, and the rise of social media is further exacerbating a potentially negative pattern. The waves of information washing over us are becoming a major cause of anxiety and depression among young persons. In the field of public health, developmental epidemiology examines conditions such as digital addiction as a mental-disorder risk factor in young people, whether triggered by digital overload or other reasons.[1] These include family dysfunction, poverty, racism, and social noncohesiveness, daily conflict with others, sexual abuse, or an environment that offers an inadequate safety net.[2] Epidemiological approaches compare and contrast specific populations.

The aim is to learn more about developmental psychopathologies and to be able to prevent adverse mental and behavioural outcomes.[3] Cyberbullying, for instance, is often symptomatic of social stigmatization, isolation, or racial discrimination, which in turn can lead to an increased risk of premature death through suicide in young persons. Approximately 75% of adults with a diagnosed mental disorder first experienced their symptoms prior to the age of 24, and an undiagnosed mental disorder in a young person will likely have a substantially adverse impact in adulthood and may be of lifelong duration.[4] Long-term research studies corroborate this, with over half of disorders first diagnosed in adulthood preceded by a psychiatric disorder in childhood or adolescence, such as attention deficit hyperactivity disorder (ADHD) and autism spectrum disorder (ASD).[5]

Despite mounting statistical evidence on the importance of applying more holistic psychosocial and pharmacological approaches in identifying and treating mental disorders in young people, the public at large, in general, remains indifferent. Even in relatively wealthy countries with established child and adolescent mental health services, access to care for young persons remains poor.[6] Also, looks can be deceiving. If a young person appears, outwardly, to be physically healthy, when that person seeks a psychological diagnosis, subsequent treatment may occur too randomly or not at all. Engaging a young person to seek out treatment requires special skills and this is what often is so glaringly absent at the community level. And when this occurs, the type of intervention, from a facility standpoint, may be entirely inappropriate. This public indifference was spotlighted in the United States when the federal government recently sued a state (Louisiana) for illegally housing an excessive number of its under-18 mental health patients in nursing home facilities, surrounded by generally non-psychiatric, aged residents.[7] In this case, nursing homes are being substituted for a chronic lack of psychiatric care facilities, a practice that occurs in many places across the United States.

The illegality of prematurely institutionalizing young persons with mental health disorders was reaffirmed in 1999, in the US Supreme Court's decision in *Olmstead v. L.C.* This ruling held that the institutionalization of young persons with mental or behavioural disabilities, when denied appropriate at-home or other appropriate residential care options, is a form of civil rights discrimination.[8] This practice remains particularly problematic considering that among visits to physicians by adolescents in the United States, depression diagnoses increased from 1.4 million to 3.2 million between 1995 and 2002.[9] Recent surveys in multiple regions of the United States have shown repeatedly that approximately 1 in 3–4 children experience a mental disorder and about 1 in 10 suffer from a serious emotional disturbance. Another recent study found, with respect to the early onset of such disorders among affected adolescents, 50% had first onset by age 6 for anxiety disorders, by age 11 for behavioural disorders, by age 13 for mood disorders, and by age 15 for substance addictions.[10]

Globally, it is estimated as many as 20% of children and adolescents suffer from a disabling mental illness at some point during this stage of life.[11] Tragically, suicide is the third leading cause of death among adolescents.[12] Alcohol and controlled substance addictions are major health problems that confront young people, and as just mentioned, it is this time in life when most such problems first appear.[13] While rates of diagnosis have increased substantially in recent years, too many young persons fail to receive proper pharmacological and psychotherapeutic treatment; this is largely because early detection warning systems remain so sporadic and fragmented.[14] One recent meta-analysis was conducted on 41 recent research studies on this subject, representing 27 countries. The findings underscored, yet again, the urgent need for early detection and intervention.[15] In the United Kingdom, early detection and intervention in young persons has recently risen in stature, becoming a core ingredient in the National Health Service's (NHS) initiative called a Framework for Children,[16] with a sustained focus on outpatient treatment programs in order to minimize the traditional reliance on hospitalization and its deleterious impacts on young persons.[17]

Learning environments are uniquely positioned to play a central role in early detection and intervention. In the United States in 2002, The New Freedom Commission's final report (the work of a presidential commission) recommended several goals to set, nationally, related to school-based mental health services, including the need to reduce social stigma and bullying, programs to detect and prevent suicide, the early screening and treatment of co-occurring disorders, and the dire need for increased funding support at all levels.[18] Measures such as these are increasingly viewed as providing the needed infrastructural support to conventional psychoanalytic and psychopharmaceutical approaches, which often have been dismal failures in helping troubled persons bridge the gap between adolescence and adulthood.[19] When this safety net is absent, or unsustainable, over a period of years, the consequences may be lifelong:

> *A few days ago I received a text from my older sister saying that she lost her job again. This is probably the third job she has been fired from in the last few months. You see, both of my older sisters (identical twins) suffer from bipolar disorder. One of them was diagnosed within the last couple of years; the other was diagnosed around ten years ago. Looking back, their issues were apparent for many years before they were diagnosed . . . these days, I hear about their lives from the sidelines, usually from my mom or sometimes my brother. It's not their fault that we rarely communicate, as I am the one who distanced myself from them several years ago. I just couldn't ride the mental illness roller coaster any longer. They took advantage of my parents and ruined their relationship with their kids. They misused their medicine and blamed others for their unhappiness.*
>
> *When I was only 9 years old, I saw my father cry for the first time. We were at a family therapy session with one of my sisters who had recently attempted suicide. I didn't know at the time what 'suicide' really meant or why we were there. I just knew that I was angry at my sister for making my dad cry. Unfortunately, it wasn't her last suicide attempt. The most memorable one happened the night that I went into labor with my first child. My parents had chosen to come to be with*

me in Austin (Texas), feeling very torn to say the least, while they were getting updates from my other sister. Thankfully, my missing sister was found (alive but unconscious) in a hotel room, having nearly overdosed on sleeping pills.

After my father passed away three years ago, one sister had what I would call a mental breakdown . . . there were nights she unknowingly left her apartment on foot and wandered around Houston in the middle of the night. I'm just thankful she was never injured (or worse). Throughout the years, we've seen their marriages fail and jobs come and go. Friendships have changed, and there have been car wrecks, AA meetings, impatient and outpatient psychiatric care, denied disability claims, countless financial issues, abusive boyfriends, and bankruptcies . . . on top of all that, they've been scammed by online predators from a dating website and burglarized by neighbors in their own apartment complex. The last few years have been a terrible ride for them, to say the least. I feel guilty that there's nothing I can do to help them.

If there's one thing I could wish for them it would be that they can find happiness . . . but unfortunately, the only thing I can do is to let them know they're loved. I can't make their:

- *medicines work like they're supposed to.*
- *brains function like they're supposed to.*
- *decisions for them.*
- *bosses understand their limitations.*
- *relationship healthy and true.*

But I can love them.

To my sisters . . . no matter how many bumps in the road you may encounter, I'll always love you.[20]

What types of treatment did these sisters receive in their youth? Was the emphasis always on conventional therapy? Was there a willingness to try alternative approaches? Perhaps this would have yielded a different outcome. Alternative therapies are available to treat pediatric patients, and it has often been said that music, for one, has the power to heal. Young people respond to music quite differently than adults and its therapeutic uses hold promise in the treatment of mental and substance addiction disorders. This is because music functions on a sociological, psychological, and physical level.[21] It is a sensory experience. For the young person who experiences a mental illness or addictive disorder in youth, the focus must remain consistent, as a consistent focus can result in a more adjusted and successful adult life.

The aged

In his description of the first psychotherapy clinic solely devoted to the mental health needs of the aged in Australia (in Melbourne), Vahid Payman spoke of the importance of mental health intervention.[22] He cited Sigmund Freud, founding father of psychoanalysis, and his skeptical view of the benefits of psychotherapy for persons in the later stages of life: 'Near or above the age of fifty,' Freud wrote in 1905, 'the elasticity of mental processes, on which treatment depends is, as a rule, lacking – old people are no longer educable.'[23] Freud believed the aged simply accumulate too large a mass of unconscious 'blocking' material for effective psychoanalysis. His contemporary, Karl Abraham, held a more optimistic view. In 1919, Abraham asserted a favorable prognosis is predicated not on the chronological age of the patient *per se*, but on the nature of the mental disorder harbored within.[24] If intervention can occur early (in old age), the patient has a greater probability for improvement. Echoing in some ways Freud's dire predilection, Carl Jung, writing in 1931, believed it the duty of the aged individual to 'devote serious attention to himself'. How many, he reasoned, are really prepared for the second half of life, for old age, death, and eternity?[25] Later, Erik Erikson, in his classic 1950 book on the eight ages of humankind, foresaw cognitive development continuing throughout the human life cycle including into old age, with persons in late life reaping the reward of psychologically well-negotiated prior life stages.[26] In many respects, this has been the case with my own mother, age 93:

Helen (Musso) Verderber was born in Chicago, Illinois, in 1924. A child of the Great Depression, she and her family were relatively well-off compared to many. Her father had become prosperous enough to purchase a row of detached three-flats in the West Garfield Park neighborhood on Chicago's burgeoning West Side, a half block from the city's impressive Garfield Park. This street, West Monroe, was lined with walk-up, multifamily gray-stone flats, only a block away from the bustling Madison Street corridor with its shops, restaurants, hotels, and the opulent (but long-gone) Paradise and Marlboro movie palaces, two grand theaters built in the 1920s. Her flat featured elaborate ornamentation, wood floors, chandeliers, rugs, and fine furnishings. Her father and mother immigrated through Ellis Island in New York from Palermo, Sicily, around the turn of the century. By the 1950s the Madison Street commercial district and the surrounding residential neighborhoods would fall prey to suburban 'white flight', and decades of severe economic disinvestment would follow, further fueled by the civil rights riots in the 1960s.

As the youngest of five, she benefitted from a stable and comfortable childhood and adolescence. After marriage my parents moved to the suburbs, like so many of their generation. As a full-time homemaker, she first exhibited symptoms of anxiety disorder at this time. She never learned to drive but nor was she interested, in part because she had previously relied on public transit. Curiously, her relative isolation in the suburbs never appeared to disturb her. She was unlike her siblings in this regard. Mom seldom left the house alone, and my father overcompensated for her rather reclusive ways. Mom preferred to stay home, and would make excuses for not venturing to unknown places. A summer vacation to a new place was a challenge for her.

The Diagnostic and Statistical Manual of Mental Disorders *(DSM-5) states the criteria for an agoraphobia diagnosis include anxiety or fear associated with at least two of the following situations – being in places that are difficult to escape from or find help in, such as on public transport or an airplane; being in an open and unfamiliar space; being in an enclosed space; being in a large crowd or queue; or being away from home in unfamiliar places whether alone or with others. Additional diagnostic criteria include anxiety or fear associated with exposure to a particularly disliked place, and the avoidance of a destination requiring a companion. Regardless, she was always a wonderful mother. My sister and I have remained patient with her rather unusual ways in this regard, especially in the years since my father passed away (1989). At age 88 (2013), mom was diagnosed with midstage dementia. She remains at home, and we provide an in-home caregiver, as mom increasingly needs assistance with the activities of daily living. Her longtime home now more than ever functions as her total 'world' and her comorbidity – dementia, with an anxiety disorder – requires special attention and care.*

Aged individuals with a mental health comorbidity, perhaps due to diabetes, arthritis, heart disease, hip replacement surgery, or osteoporosis, are putting considerable strain on the healthcare systems of countries around the world. Despite the dire warnings of a looming Alzheimer's disease epidemic (whose victims are expected to triple in number by 2050), inadequate research attention is being devoted to aged persons with comorbidity (i.e., depression, post-traumatic stress disorder [PTSD], bipolar disorder, and psychosis).[27] A lack of specialists is contributing to this crisis. Relative to the growing demand, few psychiatrists, specialized social workers, and psychologists are being trained to treat this population. Making matters worse, elderly persons are often reluctant to discuss their emotional difficulties with anyone, and especially a stranger, out of fear she or he will be perceived as weak. Clinicians, for their part, often fail to properly diagnose a psychological or substance addiction problem, as these disorders are less obvious to detect compared to more readily detectable physical ailments, such as physical immobility, the effects of falls and other types of accidents, and sensory loss. In a 2012 report, the Institute of Medicine (IOM) in the United States estimated that between 5.6 and 8.0 million elderly persons aged 65 and older had a mental illness or a substance addiction disorder, a number predicted to increase to 10.1–14.4 million aged persons by 2030. The main problem is that even in a wealthy country like the United States, the number of trained geriatric psychiatrists and allied specialists remains minuscule. This IOM report concluded by calling for a redoubled effort nationally to greatly increase the number of eldercare specialists.[28]

Because more elderly persons than ever before are living longer, with comorbidity, the need is great to learn more about how one or more physical ailments, combined with one or more mental health disorders, influences an individual's quality of life.[29] In another recent study in the United States, elderly individuals suffering from schizophrenia, recurrent manic depression, and bipolar disorder were found to have significantly lower rates of hypertension but a significantly higher rate of physical falls. Second, persons with comorbidity more frequently make emergency visits to a hospital emergency department (ED) and are hospitalized at a significantly higher rate compared to those without. Third, diagnoses of substance abuse and alcoholism are more frequent among seriously mentally ill elderly patients.[30] These patterns have been corroborated in numerous other research investigations on the relationship between mood and outlook, anxiety levels, and substance addiction disorders among older adults.[31] Unfortunately, lingering social stigma often keeps these persons from seeking proper diagnosis and treatment, and this is especially problematic for the elderly with physical-psychological comorbidity.[32]

The prevalence of major depression among adults aged 65 and older is currently about 15% in the United States. Among the elderly with comorbidity such as depression, together with diabetes, hypertension, emphysema, or osteoarthritis, this number increases to 25%.[33] Although older adults are frequently unwilling to confront their psychological problems with a professional caregiver, psychotherapy has proven effective with the comorbid elderly.[34] Simply walking in nature, or engaging in a physical therapy program, can help reduce symptoms of depression.[35] Problems can become magnified and compounded if not properly addressed. In long-term residential care settings, physically inactive aged patients with a diagnosed mental disorder are likely to experience weight loss, weakness and fatigue, and a poor nutritional regimen.[36] As for the situation in developing countries, mental disorders among the aged are seldom diagnosed or treated. In Nigeria, the aged mentally ill are dismissed outright because psychiatric care for schizophrenia, bipolar disorder, and other illnesses is simply unavailable in a nation of 168 million and with less than 200 trained psychiatrists. One facility in Nigeria, the Ademola Mental Hospital, is a traditional faith-healing center that currently practices diagnosis by incantation – the recitation of folk verse to invoke the retreat of demons responsible for causing mental illness. Here, the patients are chained to pillars on the front porch, often for hours on end.[37]

The health sciences literature has recently devoted more attention to examining the role of the built environment in improving aged persons' overall emotional outlook and satisfaction.[38] For aged persons with physical-psychological comorbidity, the built environment and nature in particular can have a positive, therapeutic impact on mental health. One recent study found that aged persons' engagement with nature vis-à-vis frequent walks through a tranquil garden, immediately followed by an art therapy session, had a demonstrably positive effect on their self-reported assessment of mood and emotional outlook.[39] In the years ahead, innovative therapy protocols such as this will be required to blend conventional with unconventional treatment approaches.[40] To this end, professional caregivers will be needed to respond to the challenges of caring for an increasingly older comorbid population, with a greater percentage in need of mental health and substance addiction treatment.[41] This is an ongoing process and its growing importance is reflected in the most recent edition of the *Diagnostic and Statistical Manual of Mental Disorders* (DSM-5).[42]

The displaced

Military conflicts, political and religious persecution, earthquakes, and the consequences of global climate change are forcing more people than at any prior time in recorded history to flee and seek refuge outside their home country. The United Nations High Commissioner for Refugees' (UNHCR) annual *Global Trends Report: World at War*, released in 2015, concluded worldwide displacement to have reached its highest level in recorded history; the number of persons forcibly displaced at the end of 2014 had risen to a staggering 59.5 million compared to 51.2 million just a year prior, and 37.5 million a decade earlier. This dramatic increase represents the greatest year-over-year increase ever, and in the time since the release of this report this crisis has further intensified. By the end of 2016, 4.8 million Middle Eastern refugees alone had fled to Turkey, Lebanon, Jordan, Egypt, and Iraq, and 6.6 million had been internally displaced within Syria. Meanwhile, about one million had requested asylum in Europe and North America. Globally, 1 in every 122 humans in 2017 was a refugee, an internally displaced person (IDP), or an individual seeking asylum elsewhere, many with PTSD. If this were the population of a single country, it would be the world's 24th largest.[43] This mass displacement of populations represents a descent into uncharted territory, characterized by the need for massive humanitarian responses on a level that clearly outstrips anything witnessed before.

In her own words, Suzanne Kawmieh, as translated by Hadia Zarzour,

> *In early 2014, I took a short trip to the Syrian-Jordanian border, specifically the Zaatari refugee camp (in Jordan) for the first time. I had been working on various humanitarian*

projects related to Syria; however, the focus had not been on the refugees but on those who were still trapped in Syria. The Zaatari refugee camp is now the forth-largest city in Jordan and is home to over 150,000 Syrian refugees. A winter storm hit the camp the week before we arrived, flooding and collapsing all of the tents. Refugees were literally left homeless (or tent-less). What little clothing and food supplies they had were destroyed. Our trip was an emergency relief trip to provide winter jackets, food aid, portable heating units and medical supplies. The refugee camp is in the middle of nowhere – far from any city or inhabited area. Tall barbed wire fences surround the camp and guards would arbitrarily open and close the camp to incoming refugees, and to volunteers and visitors. When we arrived, the guard would not allow us entry . . . those who arrived on foot and were Syrian, such as us, and who had nothing but our backpacks, were refused entry. We were finally allowed in after being forced to wait an entire day. Soon, residents from our former village back home gathered around our crowded tent. They shared with us their hardships and pleaded that we do something – anything. They showed us an expired can of lunchmeat they were given as their food ration for that entire week and how their children became ill upon eating it.

One mother showed me her young son who was having convulsive 'episodes' and asked me what was wrong with him; if there was anything I could do to help him . . . the boy hadn't been able to forget his traumatic experiences. He could only scream to drown out memories of past sounds and events. I knew we couldn't do anything; we weren't equipped with the necessary medications and didn't have a mental health professional on our team. A young girl took me aside to her tent and told me about the many girls who had been raped in Syria. How they were seized from their university campuses or homes and now required medical and mental health treatment. She described how they were now inconsolable and many had given up on life. Some had committed suicide . . . their families shamed, because they no longer had a future in their tribal families and hometowns; how they were now disowned . . . As we left, we passed back through the same military checkpoint. Guards with their automatic weapons held them visible and a large tank sat to one side . . . it was one big open-air prison. Once we passed through the checkpoint our passports were returned and I could not bear to look back . . . it was a long dirt road that led us away from the barbed wire, the tragedies, and the hushed pleas.[44]

In 1951, the UN Convention Relating to the Status of Refugees (the first Geneva Convention) was where the term refugee was first defined – a person with a 'well founded fear of persecution for reasons of race, religion, nationality, membership of a particular social group or political opinion' (UNHCR, 1951).[45] Every day in 2016, an average of 42,500 people became refugees, asylum seekers, or IDPs, a four-fold increase in a mere 4-year time frame. As for those responsible for starting and perpetuating armed conflicts, the perpetrators continue to enjoy relative impunity while much of the international community remains on the sidelines. Meanwhile, peace remains a rare commodity. Since 2010, at least 15 conflicts have erupted or reignited, including eight in Africa, three in the Middle East (Syria, Iraq, and Yemen), one in Europe (Ukraine), and three in Asia (Kyrgyzstan, Myanmar, and Pakistan). A 2014 UN report noted only 126,800 refugees were able to return to their home countries, the lowest number in 31 years. Meanwhile, decades-old instability and conflicts in Afghanistan, Somalia, and elsewhere ensured that millions will remain nomadic, often stranded for many years in refugee encampments. The ongoing plight of refugees braving harsh weather and treacherous seas has been well documented in the mass media. The UNHCR estimates, worldwide, in 2015 there were 19.5 million refugees, including 38.2 million displaced inside their own countries, and 1.8 million awaiting outcomes of claims of asylum. Shockingly, approximately half of these refugees are children and adolescents.[46]

The World Health Organization (WHO) guidelines for the provision of mental health assistance after a disaster event define three groups of distressed persons, each requiring a different mode of response: (1) those with mild psychological distress that resolves in a few days or weeks and needs no specific intervention, estimated at 20%–40% of the impacted population; (2) those with moderate to severe diagnosable psychological distress, and warranting intervention, estimated at 30%–50% of the impacted population; and (3) those with a prediagnosed mental disorder, the acuity of which typically doubles in intensity after a disaster, impacting 10% of the affected population, with outcomes including depression and severe psychotic disorders estimated to affect a further 2%–4% of an impacted population.[47] Following the Asian tsunami in 2004, when relief aid agencies were criticized for mismanaging the humanitarian response, an organization called the Inter-Agency Standing Committee (IASC) was established. Its charge is to develop a single set of guidelines to ensure the provision of proper mental health clinical intervention in such emergencies. Representatives from 27 nongovernmental organization (NGO) and non-NGO entities, academic institutions, and professional organizations were involved in launching this organization. The resulting *IASC Guidelines for Mental Health and Psychosocial Support in Emergency Settings* represents for the first time an international consensus on this area of focus.[48]

With the need growing for mental health services to care for the displaced, the disenfranchised, and the marginalized, more initiatives such as this will be needed. Persons with refugee backgrounds, many of whom have experienced persecution and forced migration from their country of origin, experience further discrimination and hostilities after arriving to resettle in a new place. These individuals and families confront mental health specialists with unique sets of challenges. The harsh, inhumane treatment and emotional trauma typically endured by the forcibly displaced can result in deep psychological disorders. These can develop prior to the actual flight from the home country as well as en route to an unknown destination. Beyond this, refugee resettlement camp workers often struggle to provide mental health services of any type in light of the sheer heterogeneity and diversity of the incoming refugees – and especially in a way respectful of their religious and cultural beliefs and traditions.[49] Much more knowledge is needed on this facet of the total experience, and specifically the impact of predisplacement factors relative to the postdisplacement experience of refugee populations of all ages.[50]

As for the plight of forcibly displaced children and adolescents, much more knowledge is needed concerning their mental health needs. A recent study of 102 young incoming refugees who were referred to a community-based mental health clinic in the United Kingdom found, after 1 year, that three quarters of young persons experienced a significantly improved psychological condition, while 25% remained the same or were now worse off than at the time of their arrival. Within this same cohort, encouragingly, however, for 90% of the group of young refugees who had resided in Britain for more than two years, their psychological health status had improved significantly.[51] This finding points to the importance of the functions of time and of stability. For young people, in particular, the premigration (predisplacement) and postdisplacement trauma associated with this experience often leaves lasting scars, especially among those who arrive at a resettlement center in a new country without a parent or guardian by their side.[52]

Earthquake and hurricane victims

An estimated 220,000 people were killed and 1.5 million persons displaced in the 2010 Haitian earthquake.[53] Many Haitian religious beliefs persistently revolve around voodoo traditions and demonic spirits, and this is why mental illness has traditionally been only marginally addressed in Haitian culture. Compounding matters, prior to the earthquake, the country was plagued by chronic understaffing issues, a lack of properly trained mental health specialists, and a virtual absence of psychotropic medications.[54] The scope of the postdisaster crisis in Haiti was of such magnitude that the only two state-run psychiatric hospitals in the entire country were completely overwhelmed by the disaster, and both shut down completely. This lack of inpatient psychiatric and addiction disorder care was exacerbated by an absence of community-based outpatient mental health clinics in the nation's towns and villages. Afterward, a number of mobile vehicular clinics were established in 2010 by international NGOs to treat the medically underserved, and open-air emergency tent clinics were set up at the two shuttered psychiatric hospitals.[55]

A body of evidence-based knowledge is accumulating on how disaster events give rise to mental health disorders, including the abrupt loss of home and neighborhood due to forced displacement, and its cumulative impacts on populations who reside in places repeatedly struck by disasters. In the United States, only recently has the Federal Emergency Management Agency (FEMA) opted to systematically provide mental health counseling and treatment services on-site in the immediate aftermath of a disaster event.[56] Hurricane Katrina resulted in higher rates of depression, domestic violence, suicide rates, and diagnosed cases of PTSD; these were all outcomes attributed not only to the event itself but also to persons' subsequent long-term displacement, unemployment, family disruption, and unhealthful emergency housing, such as the infamous, illness-inducing FEMA travel-trailer program and other types of mobile homes.[57] Disaster management specialists refer to these aftereffects as the 'disaster after the disaster'. Immediately after Katrina, in September 2005, Operation Assist was launched by the Children's Health Fund (CHF), a national NGO in the United States founded in 1987 in association with the National Center for Disaster Preparedness (NCDP) at Columbia University in New York City. Operation Assist used the CHF model of mobile medical units, essentially clinics on wheels staffed by physicians, nurses, and mental health and social service professionals. Several such mobile units were deployed to the disaster strike zone in the fall of 2005 and many who received care at these clinics screened positive for a range of anxiety and depression disorders.[58]

Young persons' attempts to cope with a mental disorder after Katrina were heart-wrenching (including my own then-14-year-old daughter's post-Katrina challenges with anxiety).[59] One important lesson learned was the value of pediatric mental health services being colocated with primary care services.[60] This is because young persons, not unlike aged individuals, dispossessed or otherwise, often are afraid to reveal their psychological symptoms to a stranger.[61] Nonetheless, the adverse consequences of climate change are not expected to subside anytime soon and are predicted to adversely impact upward of 200 million persons by the year 2050.[62] This begs the question, what are highly vulnerable communities (and their special populations) doing, architecturally and otherwise, to render themselves more resilient in the future to successfully rebound from built environment–induced adversities?

Designing for special populations

Architects often commiserate about being brought on board in a project after most of the really important decisions have already been made about site selection, urban infrastructure, project financing, budget, scope, and so on. In an age of instantaneous communications and burgeoning social media it is incumbent upon each of us to be proactive as to our role and contributions. But more to the point, waiting for politicians, attorneys, multinational corporate CEOs, disaster capitalists, and others to define and shape what is to be built or rebuilt is not a productive strategy in and of itself. When working with medically underrepresented special populations in the planning and design of mental health and substance addiction treatment environments, one should strive to achieve the following:

Early immersion – A recent report by the US Department of Veterans Affairs (2016) concluded that between 20 and 22 military veterans commit suicide every single day.[63] Learn about your local community's mental health care support infrastructure and become actively involved in grassroots organizations that promote special patients' and refugees' fundamental human rights. Become versed in their legal protections at the local jurisdictional level and get involved. Follow through with effective actions and with effective architectural interventions. Work to engage support for design initiatives in the public and private spheres. Support the mental health and addiction disorder needs of medically underrepresented people and groups by becoming a rapid responder. Work to have a positive influence on what gets built, for whom, and when.

A voice in policy making – In the current climate of distrust of government, the public's confidence in elected politicians has reached historic lows. Sadly, many politicians, in reality, actually accomplish relatively little in terms of genuinely improving the quality of the built environment. This tendency is especially so in communities where the local architectural community remains silent. Exceptions can be found, of course, but frequently a minimum acceptability (mediocrity) in planning and design quality – and especially for special populations such as those discussed previously – is considered good enough. This can particularly be the case when it comes to addressing the needs and aspirations of special and medically underrepresented populations. In times of crisis and dislocation, do not assume the voices of the dispossessed and marginalized, who even in normal circumstances are often ignored, will be heard.

Inclusion and normalization – Behavioural health environments need to be inclusively attuned to special populations and their concerns, including indigenous cultures, minorities, the elderly, children and adolescents, and persons displaced by human and natural catastrophes. How is their mental health and healthfulness (vs. illness) to be collectively defined and addressed? Cultural norms at the local level are shaped by historical precedent and tradition, and because of this the will to overcome past prejudices, biases, and patterns of discrimination must be of utmost priority. Discrimination by (architectural) design cannot be tolerated and in the absence of strong advocates, things can go awry quickly. In cases of population displacement, compassionate planning and design strategies are essential, requiring the architect to be prepositioned to adroitly design places and buildings of both direct (emergency) and long-term (permanent) consequence.

Avoid paralysis by overanalysis – In behavioural healthcare environments for special populations, stakeholder constituencies with competing agendas will cancel one another out if allowed to do so. This can lead to intractable gridlock where conflicting priorities interminably delay decision making. If unchecked, this will delay a worthwhile project, even shut it down, as often occurs when NIMBY-ism intersects with proposals to build 24/7 mental health and addictive disorder treatment centers. Worthwhile, much-needed treatment facilities are derailed each and every day due to grassroots resistances rooted in fear. Remain a 'cautious skeptic' when it comes to the input and advice of politically correct 'experts' from afar, especially in the immediate aftermath of a disaster.[64]

Inclusivity and performance assessment – Designing behavioural health environments for special populations requires sensitivity and compassion. Work to bring individuals and groups into decision making historically marginalized due to age, gender orientation, income level, and ethnic or racial background. Be attentive to their immediate needs and concerns as much as their broader aspirations. Work alongside healthcare professionals, including healthcare administrators, physicians, nurses, and counselors and patients' rights advocacy groups, and use proven participatory planning and design processes. In cases involving the retrofitting of an existing facility, identify its strengths and shortcomings to improve its daily and long-term performance. Following occupancy, apply evidence-based methodologies to carry out a systematic performance assessment (see Chapter 5).

The custodial psychiatric institutions of the 20th century thoroughly subjugated their special populations, and the lessons learned from this experience need not be repeated in the 21st century. To this end, the community mental health promotion framework developed by the Victorian Health Promotion Foundation (VicHealth) in Australia in 2005 calls for a humane, compassionate perspective and specifically addresses the needs and concerns of special populations. Its manifesto states, in part,

> Mental health is not merely the absence of mental illness. Mental health is the embodiment of social, emotional and spiritual wellbeing. Mental healthcare provides an individual with the acceptance and support necessary for active living, to achieve goals, and to interact with others in ways respectful and just.[65]

Beyond this, medically underserved special populations with mental illness and substance addiction treatment needs deserve a dignified and productive quality of life. For the architect, the question is simple: how can architecture contribute most meaningfully in the provision of therapeutic support for these individuals and the special interests they represent?

PART 2

Design

Reinventing an asylum

CHAPTER 4

In the wake of reform movements inspired by civic and religious impulses, North Americans began constructing a new generation of lunatic asylums in the late 18th century. The physicians of this era sought to contrast 'moral treatment' of the insane against the sheer brutality that had dominated the earlier, prereform period in Europe. The opportunity presented itself to construct new state-run hospitals, for physicians specializing in treatment of the insane who rejected the widely condemned inhumanity of the past. They turned toward the experimental theories and practices then gaining ground in England, and to a lesser extent, in France. By the late 1840s a new North American architectural type had been formulated – the Kirkbride asylum. Architecturally, it symbolized less oppressiveness and the calming, therapeutic effects of nature. To appreciate these reforms and the resulting architecture, it is first necessary to know a bit of the history of the earlier generation of asylums, places that would be vehemently rejected by the moral reformists.[1]

London's Bethlehem Hospital is considered to have been among the most inhumane and notorious asylums in the English-speaking world. By the end of the 19th century, 'Bedlam' was the oldest psychiatric institution in Europe, dating back 650 years to the Priory of St. Mary of Bethlem. It was founded in 1247 in the City of London as a means to fund-raise for the Order of Bethlehem, crusaders in the Holy Lands. The priory was located on Bishops Gate Street, on the north-south road leading to London Bridge.[2] It was designed specifically as an asylum rather than an adaptation of another building type, and its exterior appeared palace-like. A second and more elaborate asylum (of the same name) was designed by Robert Hooke (1674–1676) and built near Bishops Gate in Moor Fields, one of the largest remaining open spaces in the city. This institution featured attractive lawns, symmetrical rows of trees, and a prominent path leading to the main entrance. Absolute symmetry prevailed, with males housed in one wing and females in the other, on four levels. To the casual onlooker this 'palace hospital' would provide no hint of the horrors within.[3]

Patients were often constricted in arm shackles and leg locks. Despite its interior horrors it garnered praise for its outward appearance and the surrounding grounds. This overcrowded, unsanitary, chaotic, corrupt institution would become known by the public simply as Bedlam. Hellish back rooms, torture, and mistreatment on principal were the norm, in time inspiring observers to search for a more humane alternative. New Bethlehem Hospital, designed by James Lewis, opened in 1815. By the 1840s, North American visitors had nearly universally rejected even it for its institutionalism.[4] The asylum, as a type, had begun to present an architectural conundrum: was it to be strictly utilitarian, or a grand civic expression of higher societal aspirations? Would not an image of grandeur and dignity encourage more well-off families to admit their loved ones? In rural areas, its counterparts looked like large manor houses with manicured grounds and staff attendants. In the early North American asylums, a few rooms featured decorative wall surfaces, ceilings, and furnishings, all done for the benefit of visitors. However, most other spaces remained strictly off-limits to the public. By the end of the 18th century, British asylums' polarity between their opulence and their inhumanity remained unresolved architecturally. Noteworthy examples of this deep contradiction included St. Luke's Lunatic Hospital, in London (1787), and the second iteration of St. Luke's, designed by George Dance the Younger, a place where the corridors became, in effect, dayrooms.[5]

During the concurrent Scottish Enlightenment, the rival cites of Glasgow and Edinburgh competed to build the most advanced lunatic asylums in the world. This resulted in the Edinburgh Lunatic Asylum, designed by Robert Reid (1807), with its first patients admitted in 1813. It was a quadrangle in plan, composed variously of three- and two-level blocks of rooms and support spaces. This institution clearly separated patients by social class, as well as severity of illness. Its exterior was modest although various interior rooms and wards were ornamented according to the social class of their inhabitants.[6] By contrast, the Glasgow Lunatic Asylum, which opened in 1814 and was designed by William Stark, was configured as a four-level structure with biaxial wings, with a glass dome at the center, and with exterior courtyards occupying the spaces between its axial wings.[7]

The North American social reformers aimed to thoroughly redefine society's civic institutions, including its schools, universities, medical hospitals, and insane asylums. The rise of moral treatment as an alternative to prison-asylums is traceable to two specialists working independently of one another, William Tuke, in England, and Philippe Pinel, in France. Pinel had founded the two major asylums there, the Salpêtrière, and the Bicêtre. These places served as therapeutic exemplars in the way that Bethlehem had to earlier generations. New therapies were to be applied solely to the mind, not to the body, within a more benevolent custodial regimen, whereby patients would be treated so as to develop self-control under the careful guidance of a medical staff. During this period, straitjackets and leather muffs would replace prison-like chains and shackles in an effort to reinvent these places as curative, not punitive institutions. The patient would be separated from one's 'distractions' – through isolation within a 'normalized' care regimen far from the stresses of urban life.[8] The work of these two physicians in time profoundly influenced North American asylum physicians, superintendents, and their architects.

The British Retreat at York (1796), designed by John Bevans, greatly influenced William Tuke. The aim was to return the patient to society once 'cured', and use of bloodletting and physical restraints such as straitjackets and chains was rejected. It looked from the exterior like a manor house, and livestock grazed on the grounds. Its double-loaded corridors were ultimately rejected for disallowing sufficient natural light into the interior spaces.[9] Tuke is considered the father of modern British psychiatry, though many of his precepts (i.e., geographic separation of village from urban life, a strict daily regimen, and avoidance of punitive mechanical restraints) were accepted in practice prior to construction of the Retreat at York.[10]

Early North American asylums

In Philadelphia, the Pennsylvania Hospital (1755–1760), designed by Samuel Rhoads and Joseph Fox, housed the first US inpatient ward for the insane. Patients were housed in the basement until 1841, then relocated to a replacement facility in west Philadelphia. The original hospital had been constructed in phases and by 1832 the core facility housed 249 patients, 126 of whom were classified as insane.[11] It was lauded as an architecturally inspired design. Later, a much smaller, by comparison, public hospital in Williamsburg, Virginia, was built (1771–1773), designed by Robert Smith.[12] Its single-loaded plan configuration featured natural ventilation and the presence of a billiard parlor and croquet courts on the adjacent outdoor lawns, symbols of advancements in moral treatment.[13] Another influential American precursor of this period was the South Carolina Insane Asylum, by architect Robert Mills (1821–1828), built in Columbia, South Carolina. The design of this asylum was based on the precepts of moral treatment. The main façade of this symmetrical, three-level institution conveyed a

Palladian image. Outdoor exercise yards were subdivided into various programmed activities, and the facility was designed for multiple additional wings to be added over time. Among its amenities were the first roof garden for recreational use in the United States. It was praised for its speciousness, for its adoption of recent building technology innovations, and for the single-room cells that lined single-loaded corridors.[14] Shortly thereafter, however, this asylum was eclipsed by the rising influence of America's preeminent asylum physician, Thomas Story Kirkbride.

Carla Yenni writes,

> Kirkbride, a physician and member of the Society of Friends, believed fervently that establishing a new building type was essential for affecting a cure. He supervised a high-profile hospital (the first Pennsylvania Hospital, 1833–1841), advised many doctors and architects, influenced the architectural guidelines published in 1851 by the AMSAII, and wrote a book on the architecture of insane hospitals in 1854. For most of the nineteenth century, from about 1840 to about 1880, he was the single most important nineteenth-century psychiatrist when it came to matters of architecture . . . Kirkbride was devoted to moral treatment, which required a change of daily habits – regular schedules were intended to make patient internalize self-control. Not surprisingly, the spaces within hospitals and the circulation patterns reinforced this control. Patients would live a regimented life, eat healthy food, get exercise, avoid the vicious city, and visit daily with the superintendent or his wife . . . patients should be unchained, granted respect, encouraged to perform occupational tasks (such as farming, carpentry, or laundry), and allowed to stroll the grounds with an attendant . . . patients were inherently good, despite their outward behavior; and the mentally ill (were provided) the promise of returning to society after a stay in the purpose-built asylum.[15]

The interiors were well furnished and spacious, with corridors 12 feet wide with some even 14 feet in width. From the exterior, they were to appear opulent, with prominent domes containing large iron water tanks for water distribution and observation decks affording views of expansive grounds.[16] Emphasis was placed on natural ventilation as a defense against infection and disease; this give rise to the pavilion – one of the most significant advancements in the history of hospital architecture but one that itself would be rejected, in time.[17] The moral treatment movement was blooming. This required flanking male and female wings (short enough to facilitate effective natural ventilation) around an open-air quadrangle. Two state-run asylums in the United States were built in this manner, in Massachusetts and in New York State. Each was based on quadrangle plans, and in this regard they contrasted from Dr. Kirkbride's favored linear footprint of his recently opened asylum in Philadelphia. Indigent patients were relocated to these state asylums from the various almshouses and prisons, whereas patients from the upper social classes paid a fee for their psychiatric care. The asylum at Worchester, Massachusetts, was U-shaped in plan and most patients there were poor; it was built assuming the cured individual would eventually return to society as a contributing citizen.[18]

The New York State Lunatic Asylum in Utica (1842–1844), designed by William Clarke, was also a modified quadrangle campus, with three sides enclosed by wards and a fourth wing housing support functions. Clarke was not an architect by profession; he was a successful local entrepreneur who had achieved the rank of captain in the US Army and thereafter became financially successful running a gambling lottery in Utica.[19] This asylum housed 380 private rooms and 20 open wards – large spaces housing six to eight beds. As was common at the time, the mixture of open wards and private bedrooms was to attract a broad range of social classes by offering a range of patient room options.[20] When the influential British asylum physician John Charles Bucknill visited the Utica asylum, as part of a tour of other recently built North America mental institutions, he was impressed by its neoclassicism.[21]

When Utica's chief physician, John Grey, was subsequently offered the opportunity to build a lunatic asylum from scratch, he opted for a concept completely different from Utica and would work closely with H.H. Richardson on the design and construction of the Buffalo, New York, State Hospital for the Insane. This asylum was built in geographic proximity to the future Ontario Provincial Lunatic Asylum in Toronto. The focus of the following discussion is to focus on the provincial asylum built in Toronto within the context of the preceding discussion of its precursor institutions. It was a grandly conceived institution built to express the highest civic ideals of the benefactors. Its history parallels North American advancements in psychiatric care. The following discussion, first, traces the historical time line of this institution and its important

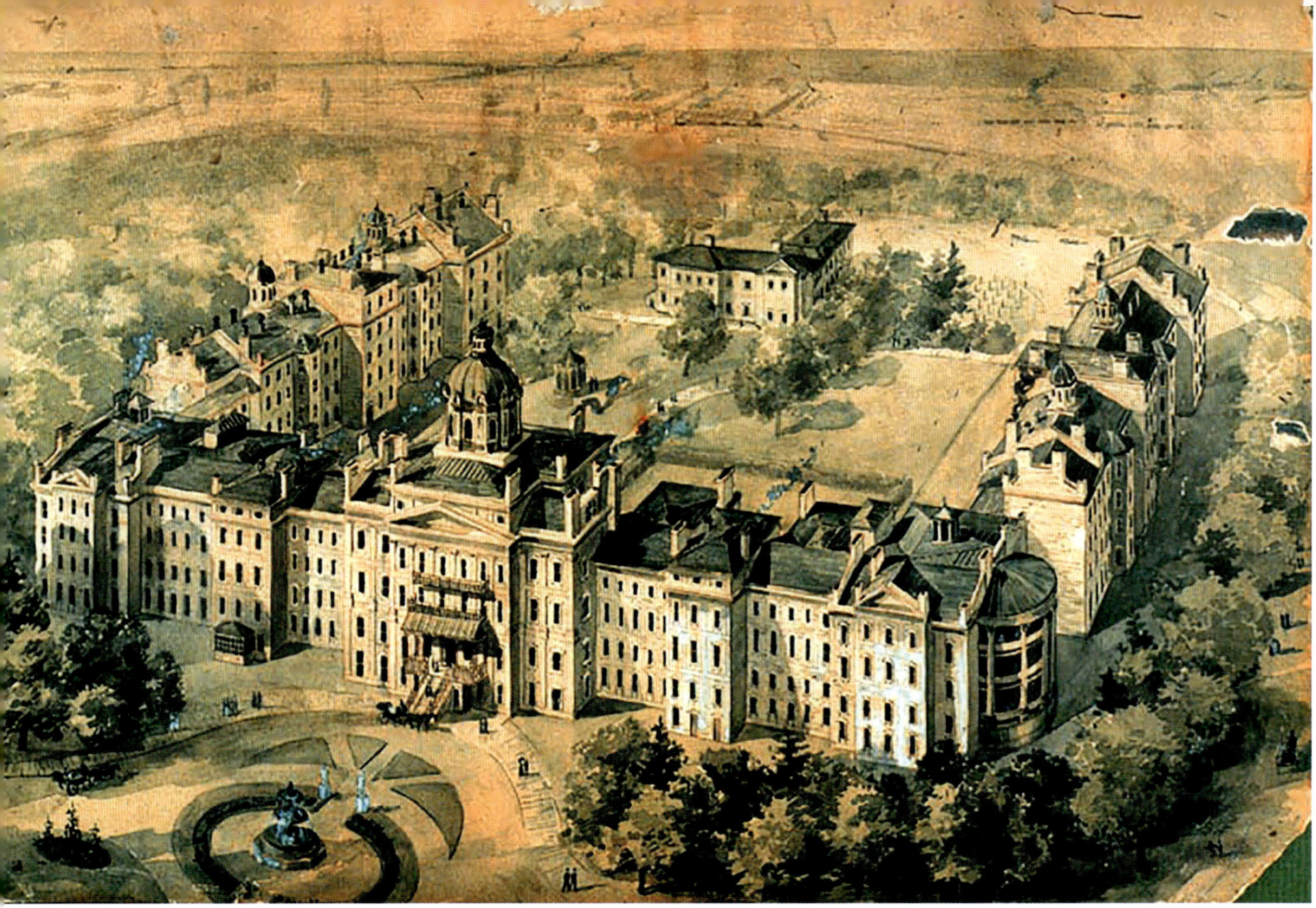

4.1 Provincial Lunatic Asylum, Toronto, 1871. Watercolor depicting the two Tully Wings added later to the 1850 main building that fronted Queen Street West.

role in the community. The second aim is to analyze the current plan to redevelop its main campus in Toronto. In response to this, an alternative redevelopment plan is presented, an alternate vision cognizant of the 165-year history of this institution.

The Provincial Lunatic Asylum in Toronto

The original buildings of the Provincial Lunatic Asylum in Toronto at 999 Queen Street West (1846–1849) were built to the design of John George Howard and considered the most prominent commission of his long career. At the time, he wrote,

> The instructions I received from the Building Committee were to design a building for the care – not incarceration – of about 500 of the insane of Upper Canada, and I made a tour of the United States in search of the best information upon that subject. The present building was designed and the plans were submitted to the medical men at their annual meeting at the Astor House, New York. After examining them, the said gentlemen expressed themselves highly pleased with the arrangements and pronounced them the best for the purpose on the Continent of America.[22]

Howard established a successful career as an architect of residential, ecclesiastical, and public building commissions built directly for or sponsored by Toronto's rapidly growing elite social class. He emigrated from England with his wife in 1832 and shortly after arriving in Toronto changed his legal surname from Corby to Howard.[23] In 1848, the British physician John Connolly had recommended to the founders of the Toronto asylum that every patient be treated kindly, with proper custodial surveillance at all times and with patients classified by symptom and shielded from being placed on public spectacle. No restraints were to be used and alternatively all patients should be encouraged to mix socially with other similar types of patients in a therapeutically restorative, aesthetically uplifting, morally grounded treatment environment.[24] The architectural response deemed best suited to address Dr. Connolly's provisos would be a building that emphasized its pastoral campus setting. Howard's proposed building and campus plan for Toronto was strongly influenced by the institutions he had visited

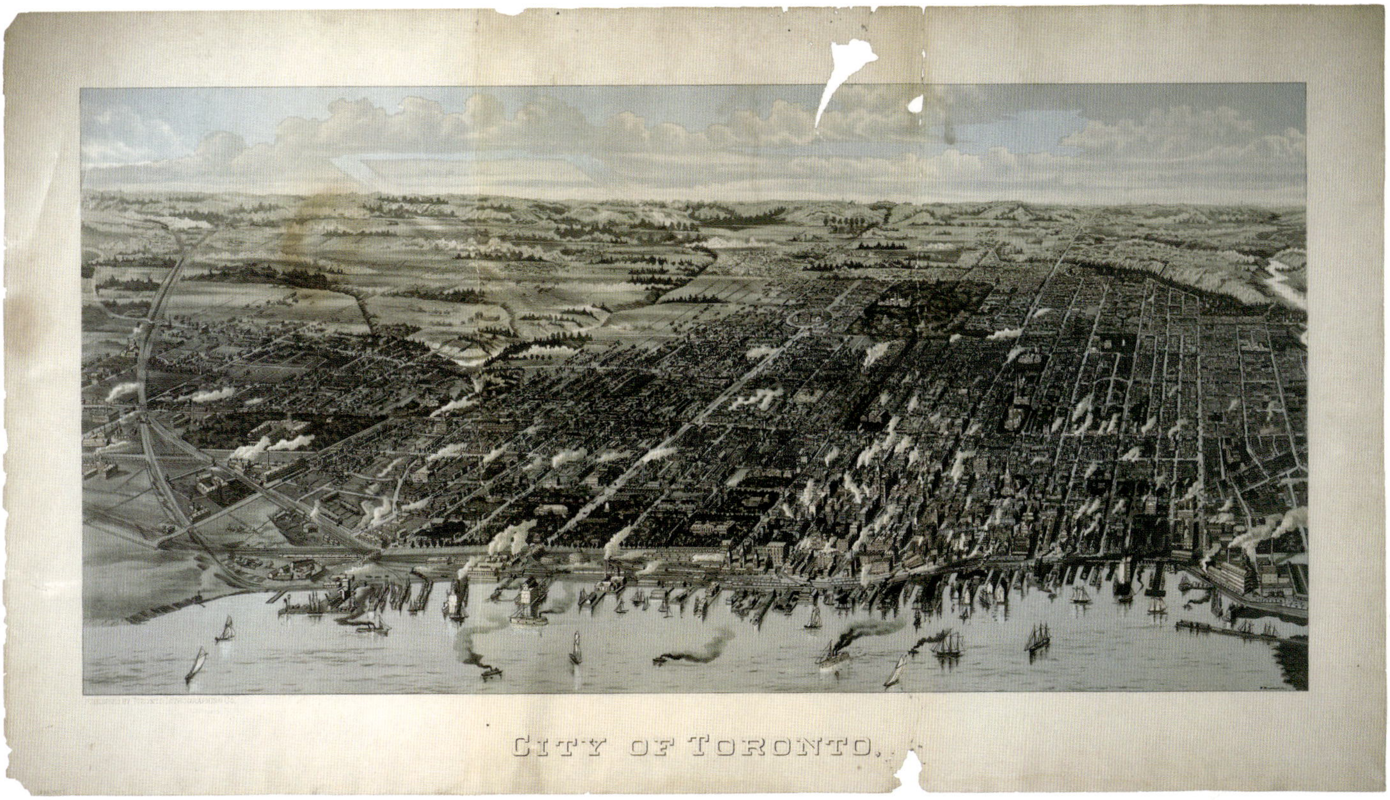

4.2 City of Toronto, view to the north, 1855 lithograph.

on his British and American tour of asylums. These included Hanwell Asylum in Middlesex, United Kingdom; the Island Retreat and Pauper's Lunatic Asylum on Blackwell Island, New York; and the aforementioned Utica Hospital in New York State and the Worcester State Hospital in Massachusetts. He also toured the (second) Pennsylvania Hospital, in Philadelphia.[25]

The site was purchased in 1844; it was a low-lying parcel of land lacking any notable natural features and previously the site of the Garrison Military Reserve. It extended south of Queen Street West all the way to the Lake Ontario shoreline. There were no ponds or streams on the site although the institution would rely on the lake itself for its fresh water supply. Since the institution would likely be expanding in time, Howard elected to locate the main building near Queen Street without being too near, so patients could maintain a modicum of privacy distant from curious passersby. Inspired by the asylum he had toured at Utica, Howard decided upon a U-shaped campus footprint for a facility initially housing 400 beds, with a double-loaded corridor, 14 feet wide, a space wider than at any American asylum at the time. The first building was set back 300 feet from the street, sited parallel with the lake to allow for direct views of the nearby waterfront, as illustrated in 1890 by W.H. Thompson (Figure 4.1) amid a city that was rapidly expanding (Figure 4.2).

Its attributes included two circular, semi-enclosed verandas, one at each end of the main building. As for plumbing, hot and cold water was available from the asylum's opening day in 1850 and potable water was pumped from a large reservoir situated 90 feet above street level to a holding tank inside the large dome directly above the main entrance. A system of interconnected staircases allowed patients to circulate independently. The facility was four levels in height plus an attic, symmetrical in plan, with men housed to one side and women to the other according to social convention. The Toronto asylum functioned uninterrupted up to World War II, with few alternations while retaining its grounds, farming plots, and various outbuildings, including its employment workshops (Figure 4.3, Figure 4.4, and Figure 4.5a–b). Soon after the asylum opened in 1850, a 12-foot-high,

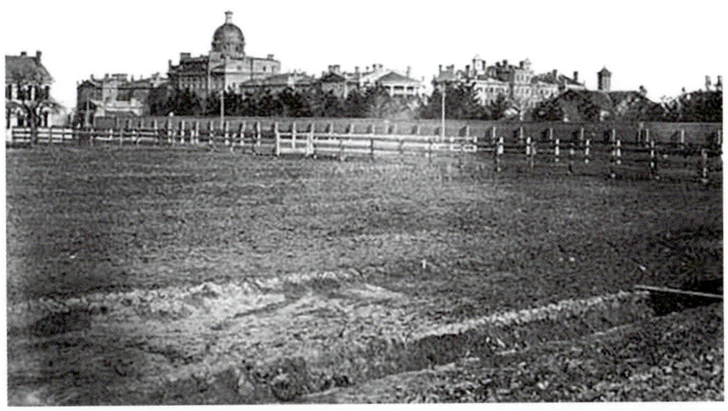

4.3 Agricultural land on the grounds of the Provincial Lunatic Asylum, Toronto, circa 1870.

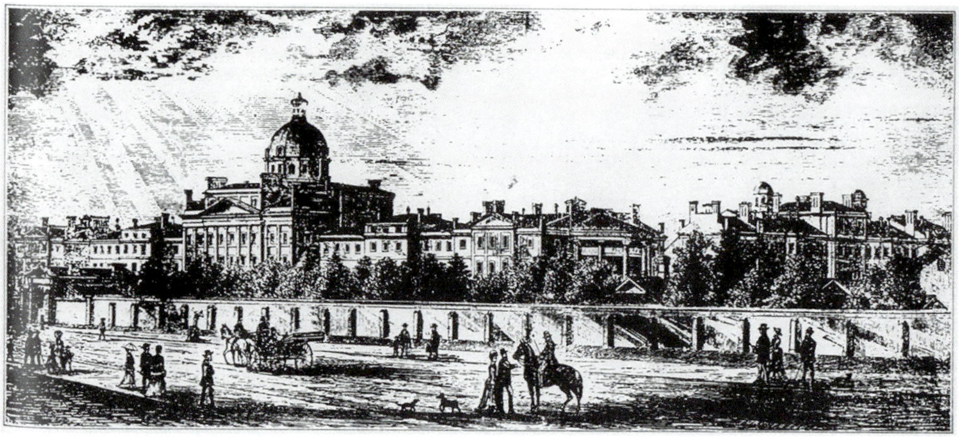

4.4 View of the perimeter wall and main asylum building from Queen Street West, circa 1870s.

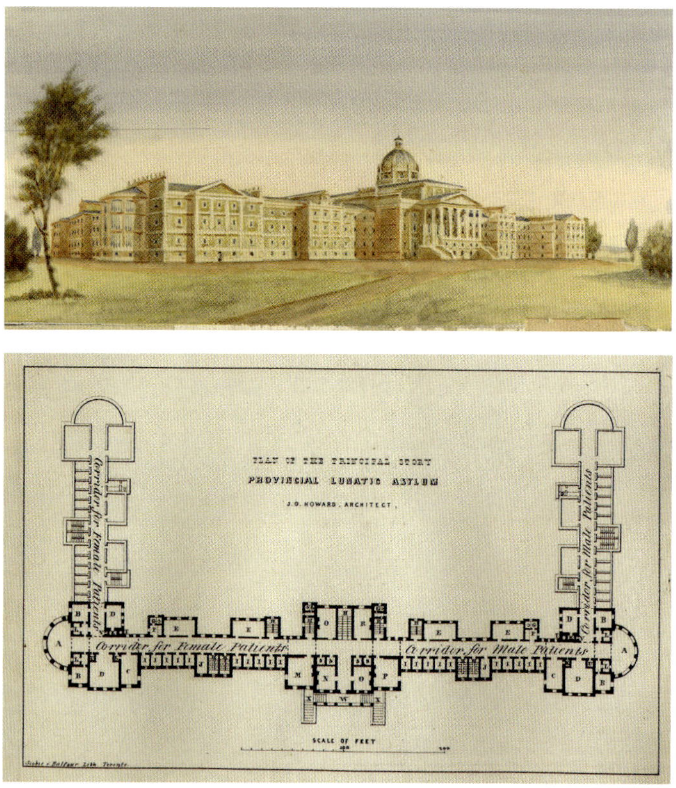

4.5a–b Architect John Howard's 1850 main asylum building, with the two Tully Wing additions depicted (top and bottom).

thick brick wall was erected around the perimeter (in part with patient labor), and this posed a formidable barrier between the asylum and the burgeoning city around it. By the early 20th century, the asylum was surrounded by a mixture of industry and working-class residential neighborhoods (Figure 4.6 and Figure 4.7).[26]

By the 1930s, the facilities were in precipitous decline. A study produced by American experts concluded the Ontario hospital network overall had sunk 'to a lamentable plane of incapacity'. At the Ontario Hospital, Toronto (OHT), as the asylum was known from 1919 to 1966, severe, chronic overcrowding was observed. Worse, the negative stigmas surrounding mental illness in Toronto had correspondingly grown in the public's view. The consultants' 1937 report concluded, 'The unpleasant feeling that many citizens have about this old hospital can hardly be dissipated.'[27] Following World War II, by the mid-20th century, the Toronto asylum marked its first 100 years of service (Figure 4.8). A *Special Committee Report* in 1950 noted severe problems throughout the province-wide network of 14 hospitals, leaving no room for complacency to persist any longer. The OHT by this time was the most overcrowded of all in the provincial network, with an inpatient population of 1,167 that exceeded its legal bed capacity by 56%! Significant renovations were recommended, and the facility was described as drab and depressing.[28] Interestingly, 6 years later, a subsequent report praised the landscaped grounds without commenting directly on the condition of the facility itself. Regardless, deferred maintenance had taken its toll and was now at a critical stage.[29]

This resulted in the construction of a new Administration Building (1954–1956), designed by Mathers and Haldenby. It was constructed right in front of and in proximity to Howard's 1850 building. Much-needed new space was now housed in this rather austere, modernist block building, three levels in height and 600 feet long. It ran parallel to the Howard building and completely dominated it visually, and unfortunately, it also blocked the street frontage along Queen Street West. Beautiful open lawns were paved over for parking. The decision to site the new building in this manner signaled the death of the 1850 building and the subsequent Tully Wing additions. However, to its critics, other site options were available that would have left the Queen Street face of the institution unscathed. Regardless, the message conveyed to the public was now crystal clear.[30] John Court speculates on these events:

> After the Second World War many aspects of life were influenced by a firm belief in modernity . . . The *new*, it was held, could almost single-handedly achieve social

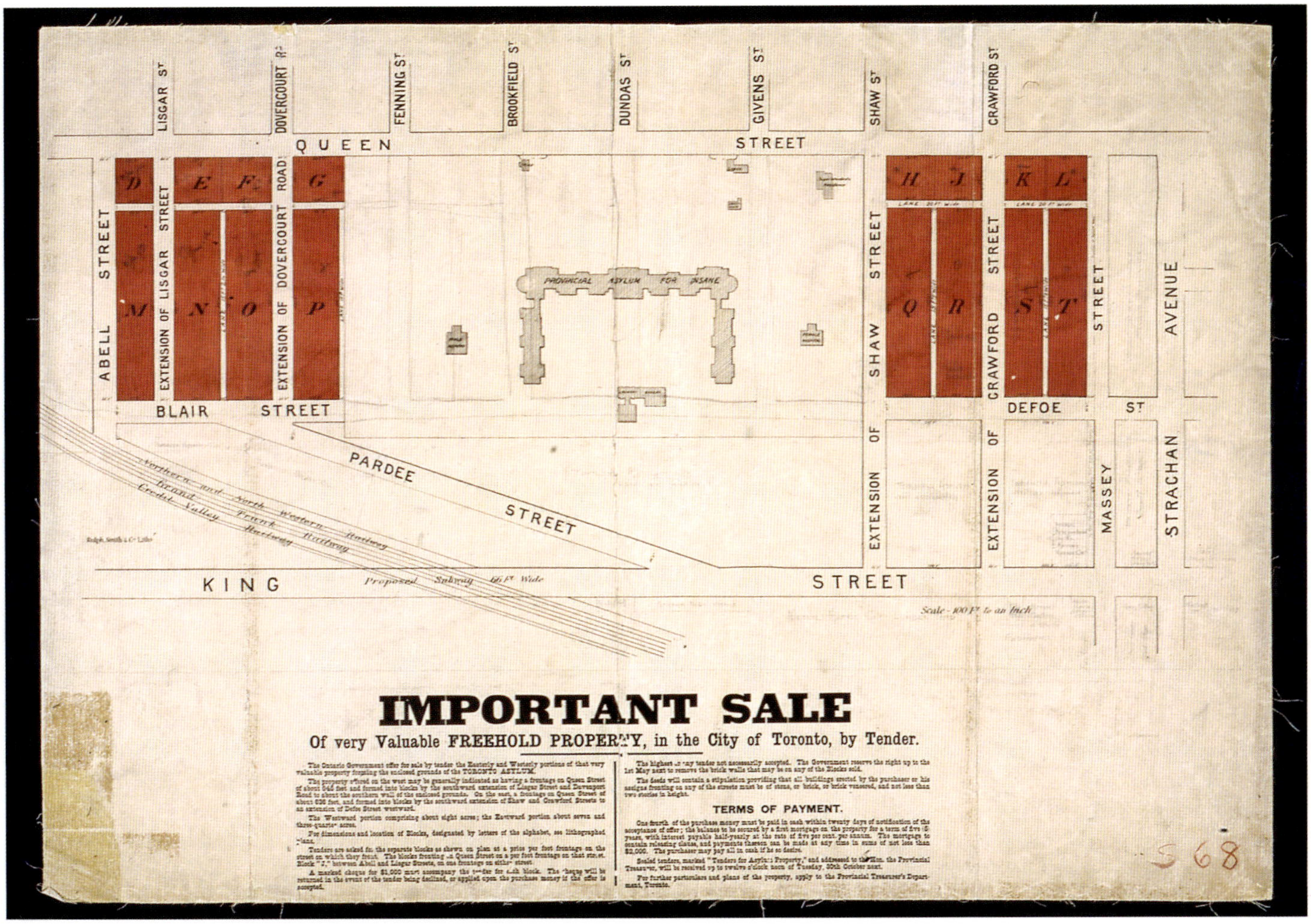

4.6 Plot plan indicating the asylum's (province's) sale of its former agricultural land holdings for urban development, 1883.

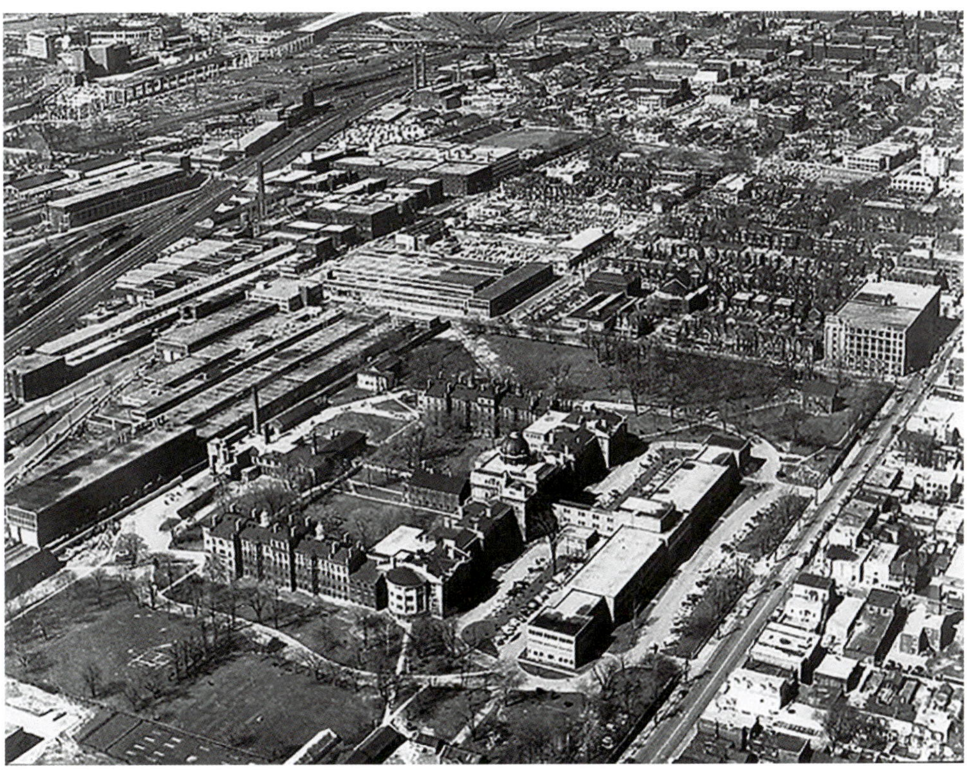

4.7 Aerial view of the old Provincial Lunatic Asylum campus in Toronto, 1957.

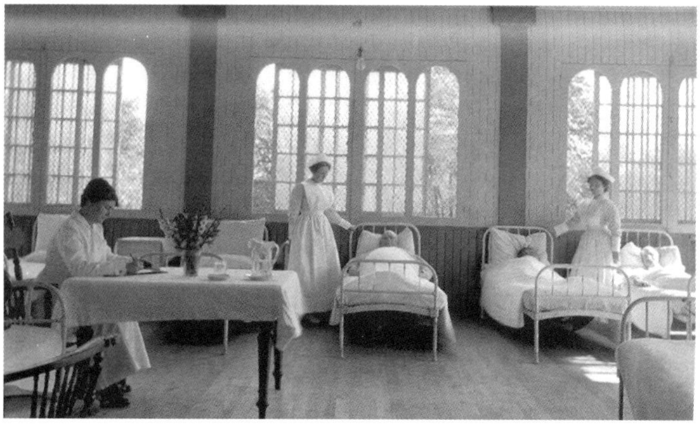

4.8 Infirmary ward at the provincial asylum in Toronto, circa 1880s.

> improvements . . . Secondly, commencing in 1951, there was a dramatic change in the clinical technology for treating and managing mental illness through the widespread introduction of tranquilizing drugs (psychotropics and neuroleptics). In addition to bringing great improvements in the prognosis for schizophrenia and other psychoses (representing a significant majority of the patients at Queen West), this advancement allowed a shift away from the earlier emphases on the confinement of patients for extended lengths of time and the need for strong physical security within institutions. . . (also) technology was (now) less radical in application than the preceding decades of experimentation with interventions like insulin coma, metrazol convulsion therapy, prolonged narcosis, electroplexy and psychosurgery. The benefits of the newer pharmaceuticals encouraged public general hospitals to overcome their resistance to establishing community psychiatric units, spurred on by Federal and Provincial policy changes.[31]

These events resulted, from 1952 to 1972, and as discussed in Chapter 2, in a substantial reduction in the centuries-old policy of constantly increasing inpatient admissions with large, long-term inpatient populations. The practice of custodial care had constantly caused overcrowding in the province's inpatient psychiatric hospitals.[32] By 1972 the inpatient residential population at Queen Street West had declined from a high of 1,200 in the early 1950s to only 440 inpatients.[33] Back in 1960, Dr. Burdett McNeel, the province's chief mental health official, posited the existence of four distinct eras in architecture for mental health care: first, large institutions erected in the latter half of the 19th century; followed, second, by smaller communities of detached cottages, citing the Whitby, Ontario, asylum (1913–1920) as a prime example (Chapter 2);[34] third, facilities built just before and after World War II with their large, open expanses of glass and long corridors; and fourth, a new, modernist phase based on decentralization and deinstitutionalization resulting in smaller, mostly outpatient mental health facilities built in community-based settings.[35] As it turned out, McNeel would reiterate his position throughout his tenure (1958–1968) that the old buildings at Queen Street West were hopelessly obsolete because the stigma associated with mental illness was as much based on the antiquated image of old asylums as anything else (Figure 4.9a–b).[36] By 1961, the facility still remained severely overcrowded and too overcentralized in an era when new psychiatric hospitals were best thought to house no more than 250–300 beds.[37]

In 1965, a comprehensive redevelopment plan of the Queen Street West campus was publicly announced with all existing structures concluded to be in need of immediate demolition and replacement.[38] In that year the old 1850 asylum housed nearly 750 patients and the name of the institution had been changed to the Queen Street Mental Health Centre. In early 1967 the architectural firm of Somerville, McMurrich & Oxley completed a master plan for the campus. As it turned out, the campus and architectural plan proposed by this firm was greatly influenced by the Saskatchewan Psychiatric Centre in Yorkton, designed by a Dr. Humphrey Osmond and his architect, Kyo Izumi, prior.[39]

The architects' master plan for redevelopment was premised on four main provisos: (1) new construction was to be phased in to maintain patient accommodation, treatment, and services throughout the entire construction period; (2) patients were to be treated as individuals or in small groups with close engagement with staff; (3) amenities were to be provided for a far wider range of therapeutic and recreational activities than had been possible to accommodate in the old building; and (4) interaction with the outside community was to be encouraged as much as possible both to destigmatize and to provide patients meaningful contact with the outside world on a daily basis. Additionally, the campus plan would decentralize patient residential care while centralizing all support functions (i.e., laundry and facility management services and diagnostic and treatment functions). An extensive underground pedestrian circulation and materials transport system was to be provided connecting all buildings on the campus. Also, outdoor space for sports activities, gardening, and tree-shaded paths were to be provided.

Architect Loren Oxley described the Toronto campus's new architectural centerpiece:

> The Community Centre will become an important element in the overall treatment program. Along with the recreational and therapeutic facilities that it contains (swimming pool, gymnasium, etc.) it will also feature a bank, beauty parlor,

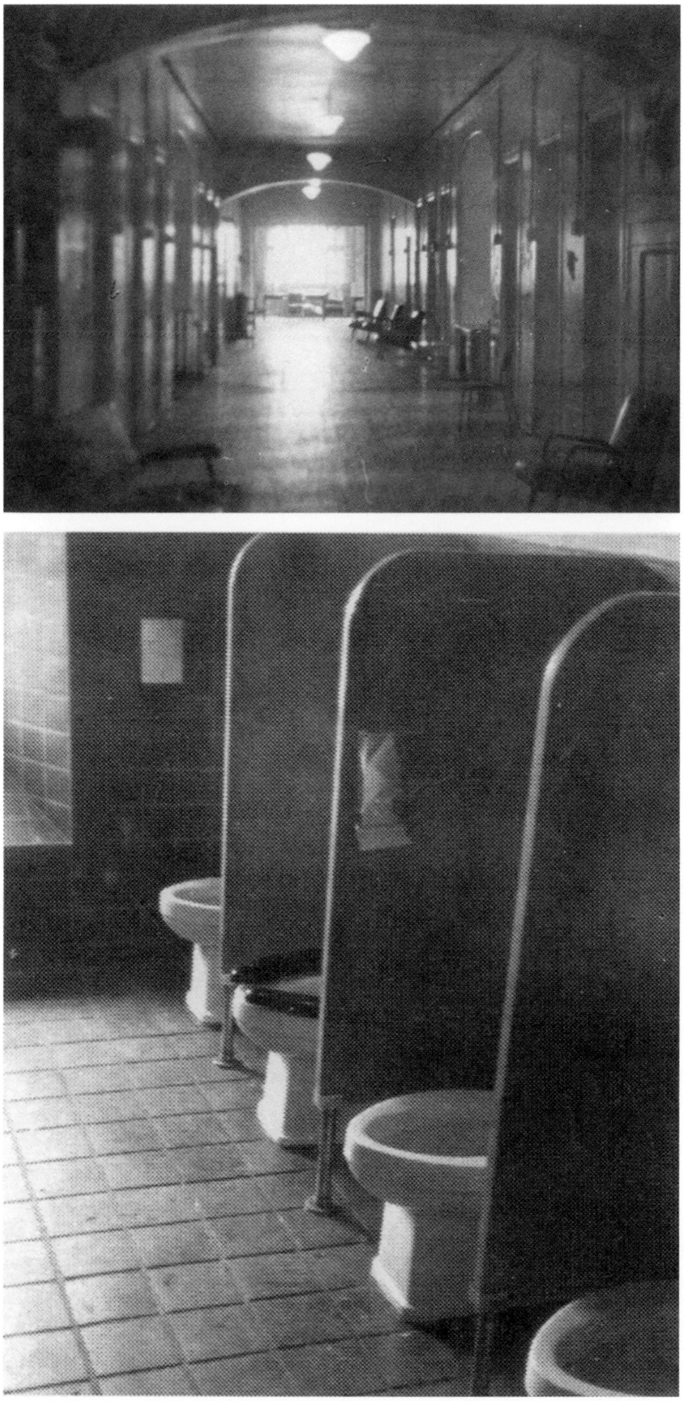

4.9a–b Main corridor in the provincial asylum ward (top) and communal toilets (bottom), 1972 photos.

> sidewalk café and other services – all in an enclosed 'shopping mall' setting. All of these facilities will be for use by the patients. Because it will so closely approximate the world outside, and because of the regular contact with outside local residents using the facilities, the patients will be introduced back into the complexities of social relationships in a controlled environment.[40]

The approved campus plan included a set of four independent, dormitory-like residential treatment unit buildings, each an autonomous entity yet interconnected at grade by a pedestrian street, supplemented by the aforementioned underground circulation system that connected every building on the campus. This back-of-house, or more appropriately, 'beneath-house' subterranean system featured unmanned battery-powered vehicles (referred as AMSCARs) for transport of supplies and equipment. This decision was made to avoid the most institutional aspects of the old asylum. Each new 'pavilion' was able to be built without having to demolish the original main asylum building at the center of the campus. However, the two later neoclassical Tully Wing additions were demolished prior to the commencement of construction.When the four new residential pavilions opened in 1974, each five-level treatment unit (Units A, B, C, and D) housed 175 beds, and each functioned as the *home base* for the patient, where inpatient and outpatient care was provided. The first floor housed the unit administrative office, admitting, emergency intake, and a 16-bed short-term patient assessment unit. The four upper floors each housed 34 beds plus dining and hygiene spaces (communal bathrooms and showers); a nursing station; group therapy and dayrooms; and offices for staff psychiatrists, psychologists, and related personnel. The lower level (basement level) directly beneath each unit housed classrooms and staff support amenities (i.e., lockers and meeting rooms). These buildings allowed for strict control of the patient at all times. The four buildings were connected to the new Community Centre vis-à-vis the aforementioned central circulation system (Figure 4.10 and Figure 4.11).[41]

The 1956 Administration Building housed a library and offices on the ground floor; an auditorium was added to the front façade in 1980. The second floor housed offices and the third floor housed 60 patients; each patient room had its own washroom. This unremarkable building rendered the 1850 Howard building virtually dismissible, although it had garnered no architectural awards in its time itself. By now, it appeared the staff had become far more negative – even hostile – toward the 1850 building (although patients at times appeared to be more afraid of the staff than the building itself). Among the staff, the unspoken fear was that the total institution was doomed unless new buildings were built, and soon.[42] This was attributable to broader events occurring in the modern history of psychiatry insofar as obsolete 'scientific' treatments of the old asylum era were now rejected, although it was now impossible to dissociate this stigma from any associated stigma.[43]

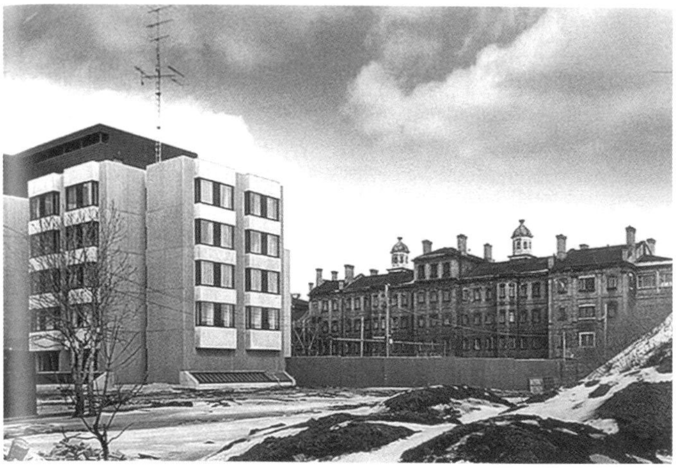

4.10 View of a 1974 residential pavilion building with the 1850 John Howard original asylum building in background.

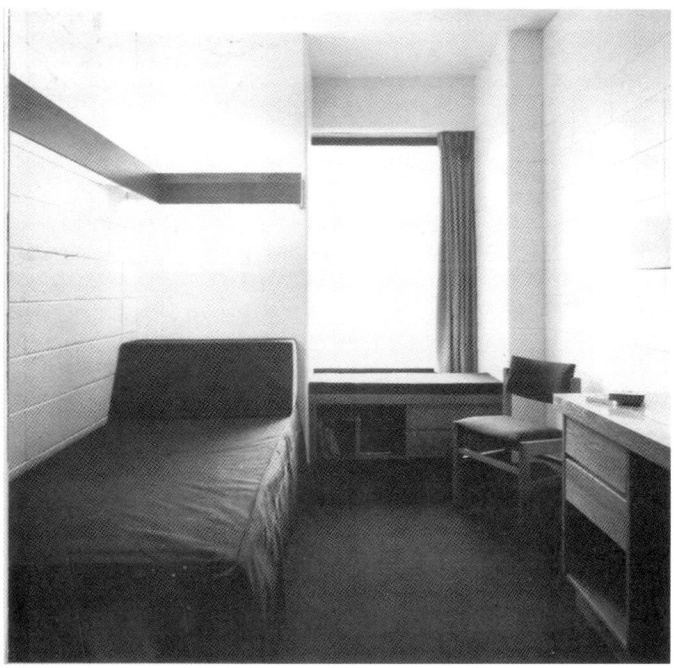

4.11 Interior of a patient room in a 1974 residential pavilion.

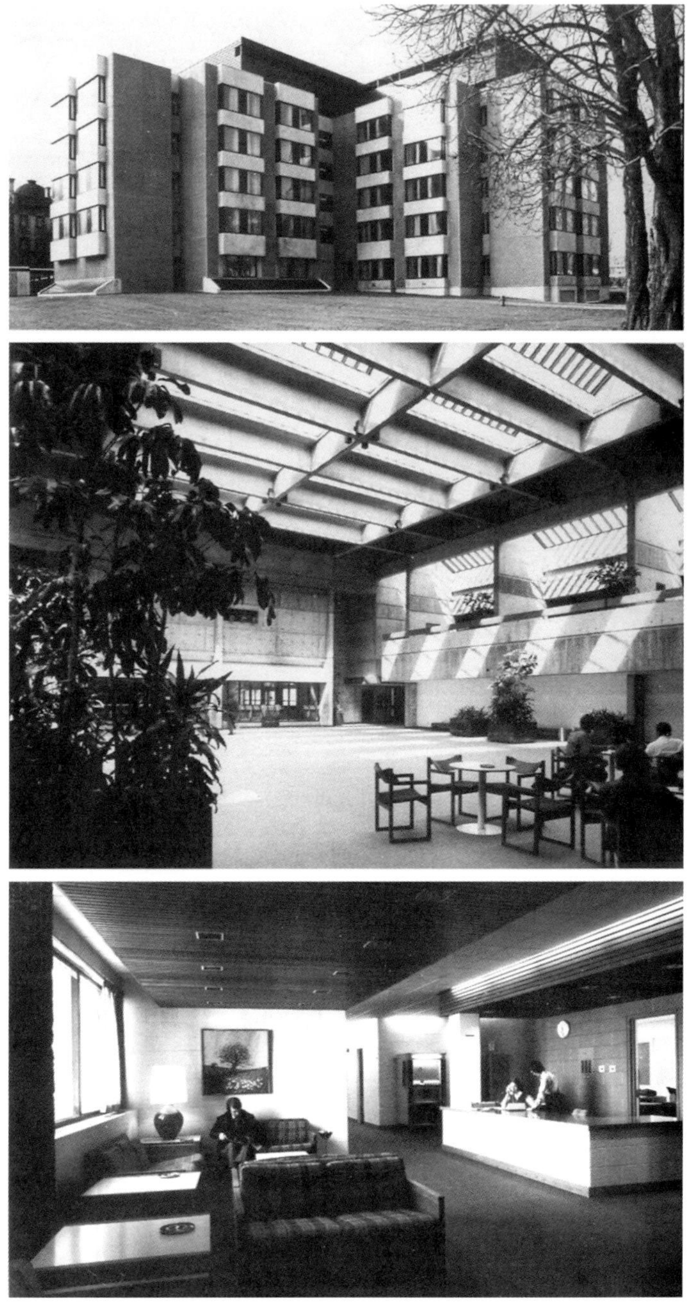

4.12a–c Exterior view of one of the four 1974 pavilions (top), interior of the commons building public atrium (middle), and a dayroom in a residential pavilion depicting an open nurses' station, later enclosed with glass (bottom).

A postoccupancy assessment was conducted to compare the pre-relocation and post-relocation experiences of patients and staff on this 27-acre campus. A three-person research team began work in 1972 and in the following 12 months the inpatient census continued to fall, and this was attributed to the 'revolution' then unfolding in new drug-based therapies, as discussed in Chapter 2. Among the team's findings in its report of 1973, the staff, patients, and the general public were all described as nicely embracing the new campus buildings (Figure 4.12a–c). As for the new dormitory-like accommodations, in postmove interviews one patient referred to newfound pride compared to when friends had visited him in the old asylum, remarking, 'When you had visitors you felt so uncomfortable to have them see you in a place like that.'[44] It was also observed by the team that patients were ratcheting up their personal appearance and hygiene level compared to before, with their new surroundings 'clearly serving to enhance their sense of self-worth'.[45]

Specifically,

> The patients' behavior had changed. They were calmer and less bizarre. This can be explained in part by the crisis intervention unit on the main floor . . . when disturbances did occur on the upper floors they were much easier to contain (and it was) easier to diffuse disruptive incidents . . . the new building was perceived by staff and patients as providing a more normal environment. Most patients expressed approval . . . in its relative luxury, freshness and brightness . . . there was much less property damage and the cleaning staff reported that people tried to be neater. . . (but) contrary to some pre-move predictions the attractive and comfortable new environment did not make patients less willing to leave the hospital. Almost all the patients said they would be happy to get out of the hospital in spite of the changes.[46]

As for the staff's assessment, the move to the new buildings coincided with the introduction of new treatment programs and administrative policies. As a result,

> Changes in staff behavior and attitudes, therefore, cannot be attributed solely to the new programmes nor solely to the new architecture . . . prior to the move most of the clinical staff were dubious about the extent to which a new physical structure could influence the quality of therapeutic care. They anticipated a wide range of problems associated with the design of the building . . . many of the staff (at first) expressed feelings of resentment about the intended final outcome . . . claiming their suggestions and briefs were largely ignored by the architects and many said they felt as though they had been 'talking to the wind' . . . After the move, however, most staff members expressed positive attitudes . . . enjoying their work more with some adding their attitude towards patients had also changed for the better. . . (staff) reported they had felt somewhat ashamed and defensive about the old building in comparison to their colleagues at up-to-date psychiatric hospitals elsewhere . . . the new architecture combined with the new programmes it stimulated generated a sense of pride among staff and increased morale.[47]

In terms of patient privacy, some social spaces on these new residential units drew nearly every patient while other larger social spaces remained underused, by comparison. However, the architects' essential concept had been realized, with patients generally moving from their private retreat (bedroom) to interact with increasingly larger groups of people in larger social spaces, whereas in the asylum building they had been forced to share bedrooms and thrust into nonprivate spaces without any graduated hierarchy of modifying, *in-between* spaces. The task was now to administer four decentralized yet interconnected mini-psychiatric hospitals. For example, the former central admitting function was now decentralized to each of the four treatment unit buildings. Second, a spirit of friendly rivalry ensued after the move, as each unit *competed* with the others. With regards to the Community Centre built at the center of campus, directly behind the 1850 asylum, the research team concluded the following:

> The Community Centre was designed to counteract the anticipated (social) isolation in the four treatment towers . . . but it did not realize its full potential . . . the staff often did not use it for their meals and neither was its grand scale conducive to relaxed mingling or private conversations. Meeting and talking informally with other staff members instead usually took place within the individual treatment towers . . . where the scale of the architecture was more intimate . . . had the four treatment towers been designed today (1975) it is entirely possible (they) would have been located in different areas of the city, each within its own community context.[48]

The scale and ambiance of the community center's 'mall' concept was found to be lacking in subsequent years.[49] The postoccupancy assessment was criticized at the time for its singular promotion of the virtues of modernism over heritage architecture.[50] For its part, the province sought to transform the place, essentially, into a center for psychiatric care, in a serious effort to fully shed any stigma associated with the term 'insane asylum'.[51] In 1999, the campus was rechristened the Centre for Addiction and Mental Health (CAMH), and it was designated by the World Health Organization (WHO) as a center of excellence. CAMH had been formed through the merger of the Queen Street West campus with the Clarke Institute of Psychiatry, located on College

1853: Northern Railway of Canada opens

1850: Provincial Lunatic Asylum, 211 patients transferred from Temporary Asylum (former jail on King Street)

1861: Queen Street West streetcar begins operations

1860: Queens Park opens

1871: Name changed to 'Asylum for the Insane, Toronto'

1858–1879: Crystal Palace Exhibition Hall occupies south half of asylum site

1914–1918: World War I

1909: Institution's name changed to 'Hospital for the Insane, Toronto'

1941–1945: World War II

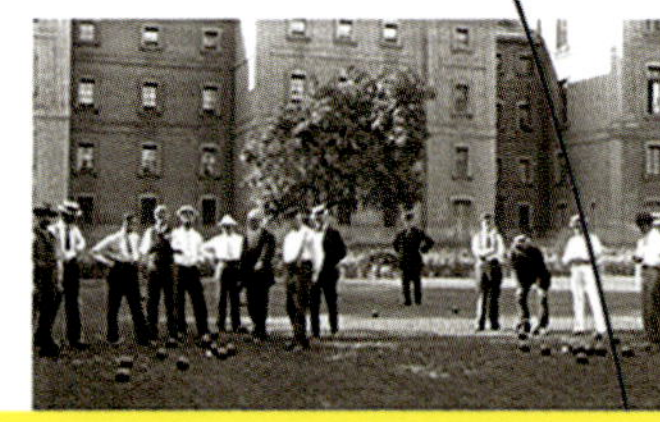

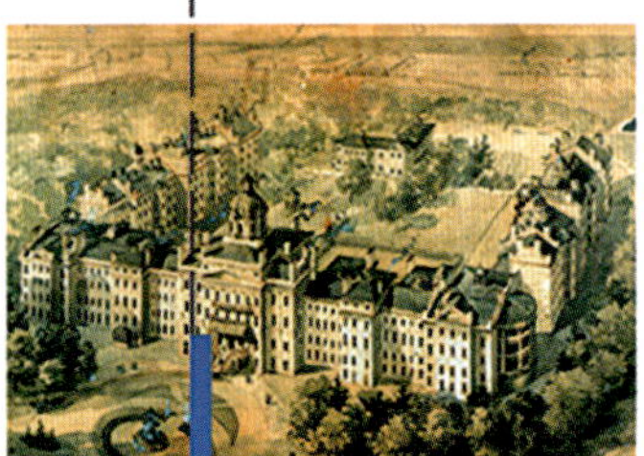

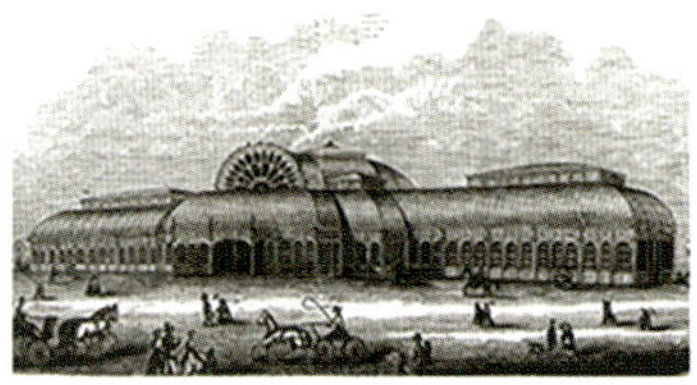

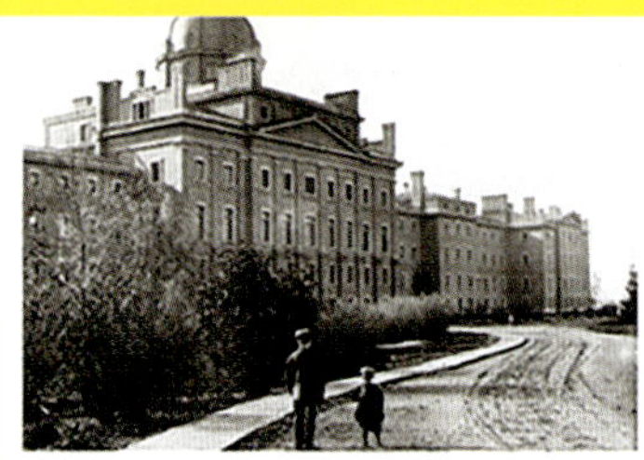

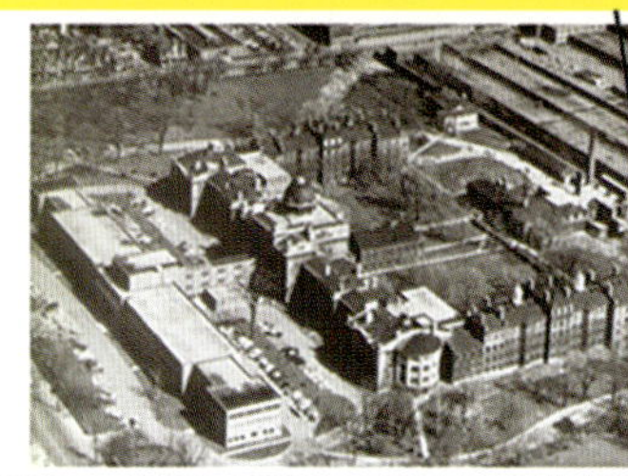

1853–1875: Dr. Joseph Workman appointed first Medical Superintendent

1873: John and Jemima Howard sell private estate to City of Toronto – rechristened as High Park (3.8 km away) in 1876

1891: 'Asylum for the Insane, Mimico' opens as branch of Queen West asylum

1919: New asylum in Whitby opens, intended to replace Queen Street campus. However, both continue to be utilized by province

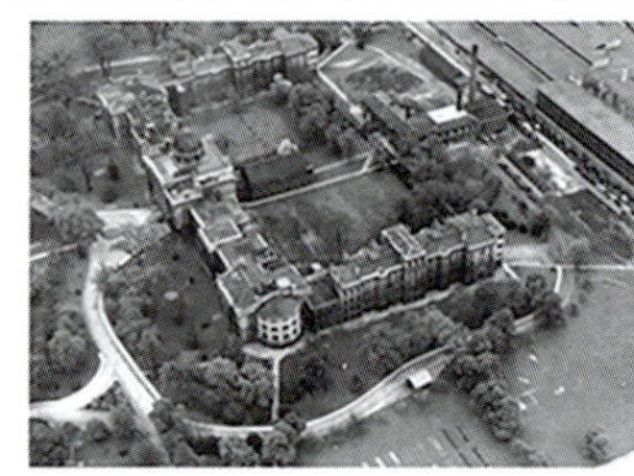

1919: Totonto hospital's name changed to 'Ontario, Hospital, Toronto'

1846: 'Provincial Lunatic Asylum' construction begins on 50 acre parcel on the Garrison Military Reserve. Architect: John Howard

1889: Government sells 23 acres of open land. East and West perimeter walls rebuilt using original materials. Site reconfigured to present boundaries

1912: City of Toronto purchases Trinity College Campus on Queen Street West. Land combined with Bellwoods Park to form Trinity-Bellwoods Park

1949: Alcohol Research Foundation established (later named Addiction Research Foundation)

1853: Perimeter wall complete, built by inmates

Horse carriage patient transport vehicles replaced with trucks

1850 1900 1950

4.13 Time line/chronology of CAMH in Toronto from 1850 to 2020.

1964–1966: Clarke Institute of Psychiatry opens (College Street)

1967: Donwood Institute opens (Brentcliffe Road)

1976: 1850 asylum building demolished

1998: Metro Toronto municipalities amalgamate into City of Toronto

2001: Vision and Master Plan outlines Queen Street site's transformation into 'Urban Village' – mixed-use with new public vehicular thoroughfares

2010: CAMH contest to name five new public vehicular thoroughfares to bisect Queen Street West campus

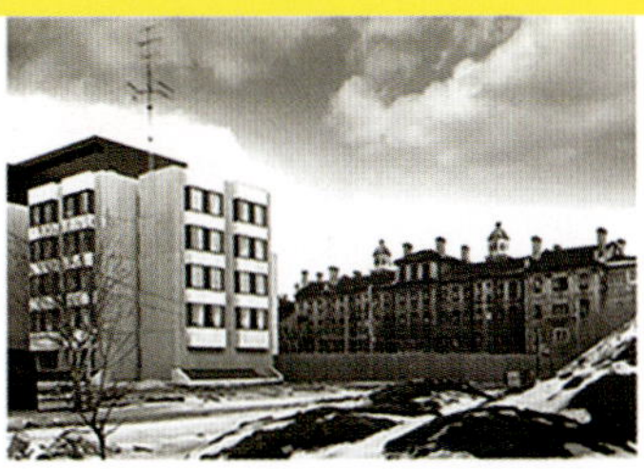

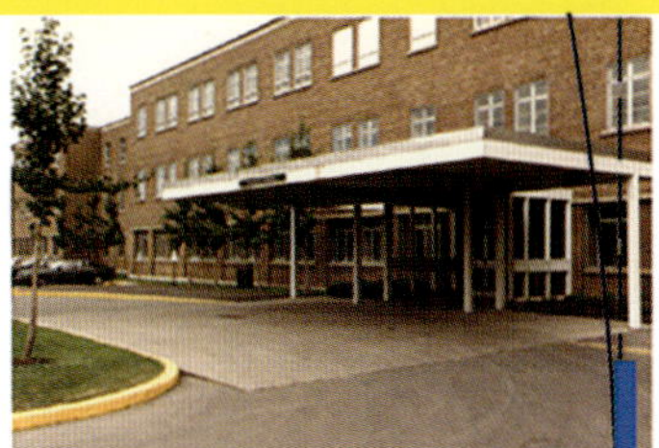

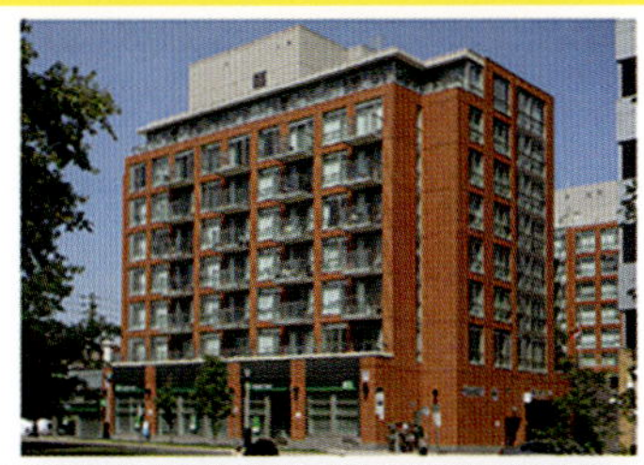

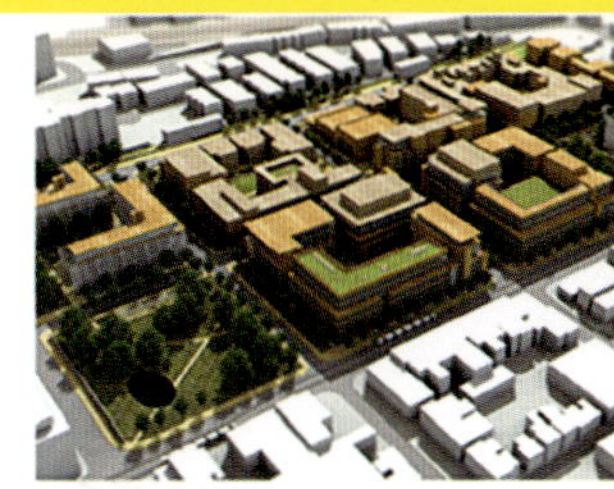

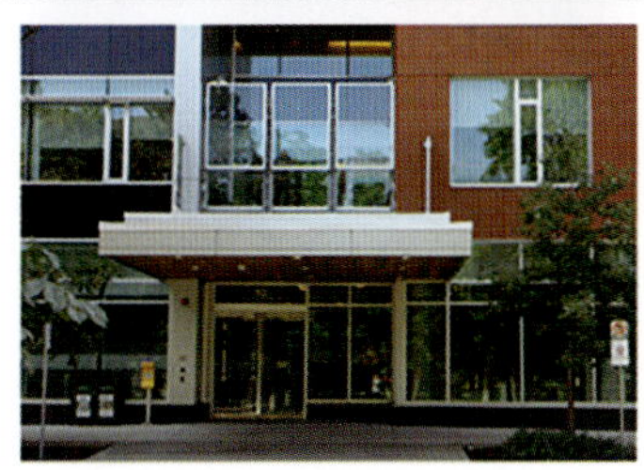

1966: Name changed to 'Queen Street Mental Health Centre'

1954: Yonge Street Subway opens

1953: Municipality of Metropolitan Toronto created

1956: New Queen Street West Administration Building opens

1978: Former Superintendent's Residence (later Nurses' Residence) demolished

1972: Inpatient Treatment Units 1 and 2 and Paul Christie Community Centre open

1998: CAMH formed from merger of Queen Street Mental Health Centre, Clarke Institute of Psychiatry, Addiction Research Foundation, and Donwood Institute

1974: Inpatient Treatment Units 3 and 4 open

2004: The Ministry of Health approves CAMH's updated Functional Program and campus redevelopment plan

2015: College Street CAMH campus threatened with demolition to construct four 40-level condo towers on same site

CAMH adjacent neighborhood gentrification accelerates

2000

2015

Street across from the University of Toronto's main campus; the Addiction Research Foundation; and the Donwood Institute. The board elected to remain at the Queen Street West site while maintaining day-to-day operations there. Shortly thereafter, the CAMH board of directors announced its intent to reconfigure its operations, retaining the Queen Street West campus of the 'hub' of an in-place reinvention. This history is visually represented in Figure 4.13 as a chronology of events having occurred across four major periods: 1850–1899, 1900–1949, 1950–1999, and 2000–2015.

The approved redevelopment plan for CAMH

The formally approved CAMH Vision and Master Plan of 2001 set the stage for how the campus would be transformed. Based on the outcome of an international design competition, the C3 Consortium was selected to guide this process. This selected team consisted of Montgomery/Sisam Architects, Kuwabara Payne McKenna Blumberg Architects (now KPMB), and Kearns Mancini Architects. In 2002 CAMH received approval from the Ontario Ministry of Health and Long-Term Care for the C3 Consortium's master plan and in 2004 the ministry granted final approval for CAMH's 'Functional Program' for the future. An *urban village* was to be created through the fusion of CAMH and non-CAMH land uses by way of a number of public-private mixed-use buildings, and new public city streets extended into the campus. That same year the chosen architectural/engineering (A/E) team received awards from the Canadian Institute of Planners as well as the Ontario Professional Planners Institute for its CAMH work. In 2005, CAMH and the firm Urban Strategies received a City of Toronto Architecture and Urban Design Award (Honorable Mention), and the province announced approval and funding for Phase 1A of a four-phase redevelopment project. At the time, there were 485 beds on campus and this number was to remain about the same when all four project phases are complete in 2020.

The four phases were as follows:

Phase 1A – By the spring of 2008, the first four buildings were complete and occupied. Montgomery/Sisam, the lead architectural design firm, stated in 2015 its overarching goal was to 'dematerialize the concept of a big hospital'.[52] These new buildings were Buildings E1, E2, E3, and E4, all identical in appearance. One housed outpatient addictive disorder programs, another housed 24 patients in treatment for addictive disorders. This program had been relocated from the Donwood Campus (located in a residential neighborhood north of Eglinton Avenue East). Another housed patients undergoing treatment for mood and anxiety disorders. These four-level buildings were residential-like, not unlike college dormitories. Each floor housed six private bedrooms with a private bath/shower, a living room, dining room, courtyard gardens at street level, and a bay window at the end of each corridor with an L-shaped window seat.

Phase 1B – In 2009, following a request for proposals, the first non-CAMH building was built by a private developer; it was a mixed-use building with market-rate housing and street-level retail.[53] In 2010, the 1956 Administration Building was demolished, clearing way for Phase 1B and subsequent construction phases. A street naming contest was held at this time to name the five new city streets to be built. By 2012, all three new Phase 1B structures were occupied and the CAMH Foundation announced it had raised US$108 million from the private sector for its Transforming Lives capital campaign. The new buildings housed patient services, including a geriatric mental health unit of 28 beds, consisting of 20 private rooms and 4 semi-private rooms, plus an adolescent treatment unit of 12 beds (all private rooms), for an age cohort somewhat more acute than in the past.[54] New street-level retail included a full-service pharmacy, and an auditorium for community outreach programming.

Phase 1C – In 2011 the Ministry of Health and Long-Term Care approved funding for Phase 1C of the CAMH campus redevelopment plan. This consisted of two additional new buildings – a non-CAMH building fronting Queen Street West housing retail at street level, with market-rate housing units above (C1), and a CAMH-use-only building of eight levels of outpatient services, administrative spaces, and the family support program, situated directly above street-level retail (C2). Parking is provided beneath these two structures. The architects' goal, as in Phase 1B, was to establish maximum transparency at street level with CAMH functions occupying upper floors. The neighborhood by this time experienced rapid gentrification with many longtime property owners and renters having been pushed out due to skyrocketing land values.[55]

Phase 1D – The major construction in Phase 1D will house the Acute Care Inpatient Treatment Unit (120 beds) plus 10 specialized diagnostic units, on five levels, with street-level retail. In this building, each inpatient unit will have a double-loaded corridor in a racetrack configuration, and a small, open-air balcony with a 12-foot glass perimeter wall. This building, or Block H, will house the partial hospitalization program for 'borderline' patients who may episodically require 24/7 care. The small balconies, combined with the absence of a street-level courtyard, or roof terraces on the upper levels, are key features. When this phase is complete all of the 1974 structures will have been demolished. The CAMH emergency and trauma care unit will be relocated from its current College Street site to the lower level of this block building and accessed via a driveway connecting to the existing below-ground parking deck.

An alternative proposal for reinvention

Documenting the history of CAMH and its neighborhood is a fascinating opportunity in and of itself; so much has occurred there over the past 165 years. Successive waves of urban growth, decline, and rebirth have visibly impacted the 27-acre CAMH campus. The tracing of this historical trajectory can be represented as six distinct periods, or intervals, of development. Base maps were subsequently developed (by the author) in an effort to capture major changes that have occurred on the CAMH campus and its surrounding neighborhoods from 1860 to the present – and projected to 2020. For each interval, a series of six base maps are presented documenting the status of the campus and its urban context. These intervals represent the years 1860 (1), 1900 (2), 1960 (3), 2000 (4), 2015 (5), and 2020 (6). This information is presented as an urban morphology of CAMH since 1860 (see Appendix). The base maps address these six themes:

1 Figure-ground relationships
2 Land use patterns
3 Landscape amenities
4 Landmarks and anomalies
5 Sound/circulation patterns
6 Transportation amenities

Collectively, the 36 base maps (six urban analyses, each over six time intervals) and their accompanying narratives in the Appendix make a compelling case. Sadly, the formally approved campus redevelopment plan for 2020 obliterates more than 80% of the remaining open green space, and by the end of Phase 1D in 2020 new construction at CAMH will have totaled nearly 2 million square feet. As for its creators' urban village concept, the quality of the outcome will be mixed, at best. Overdevelopment is problematic on many levels and especially the superimposition of an urban street grid onto a once-pastoral campus. To this end, a series of five photomontages are presented with the aim of further communicating the current vibrancy, diversity, and eclecticism of this part of Toronto. The immediate area is a rich mosaic of small commercial businesses, semidetached townhouses, repurposed industrial lofts, condo towers, and CAMH (Figure 4.14a–b through Figure 4.18a–b).

In the formally approved redevelopment plan, a number of inconvenient truths will quite likely have been revealed. In response, the following discussion presents an alternative vision for the redevelopment of CAMH. This vision for reinvention is called the 'Alternative Proposal for CAMH in Toronto', or APT. For one, most of its attractive grounds and places for respite and quiet contemplation will have been lost (Figure 4.19). To the patient, CAMH will have become nearly invisible although, paradoxically, this was a main design objective of the master plan and architectural team. The net outcome will very likely be disorienting. That is, many individuals with mental health and substance addiction disorders will have difficulty in wayfinding, and become disoriented. If the building she or he needs to get to for, say, an 11:00 a.m. appointment is difficult to find, it renders the urban journey to and from all that much more challenging. Beyond this, the entries and lobbies of the two already-built new structures are rather unwelcoming and corporate-like. The first impression of having arrived at an office building will be surreal for many. Lacking a sense of having arrived where one needs to go, especially in a mental health and addictive disorder treatment facility, is needlessly stressful. The APT acknowledges the reality that approximately 50% of this plan has already been implemented (2018). These new buildings, because they

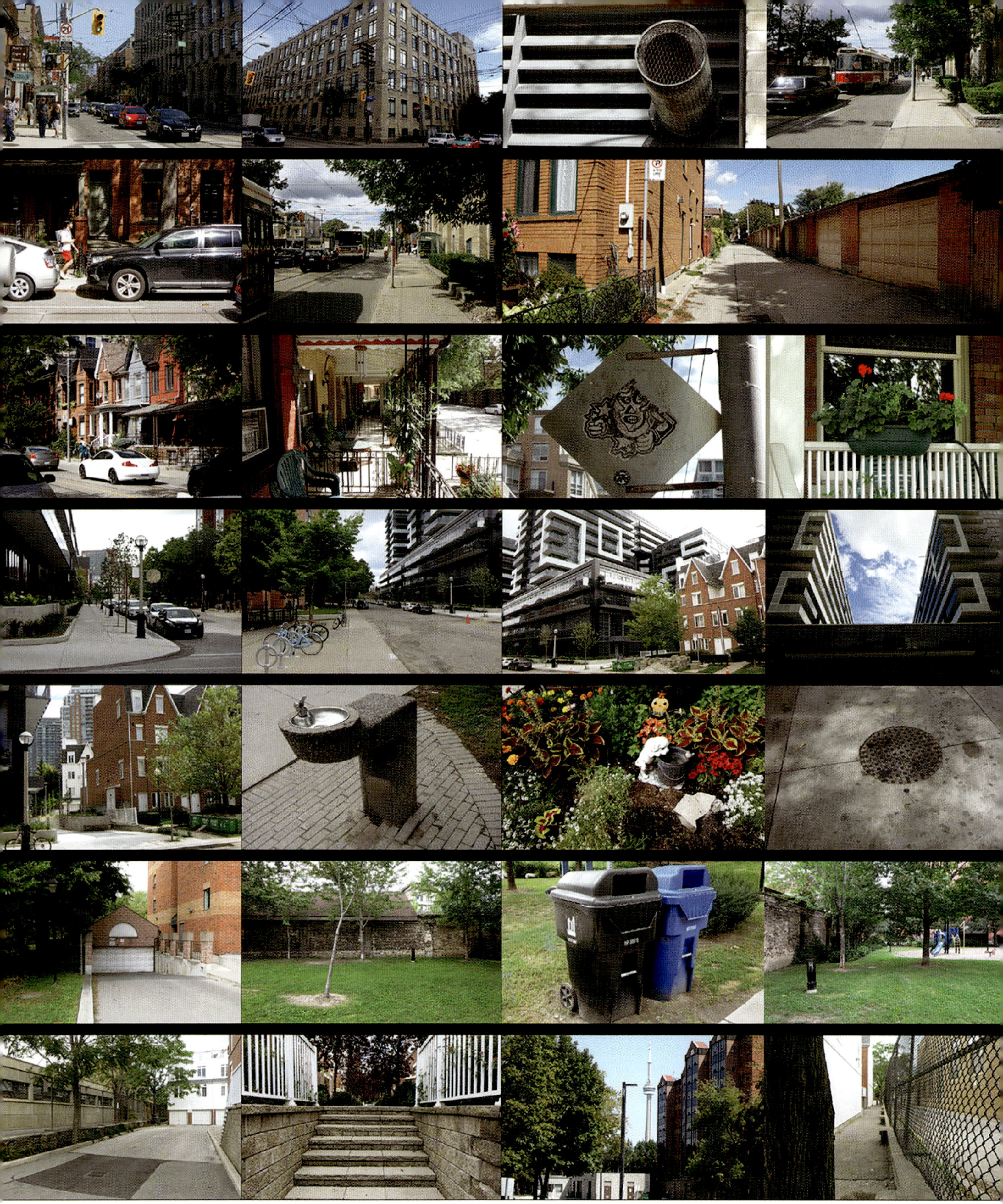

4.14a–b CAMH urban fabric analysis 1.

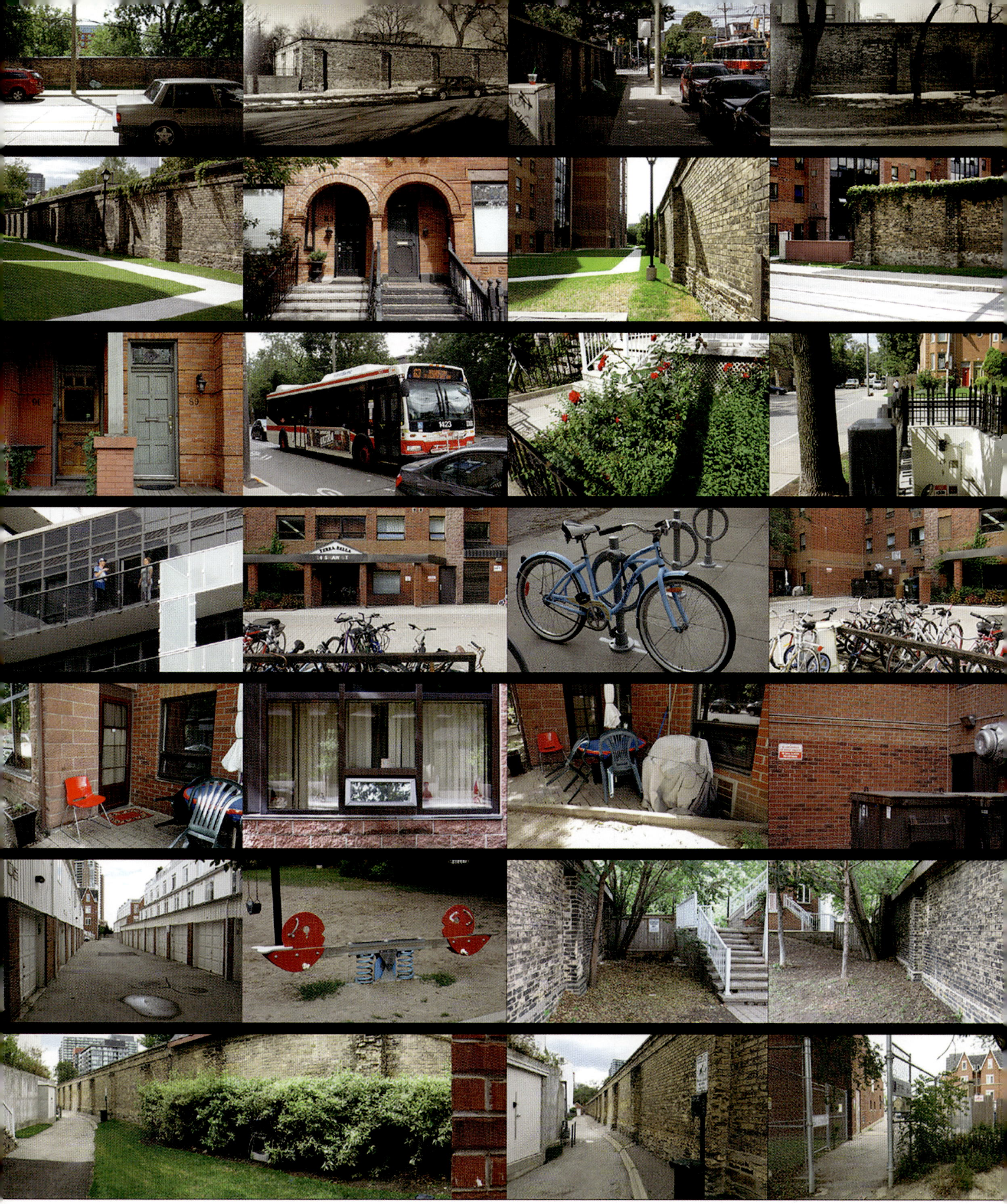

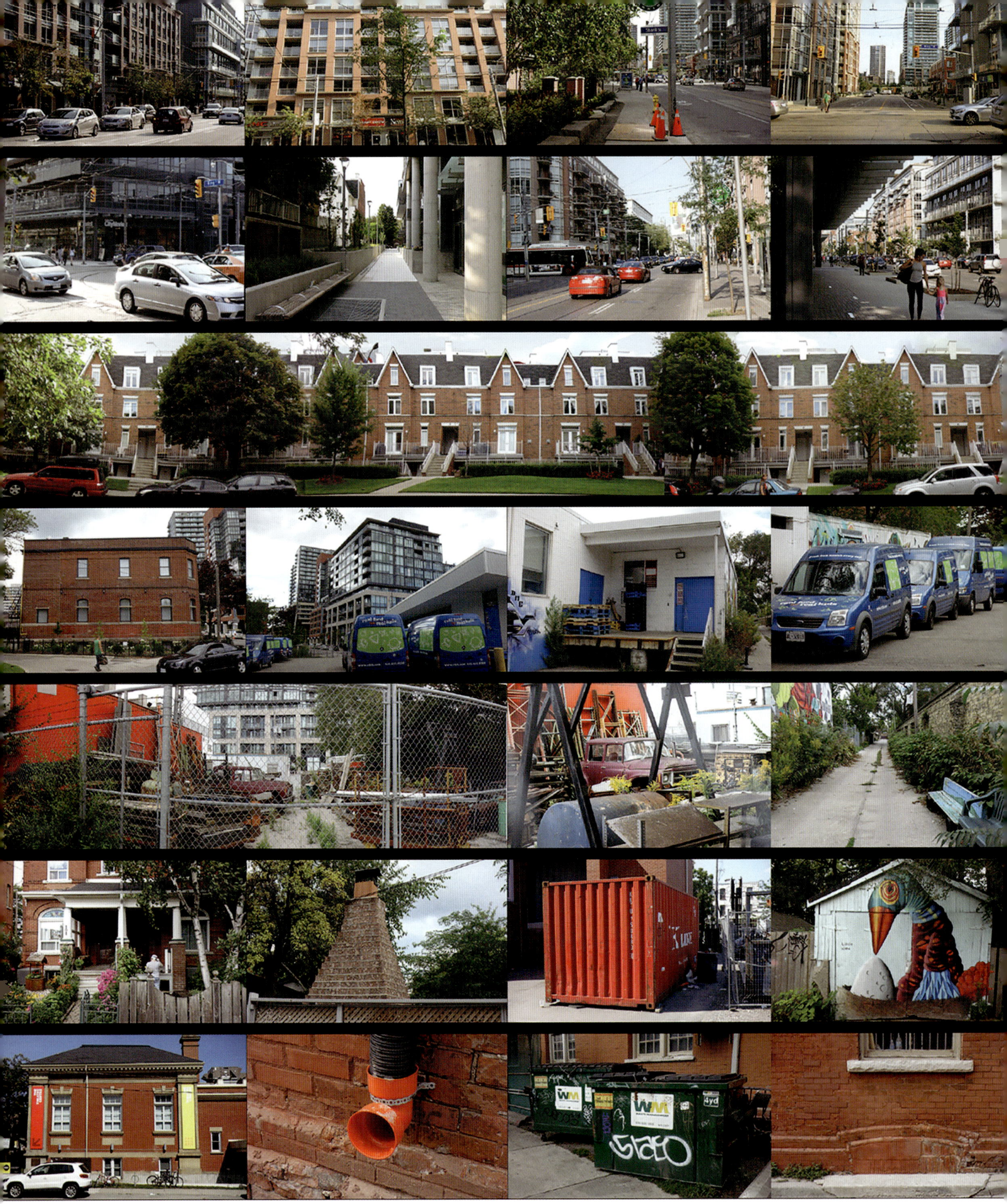

4.15a–b CAMH urban fabric analysis 2.

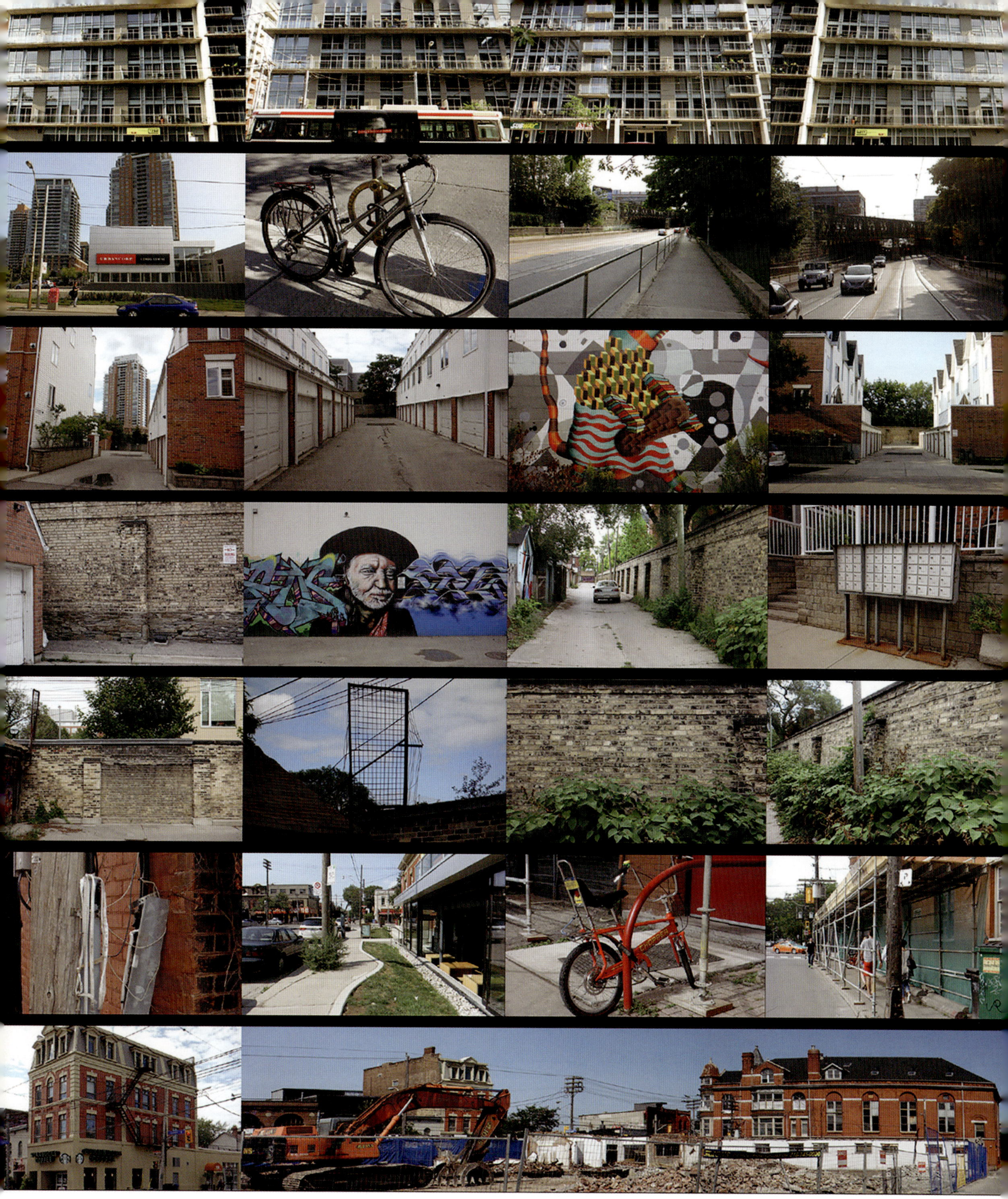

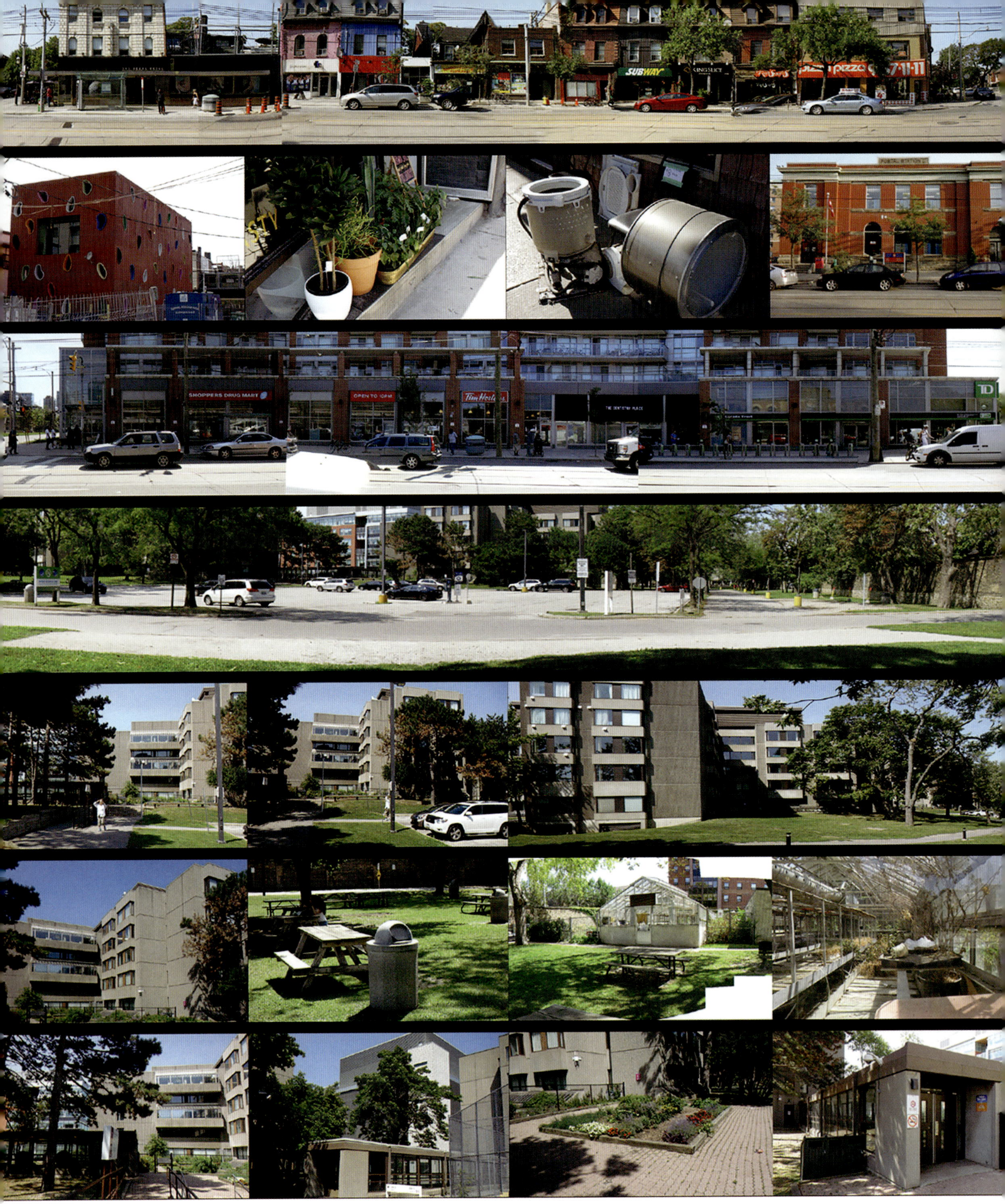

4.16a–b CAMH urban fabric analysis 3.

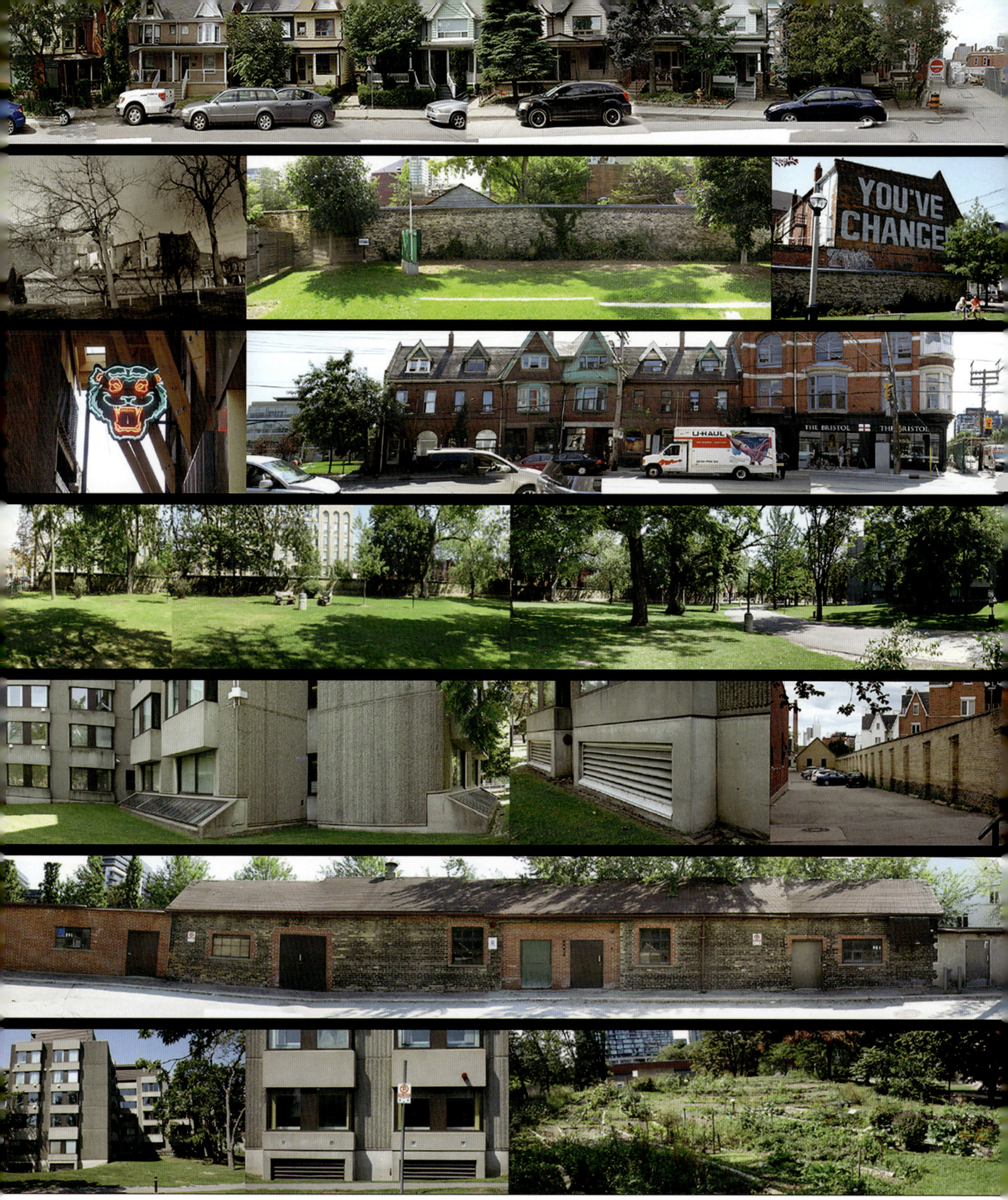
YOU'VE
CHANGE
U-HAUL
THE BRISTOL
THE BRISTOL

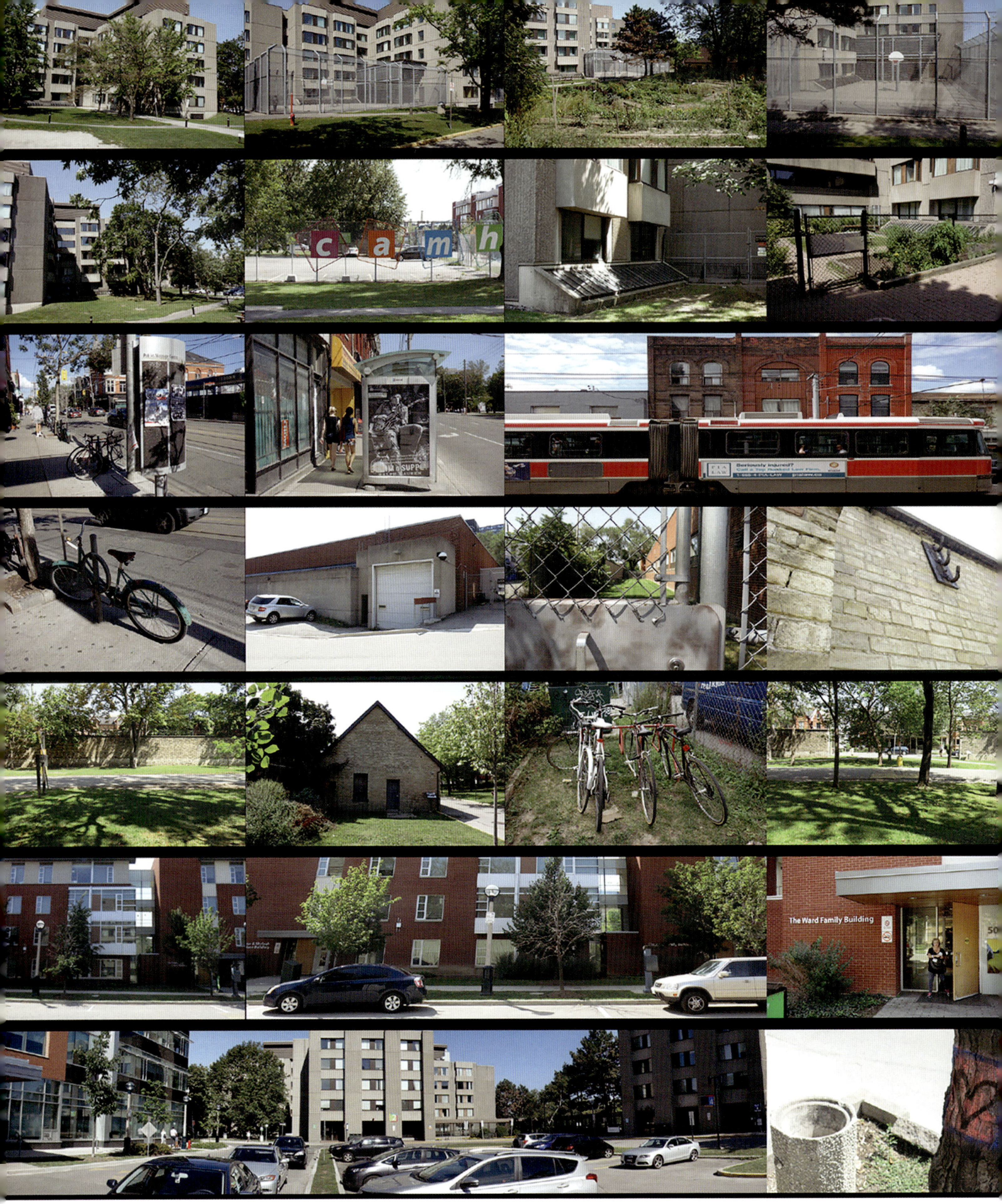

4.17a–b CAMH urban fabric analysis 4.

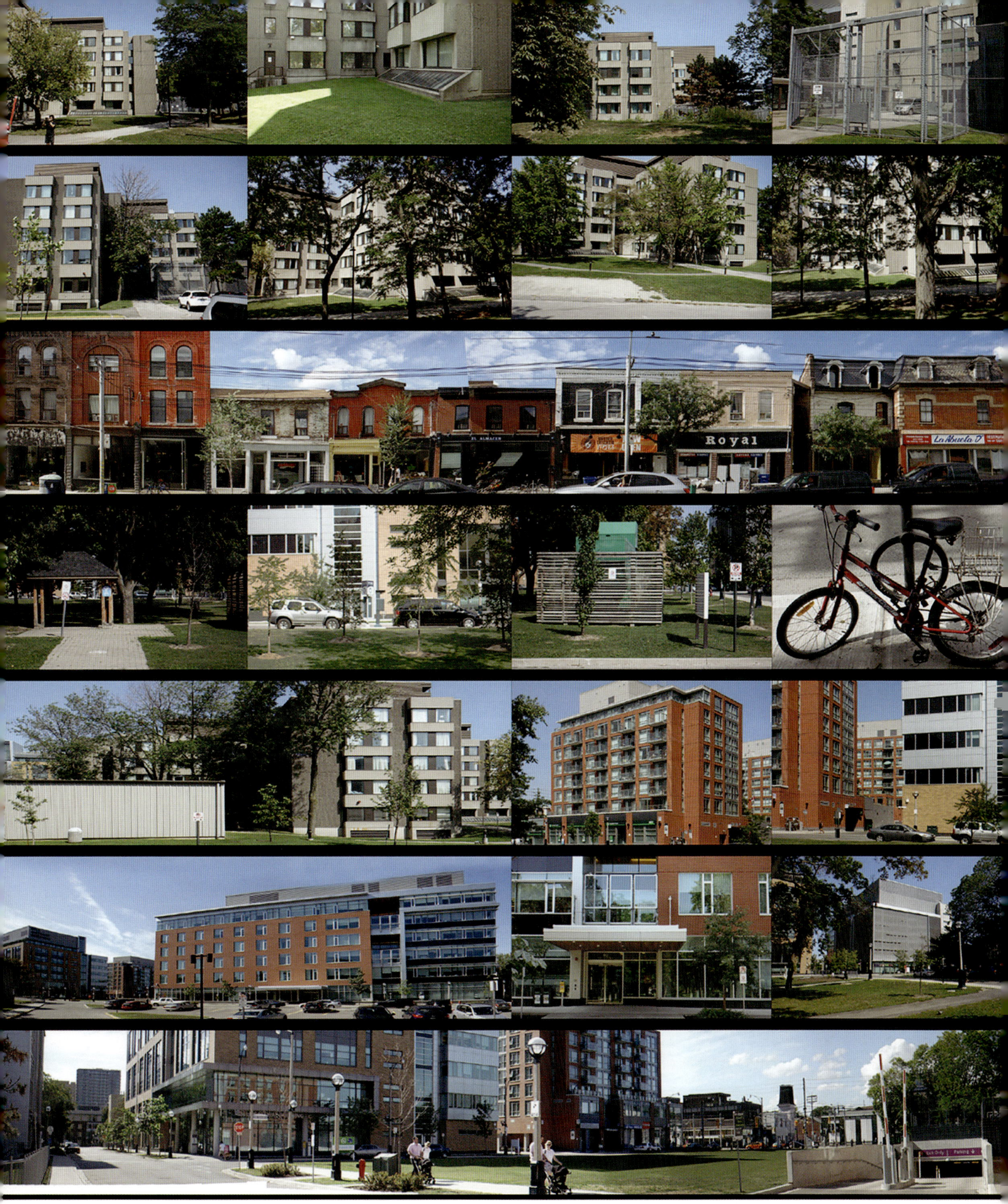
Royal

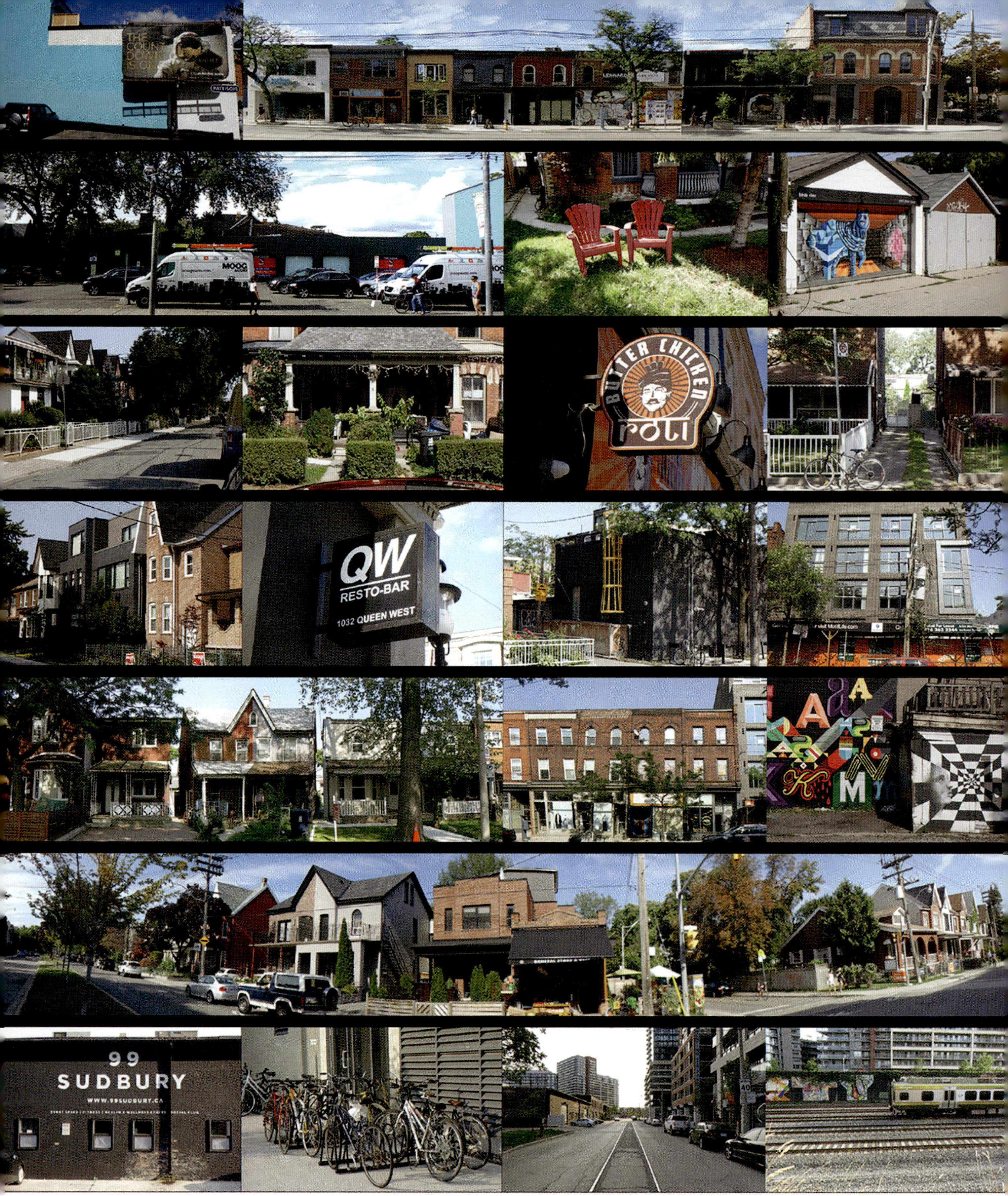

4.18a–b CAMH urban fabric analysis 5.

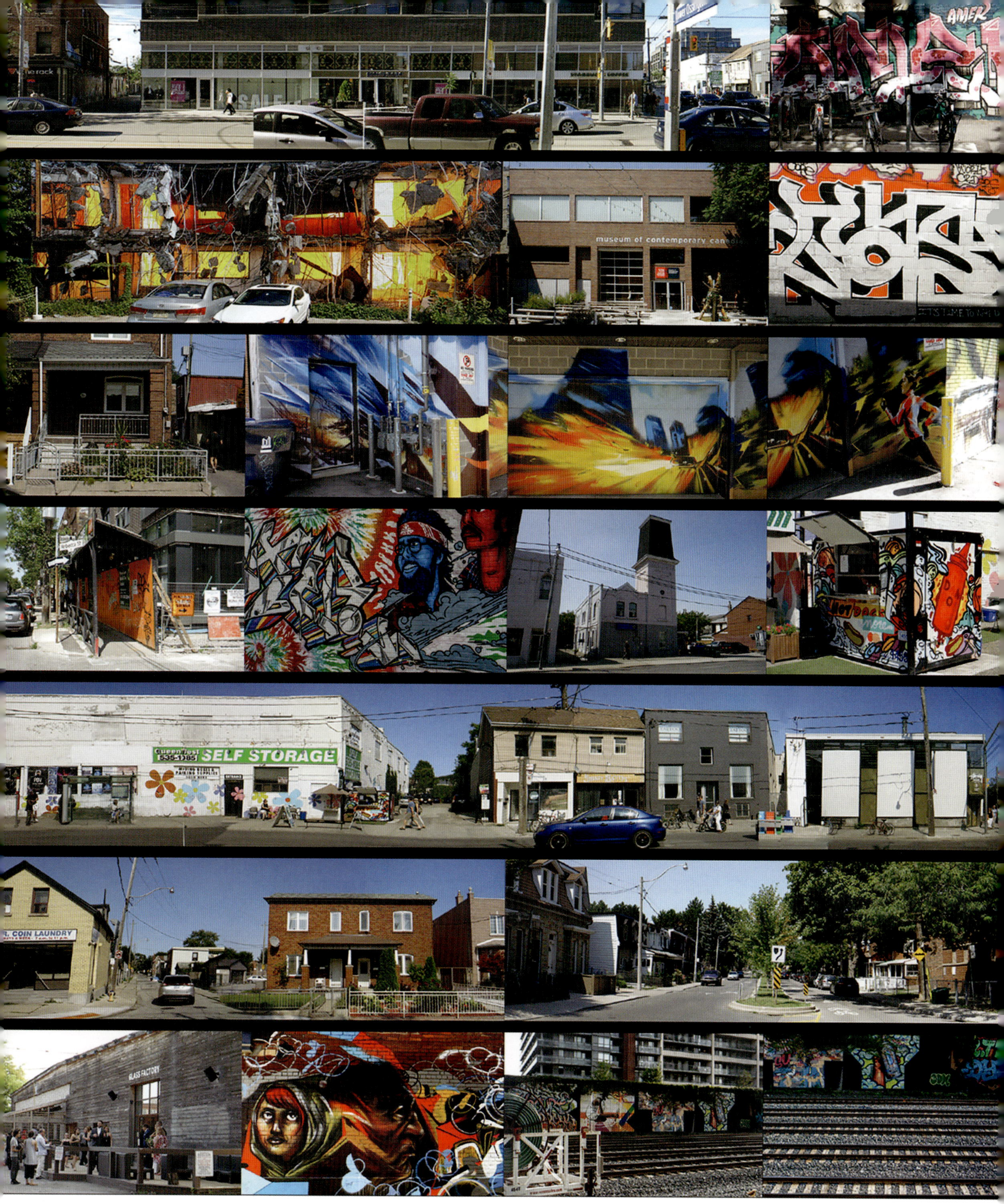
AMER
museum of contemporary canada
SELF STORAGE
COIN LAUNDRY
GLASS FACTORY

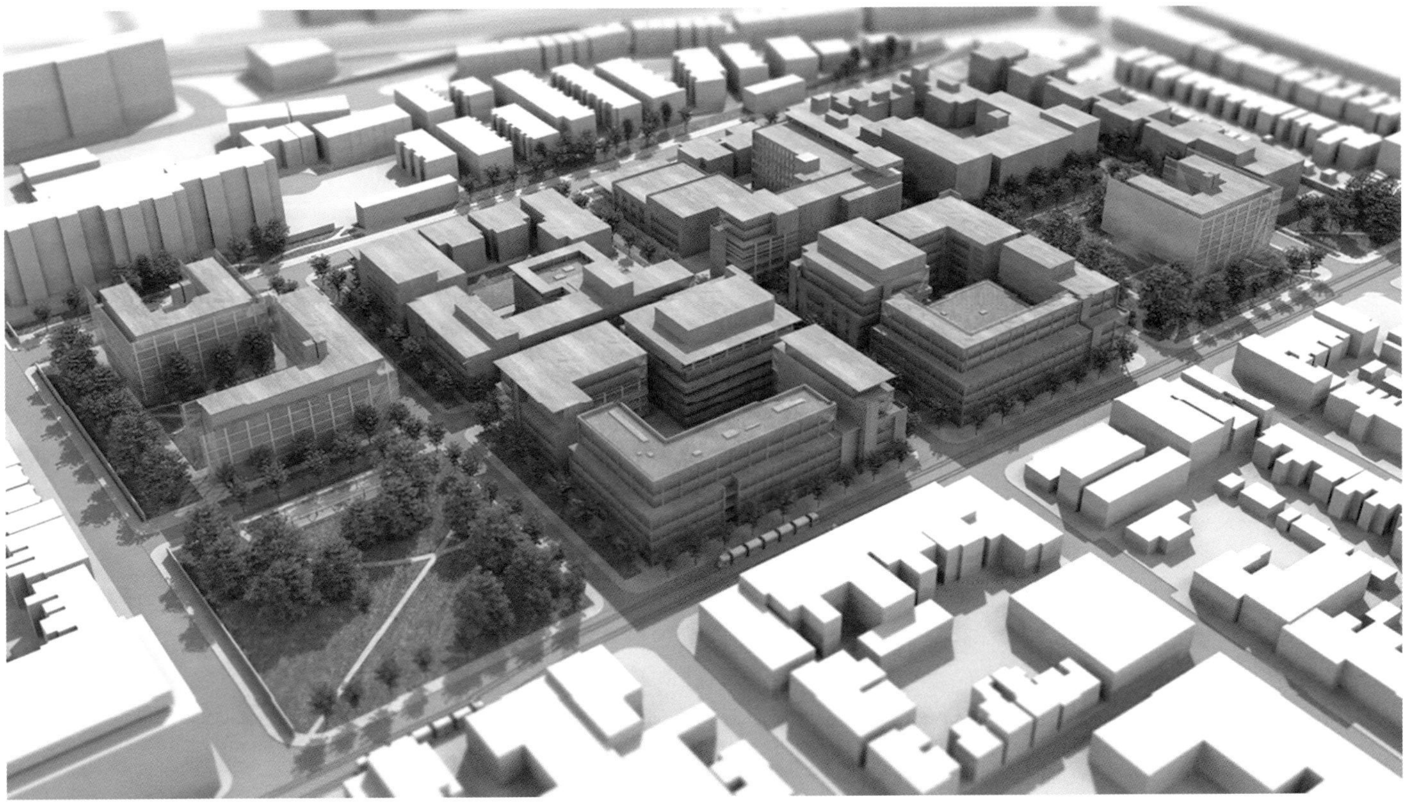

4.19 Rendering of approved redevelopment plan for CAMH, 2007.

already exist, are therefore woven into the APT. The APT functions as a narrative and its fundamentals are expressed within the structure as same as the compendium of planning and design considerations presented in the following chapter (Chapter 5).

1. *Site, context, and sustainability*

The formal, approved CAMH redevelopment plan leaves something to be desired in terms of creating a genuinely salutogenic, health-promoting environment. Too large a percentage of the remaining open space on the campus will have been lost, paved over, or replaced by generic mixed-use 'block buildings'. Meanwhile, psychiatric treatment philosophies, psychiatric care provider organizations, public health agencies, and patients' rights advocates are recognizing the value of proactive engagement with nature/landscape. This is impossible to retain, let alone sustain, if the therapeutic functions of nature/landscape are minimized or, worse, obliterated. Professional caregiver teams will thus have less space of this type to work with, therapeutically, on a daily basis, in caring for their patients. The APT retains two large remaining open parcels of land fronting Queen Street West. This set-aside measure is of necessity, in direct reaction to the overpowering presence of the recent (2012) addition of the Bell Gateway block building and a second, large block building currently planned for the other open space fronting Queen Street West (immediately to the west of the 2012 building). In addition, the remaining fragments of the 19th-century masonry asylum wall would be retained (vs. demolished, as planned). Next, the city street grid currently planned to inanely cut through the CAMH campus – dissecting it into nine squares of roughly equal size – should be immediately canceled. The two new city 'streets' already built and operational are more than enough, and therefore the APT calls for no additional new city streets to senselessly carve up the historic CAMH campus.

Two new inpatient pavilions are proposed in the APT, to be built on opposing corner infill sites at the back side of the campus (Figure 4.20). These are the Residence West and Residence East buildings, each six levels in height and each able to be expanded in height by three additional floors in the future. The bed capacity in each tower upon initial construction is 80 beds, and expandable with an additional 64 beds. The intent is to carefully insert each structure into the existing ensemble without further disrupting the front side of the campus or any existing exterior green spaces. Pathways and green spaces are created around these new pavilions, made possible largely due to raising – lifting – the entire structure up from the ground plane. The aim is to transform otherwise *lost* green space into an urban oasis for the benefit of both CAMH and the surrounding neighborhood, not unlike the grounds at Ontario Shores, in nearby Whitby (see Chapter 2). A microfarm, new gardening plots, and ground-level recreational activity spaces are created as a result, amenities otherwise not present in the formal, approved CAMH campus redevelopment plan (Figure 4.21a–c). The preservation of what remains of the landscaped grounds and outdoor activity spaces is of high priority in the APT, because this was a major point of contention at the heart of the local neighborhood's opposition to the approved CAMH redevelopment plan (see Figure 4.22 and Figure 4.23).

2. *Arrival, public, and semipublic spaces*

The four 1974 inpatient units and the existing community center are to be retained, repurposed, and linked by the existing continuous street-level circulation spine, and also at below-street level, by the existing corresponding tunnel system. At grade, this element is highly transparent with full-height windows spanning the entire length; it is therefore highly feasible to retain these current amenities. The campus's central power plant is also to be retained and renovated. Two new inpatient pavilions are connected to this existing network at the street level and also below ground. As mentioned, the four 1974 units are to be repurposed for use as counseling, programmed group therapy, and staff support functions and are linked, physically, to the new arrival lobbies and vertical circulation cores of the two new residential structures. The arrival/circulation element of each pavilion features externally mounted horizontal louvers and a vegetated greenwall. The 1974 community center is retained and renovated – preserved with its atrium and soaring ceiling, clerestories, interior cantilevered perches, and the swimming pool. A new campus-wide directional wayfinding system will integrate the repurposed 1970s buildings with new

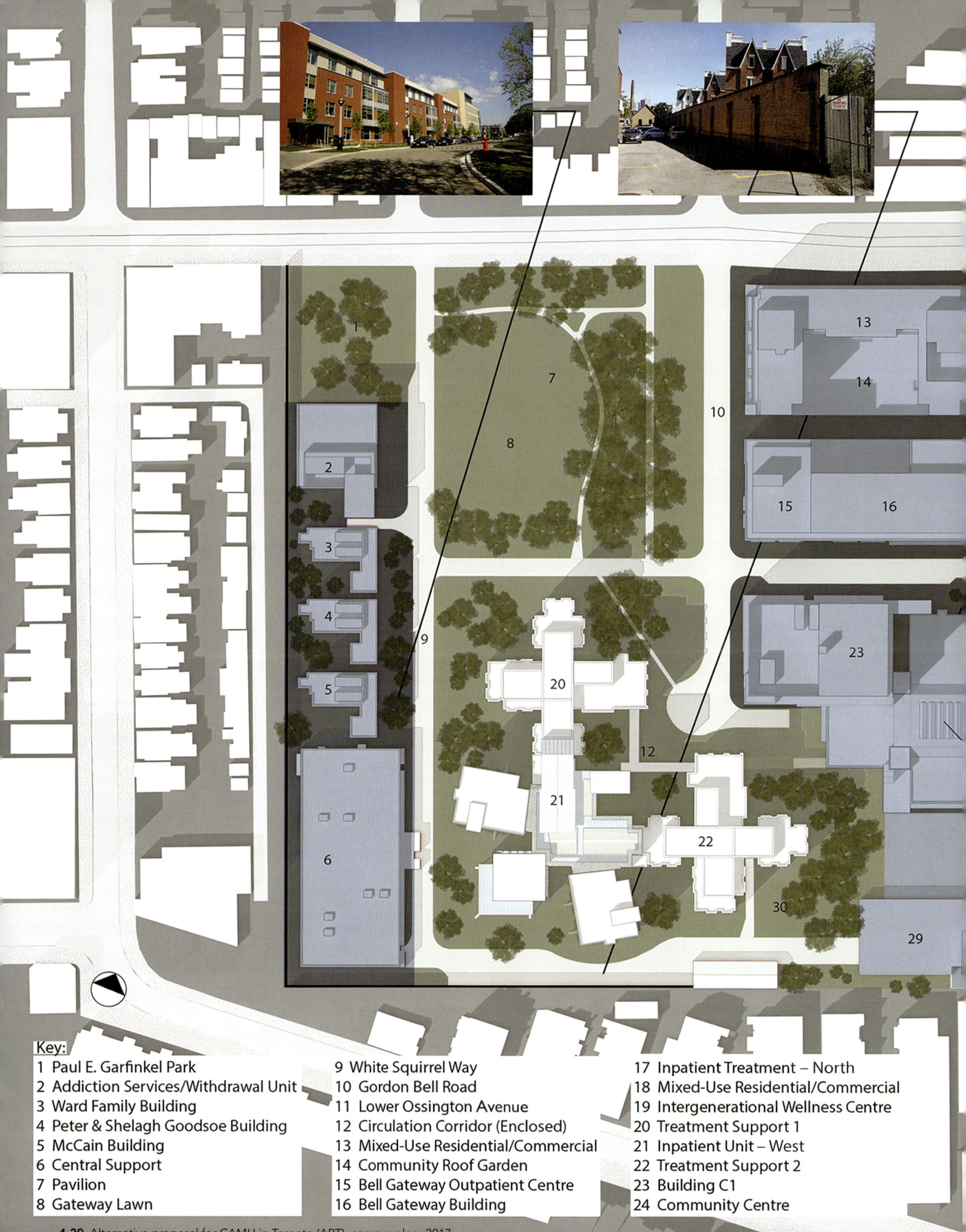

4.20 Alternative proposal for CAMH in Toronto (APT), campus plan, 2017.

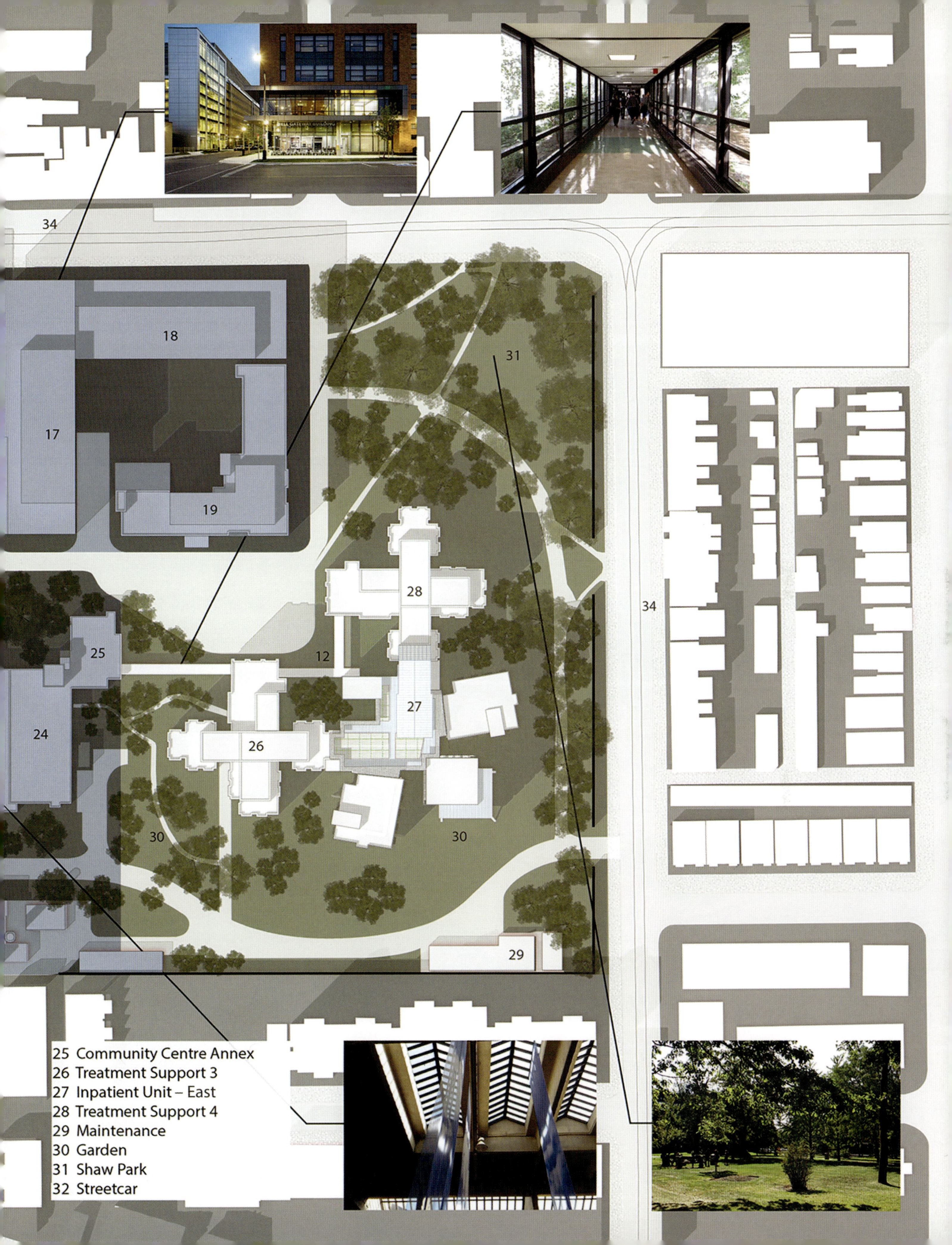
34
18
17
19
31
28
34
25
12
27
24
26
30
30
29
25 Community Centre Annex
26 Treatment Support 3
27 Inpatient Unit – East
28 Treatment Support 4
29 Maintenance
30 Garden
31 Shaw Park
32 Streetcar

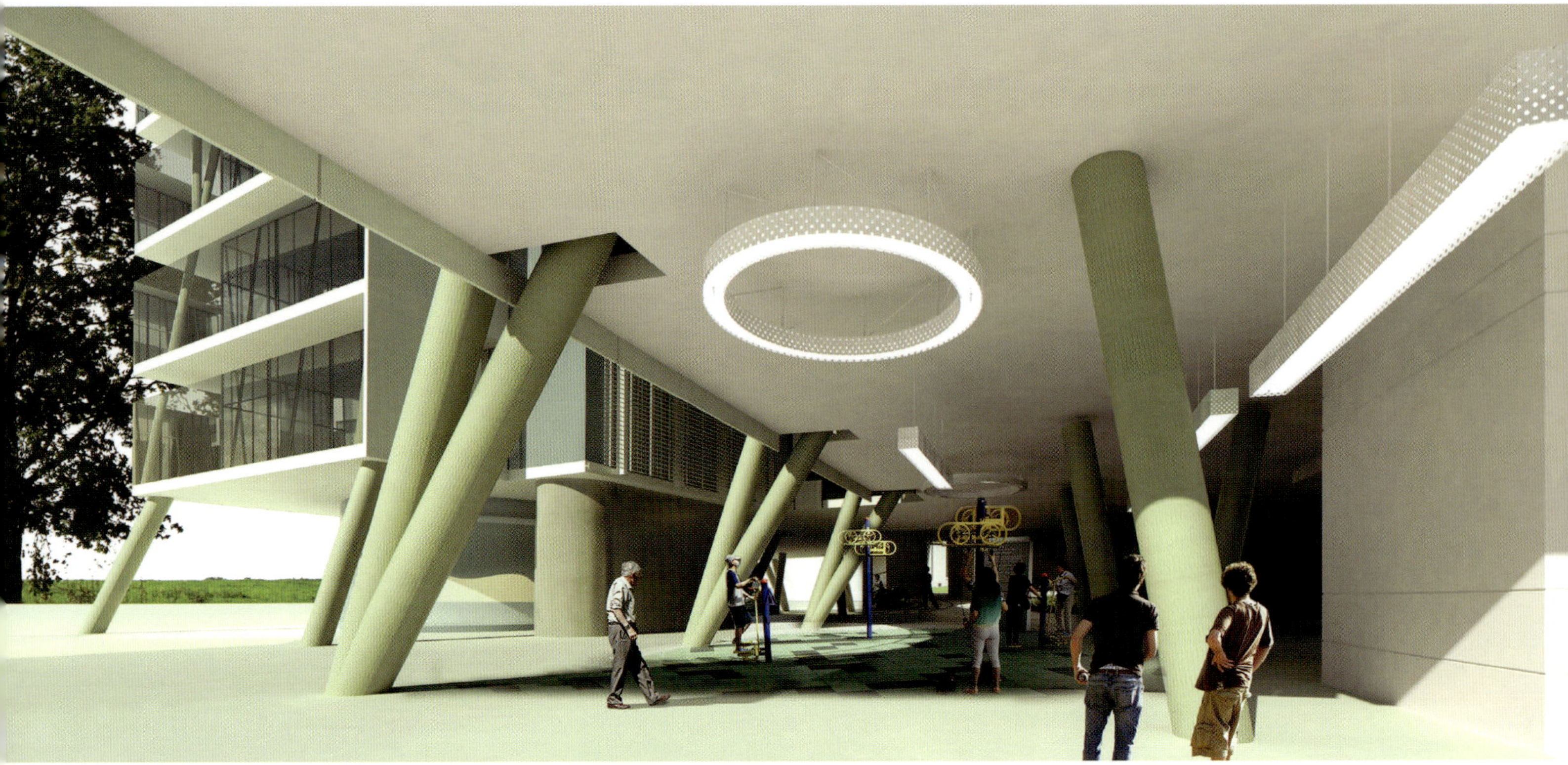

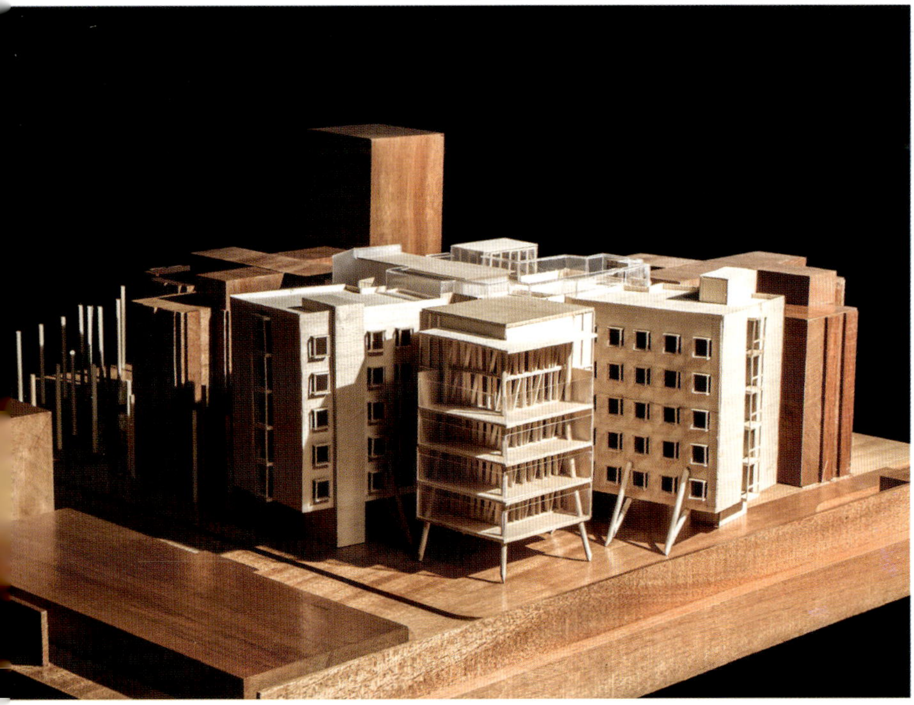

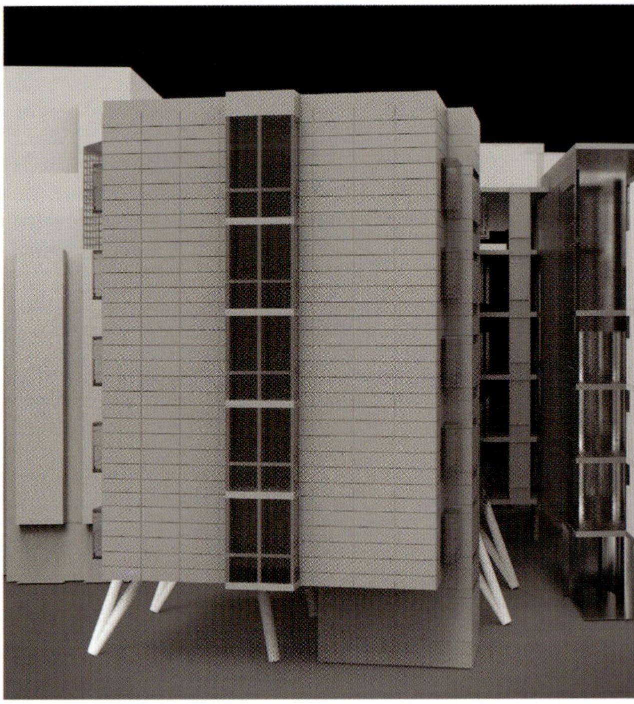

4.21a–c APT, 2017, ground-level view of sheltered activity space beneath one of two new residential towers (top) and an exterior view of one tower (bottom). Architect: Stephen Verderber.

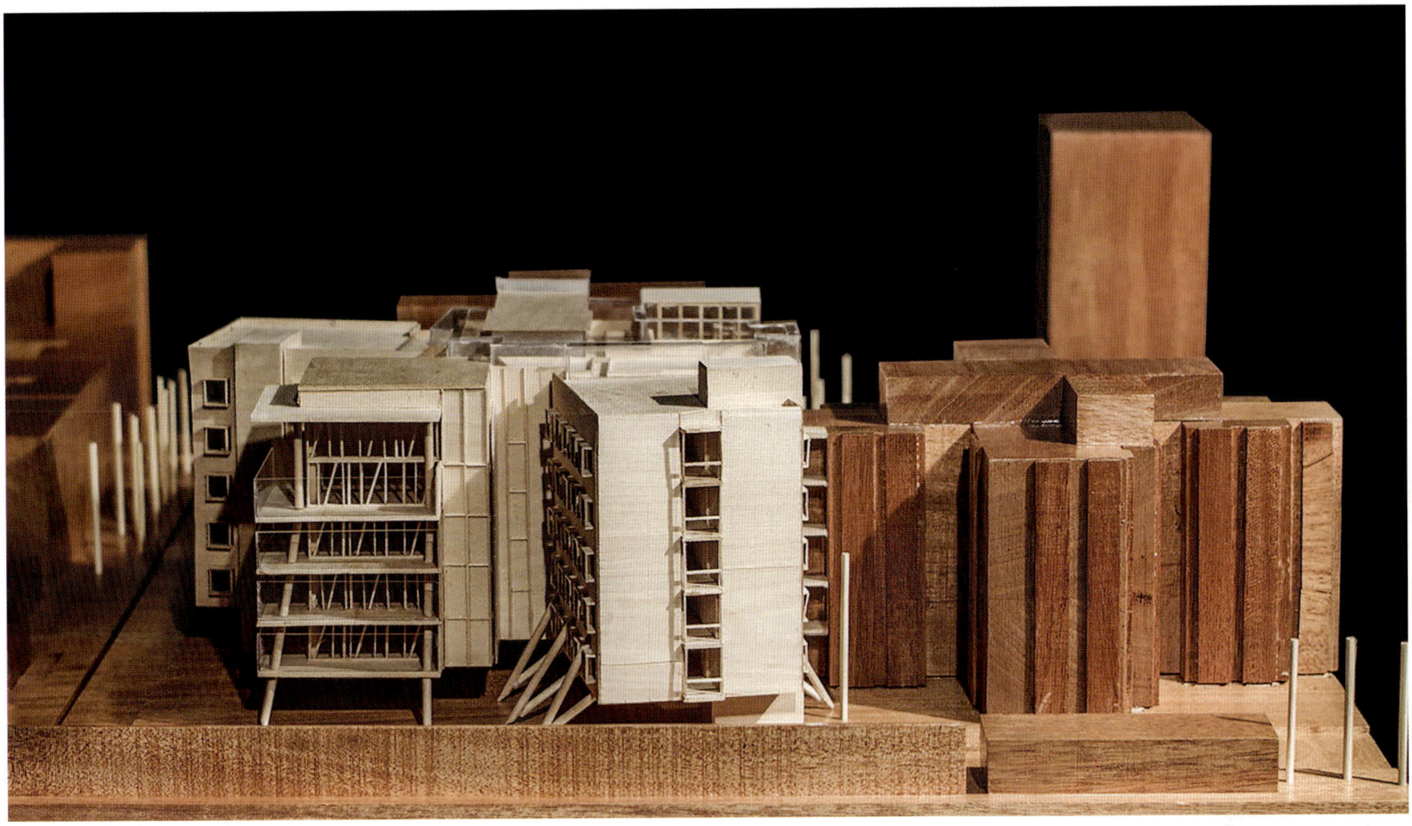

4.22 APT, new residential tower (east), model photo, 2017. Architect: Stephen Verderber.

construction in a seamless blend of 'old' with new, with the aim of establishing a series of welcoming, aesthetically rethought arrival spaces (Figure 4.22 and Figure 4.23).

3. *The inpatient care unit (PCU)*

The two proposed residential towers occupy prominent corner sites, at the rear of the campus, in the APT, their configuration and appearance informed by the concept of patients' graduated territoriality, as this corresponds to a gradual increase in an individual's freedom of choice and spatial movement in terms of independent circulation about the campus (see Chapter 5). The restrictive footprints of these two infill sites resulted in the decision to elevate them above the ground plane by means of diagonalized structural columns, or *legs*, as this results in a far higher degree of horizontal connectivity with the adjacent open landscaped spaces. The added exterior space this strategy yields beneath each tower supports diverse programmed activities, from counseling, lectures, and concerts, to a weekly farmer's market (Figure 4.21a–c). Seating areas and small plots for gardening are provided, as is a water-wall. A circular, multipurpose event space supports programmed CAMH activities and is also available for use by the local community (Figure 4.24a–e).

Patient rooms – The residential units on floors 2–5 each house 16 beds in two clusters of eight bedrooms. All patient rooms are private with a private, wheelchair-accessible bath/shower. Each features hardwood floors, color-accented walls, and a recessed ceiling grid, allowing for varied visual atmospheric effects achievable vis-à-vis fiber optic technology. A panelized headwall and a window seat are provided with a private built-in reading light. A window in the seating niche element is operable. The dual doors to the patient room are double leafed in a major/minor configuration – with the major door allowing access from either side, and the second, or minor, door allowing staff access to the bedroom in the event of an emergency. A wood desk, bed, side table, and built-in closet are also provided.

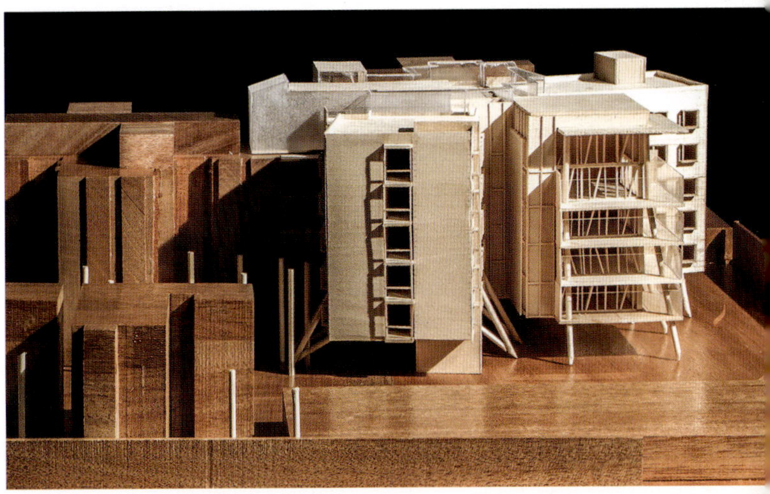

4.23 APT, new residential tower (west), model photo, 2017. Architect: Stephen Verderber.

4.24a–e APT, exterior view of extruded 'rehabilitating' legs of the n residential towers, ground-level plan of one new residential tower (le inpatient units levels 2–5 (plan), view of dayroom terraces with prot tive security barrier, and horticultural therapy roofscape (right), 201

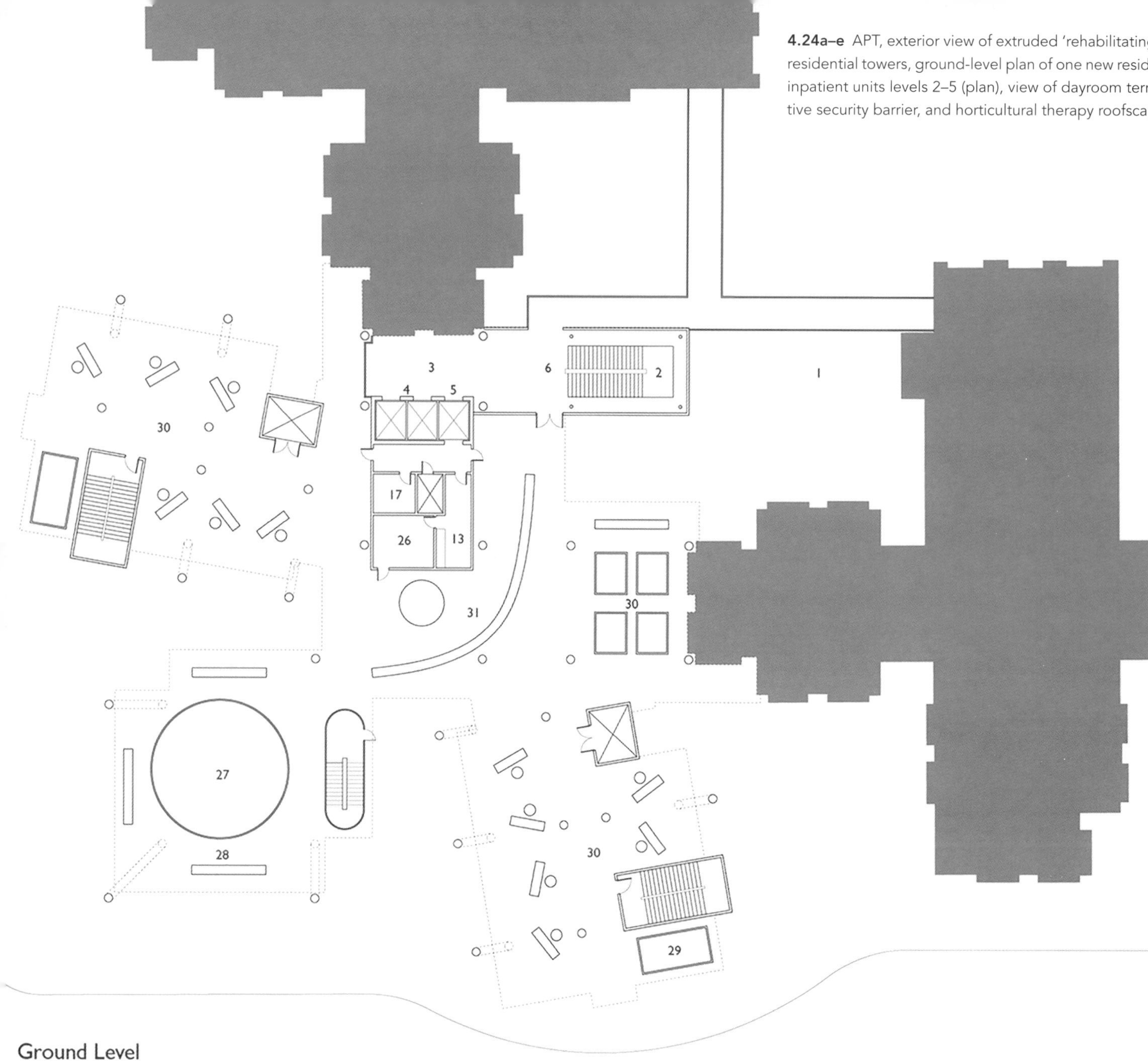

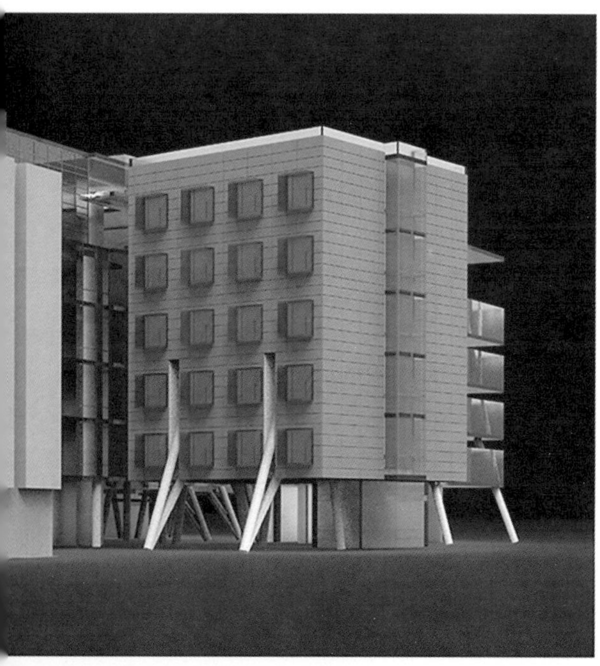

Key

1 Lawn (existing)
2 West stair tower
3 Foyer
4 Elevators 1–2
5 Elevators 3 (staff priority)
6 Inner lobby
7 Staff restroom
8 Staff breakroom/kitchen
9 Staff corridor
10 Nursing/observation
11 Storage
12 Flex office
13 Nursing support
14 Workstation
15 Unit coordinator
16 Seclusion
17 Restroom
18 Clean/soiled linens
19 Dining
20 Mechanical
21 Dayroom
23 Group counseling
24 Exterior terrace
25 Media wall
26 Comfort room
27 Multipurpose pavilion
28 Seating
29 Garden
30 Multipurpose (exterior)
31 Waterwall
32 Winter garden

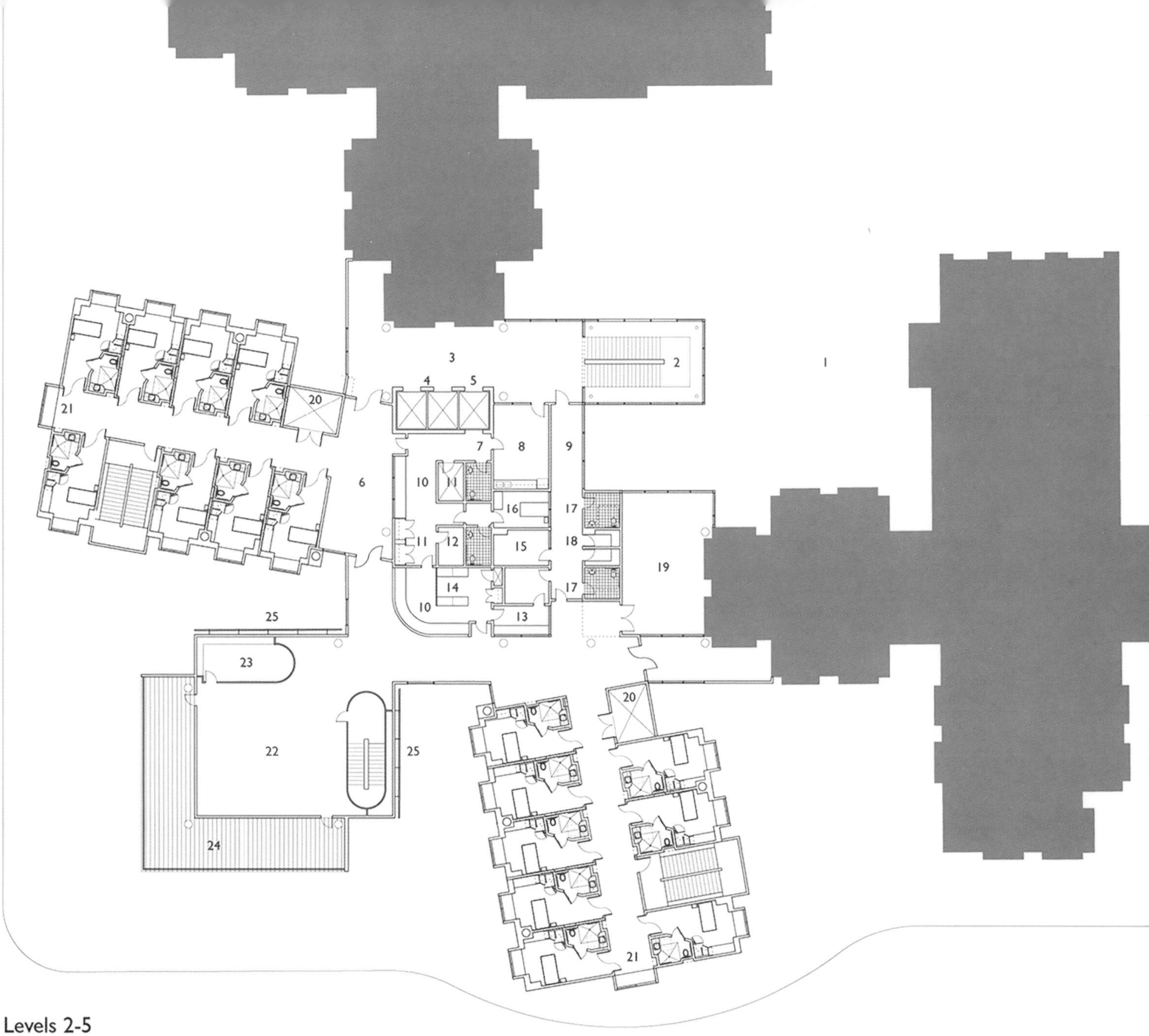

Levels 2-5

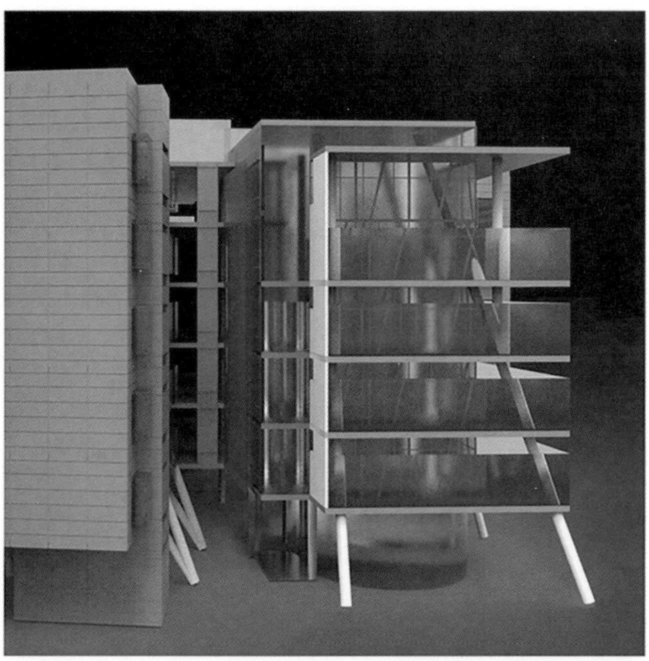

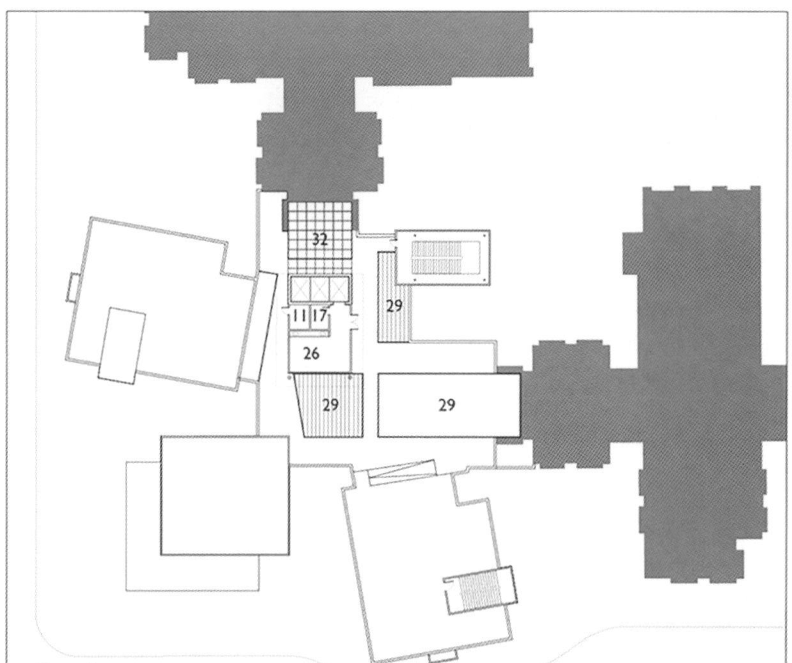

Roofscape

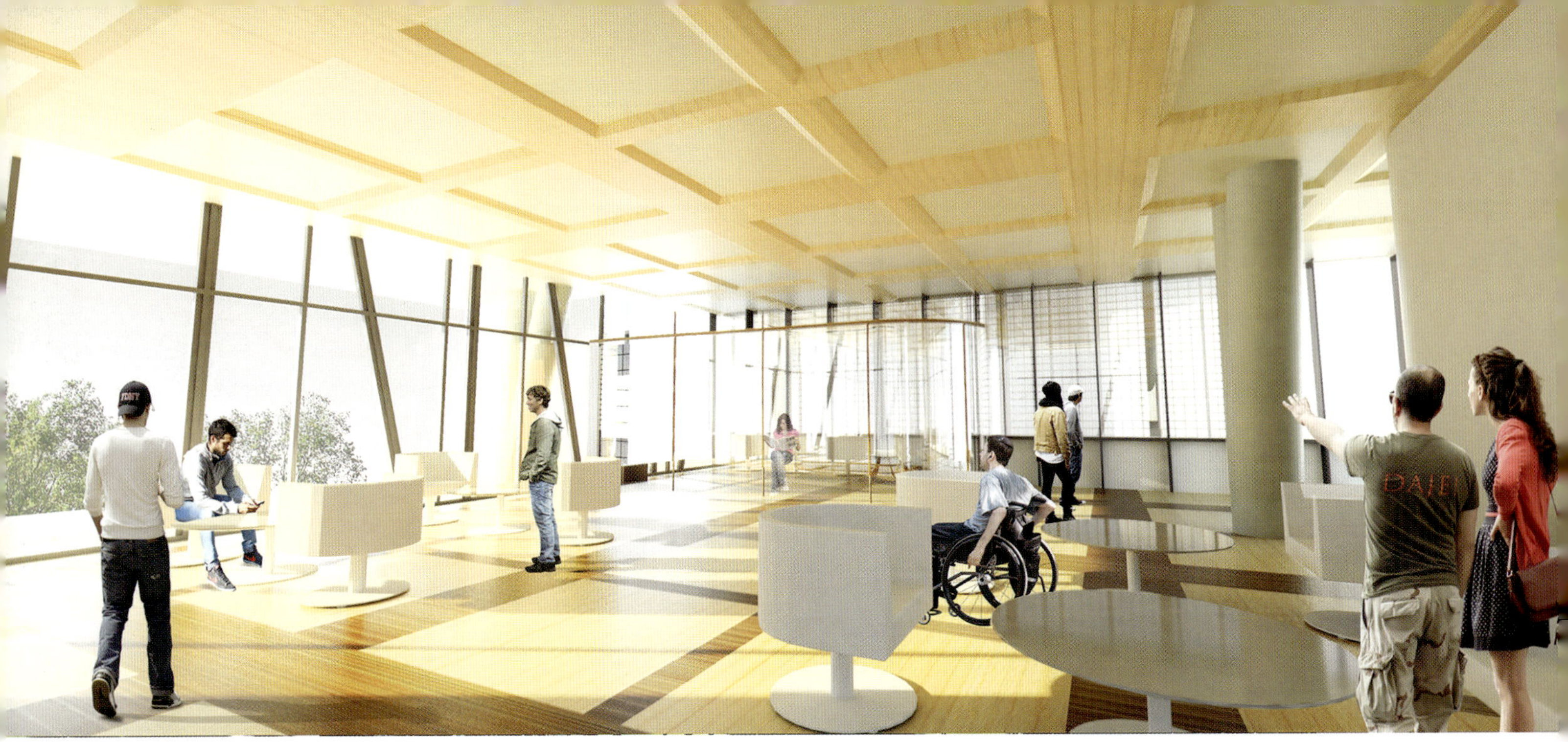

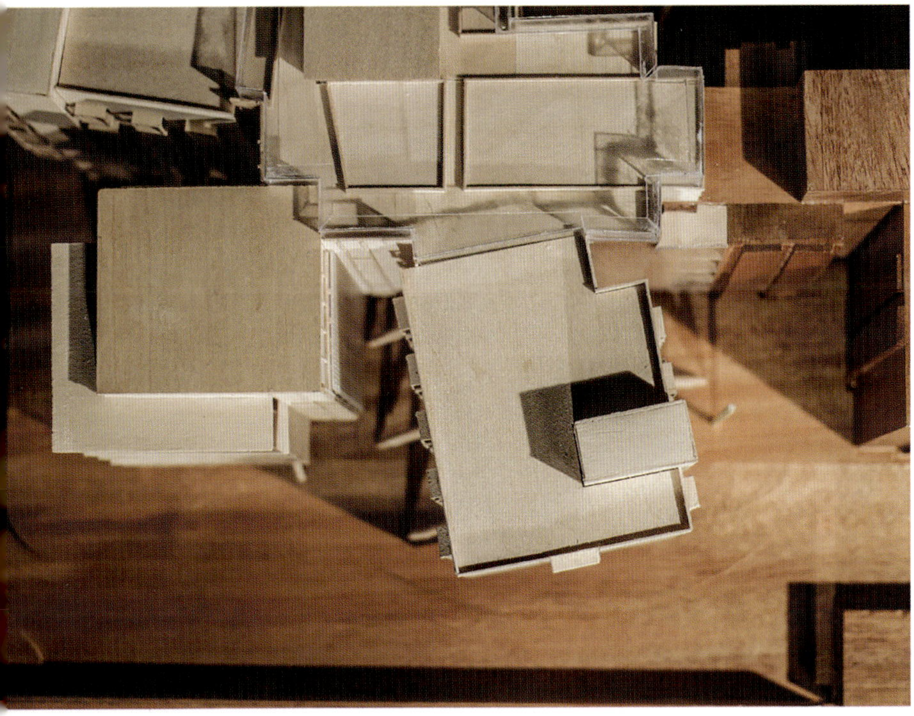

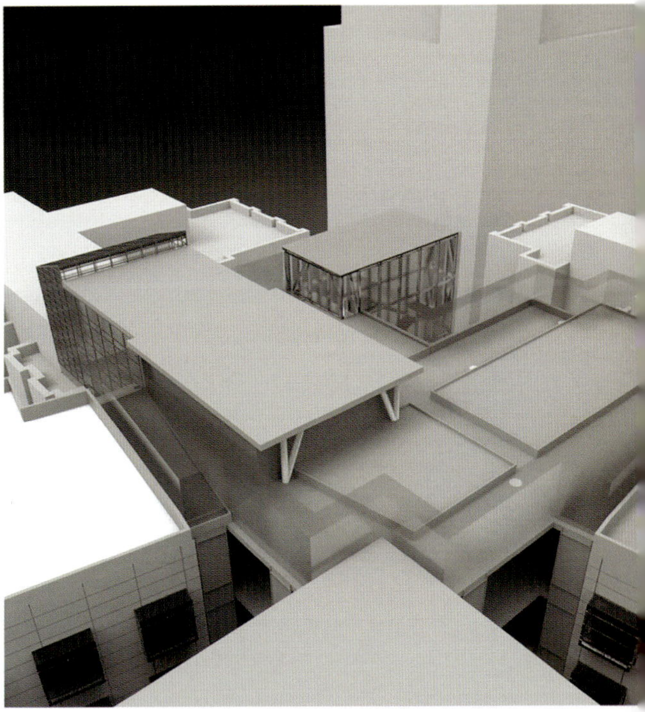

4.25a–c APT, 2017, interior of day/activity room and breakout consult room in a typical new residential unit (top), and the horticultural therapy roof terrace, model photo and rendering (bottom), 2017.

Staff workspaces – The staff workstation functions as a hybrid element in its configuration and in its appearance, featuring strategically positioned windows, access points, and a feeling of relative openness, yet with securable spaces immediately nearby. The residential unit dining room is located directly across from this central staff work zone; the exterior façade of a retained 1974 residential unit is repurposed, now to function as one of the four 'walls' in the dining room, on each unit floor. Food is transported from the central kitchen (the existing facility housed in the community center is retained and renovated). The specific calibration and amenity of the staff work zones on each residential unit in the APT is referenced in Chapters 5 and 6. The two patient room clusters of eight bedrooms are semiautonomous from a security perspective, and a back-of-house, staff-only corridor affords safe passage to and from the unit. All three primary occupied zones on the unit – patient bedrooms, staff work zone(s), and communal staff/patient spaces – can be locked down as required.

Multipurpose room and unit terrace – The residential unit on each floor features a multipurpose dayroom/activity space and an adjacent exterior terrace. These spaces are located at the center of the unit, in plan. The exterior terraces overlook the surrounding neighborhood and are bright and spacious, with natural ventilation

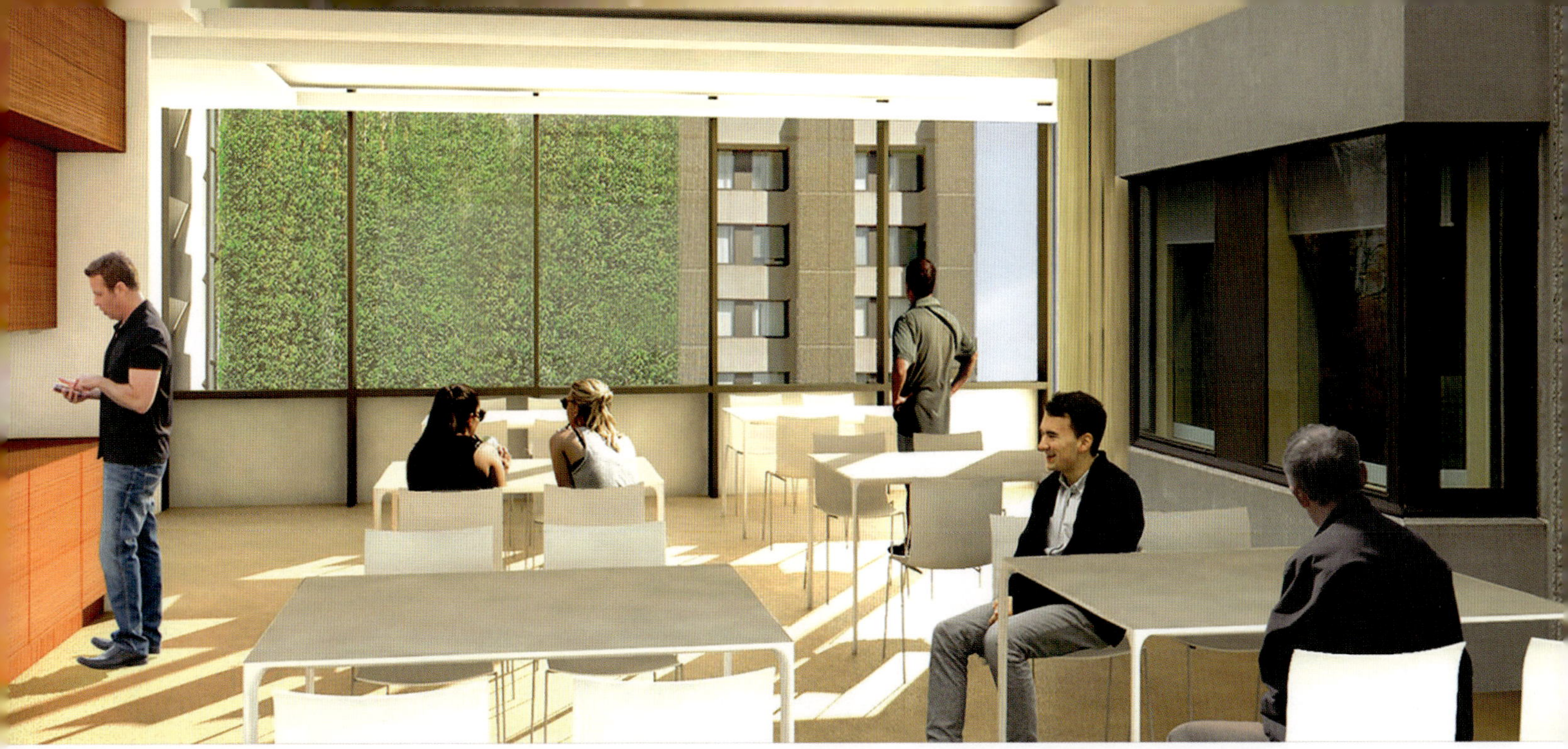

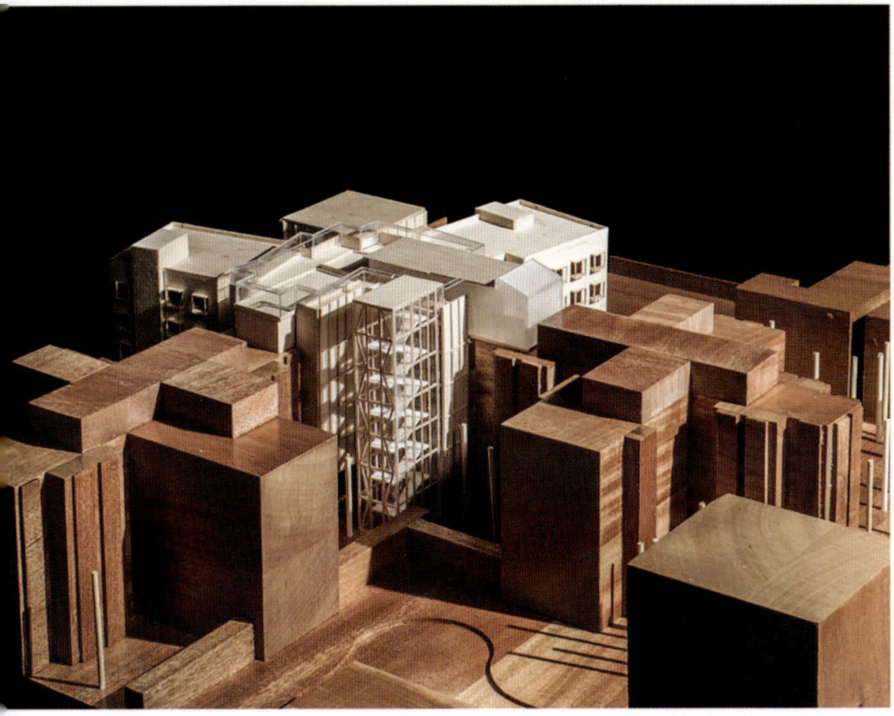

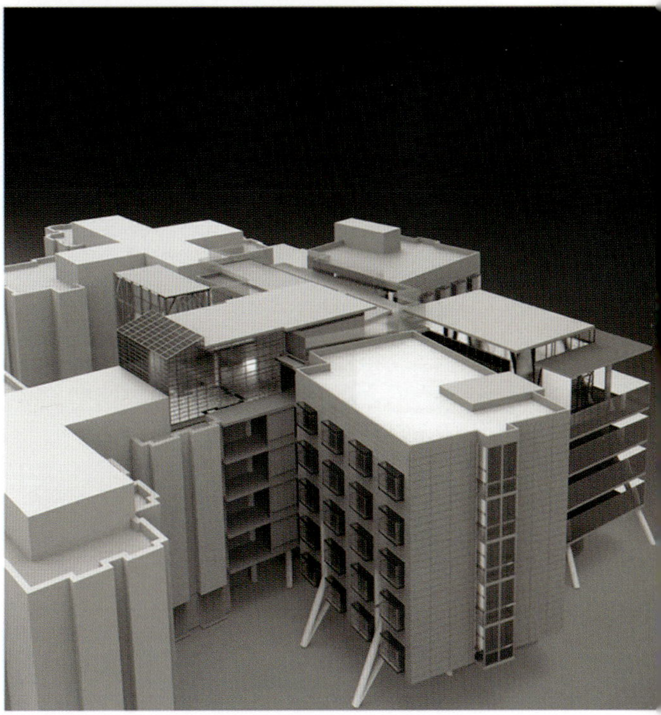

4.26a–c APT, 2017, dining room, new residential tower inpatient unit incorporating repurposed 1974 pavilion, with view of new 'green' stair tower (top), and exterior view of new arrival stair tower, model photo, and extruded legs and window seat bays of the new residential towers, rendering (bottom).

and a capsule-shaped group room/chill space. All access points are monitored audiovisually 24/7. The sheltered exterior terrace enables patients to spend time outdoors and are for use throughout the year, as weather permits; an encompassing 9-foot-high transparent high-security wall membrane is provided. Specifically, this element is able to withstand blunt-force impacts and disallows patients from climbing over the top (Figure 4.25a–c).

Roof terraces – The roof level of each new patient pavilion houses a horticultural therapy garden, indoor classroom/workshop room, adjacent comfort/chill room, a gardening equipment supply room, and restrooms. Nearby, on this same level, an all-season horticultural therapy greenhouse is provided. A 9-foot-high transparent glazed-panel wall, similar to that of the aforementioned multipurpose/dayroom terraces, functions as a high-security protective membrane, and this device encloses the patient-accessed portions of the roof terrace (Figure 4.24a–c). The roof terrace is accessed from all floors by means of the seven-level stair tower and elevators (Figure 4.26a–c).

View Simulation/Mediamesh system adapted to healthcare attuned micromesh system – The emergence of advanced virtual imaging technology enables the patient to experience an enhanced relationship with the exterior physical world from within the interior

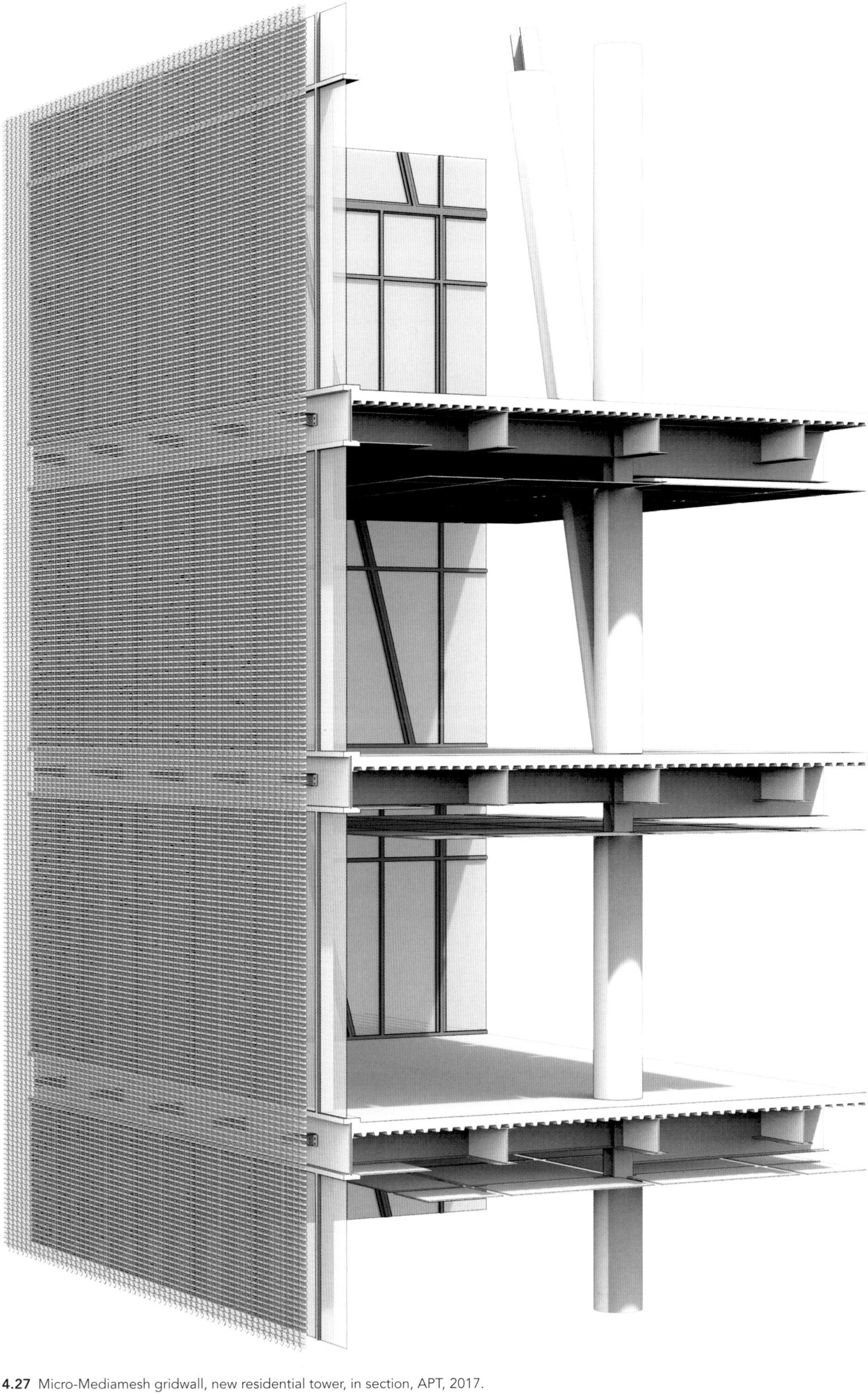

4.27 Micro-Mediamesh gridwall, new residential tower, in section, APT, 2017.

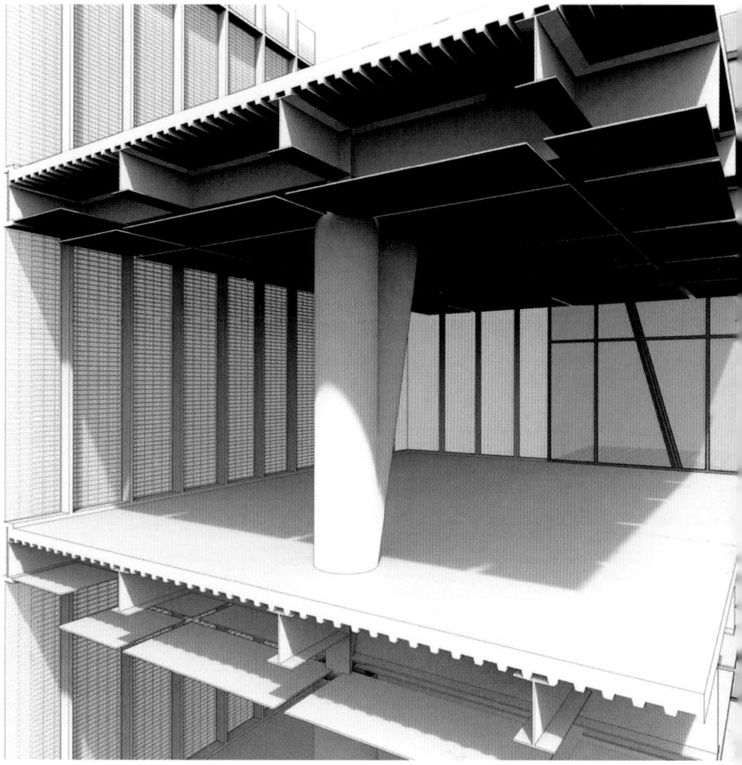

4.28 Micro-Mediamesh gridwall, as viewed from interior of the day/living and breakout consult area, in section, APT, 2017.

of a healthcare facility. It has become possible to attain virtual immersion in 'other realms' beyond the immediate realm through self-selected or 'prescribed' representational imagery, on either nearby walls and ceilings, or through a view of informational content perceivable through the window aperture – all now becoming blank canvasses to be 'repainted' as therapeutic amenities. In this regard, first, each patient room in the two residential pavilions in the APT would be equipped with a programmable internal ceiling grid, and second, a number of patient rooms would be equipped with a programmable, externally mounted image-viewing grid. The ceiling grid in each bedroom is installed directly above the patient bed and is controllable by the caregiving staff or the patient (where deemed appropriate). This smart ceiling allows for variable view content, ranging from a morning sunrise to a bright blue afternoon sky with passing clouds to a crimson sunset, to the projection of sequentially themed views of highly varied informational content.[56]

A recent commercial technology, widely known as the patented Mediamesh system, has become an integral part of urban commercial districts from Tokyo to New York to London to Sao Paulo and many points in between. During my first trip to Japan, I was mesmerized by the vast assemblages of electronic billboards in the Ginza District. I stood in the middle of the street, gazing upward in every direction, absorbing the myriad types, sizes, and shapes of installations. They were iconic and left a powerful impression. Typically, these e-billboard installations are found in dense urban settings, are large in scale, and are typically deployed to hawk Coca-Cola, the latest Ford F-150 model, films, fashion brands, and the like. They are installed on and above buildings of varying height and volume as digital billboards, at times becoming building-like, frequently in densely packed grid-like arrangements, commanding attention. This technology currently allows for the projection of large-scale compressed, or flattened, highly iconic, stunning informational content, although Mediamesh technology has seldom been utilized to project normative 'views', per se. This technology holds tremendous promise, however, for the projection of iconic *surrogate* view representational content. Interestingly, this type of application has yet to be field-tested anywhere in an actual healthcare treatment-facility setting, and the time is right to extend its applicability into this milieu. In response, an adaptation of the generic Mediamesh system is proposed for CAMH, and is therefore incorporated in the APT. Regarding its specific application here, a *micromesh* projection grid is installed on the exterior façade, directly facing a subset of patient rooms housed in the residential pavilion that would otherwise likely experience a somewhat restricted view sight line from the patient's bedroom window (Figure 4.27). With regard to the impact of the micromesh projection grid on the living/dayroom element upon which it is installed, natural light is transmitted to the inboard side, and interior-side glazing of the gridwall plane is translucent so as to not compromise patient confidentiality in the form of anyone in the dayroom being able to peer directly across into any patient bedroom (Figure 4.28).

The therapeutic amenity of nature-themed view informational content, taken in from hospital windows, whether this content is simulated or real, is well established in the empirical research literature.[57] And patients' direct exposure to informative, sufficiently interesting views has been associated with a shorter length of hospital stay and an overall higher level of satisfaction.[58] Window-view representations – that is, surrogate 'views' installed in physically windowless hospital rooms, including wall murals and the representation of indoor plants – have been found to be effective substitutes for a real view during hospitalization.[59] Here, the subset of two to three inpatient rooms per floor level that looks directly out to the Mediamesh projection grid (of the 16 beds on the unit) would therefore be provided with something a conventional patient room does not have – accentuated, highly variable view information content able to be tailored to an individual's needs and preferences. Images may be passive or active

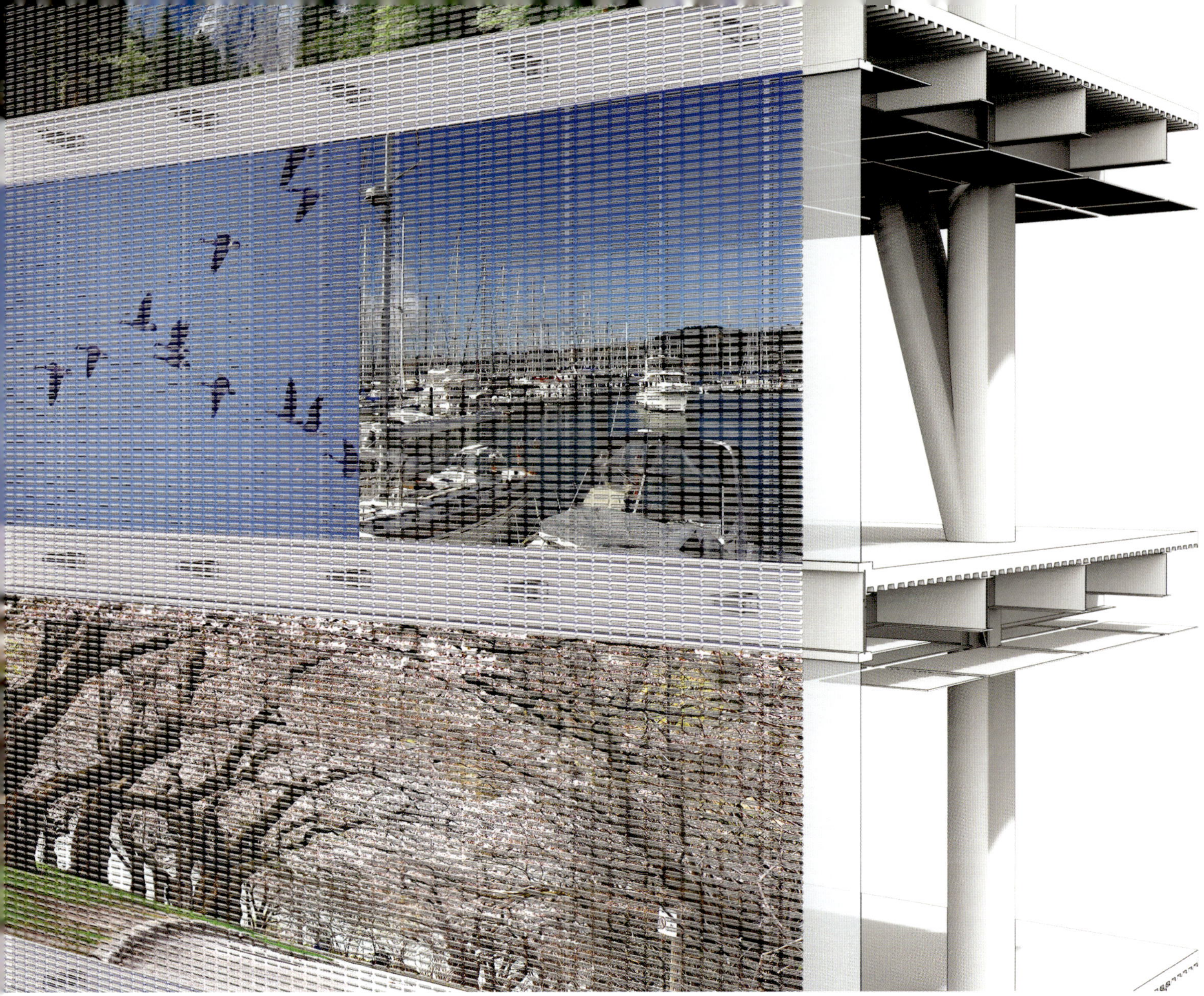

4.29 View-activated micro-Mediamesh gridwall, APT, 2017. Architect: Stephen Verderber.

in informational content and able to be digitally enhanced. This adaptation of current Mediamesh technology holds much promise in healthcare applications, for it allows for 'prescribed' image content in a premeditative, choreographed manner. More specifically, the term *micromesh* is introduced here as a result of the densification of the grid element to now hold as many as four times the number of horizontal tubes, or rods, resulting in a far higher degree of image resolution than is typical in current Mediamesh systems.

When the perceivable view plane and its informational content are considered holistically as a single therapeutic intervention – almost as a type of medication – much is possible. A patient is prescribed, for example, a specific view type or theme for, say, three hours daily. This prescription from this point on becomes modifiable as deemed necessary by the caregiving team, perhaps in close consultation with the patient. View content is therefore *designed*, or tailored, with regard to each patient's unique conditional needs and preferences. The *adapted micromesh-grid* technology makes it possible to attain a high degree of flexibility in this regard. View informational content is interchangeable and malleable in response to patients' circadian rhythms, conditions, ages, lifestyles, and so on under the supervision and purview of the interdisciplinary caregiver team (Figure 4.29).

The patient rooms in the APT feature varied, color-accented outer walls in each room. The simulated views visually accessible from within the room, as projected on the mesh grid, can be patterned and synchronized to the rhythms of the day as it becomes night, from urban to rural scenes, the changing seasons, varied weather conditions, and so on (Figure 4.30a–f). In theory, the degree of simulated 'view personalization' is unlimited, and the

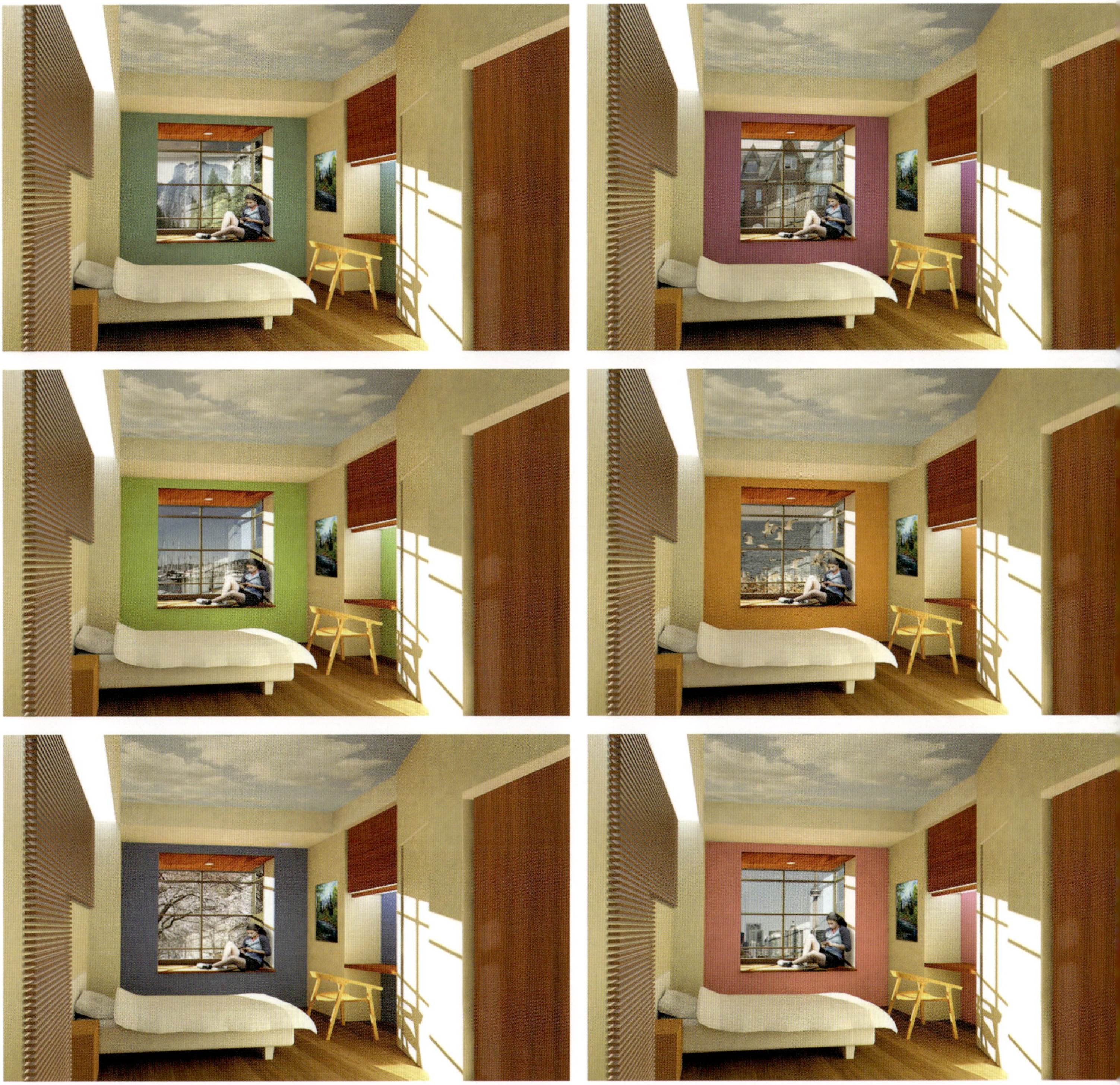

4.30a–f Patient room depicting cantilevered window seat bay; varied surrogate view representations; LED-controlled ceiling depicting 'blue sky mode'; modulated perimeter wall colors; and built-in desk, storage unit, and recessed bed/headwall, APT, 2017.

prescription for one's therapeutic view content is flexible, able to be 'designed' in coordination with the patient's progress while in treatment. A single view is projectable on the micromesh surface grid to multiple rooms or multiple views are projectable to multiple rooms simultaneously. As for the projection grid itself, it is lightweight, see-through element simultaneously allowing light to enter adjacent interior spaces (on the inboard side) and, in this case, the residential unit multipurpose activity space on each unit floor.

4. Diagnostic and therapy/treatment realms

The 1974 residential units retained in the APT are to be repurposed to *non-patient-housing* functions, with residential units relocated to the two new towers. Inpatient units would also be housed in a third location – one of the two 'block buildings' (part of the formally approved plan) fronting Queen Street West. The 1974 buildings would house comprehensive support programs,

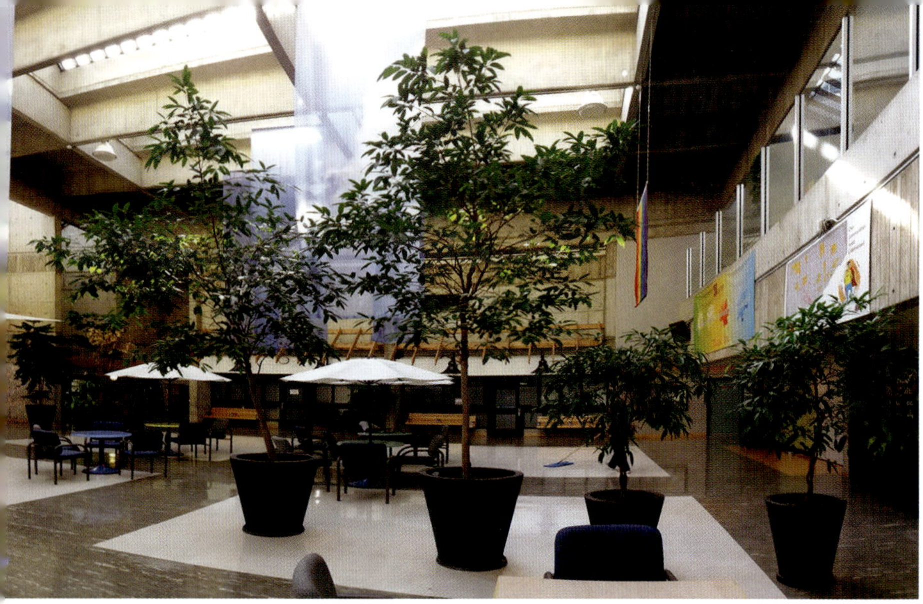

4.31 Repurposed public commons building atrium, CAMH, APT, 2017.

including administration, community outreach, staff training, group and individual counseling, and patient activity areas, including art therapy, music therapy, and occupational therapy, as well as portions of the partial hospitalization program. Recreational therapy programs would be provided at multiple sites on the campus. The modernist heritage buildings' size and quality of construction make them well suited for adaptation to non-patient-housing uses. The CAMH emergency trauma unit would continue to be based at CAMH on College Street (whereas the formally approved redevelopment plan calls for its relocation to Queen Street West).

5. Outpatient treatment environment

The APT recommends the majority of outpatient services at CAMH be housed in the future in the two 'block buildings' (part of the formally approved plan) fronting Queen Street West, together with ground-level exterior space for an outpatient therapy garden and play yard. These services, by being in proximity to the main arrival point to campus, will facilitate patient and visitor wayfinding. As for the community outreach program, a staging area is provided in the sheltered parking deck for two mobile mental health clinics that will travel throughout a network of program sites in the Greater Toronto Area (GTA). Existing partnerships with schools in the GTA would be expanded, and these mobile clinics would facilitate further partnering opportunities in the community. This will expand services in many neighborhoods that remain underserved at present. This is compounded by the fact that many patients and their families experience difficulty traveling to and from the CAMH main campus.

6. Landscape therapeutics

Gardening and horticultural therapy programs in mental health and addictive disorder treatment have been shown to foster psychological benefits (discussed in the next chapter). Simply providing something 'nice to look at' such as a small lawn parcel is insufficient because exterior space design strategies can achieve so much more. The 'lifting up' of the two proposed patient pavilions allows for a greater degree of spatial transparency in this regard – that is, thera-serialization – than if these two structures sat entirely on the ground. The exterior space this strategy yields supports group therapy, quiet contemplation, community engagement, and horticultural therapy, resulting in a significantly greater amount of exterior space on the ground level and for greater interconnectedness as opposed to multiple smaller parcels remaining visually and spatially noncontiguous. Walking through attractive grounds is an important activity, but *active engagement* through encountering nature firsthand in various ways affords greater therapeutic possibilities. This can also yield a greater degree of automaticity – that is, the power to draw occupants to these spaces repeatedly because they are inherently interesting places to be. The APT proposes advancing nature and landscape to the forefront in both indoor and outdoor contexts – that is, landscaped exterior spaces – together with the repurposed 1974 CAMH community center and its large central atrium. This atrium is currently relatively lifeless, and yet it receives plentiful natural light; this space would be transformed into an all-season therapeutic/winter garden. It is ill-advised to demolish this heritage-quality structure. With its current abundant light, further complimented by new, full-spectrum lighting, much more than at present is achievable in this building, as well as across the CAMH campus (Figure 4.31). A bird sanctuary would also be established at CAMH in these newly created open green spaces.

7. Administration and total environment

The APT encourages CAMH to promote environmental stewardship best practices by becoming (1) a recognized leader in ecological sustainability by advancing a genuinely empathic community public relations campaign in this regard; (2) a recognized leader in patient and caregiver safety by promoting patient and family empowerment through the ongoing enhancement of the therapeutic affordances of its historic built environment;

(3) a leader for having protected and enhanced a portion of its heritage-quality landscape, in establishing life-cycle assessment metrics to document the ongoing well-being of these amenities, and in promoting a sustained program in evidence-based design research to examine the relationship between the outdoor environment and mental health outcomes; and (4) a recognized leader in best practices in environmental sustainability in total campus resource management, including the retrofitting not only of its site/landscape resources but also of its heritage-quality modernist buildings, while striving to become a de-carbonized campus (see Chapter 5).

History repeats itself

A peculiar and, in a way, eerie chain of events is unfolding in Toronto, for the wheels of destigmatization are once again in motion. In 2007, John Bentley Mays, writing in *Canadian Architect*, characterized the approved redevelopment of CAMH as a sweeping CA$382 million recreation of an historic site, unprecedented in Canadian psychiatric hospital history. He saw it as an effort to eradicate any lingering reminders of psychiatry's dark past and the (by then) 30-year trend in psychiatry toward psychopharmaceutical treatment. A consortium of architects and planners led by Montgomery Sisam Architects, KPMB, and Urban Strategies together had arrived at a 'pioneering approach' with its *urban village* concept. Yet in doing so they inadvertently rejected an historic landscape.[60] Mays described the first phase (Phase 1A, including the Fennings Street extension into the campus) as bland and conservative, while going to extremes to eradicate remaining vestiges of its once-spacious landscaped grounds. In his words,

> In 19th century Britain and North America, democratic and populist tendencies in the culture at large led to drastic changes in official attitudes toward the insane. A new psychiatric elite, disgusted by the old regime of chaining the mad in dangerous prisons and filthy dungeons, called for a new hospital architecture to express the spirit of the times: open to fresh air and sunlight, in peaceful rural settings, from which cruelty and neglect had been banished in favor of good diet, sensible recreation and humane, individual care for the ill. In 1846, when its cornerstone was laid. . . (Howard's) asylum promised to be a great architectural incarnation of this new era . . . its walls and long galleries rose on a marshy plot reclaimed from the Fort York military reservation in the still sylvan countryside . . . This early optimism . . . would soon be dimmed by a generally gloomy recognition that the mental disorders that doctors purported to treat were more intractable and insidious than an earlier generation of fresh-air adherents (led by Dr. Kirkbride) had believed. . . (and also) beneath the surface ran the question of social class: early Victorian avant-garde psychiatrists, trained to treat maniacs from genteel, literate, and religious backgrounds, were suddenly confronted by waves of seriously disturbed people thrown into the medical system by immigration, industrialization, and urbanization . . . by the 1970s, Howard's asylum was widely hated by patients, doctors and ordinary Torontonians. It had come to symbolize the ghostliest aspects of past psychiatry . . . but by then new ideas were in the air – deinstitutionalization . . . and a devolution from large centralized hospitals into smaller units . . . In 1976, the last remnants of Howard's asylum fell under the wrecker's ball despite a preservation effort championed by Toronto architect A.J. Diamond, after a psychiatric and political establishment determined this hospital must go.[61]

Mays now feared the prevailing architectural winds would differ little from those of 50 years earlier:

> In (the asylum's) place rose four treatment units, by Somerville, McMurrich & Oxley, which seemed to observers at the time and since to resemble college dormitories . . . all four of these are to be bulldozed. It's worth noting that these buildings, now doomed, were much admired when they were completed. In a 1975 article in *Canadian Architect* about the just-finished project, we read about the delight of patients and staff with the new facilities' comfort, beauty and modernity. . . (while) in 2007, the medical director and CEO (Dr. Paul Garfinkel) declared the 1970s units that pleased so many 'are unacceptable in the 21st century of health care; they are cramped, undignified, disrespectful of the needs of individuals, and hardly inspiring of hope.' So what makes

> CAMH so sure they're not recasting into brick and mortar merely the newest fad in psychiatry in a never-ending cycle of 'breakthroughs' and disappointments that have been ongoing since the early 19th century?[62]

As it turns out, Mays was not alone. Soon after the project's unveiling, grassroots community groups assailed the urban village model on multiple fronts. To them, it was a false dichotomy to bring city streets into the campus merely as a means to normalize it. Harsh critiques soon surfaced within the Toronto medical establishment, who lamented the near-complete loss of open green space. However, the urban village had by then garnered currency within mainstream architectural and planning circles in and beyond Toronto. This signaled to preservationists and others that any disagreement would become nothing less than an arduous uphill fight. Importantly, some medical experts feared the urban village concept would strike fear into patients, who would now be at risk of public ridicule from passersby during trips to and from treatment sessions while attempting to negotiate an incoherent campus layout from a wayfinding perspective.

In 2003, a coalition of local patient activists, businesses, and private-citizen opponents brought CAMH before the Ontario Municipal Board (OMB). The OMB is a quasi-judicial body with wide-ranging powers over planning matters throughout the province. They demanded much greater transparency on the part of CAMH, additional environmental impact studies, and a thorough public review of the architectural design of all proposed buildings and especially their height and proximity in relation to the Victorian scale of the adjacent (and now threatened) Queen Street West commercial streetscape. At one point, CAMH had even proposed a 50,000-square-foot grocery store in one of the new 'block buildings' along Queen Street.[63]

Writing in 2000, Edna Hudson stated the CAMH redevelopment 'machine' had already been up and running for more than a decade:

> Any building sets a pattern of co-presence and co-awareness among its users . . . the social process of stigmatization is a prelude to a pathological community. . . (and) the contrasts between the Howard building and the (1956) Administration Building were readily used in a process of stigmatization of the old building, gathering momentum with the realization that the institution must stay at its location on Queen Street. By 1975 the residential patients were housed in four new Treatment Units, and the Howard building stood empty. When the four Treatment Units took over the core function of the Howard building, the stage was set. It was argued by the Ontario Heritage Foundation, abetted by the Toronto Historical Board, Toronto City Council, and a group of concerned citizens, that the Howard building should not be demolished, and indeed, that the Administration Building should be demolished instead. Meetings took place between government representatives and all of these groups, including the Architectural Conservancy of Ontario. An architectural proposal was commissioned that supported the view the Howard building might now be renovated and re-used . . . The direct competition between the Howard asylum and the Administration Building was now apparent and took many by complete surprise. The old building had already been publicly insulted and shamed by its propinquity to the newer (1956) building, its special qualities misunderstood, uncelebrated. The renovation proposed by A.J. Diamond Associates was superb. It proposed innovative changes . . . and retention (while) making use of its full potential . . . an historic building lost the contest for survival because most were unable to see its adaptive potential.[64]

The loss of the 1850 Howard building in 1976 was the result of preservationists' and other concerned parties' inability to prove how a stigmatized building can be repurposed and reborn. This challenge first became apparent in 1975 when the Ontario Provincial government passed a new Heritage Act. This law only heightened the ambiguities surrounding attempts to save any provincially controlled building deemed worthy of heritage protection. The alternative proposal presented by A.J. Diamond & Associates was viable and economically feasible. Despite its merits, it remained impossible to overcome intense antiasylum feelings associated with the Howard building. One elected official after another failed to defend it, and the staff at Queen Street West saw no further useful life for it. This conundrum reflected the struggle every heritage building finds itself in when caught in the headlights in the civic realm; heritage is rarely a popular cause in the moment. In Toronto, this is especially true when it

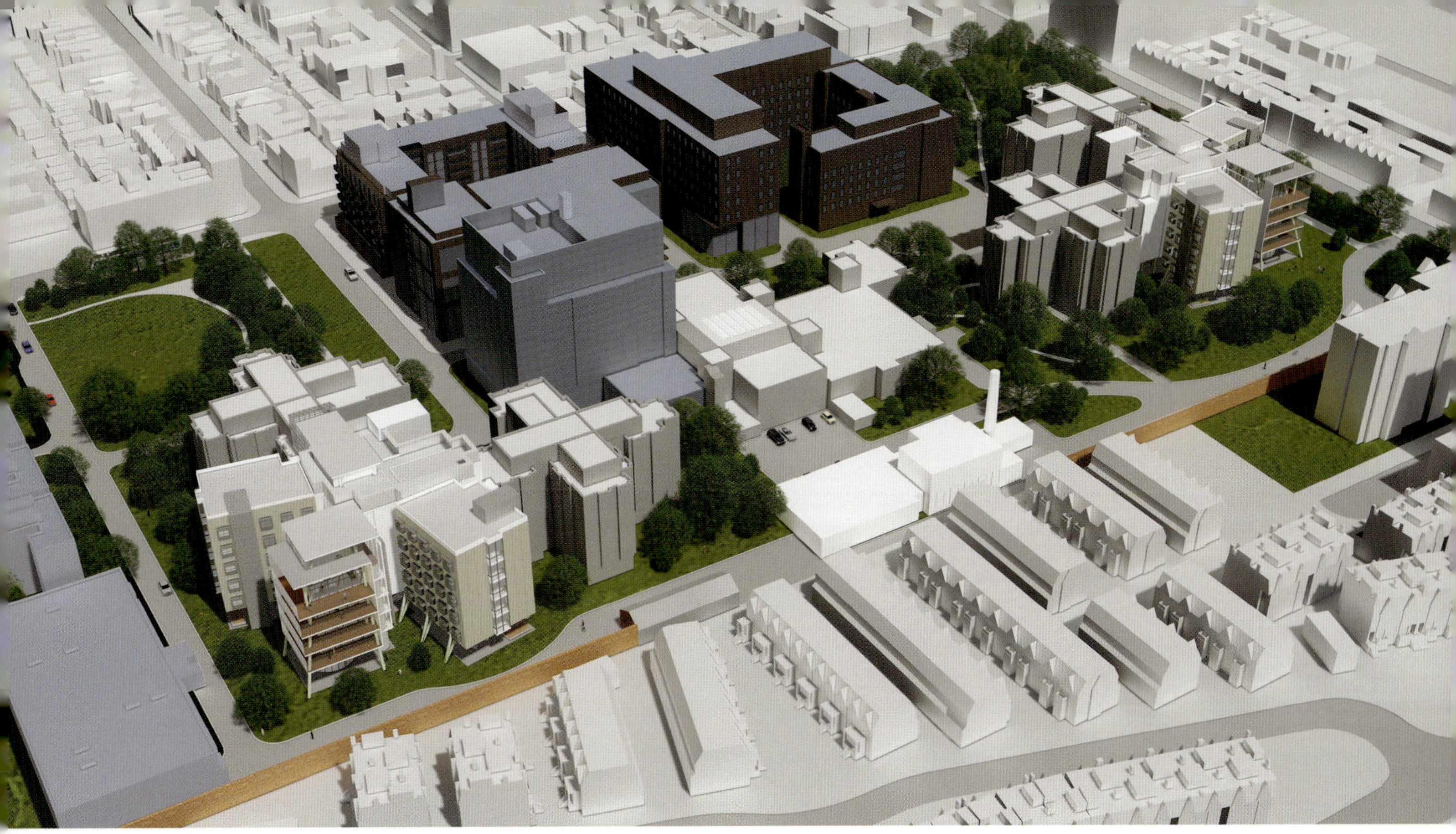

4.32 2020 redeveloped CAMH campus, incorporating completed (as of 2015) portions of approved 2007 plan (shaded in blue), the new east and west residential towers, the four repurposed heritage-eligible 1974 pavilions, public commons building and power plant, and the preserved (and enhanced) heritage-eligible open green spaces of the APT, 2017. Architect: Stephen Verderber.

comes to intensely competitive land-redevelopment pressures in the urban core.[65]

This is precisely what preservationists recently faced in their failed attempt to save the 1970s buildings from demolition on the CAMH campus. The structures sometimes had been tarred and feathered, stigmatized first by the CAMH administration and its board of directors and later by the local political establishment. Was it mere coincidence how a CAMH vice president for campus redevelopment and real estate was now on board with the new directive to maximize economic returns through leasing CAMH-owned land with 99-year leases? The main difference was that it was now a market-driven version of what occurred a generation earlier on the *same campus*.

In 2015 CAMH announced rather belatedly it had hired noted Swedish architect Stefan Lundin, the lead architect of the Östra Healthcare Centre for Psychiatry (see Chapter 6), as a consultant for its reinvented campus.[66] More broadly, some pro-CAMH plan voices might be tempted to inaccurately draw comparisons to St. Olav's Medical Center in Trondheim, Norway – where an existing street grid there was (mostly) already in place.[67] In the end, let this serve as a cautionary tale. Architectural activism is no crime (Figure 4.32). Meanwhile, the surrounding neighborhood and indeed many observers across the entire Toronto metro area remain highly skeptical of what is to come. If nothing else, the APT's vision delineates an alternative approach to the reinvention of an asylum campus.

CHAPTER 5

Planning and design considerations for behavioural health architecture

Psychiatric and substance addiction treatment environments are complex, for there exists no single definition that aptly summarizes their broad typological variability. They operate in diverse geographic, sociocultural, and political contexts and the pervasive treatment gap discussed in previous chapters increasingly overwhelms the coping capacities of existing treatment service networks. These built environments are regulated by local, regional, and federal governmental agencies with licensure oversight for the minimum compliance of health and human welfare, and their daily operation is further subject to oversight by third-party accreditation commissions, in many jurisdictions. There is therefore no sole set of facility-related issues deemed justifiably 'global' in scope, and it would be rather unrealistic to aim for this. However, many time-tested *patterns* and precedents, rooted in salutogenic concepts with regards to the planning, design, construction, and assessment of occupied facilities and their campuses, are identifiable and indeed applicable across time and space. A paradigm that would seek to capture to a reasonable degree a salutogenic planning and design perspective might encompass:

- Learning about the salient attitudes and values held by the local community toward mental illness, the role of community health promotion, and the community's responsiveness to its individuals in need of diagnosis and treatment.
- Identifying and seeking to overcome obstacles in site and facility procurement, design, construction, and life-cycle operation from an eco-humanist perspective – with human well-being together with ecological conservation concerns being of high priority.
- Responding to expectations regarding minimum code and regulatory-agency licensing performance standards in the procurement, planning, design, construction, and operation of mental health and allied inpatient and outpatient treatment facilities.
- Establishing bona fide public-private partnerships where feasible between mental health care provider organizations, nongovernmental organizations (NGOs), and appropriate governmental oversight agencies as a means to achieve positive and mutually shared goals and outcomes that are otherwise unattainable.
- Working to overcome, at the local community level, current healthcare provider organizations' strategic challenges and obstacles to more effectively serve their immediate community's mental health and addiction disorder treatment needs.

The compendium of patterns presented in this chapter consists of 74 salutogenically based issues centered on inpatient (hospital-based) and outpatient (clinic-based) healthcare environments. Each issue seeks to address a specific aspect of the mental health and substance addiction equation and is premised on exploring person-environment normalization from the perspective of site connectivity, functional planning, aesthetic concerns, environmental stewardship, local cultural norms, and the role of vernacular building traditions relative to placemaking in the cause of mental health promotion. Individually and collectively, this compendium of concerns builds on the past 50 years of architectural research.[1] The aim is to coalesce, elevate, and disseminate this discourse. Hospitalization is often a time of personal crisis. The treatment environment need not represent yet an additional barrier, source of stress, nor contribute to an individual's diminished personal integrity or self-dignity. Genuinely salutogenic support mechanisms of this type can most directly manifest in (at least) four ways: instrumental, aesthetic, emotional, and spiritual.

Aesthetic support embodies the interpretative role of built form and the meanings it communicates. *Emotional* support denotes the ability of the physical setting to promote healthfulness and to increase the competency level of the individual. *Spiritual* support manifests in the patient and in one's significant others' capabilities to proactively self-actualize so the patient can once again live a dignified, productive life out in the community. Specific diagnoses addressed in the following discussion include anxiety disorders, posttraumatic stress disorder (PTSD), obsessive compulsive disorder, panic disorder and social phobia, attention deficit hyperactivity disorder (ADHD), autism spectrum disorders, bipolar disorder, borderline personality disorder, depression, controlled substance abuse, eating disorders, mental illness associated with HIV/AIDS, schizophrenia, and risk of suicide. This compendium of 74 precepts is presented in seven parts: (1) site, context, and sustainability; (2) arrival, public, and semipublic spaces; (3) the inpatient care unit; (4) the diagnostic and treatment realm; (5) outpatient treatment environments; (6) landscape therapeutics; and (7) administration and total environment. These considerations are discussed with respect to inpatient and outpatient adult psychiatric hospitals, child and adolescent psychiatric centers, forensic institutions, and alcohol and substance abuse treatment centers.

More specifically, they address:

1. *Hospital inpatient* stays in a psychiatric hospital or the psychiatric unit of a general hospital. Inpatient hospitals treat the most acute phases of mental illness. Typically, patients requiring longer-term care are transferred to a psychiatric hospital for further treatment.
2. Psychiatric hospitals treating mental illnesses exclusively, with physicians on staff to address medical conditions such as drug and alcohol detoxification and rehabilitation, eating disorders, geriatric psychiatry, and pediatric services.
3. General medical and surgical hospitals with a psychiatric unit or substance abuse treatment unit housed on-site.
4. Residential mental health treatment centers for longer-term care. These settings provide medical care, are less hospital-like, and include residential settings for persons with chronic illness, alcohol and drug addictive disorders, and support services for the aged.
5. Outpatient treatment clinics providing day services only. Some are hospital based while others are freestanding. Some are walk-in clinics whereas others require a physician's referral.
6. Partial hospitalization programs (PHPs), also referred to as day programs, which are attended by patients for 6 or more hours per day most days of the week and provide less intensive services compared to full hospitalization programs. The focus is on psychiatric treatment, group therapy, health education, and individual counseling provided in freestanding and hospital-based facilities.
7. Intensive outpatient programs (IOPs), which are similar to PHPs but are attended for only 3–4 hours daily; patients may also meet during the evening hours to accommodate clients' work schedules during the day. This type of care may be hospital based or provided at a freestanding clinic.
8. Community mental health clinics, nonresidential settings where patients obtain individual and group therapy, and where medication management treatment is provided on-site. These facilities treat persons assessed to be below the acuity threshold for inpatient treatment.
9. Private practice practitioners, including social workers, psychologists, and psychiatrists in private individual or group practice. Appointments may be for individual, group, or family therapy. Many accept third-party insurance copayments, while others accept only personal payment for services.
10. Telepsychiatry and tele-mental-health services, which refer to the off-site delivery of psychiatric assessment and treatment via telephone, Internet, e-mail, online chat, or videoconferencing. Most often this is appropriate for individuals residing

in remote geographic locales, in medically underserved areas, and individuals who are homebound.

The 74 considerations are for broad interpretation by architects, landscape architects, interior designers, planners, engineers, sustainability and resiliency specialists, direct caregivers including physicians, psychiatrists, nurses, and their allied support staff, philanthropic fundraisers, organization administrators and their boards of directors, federal government agencies, private philanthropic foundations, grassroots mental health organizations, elected officials, health policy specialists, evidence-based design researchers, public health agencies, service providers, and staff personnel in shelters for the homeless. This compendium is also intended as a reference source for mental health and substance abuse advocacy groups.[2] It is hoped that the broad-brushed scope of this compendium allows for its equally broad interpretations in diverse contexts.[3] As for the reader's access and referral to more technical information on this subject, including specific products, an excellent reference source for architectural practitioners and others is the most recent iteration of the Design Guide for the Built Environment of Behavioral Health Facilities (seventh edition, 2016).[4]

D. Kirk Hamilton has identified four levels of evidence-based professional practice in architecture for health, with Level 3 practitioners carefully following the literature, publishing and presenting their work to others, and having acquired direct experience in conducting research in the field. Some of these individuals (whom he refers to as Level 4 practitioners) regularly conduct sophisticated field research themselves and collaborate with other specialists, including social scientists, and they commonly subject their work to external peer review in the form of professional design awards programs. Level 1 and 2 practitioners, for their part, may or may not engage in any of these specific activities. The following discussion speaks to practitioners who operate at any of these four levels, however, and these specific planning and design considerations are geared to help all in the generation of 'design hypotheses' for further testing and refinement in professional practice, as well as in environmental design research contexts.[5]

Any compendium such as this might be seen by some as too prescriptive – or 'set in stone'. But in truth, what use is it to specify, for instance, the *exact* size of a consultation room? How could any such prescription be universally applicable? Any such statement must be tempered by the realities imposed by local codes and myriad other concerns, on the assumption that every situation is unique. These considerations are therefore not to be misconstrued as a 'nuts-and-bolts' or auto repair manual–type guide of any sort.[6] Lena From, writing in *Architecture as Medicine*, similarly argues for a middle-ground position, as she notes the inherent danger of overemphasizing any single theory, research study, or finding (perhaps at the expense of other relevant research studies) and then overgeneralizing off of it, for one, because relying too much on too little data can and will very likely skew what gets built, perhaps for years or decades to come. She described how Stefan Lundin, the lead architect of the Östra psychiatric replacement hospital in Sweden, agrees with

> the sharp criticism leveled by architects the world over at the research community as a whole, and EBD [evidence-based design] research included [because] its insistence on quantifiability belittles the intrinsic worth of the creative process. Little importance, or none at all, is attached to the architect's experience-based, artistic and intuitive work of exploration, even though it is by far the most important and decisive factor for the outcome in built form . . . Yes indeed, we need a new language and new concepts will have to be developed. Architectural research needs to open up to the sensory properties of healthcare architecture. But if a new language describing the impact of architecture on we humans is to be created in earnest, the profession will also have to open up to and be prepared to assimilate the findings of its own research.[7]

And then there is the story of the American architect, who, while being given a tour of a recently opened award-winning psychiatric hospital in Europe, asked its medical director (a psychiatrist), after noticing that the patients were dining with 'normal' glassware and regular silverware, 'Why do you allow your patients to use those items?' The medical director calmly responded, 'Why would we not allow our patients to use those items?' Is the architect really capable at all of designing for people who are 'othered' as defined by Foucault (i.e., those trained professionals who exist solely by reason of their specialized training, and for no other reason than because the architectural elite is so inextricably a part of mainstream society itself)?[8] In this regard, at the end of the day, it is the frontline direct caregiver who is most qualified to address the needs of those with whom he or she works and cares for on a daily basis, not the elite architect who waltzes in and out of the scene, periodically, while hoping to acquire some degree of trust and acceptance.[9]

The psychiatrist J. Fisk has identified two inherently conflicting approaches in the planning and design of psychiatric facilities: facilities for a unique patient population, and those for a generalized patient population.[10] In her insightful 2014 book on the subject of architecture and psychiatric health, Evangelia Chrysikou identified three factors: the importance of the patient's personal safety and security, the importance of being cognizant of the individual patient's level of personal competence (here drawing directly from the work of the pioneering environmental gerontologist M. Powell Lawton), and the key function of the patient's personalization opportunities in one's physical setting and her or his associated freedom of choice within that treatment setting. She refers to this triad as the SCP Model.[11] The reader is referred to her book for further discussion of this conceptualization.

The 74 design considerations presented here are summarized in Figure 5.1. Precedents otherwise worthy of being cited were omitted due to one or more possibly questionable issues. One such example was a recently built psychiatric hospital in Japan. It lacked private bath/shower rooms for the inpatients; although communal bath/shower rooms are still culturally acceptable in Japan, they are considered counternormative in many other parts of the world.[12] An overarching intent in assembling this compendium is for others to be inspired to build upon it to improve the *quantity* of behavioural health environments, everywhere. In this regard we must do our best with the best information available at hand. Some evidence-based researchers, including Mardelle M. Shepley and Samira Pasha, seem to argue an opposing position when they assert, 'The amount of research on this topic (psychiatric facilities) is minimal and (still) insufficient to inform the design process and support the generation of design guidelines.'[13] Of course, much more evidence-based research is absolutely needed on this subject, without question. This is not a point of contention. In the meantime, architects and others must do their best with the knowledge at hand, through their work and contributions to the state of the art, to advance the case for individuals with mental illness and addiction disorders. It is a three-way street: evidence-based knowledge, the process of design, and the dissemination of research-based design outcomes (buildings and landscapes) are inextricably interwoven. That said, it is hoped the reader will think of each design consideration as a *hypothesis* for testing and refinement.

1 Site, context, and sustainability

Salutogenic environments

Aaron Antonovsky, a medical sociologist, first defined the concept of salutogenics as the confluence of multiple positive factors supportive of human health and well-being, in sharp contrast to prevailing, negativity-based definitions of sickness and disease associated with pathogenesis.[14] The term *salutogenesis* is derived from the Latin *salus*, meaning 'health', and the Greek *genesis*, meaning 'origin'. Antonovsky asserted that humans need and require cognitively supportive, meaningful environments to cope with highly stressful everyday conditions, conditions that threaten to destroy our sense of place attachment within the world. He defined 'cognitive coherence' as a three-pronged phenomenon consisting of *comprehensibility*, the belief that things occur in an orderly and relatively predictable manner that allows humans to be capable of reasonably predicting future events; *manageability*, the belief that humans possess the ability to successfully solve problems and any given situation is therefore potentially solvable and within one's range of control; and *life meaning*, a belief that life is intrinsically interesting and a source of fascination and is therefore worth living, with each human having a unique purpose and mission in life, leading to the belief that, therefore, it is worth knowing and caring about what one's eventual life outcome will be. Jan A. Golembiewski has further examined the relevance of salutogenic theory and human well-being in relation to the planning, design, and daily management of psychiatric treatment facilities.[15] He has found that in the face of adversity, individuals with mental illness are reluctant to leave that which is familiar and known. The places where we live, work, and accumulate a lifetime of memories and experiences are psychologically enduring and are fundamental to well-being. Unsupportive environments, by contrast, challenge our mental health status and our physical competency levels. Comprehensibility is the vehicle by which a psychologically disturbed individual attempts to interpret (or misunderstand) these situations and places. In a mental health facility context, this entails being capable of comprehending and to some extent accepting the meaning of why he or she is there, how to negotiate the immediate facility and its interpreted meanings, and how to function within it daily; this entails effective coping, with the assumed aim of seeking to be discharged expeditiously. This transcends 'meaning', or issues of manageability alone,

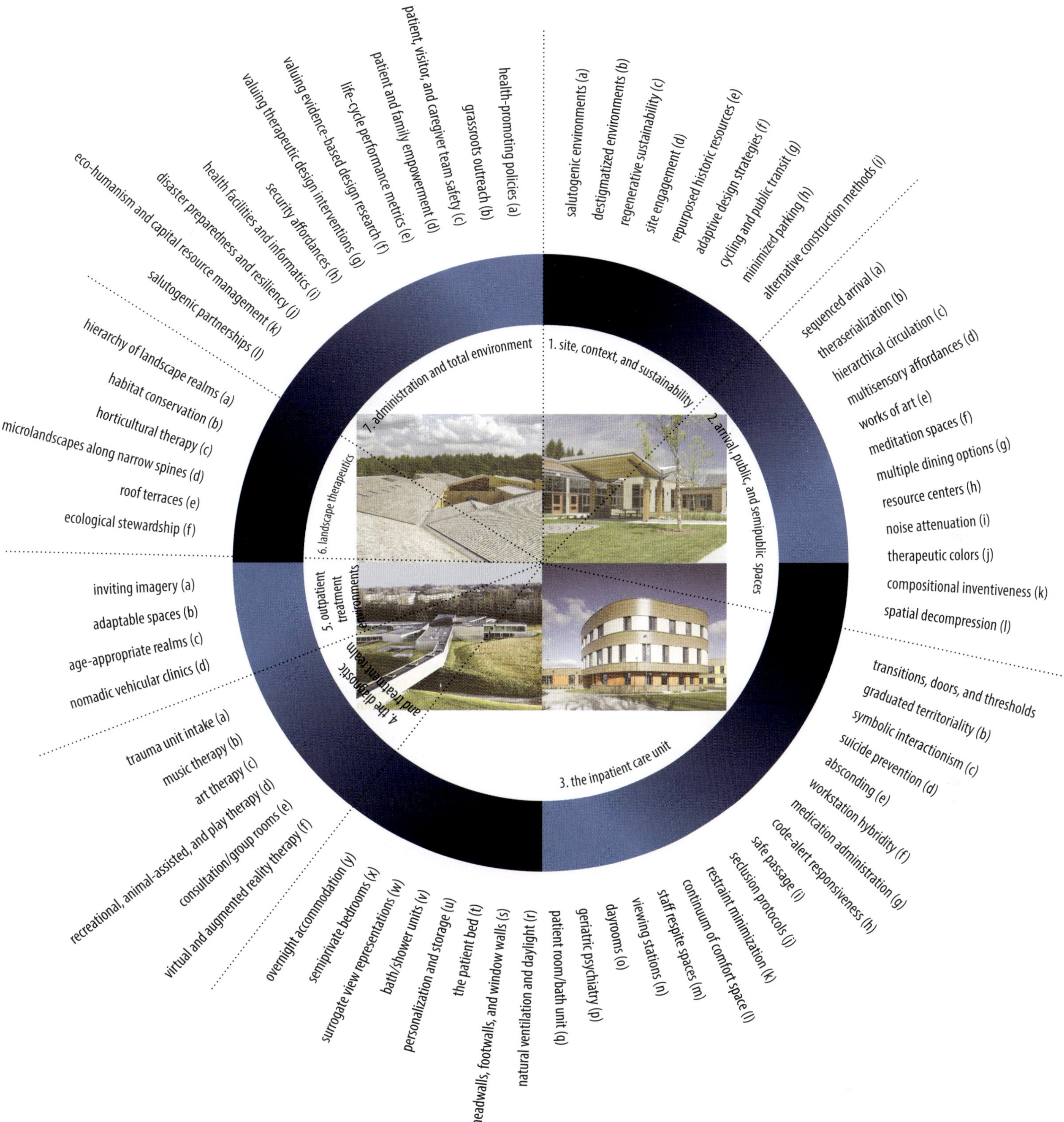

1. site, context, and sustainability
salutogenic environments (a)
destigmatized environments (b)
regenerative sustainability (c)
site engagement (d)
repurposed historic resources (e)
adaptive design strategies (f)
cycling and public transit (g)
minimized parking (h)
alternative construction methods (i)
2. arrival, public, and semipublic spaces
sequenced arrival (a)
theraserialization (b)
hierarchical circulation (c)
multisensory affordances (d)
works of art (e)
meditation spaces (f)
multiple dining options (g)
resource centers (h)
noise attenuation (i)
therapeutic colors (j)
compositional inventiveness (k)
spatial decompression (l)
3. the inpatient care unit
transitions, doors, and thresholds
graduated territoriality (b)
symbolic interactionism (c)
suicide prevention (d)
absconding (e)
workstation hybridity (f)
medication administration (g)
code-alert responsiveness (h)
safe passage (i)
seclusion protocols (j)
restraint minimization (k)
continuum of comfort space (l)
staff respite spaces (m)
viewing stations (n)
dayrooms (o)
geriatric psychiatry (p)
patient room/bath unit (q)
natural ventilation and daylight (r)
headwalls, footwalls, and window walls (s)
the patient bed (t)
personalization and storage (u)
bath/shower units (v)
surrogate view representations (w)
semiprivate bedrooms (x)
overnight accommodation (y)
4. the diagnostic and treatment realm
trauma unit intake (a)
music therapy (b)
art therapy (c)
recreational, animal-assisted, and play therapy (d)
consultation/group rooms (e)
virtual and augmented reality therapy (f)
5. outpatient treatment environments
inviting imagery (a)
adaptable spaces (b)
age-appropriate realms (c)
nomadic vehicular clinics (d)
6. landscape therapeutics
hierarchy of landscape realms (a)
habitat conservation (b)
horticultural therapy (c)
microlandscapes along narrow spines (d)
roof terraces (e)
ecological stewardship (f)
7. administration and total environment
health-promoting policies (a)
grassroots outreach (b)
patient, visitor, and caregiver team safety (c)
patient and family empowerment (d)
life-cycle performance metrics (e)
valuing evidence-based design research (f)
valuing therapeutic design interventions (g)
security affordances (h)
health facilities and informatics (i)
disaster preparedness and resiliency (j)
eco-humanism and capital resource management (k)
salutogenic partnerships (l)

5.1 The compendium of 74 planning and design considerations.

because coping with psychological and physical stress, uncertainty, and adversity is challenging enough while in treatment. Ideally, the patient can become empowered to be instrumentally in control of both his or herself and his or her physical surroundings.[16]

Destigmatized environments

The aim of healthcare provider organizations to shed any lingering vestiges of the old, antiquated custodial institutions of the 20th century is well justified. Ironically, this aim was of no less concern in the mid-19th century to Dr. Thomas Story Kirkbride. He wrote, in his time (1854), that the style and layout of the asylum building and its surrounding campus must be carefully considered: 'although it is not desirable to have an elaborate or costly style of architecture, it is, nevertheless, important that it should impress favorably not only upon the patients, but their friends and others who may visit it.' Any resemblance to a prison was to be carefully avoided: 'The means of affecting the proper degree of security should be masked,' he advised, with the 'building's custodial appearance camouflaged by ornamenting its grounds with gardens, fountains, and summerhouses.' To Kirkbride, these improvements were essential in convincing patients and their families to support the institution, because first impressions, then as today, are extremely important. He noted,

> No desire to make a beautiful or picturesque exterior should ever be allowed to interfere with the internal arrangements. Have your parlors and rooms large and airy, with high ceilings, your corridors wide, and the overall good impression of the building will be sustained.

As for the importance of an informative view,

> The surrounding scenery should be of a varied and attractive kind, and the neighborhood should possess numerous objects of an agreeable and interesting character, the building itself should be placed so that the views from every window, especially the parlors and rooms occupied during the day, have pleasant prospects and exhibit life in its active forms.[17]

Persistent stigma associated with an obsolete campus or its constituent buildings will indeed trickle down to the residential inpatient treatment unit. And retrofitting an outdated building envelope may be no substitute for a total replacement facility or a total replacement campus.[18]

Regenerative sustainability

Hospitals consume vast amounts of nonrenewable energy, and in the United States today they consume twice as much energy as office buildings, per square foot, with nearly US$3 billion expended on electricity alone annually. Tremendous possibilities exist to rectify this troubling dilemma through the expanded use of geothermal, wind, hydrogen, and solar power systems and sources. The Fachkrankenhaus Nordfriesland psychiatric hospital in Bredstedt, Germany (2004–2007), was in the first cohort of European hospitals in the EU Union of Hospitals Demonstration Project. It has reduced its overall electrical energy consumption footprint by 57%, a feat achieved by incorporating double-skin façades, solar thermal mass walls, and an integrated heat-power plant, among other carbon-reducing features.[19] Psychiatric and substance abuse treatment facilities globally must now be judged by environmental as well as human-oriented mending metrics – by their ability to heal humans as much as by their ability to help heal, if even in some small contributing way, our besieged planet Earth. A *regenerative* psychiatric hospital or clinic is self-sufficient, an entity capable of giving something *back* to the environment – not just taking from it – in the form of a net positive contribution. For instance, why remain dependent on the conventional power grid? As for recycling, the NGO Hospitals for a Healthy Environment (H2E) reported in 2007 that a small but growing number of healthcare organizations in the United States were on the verge of approaching 50% diversion rates in their operational waste streams. The GrassRoots Recycling Network's zero-waste business principles program has garnered much international interest as mental health care providers begin to explore innovative ways to reduce their carbon emission levels. Its 10 provisos, all applicable to psychiatric hospitals and related clinics, involve (1) committing to a triple bottom line of social, environmental, and economic performance benchmarks; (2) applying the precautionary principle before committing to any toxic or wasteful practices or systems; (3) directing zero waste to local or regional landfill or incineration sites; (4) assuming all responsibility for take-back packaging and avoiding all redundant packaging; (5) purchasing reused, recycled, and composted materials; (6) preventing pollution and reducing or eliminating the generation of on-site waste; (7) opting for the highest and best uses of available land and facility resources and continually reassessing policies and practices in this regard; (8) developing economic incentives for workers, patients, and suppliers to help the organization achieve a regenerative (net positive) carbon footprint quotient; (9) ensuring all products and services sold or provided are nontoxic in all forms; and (10) adopting policies that promote nontoxic production, reuse, and recycling processes at all levels.[20]

Site engagement

Some of the architectural case studies presented in the following chapter (Chapter 6) appear to organically, naturally arise from their sites. This interpretative site design strategy has too rarely been adopted in the long and checkered history of hospital architecture. A flat site was usually always preferred over a sloping one, particularly one with pronounced, irregular terrain. The result was often a structure that would appear to be platonically disengaged from its immediate site environs, to be little informed by it. Compassionate engagement of a site denotes a give-and-take dialogue; the opposite of this type of strategy came to dominate the era of the modern megahospital – as was the case with the McMaster University Medical Centre in Hamilton, Ontario (1972), where the superstructure conveyed the appearance of an automobile assembly plant that completely dominated its site.[21] As for recent psychiatric hospitals, the Juravinski Centre for Integrated Healthcare in Hamilton, Ontario (Case Study 12), responds rather successfully with regards to establishing a give-and-take relationship with the irregular topography of its site. Other case studies in the following chapter that establish a dialogue with their sites include Hopewood Park in the United Kingdom (CS 3) and the Helsingor Psychiatric and Hospital and Clinic in Denmark (CS 8), where level changes and the site's topographic variability become important ingredients within an engaging architectural and landscape equation – in a naturalistic setting that conveys a rather quiet presence, visually, with its meandering ramps, walkways, and retaining walls and an inventive redirection and reconfiguration of landform. The sensitive reconfiguration of a site can allow for semi-enclosed pockets of occupiable outdoor space near the building and yet convey a feeling of being far removed, as these types of small, protected spaces and enclosures can help reinforce a patient's positive cognitive orientation and consequently decrease the stresses and rigors associated with one's daily treatment regimen. When exterior spaces such as these are effectively woven into their corresponding, adjacent interior spaces – that is, dining rooms and their patios, or a therapy pool with a patio set apart by a low retaining wall or set into a gentle slope enabling their occupants to be partially obscured – genuine engagement with the site is achievable without compromising universal accessibility.

Repurposed historic resources

The governing boards of psychiatric hospitals at times can, and will, be indifferent to the importance of examining the benefits of preserving historic facilities under their purview. As for the feasibility of preserving and repurposing an old asylum building on the grounds, admittedly, these buildings continue to convey stigma associated with the bygone era characterized by electroshock therapy, excessive physical restraint, lobotomies, and other long-discredited treatment methods. This enduring stigma has had a few unfortunate, unintended consequences, however, as the opportunity to save an otherwise meritorious building from demolition becomes lost. Exceptions to the pattern of prematurely dismissing historic buildings from their repurposing to new uses include the transformation of the historic Devon County (UK) Pauper Lunatic Asylum into a transitional affordable housing community.[22] There, the oldest structures on the grounds continued to retain intrinsic architectural merit – apart from their now-discredited former uses in a bygone era. Unfortunately, often, obsession with 'the new' takes precedence over all else and as a consequence time is not taken to duly appraise the merits of retention. Asylum additions and replacement structures built in the 1960s and 1970s were usually aesthetically uninspiring despite featuring the latest treatment philosophies of their day. Unfortunately, this remove-and-replace mantra remains alive and well in the 21st century (see Chapter 4), as history tends to repeat itself. Regardless, work to save important and unique older structures, to non-patient-housing functions, and repurpose them in new, interesting ways. A combination of adapting the best of the old with new construction is often most prudent, and this simultaneously will serve the best interests of the surrounding neighborhood as well. Reinvention-in-place strategies need not be tantamount to wholesale

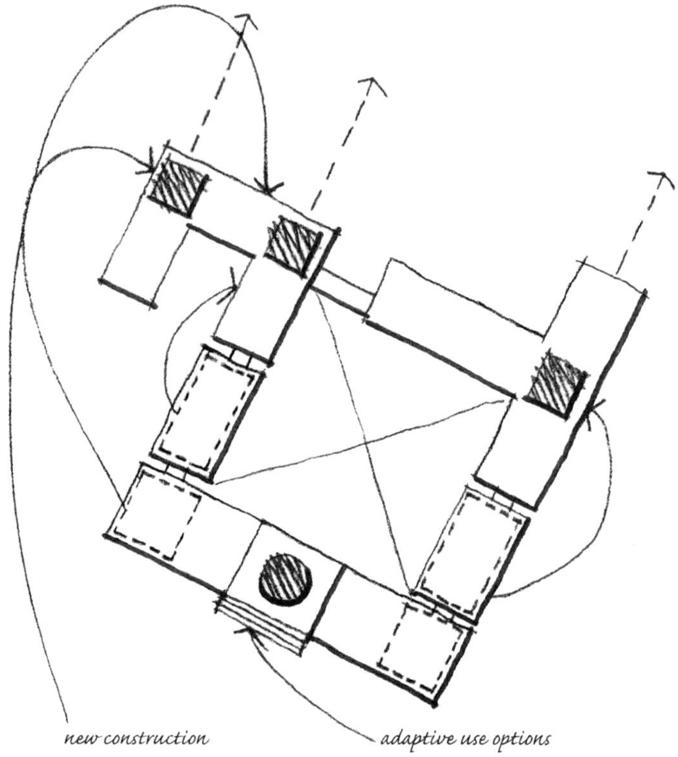

5.2 Prioritize ecological sustainability.

destruction, however. Implement a phased campus redevelopment process as soon as a decision is made to remain in the institution's current location, then proceed to explore multiple, carefully articulated repurposing strategies. The general public is in many cases uninformed of the significance of the cultural heritage about to be obliterated, unless a sincere, participatory consultative process is put in place.[23] In the case of psychiatric architecture, a new facility may be built on a portion of an existing medical campus, for example, as in the cases of the Östra Healthcare Centre for Psychiatry (CS 2) and the Marie Bashir Centre, in Sydney (CS 4). Recent examples of replacement hospitals in rural contexts on land repurposed from an old asylum include the Junction 17 campus (CS 17) and the two case studies of forensic facilities presented in Chapter 6, the Lowry Unit (CS 14), in the United Kingdom, and the Worcester Recovery Center, in Massachusetts (CS 15). The venerable Buffalo State Hospital in New York, designed by H.H. Richardson (1880), has been transformed into a hotel and conference center, with additional space available for conversion to affordable housing and other related future uses.[24]

Adaptive design strategies

Global climate change is a reality, and its existence is extensively supported by dozens of international scientific organizations, including the Intergovernmental Panel on Climate Change (IPCC). The IPCC is an intergovernmental body with a global reach, as it operates under the auspices of the United Nations. Founded in 1988, its principal task has been to provide the world with an objective, scientific overview of global climate change and its political, economic, demographic, and environmental impacts. The IPCC bases its findings on published peer-reviewed literature, and its fifth assessment report was published in 2014.[25] This report concludes that more and more populations will be abruptly displaced as a result of the many and diverse changes that lie ahead, including sea level rise and unpredictable weather patterns resulting in intense precipitation in some places and severe drought in others (see Chapter 1). Correspondingly, evidence-based net-zero and energy-regenerative site-planning and building-design strategies for psychiatric hospitals and related facilities will need to be increasingly responsive to changing local conditions within this new reality because the status quo will no longer apply. In places that will increasingly experience hotter, more humid conditions, endeavor to employ linear building configurations; enhanced cross ventilation, transoms, ceiling fans, and high windows that vent fresh air and cisterns to capture and recycle rainwater together with pronounced overhangs and sunscreens. In increasingly hotter, dryer regions, employ more compact massing, courtyards, and below-grade spaces insulated by the earth, and landscaped roofs with broad overhangs. In increasingly moderate regions, such as across the northern boreal latitudes, employ a mix of pitched and landscaped roofs to capture rainwater while accommodating snow loads, with combinations of linear and centralized massings, operable windows, enhanced thermal insulation, overhangs, and moveable sunscreens. In colder regions, employ a north-south exposure axis tempered to balance internal heat gain-loss ratios, landscaped and pitched roofs, operable windows, heavy thermal insulation, and energy-efficient landscaping and building materials. In increasingly hot, humid regions, shield the structure(s) from excessive direct sunlight by means of deciduous trees planted in related proximity (especially on the south side), together with landscaped roofs and trellises. In increasingly hot, dry regions, employ vegetated trellises, various types of opaque screening devices and shaded patios, semi-enclosed courtyards, operable windows, vented roof configurations, and recycled construction materials. For mental health facilities in increasingly moderate climatic regions, plant deciduous trees to the south and coniferous trees along the north face, and employ windbreaks without negating solar access affordances (Figure 5.2).[26]

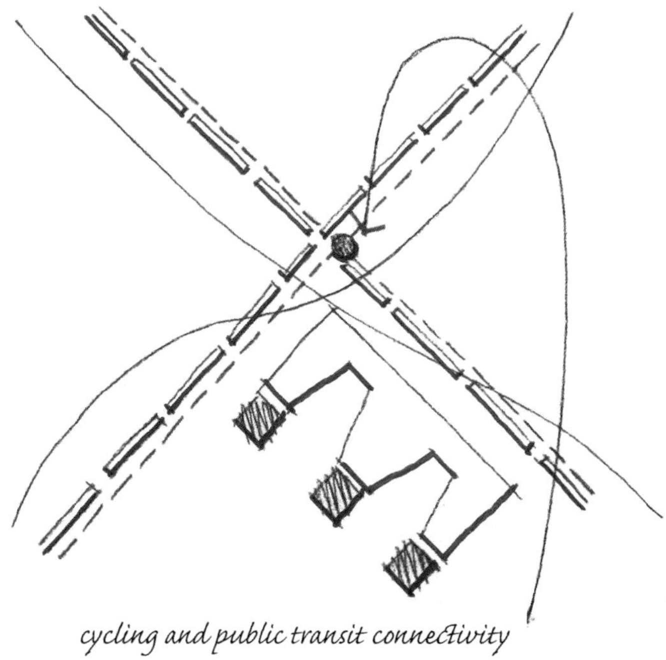

5.3 Provide transit and cycling connectivity.

Cycling and public transit

Historically, asylums were built in the countryside, far from the bustle of town and city centers. The intent was to remove the insane and all other social undesirables from the everyday environment and in so doing disassociate these individuals from normative connections in their past lives. Early on, the roads leading to the asylum were unpaved and difficult to negotiate in inclement weather, with few to no other viable transit options. Supervising staff and direct caregivers often lived near the asylum or on the grounds of the institution. With the arrival of the automobile, on-campus parking capacity was created, and while reasonable provisions were made, official institutional policy discouraged staff from driving to work. The CAMH campus (Toronto, Chapter 4) in time became integrated into the city's improved street transportation grid. These connections, with the recent addition of cycling lanes, are examples of the city's effort to further establish the district's transit-oriented development (TOD) amenities. However, numerous recent mental health hospitals have been built rather remotely from city centers, a pattern attributable to the availability of already-owned or otherwise affordable land (often on or adjacent to the grounds of an abandoned or underused old asylum complex). In these situations, auto dependency prevails (Figure 5.3). Of the Chapter 6 case studies, this was the case with the Children's Centre for Psychiatric Rehabilitation, in Hokkaido, Japan (CS 20); the Worcester Recovery Center and Hospital, in Massachusetts (CS 15); and Kingfisher Court, outside London (CS 1). By contrast, case studies with strong cycling and public rail transit-network links include the Östra Psychiatric Treatment Centre, in Sweden (CS 2); the Professor Marie Bashir Centre, in Sydney (CS 4); the Psychiatry and Behavioral Medicine Unit, at Seattle Children's (CS 19); the Sowa Unit in Saitama, Japan (CS 21); and the CAMH Village Family Health Team Clinic in Toronto (CS 22).

Minimized parking

Most medical center parking garages are aesthetically lacking, to say the least. They are intrusive, monolithic, and difficult to navigate, with the worst examples also posing severe challenges to individuals with physical and cognitive disabilities. The 1960s and 1970s were the glory years of the oversized, domineering medical center parking garage, and this was the case with many hospitals in the Toronto metro area, including North York General Hospital, with its main hospital obscured by a mammoth parking structure built directly in front of it. It is the first thing viewed when approaching the main entrance to campus. This complex was designed first and foremost for the automobile, not for pedestrians. As one winds through level after level, any visual connection with a main 'public entrance' becomes remote and eventually it is virtually lost. Psychiatric and addiction disorder treatment facilities, whether serving inpatients, outpatients, or both, should provide an alternative to a large parking deck. It is countertherapeutic to have to encounter upon first arrival a looming mega-parking deck, not unlike at a large airport, where the deck is the first and last thing encountered. Large surface lots adjacent to psychiatric care facilities can be equally oppressive, forcing long walks to the main public or staff entrance. Mega-surface lots also consume large parcels of formerly open, green space; they impede rainwater runoff and contribute to the urban heat island effect.[27] Alternatively, provide small clusters of surface parking, with a mix of stall sizes, and provide incentives for electric, hydrogen fuel cell, and hybrid vehicle alternatives. Create an unobtrusive presence for all vehicles on the campus to the extent possible through a strategy of smaller decentralized pockets of parking. These zones can be physically screened from direct view from patient treatment areas, meditation spaces in exterior courtyards, dayrooms, dining areas, and inpatient residential units by using berms, screened walls, trellises, vegetated vertical walls, as well as shrubs and trees. It is stressful to have to hear the sound of a vehicle passing in an adjacent driveway, too close to a therapeutic garden or a patient's bedroom, perhaps to the point of becoming a cause of agitation among patients. A 2012 study reported the field-testing of an 'environment of care' assessment scale for the prediction of the propensity of psychiatric patients to attempt suicide during their hospitalization.[28]

Alternative construction methods

The adoption of emerging low-tech construction methods merits careful consideration in the design and construction of mental health and related facilities. These include the adoption of rammed-earth construction methods and the use of restreamed (recycled) waste materials in construction. Rammed earth is an ancient technique employed in the fabrication of walls, foundations, and floors using raw materials such as earth, chalk, lime, and gravel. It represents a reawakening of interest in a long-dismissed method that today is appreciated as being ecologically sustainable. This type of construction is noncombustible, thermally massive, strong, and durable. However, rammed-earth walls and structures can be labor intensive without the local availability of proper machinery (powered tampers), and they are susceptible to water-infiltration damage if inadequately protected and maintained over time. Rammed-earth structures exist on every continent except Antarctica, in environments ranging from the temperate and wet, to semiarid deserts, mountain regions, and in the tropics. Excellent reference sources are available that more fully describe this promising low-tech regenerative sustainability technology.[29] As for health-related applications of these methods, a recent meditation and contemplative center constructed at Stanford University in California (2015) by Aidlin Darling Design features vertical slats and thick, rammed-earth walls.[30] The second low-tech method mentioned, recycled-waste building material technology, has barely been explored in healthcare architecture and, as with most innovations, new ideas tend to germinate in small-scale, nonhealthcare building types. One small house recently built in Ghana (2015) featured rammed-earth walls and translucent windows fabricated from reused potable water 'bladder' packaging. This residence was the winning entry in a student design competition held at a London-based art academy, for a single-family house in a remote village in Ghana's southern Ashanti region. This house, designed by Anna Webster, chose the traditional building method of compacted rammed earth.[31] Many possibilities exist in terms of alternative construction materials and methods, with immense potential to reduce the carbon footprint of architecture for mental health, and particularly in the case of outpatient clinics in medically underserved regions.

2 Arrival, public, and semipublic spaces

Sequenced arrival

An individual's perception of and attitude toward mental health and addiction disorders begins, architecturally, when one first encounters a diagnostic and treatment center. That initial approach – the first impression – is critical. A positive and welcoming image will go a long way, and that first appraisal will be negative if the built environment appears imposing, threatening, or uninspiring. The damage caused by a negative first impression can be difficult to reverse, especially for the reluctant to-be patient about to be admitted for a life-threatening substance abuse or eating disorder. One may already feel as if having 'failed' for reaching such a supposedly low point in life, and a confused or ambiguous 'message' interpreted from or through the physical setting may inadvertently function as a negative reinforcer with respect to the decision to seek out treatment ('Am I doing the right thing?'). An uninviting or inappropriate image may cause one to prematurely reconsider. As previously mentioned, if one arrives by auto, the placement and appearance of the parking area or structure should not visually dominate the arrival zone. But neither should the parking zone(s) be so far removed from the entrance to the facility that access becomes problematic. If one arrives by public transit, an excessively long walk can be equally problematic. It is advisable therefore to provide serialized, layered zones of arrival starting from the edge of campus as a means to draw one inward toward the public arrival zone and main entrance. Design for layered zones as if the building is both literally and symbolically reaching outward, as if extending a helping hand to draw one inside in a nonthreatening manner (Figure 5.4). Achieving symbolic 'outreach' can occur in many ways, architecturally. The Lowry Unit in the United Kingdom has a planar element that

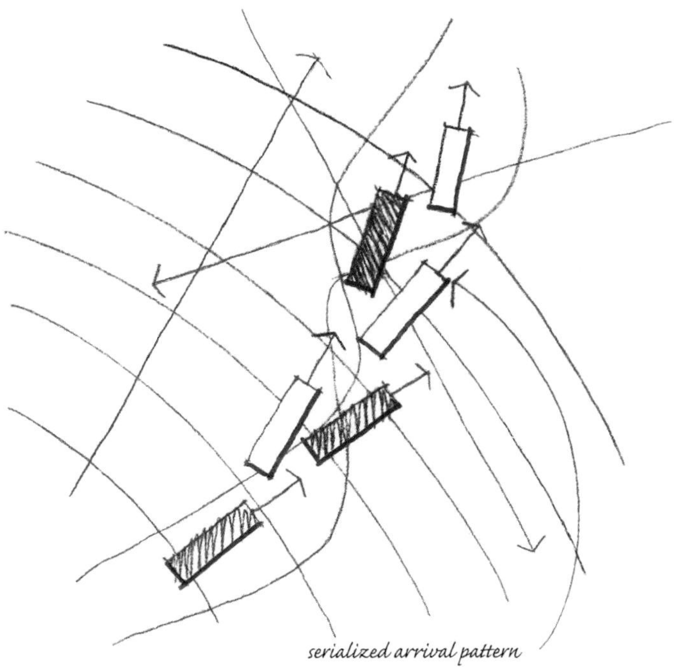

Figure 5.4 Sequence arrival zones.

extends outward, welcoming visitors while identifying its public entry portal (CS 14). The drop-off canopy at the Southdown Institute in Canada (CS 7) provides protection from the elements while aligning the visitor with the center's main arrival axis. Perhaps the boldest strategy among the 25 case studies in Chapter 6 is the large sheltered public arrival zone at the Marie Bashir Centre in Sydney (CS 4), where the entire structure extends outward above the public arrival portal. A canopy drop-off area at or near the public entrance should not be overbearing or too voluminous. The forecourts at Roseberry Park, in the United Kingdom (CS 5), and the currently in-construction psychiatric hospital in Bispebjerg, Denmark (CS 25), are effective in this regard; brick-paved vehicular access drives connect the residential pavilions and various supports with nearby decentralized parking zones. Campus arrival sequencing and interior wayfinding systems, ideally, seamlessly reinforce one another as the individual progresses from the outdoors to various interior zones leading to the inpatient unit and other destinations. Movement through the facility and grounds should not be convoluted nor perceived as stressful, a fundamental theme in the literature on healthcare architecture for more than 30 years.[32] The low-key arrival sequence at the Ballarat Mental Health Hospital, in Ballarat, Australia, by the Billard Leece Partnership (2010) achieves this (Figure 5.5).

Theraserialization

The public realm of a treatment facility and its grounds possesses considerable therapeutic potential, and a design strategy maximizing transparency can be effective, both aesthetically and psychologically, if it does not compromise personal privacy (Figure 5.6). Underwindowed and windowless circulation arteries and associated spaces, especially with incoherent directional signage and inhibited visual access with the outdoors, often result in cognitive disorientation. The directional signage system in many such situations must overcompensate for this disconnect.[33] It becomes needlessly challenging for visitors, patients, and staff, who may often spend the majority of their shift walking about the facility and grounds. A nurse may walk upward of 5 miles during an average 12-hour shift. A drab, lifeless facility, needlessly hard to navigate and visually disconnected from the outside world, can contribute to physiologic and psychological fatigue. Reconsideration is justified, as an aid, to maintain or restore the perceptual and cognitive attentional capabilities of every building occupant. Lobbies, atria, reception areas, corridors, seating alcoves, waiting rooms, and vertical circulation elements such as elevators and staircases impact occupants and can consume as much as 40% of the total facility footprint. Recently, the process has begun to reconsider alternative strategies in this regard. Prior, the corridor was not considered a zone that possessed therapeutic amenity in its own right; it was seen as purely transitory. Yet this is where walking therapies, contact with nature, and informal consults often take place. A recent research study focused on the therapeutic benefits of hallway ambulation among hospitalized geriatric patients Corridors, public seating areas, and semiprivate alcoves are now the common ground where team members are most likely to see one another and interact.[34] These spaces have been a part of the healing environment since the *asclepia* of ancient Greece, with the stoa ward flanking an open-air courtyard. Transparency and visual openness were fundamental for seeing in, and seeing out (Figure 5.7).[35] Achieve a seamless, transparent layering of interior with exterior space in a serialized manner as a continuum – linking the priorities and skill sets of the architect with those of the landscape architect within the emerging discipline of *landscape therapeutics* (Figure 5.8).[36] The Helsingor Psychiatric Hospital (CS 8) effectively expresses this strategy (see Chapter 6). Horizontal theraserialization is being explored, including strategically sloped, diagonalized wall planes that deflect and redirect transmitted daylight from above, i.e. Knittelfeld State Hospital in Austria (2005–2008) by Fasch & Fuchs with Lukas Schumacher.[37]

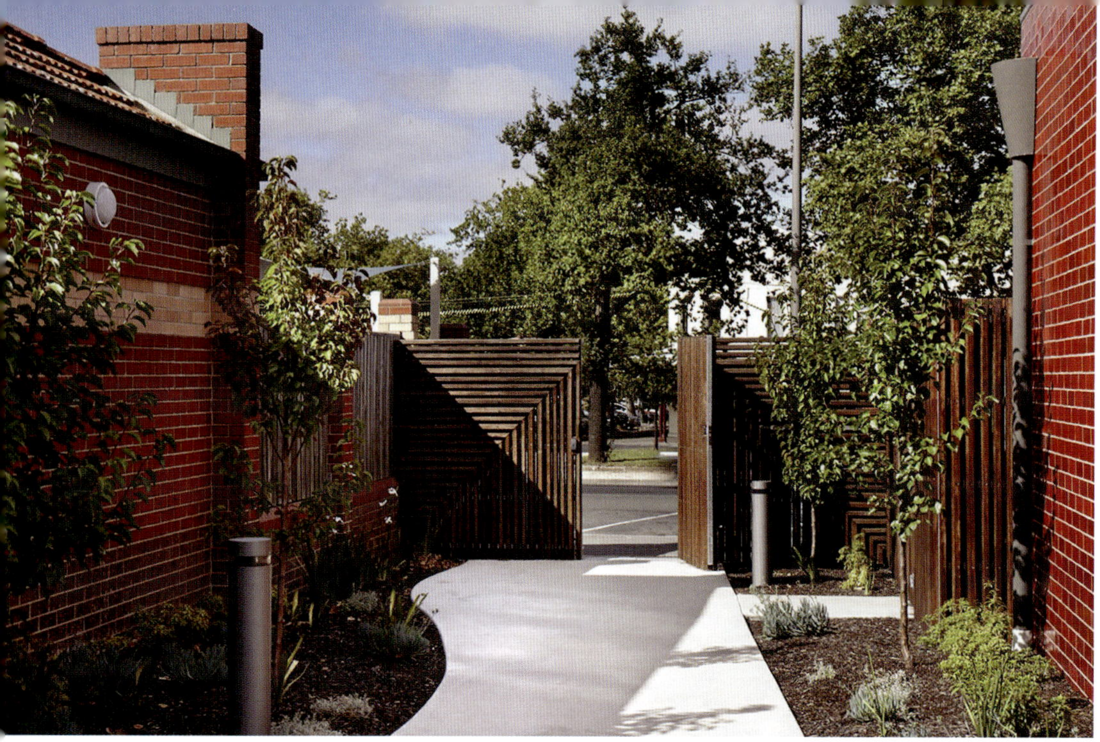

5.5 Serialize arrival spaces.

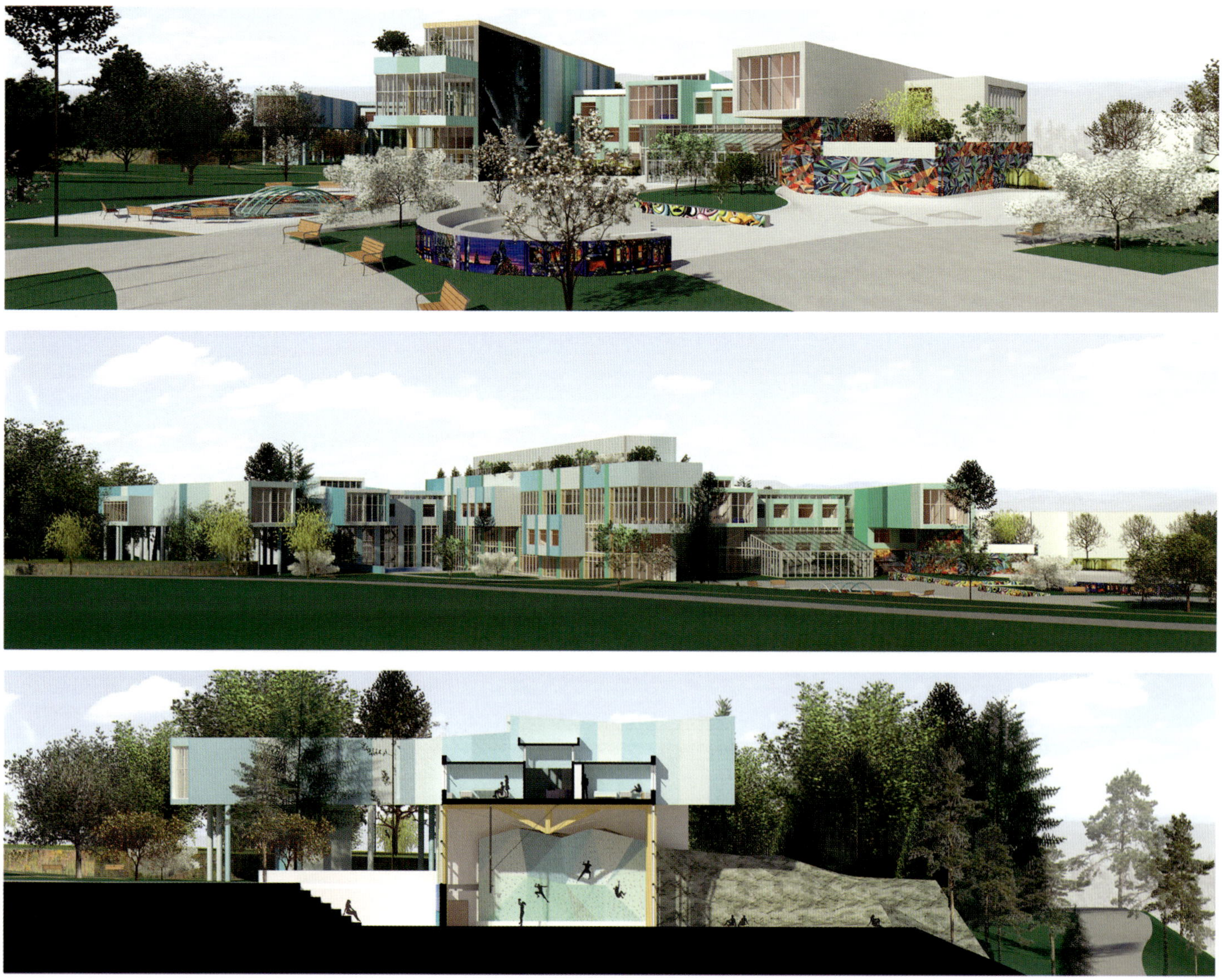

5.6 Theraserialize circulation, residential, and therapy/treatment realms.

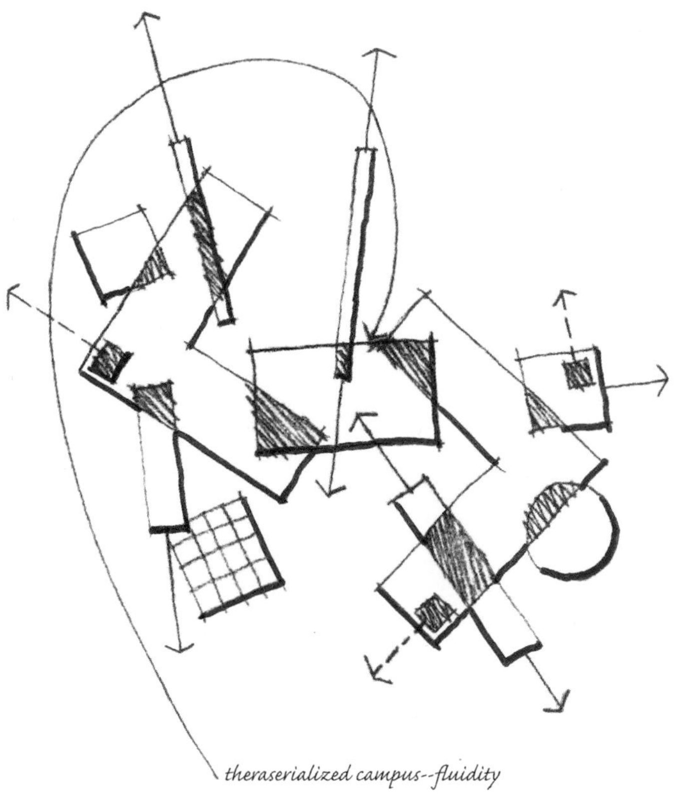

5.7 Establish interior-exterior connectivity.

Hierarchical circulation

Numerous case studies in Chapter 6 feature various 'soft', or intermediary, arrival and associated semipublic spaces. These function as attractors, not unlike symbolic bridges extending outward beyond the facility. Examples include the 'pedestrian mall' at Worcester in the United States (CS 15) and the main arrival level at Marie Bashir, in Sydney, Australia (CS 4). Nineteenth-century insane asylums' double-loaded corridors were quite dreary and forbidding, by contrast. Their harshness was depicted in numerous iconic paintings, sculpture, and engravings from that era, such as that of St. Luke's Lunatic Hospital in London, depicted in an 1808 painting by Thomas Rowlandson and Augustus Pugin.[38] These spaces were dark and utterly depressing. Today, circulation zones and arteries are able to be quite the opposite: far more commodious versus drab conduits for the transport of people, equipment, and supplies. Beyond this, the provision of multiple path options allows for greater of freedom of choice in self-selecting the most preferred route in a given situation.[39] This can be achieved while allowing for individuals' rapid transition into 'safe zones' when necessary, without shutting down an entire facility. This concept applies equally to public, semipublic, and semiprivate zones. Further, circulation network design requires assiduous planning in anticipation of an individual who may seek to abscond. A balance is possible that is safe and secure without sacrificing privacy, such as the ability to spend time in a small outdoor courtyard or walking the grounds independently, freely. Attention restoration theory (ART), a theory developed by the environmental psychologist Stephen Kaplan, postulates that humans crave the ability to engage with psychologically restorative spaces, spaces and buildings that repeatedly draw us back to them. These predilections are grounded in our interest in seeking out opportunities for positive distractions, and engagement with nature directly satisfies this basic human predilection because it is perceived as relatively effortless and is therefore highly appealing.[40] ART, in theory, calls for hierarchical circulation networks, including alternate routes, affording contact with nature without seeming restrictive or confining. Nonetheless, the safety of patients and staff must not be placed at risk.[41]

Multisensory affordances

The administrators of large, complex psychiatric hospitals and clinics are confronted on a daily basis with the challenge of providing an inviting and human-scaled treatment environment.[42] Design strategies that result in multiple visual landmarks, scalar modulations, art installations, level changes, varied ceiling configurations, color palettes, skylights and clerestories, and differentiated walls and floor surfaces can aid in this regard, creating an interesting environment from a multisensory perspective, an environment that remains interesting upon repeated encounters.[43] The layout at Östra, in Sweden (CS 2), revolves around two large courtyards; the circulation at the High Care Clinic in the Netherlands (CS 13) is a central linear spine with three fingers. The curvilinear pedestrian spine linking multiple zones of the Worcester Recovery Center in the United States is effective (CS 15), as it provides a coherent focal point for a large, complex campus. By contrast, the relentless, formal façade of Bethlehem (Bedlam) Hospital in London, United Kingdom (1647), evoked the grand European palaces and country estates of the 17th and 18th centuries. Internally, its absolute symmetry, overcrowding, and inward focus was stultifying, tantamount to sensory overload – a place to avoid due to its orthogonality, overcapacity, unyielding floor plan, and overall severity made all that much worse by patients' restricted contact with the outdoors. The recently demolished International Style Prentice Women's Hospital at Northwestern University (1975), designed by the celebrated Chicago-based architect Bertrand Goldberg, featured an aesthetic vocabulary

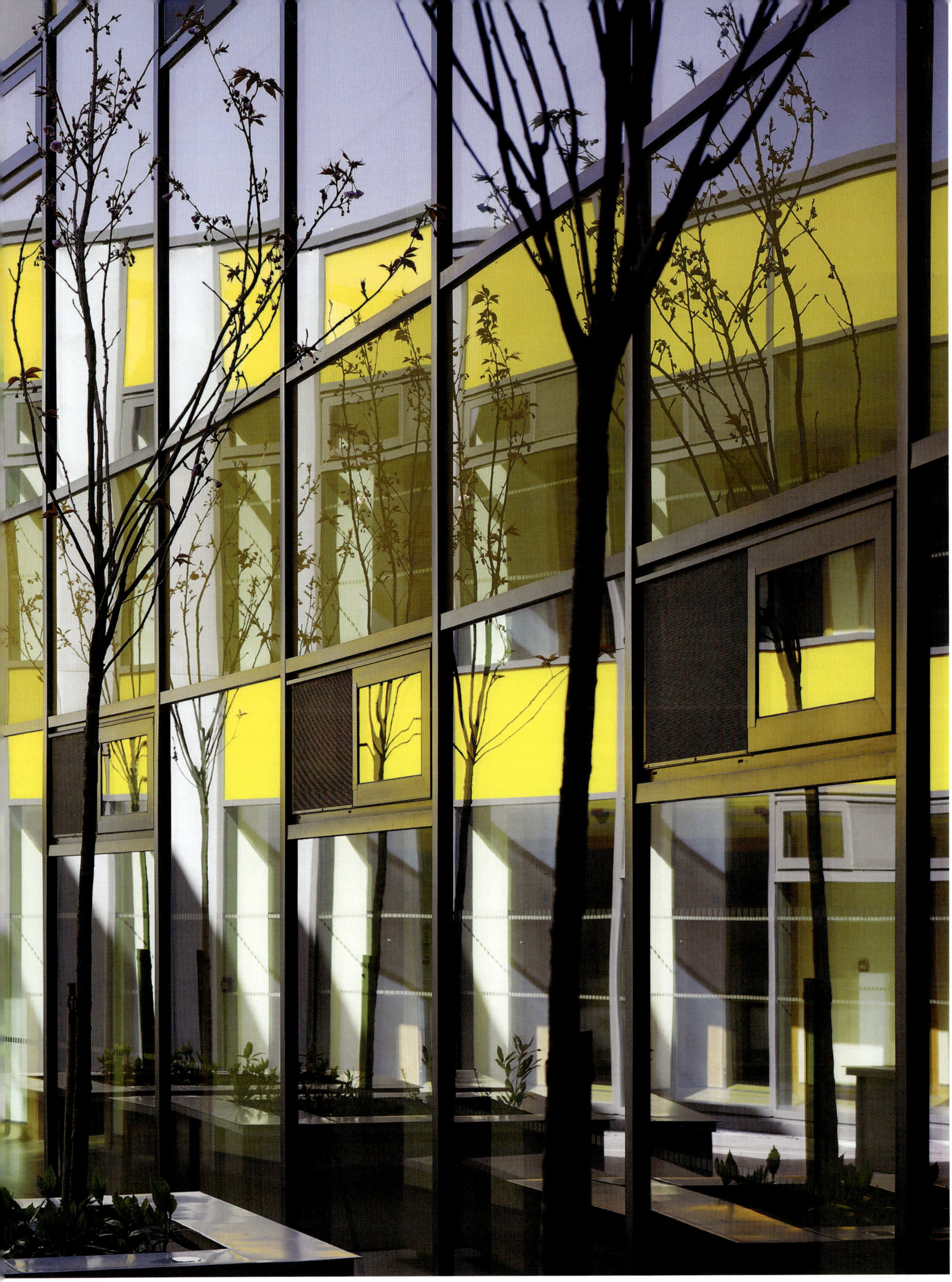

5.8 Incorporate transparency.

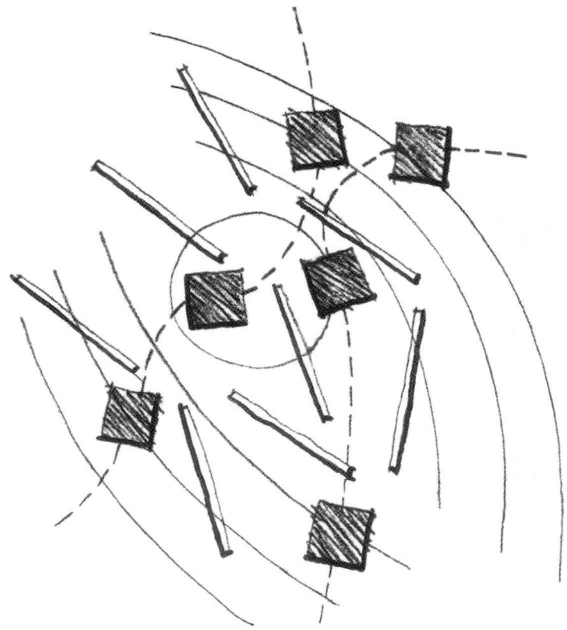

5.9 Multisensory affordances.

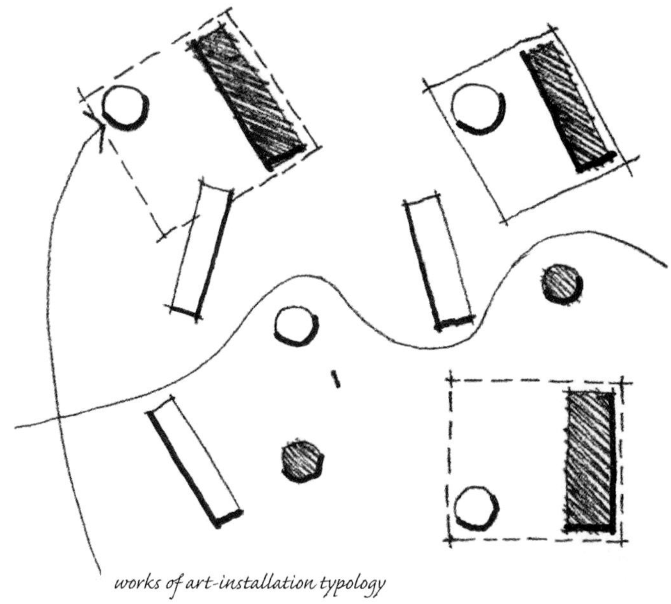

5.10 Art as therapeutic modality.

one might best describe as brutalist and understimulating. Compositionally, it was a nine-level concrete quatrefoil tower with oval windows, cantilevered to appear suspended above a rectangular black 'Miesian' podium cube directly below. The nursing stations on the patient units were located in a central core with the patient bedrooms surrounding it in a panoptical configuration arrived at to minimize walking distances and to maximize visual surveillance of every patient.[44] Patients encountered unusually shaped oval windows, and the views they framed to be psychologically disorientating. The windows in this case and their insufficient view amenity stand as an example of the importance of multisensory affordances in a healthcare environment. Avoid unintended outcomes that may become, upon prolonged exposure, spatially disorienting, such as a deficient view; high repetitiveness; inscrutable, indecipherable forms; chaotic color schemes; low lighting levels; or furnishings and objects that may invoke hostile or aggressive behaviours. Spaces perceived by occupants as psychologically (perceptually) windowless have been empirically found to be the equivalent to a sensory-deprived, physically windowless room (Figure 5.9).[45]

Works of art

Many asylums in the 19th and early 20th centuries displayed works of art and fine furnishings in public galleries and visitors' rooms. Portrait paintings, ornate birdcages, large plants, expensive draperies, and rugs were intentionally meant to contribute to a dignified, socially acceptable atmosphere. These artifacts were also incorporated as a source of comfort, and to morally and spiritually uplift the patient. At a number of institutions, this policy resulted in the accumulation of a significant art collection over time. Such was (ironically) the case at Bedlam Hospital in London, and this was apparently done there and elsewhere to visually compensate for the otherwise sensory-deprived conditions that confronted patients and staff within most parts of the facility. These artifacts were usually confined in their placement, often installed near the main entrance and the superintendent's office. As for the art itself, works were often donated by local benefactors; this usually meant there was relatively little choice as to what could be placed on public display within the institution. Beyond this, some physicians also regarded themselves as fine artists and as such they would donate their works for public display.

Asylum staff sometimes staged musical and dramatic performances, with even lowly ward attendants performing. Theo Hyslop, superintendent of Bedlam from 1898 to 1911, was himself a keen artist who exhibited at the Royal Academy (and later became a controversial art critic). He encouraged the patients there to paint, and he enthusiastically displayed their art.[46] The current trend at many institutions is to bring calming, naturalistic artworks indoors through rotating exhibits of contemporary art or through the display of an institution's own permanent art collection (see Chapter 2). Today, artworks displayed often feature nature and landscapes and expressive media include photomurals, photomontages, large paintings, elaborate textiles, and even electronic media (Figures 5.10 and 5.11). A recent evidence-based investigation found that the psychiatric patients in a community-based arts program most closely identified with art expressing positive and normative meanings – themes associated with self-discovery, hope, and acceptance – as this fostered a heightened sense of self-control and sense of purpose in life.[47] At the Village Family Health Team Clinic (CS 22) in downtown Toronto (see Chapter 6), full-height, abstracted photomurals of forests and waterfalls from the surrounding region are on permanent display throughout. These large-panel installations

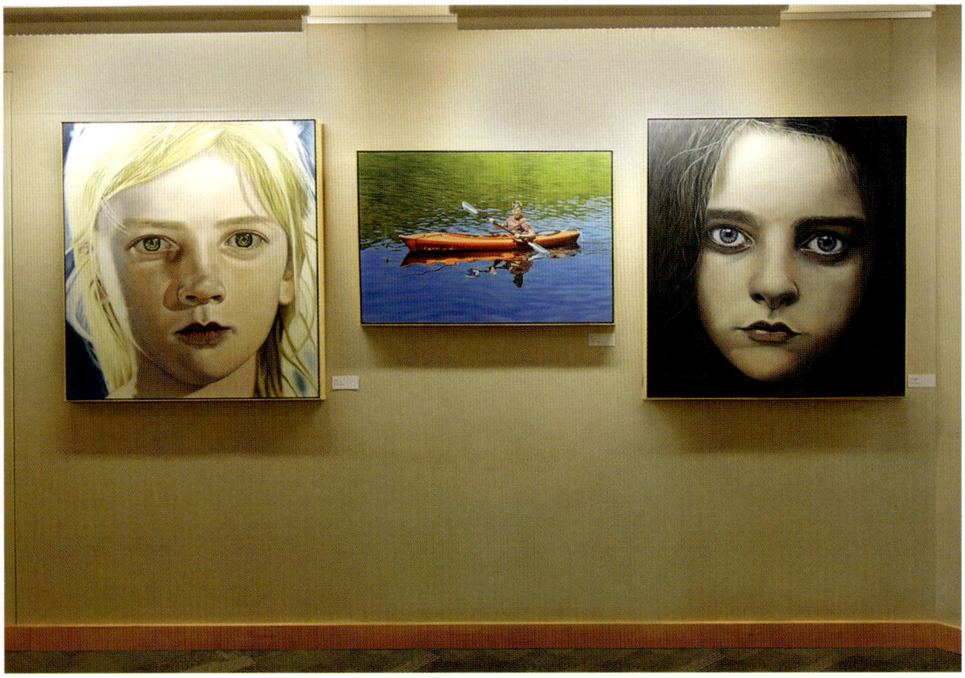

5.11 Display works of art.

are engaging and enlivening, and activate an otherwise minimalist interior decor. Art is often effective in wayfinding behaviour as well, such as at the 325-bed Ontario Shores Centre for Mental Health Sciences (1996) in Whitby, Ontario (see Chapter 2). There, colorful photomurals are permanently installed along a central circulation spine and are effective as landmarks (Figure 5.12).

Meditation spaces

The asylums operated by religious orders included a chapel either in the main building or elsewhere on the grounds. These places were located in proximity to the public entrance and were provided for use by the staff, patients, and visitors. They served as semiprivate places, places to obtain respite away from the chaos of the open wards. The campus at the London, Ontario Psychiatric Hospital (1884), neoclassical in configuration and appearance, included a freestanding chapel. This asylum, designed by Thomas H. Tracy, was modeled on Dr. Thomas Kirkbride's Pennsylvania asylum. In this case, its ornate Chapel of Hope (1884) was built in the Gothic Revival style and was constructed, in large part, with forced patient labor and was in a highly visible part of the campus next to a tree-lined lane, offering magnificent vistas of the grounds. The chapel was prominently sited so that patients strolling the grounds or working the asylum farm could easily see it. It featured a prominently pitched roof with four dormers and exquisite stained-glass windows. Much of the campus was spared demolition and is now protected by provincial heritage-status regulations. It was closed in 2014 after 144 years of continuous operation.[48] The Kalamazoo, Michigan, Michigan Asylum for the Insane (now the Kalamazoo Psychiatric Hospital), opened in 1859, was also a Kirkbride asylum and its original structures are gone, having been replaced in the 1960s and 1970s. It once featured a prominent chapel on the grounds.[49] Most recent residential mental health and substance addiction treatment centers provide a space for meditation and related activities. The meditation chapel at the Southdown Institute (CS 7), north of Toronto, is in proximity to the main arrival area (Figure 5.13). Its soaring ceiling and large windows overlook a wooded semi-enclosed court.[50] Spaces for prayer, meditation, and personal respite tend to be used frequently. Progressive inpatient and outpatient treatment centers now feature one or more such spaces for formal or informal use. Provide options, balanced with security, safety, and personal privacy provisions. Minimize intrusive noises and judiciously select and arrange the furnishings, built-in or otherwise. Include works of art where appropriate. When feasible, connect these spaces to adjoining exterior spaces by means of a patio or terrace, with vegetated screens, building setbacks, level changes, trellises, and seating to buffer unwanted visual intrusions.

Multiple dining options

In inpatient psychiatric and addiction disorder treatment settings, multiple dining areas are often provided – for patients, located on the unit; a second in a central dining room, shared by all and located in a semipublic zone; and a third, smaller-scale staff-only

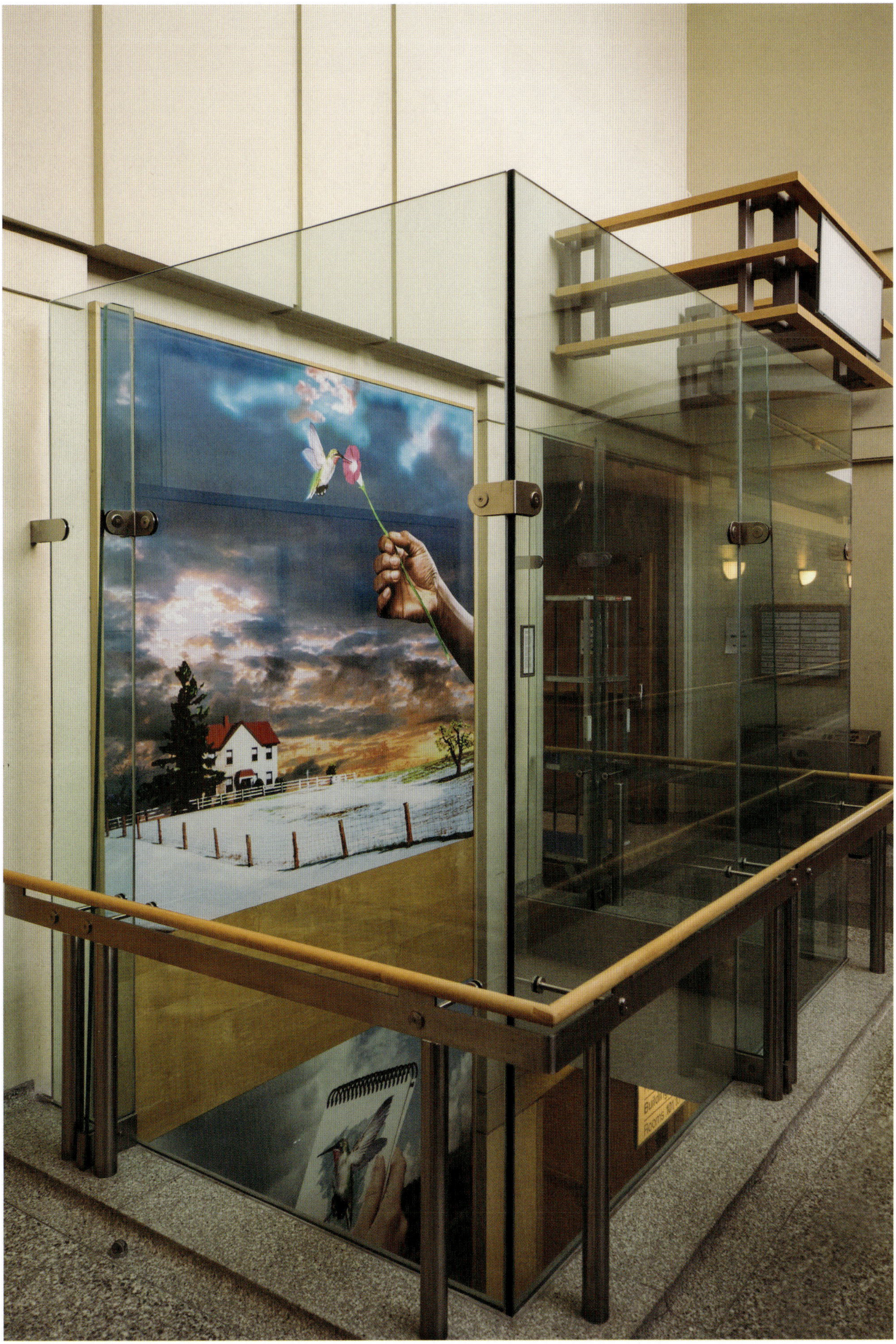

5.12 Incorporate art as a wayfinding device.

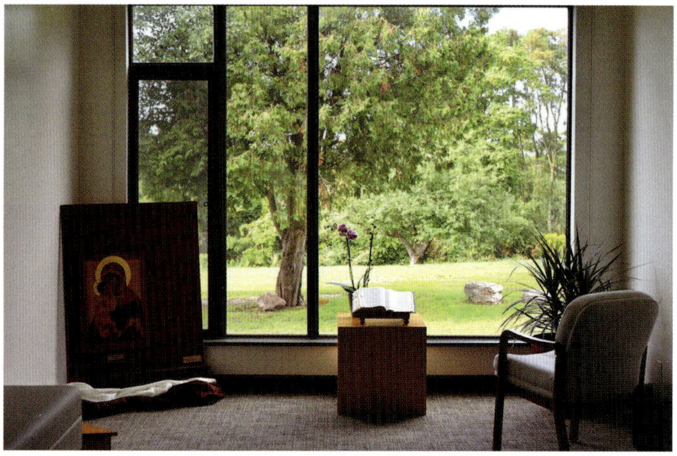

5.13 Incorporate meditation spaces.

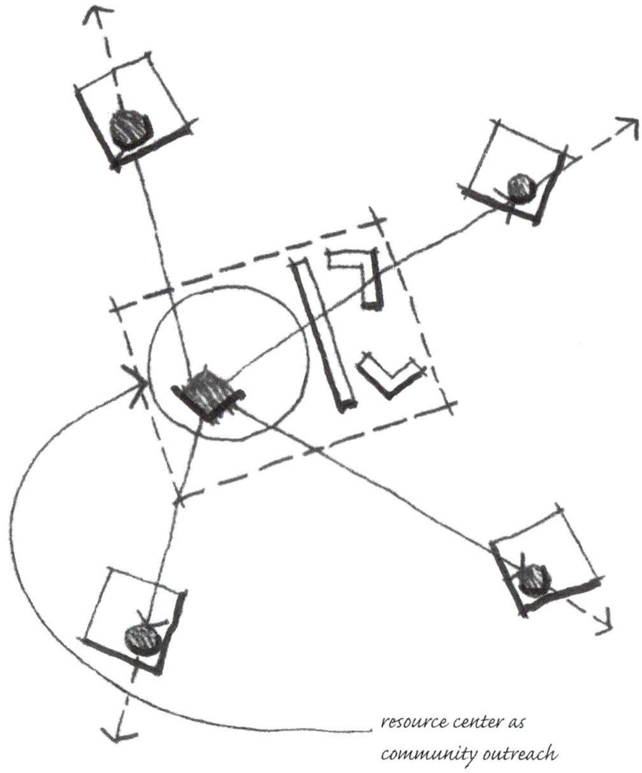

5.14 Engage the community in lifelong learning.

dining area, such as a break room located away from the residential unit. Dining is an opportunity for social interaction, although too often the facility is not designed to properly accommodate all three types of settings concurrently. They are often noisy, with floor, wall, and ceiling surfaces unnecessarily reflecting and amplifying sounds. Excessive noise levels, combined with the absence of privacy, may make it difficult to spend time in these places. This can render an otherwise attractive and well-appointed dining space unappealing to those for whom it was intended. Unfortunately, such drawbacks can overshadow aesthetic appeal, and a view overlooking a lawn or garden does not necessarily negate this functional deficiency. Similarly, being in proximity to a public lobby or recreational gym is just as undesirable. Such conditions will often result in retreat. The dining areas at Östra, in Sweden (CS 2), overlook open-air courtyards, and the main dining room at Junction 17 in the United Kingdom (CS 17) features a full-height mural of a forest scene. Variable ceiling heights can contribute aesthetically, as is the case at Junction 17, and in a larger space, a folding partition wall can subdivide it into multiple smaller spaces. Furnish these spaces to support diverse events, including musical concerts, plays, art exhibits, film screenings, and local organizations' scheduled meetings (i.e., 12-step meetings).[51] Mitigate unwanted noises and other distractions without shutting out nature (i.e., views to the outdoors or a patio or terrace). Create an inviting atmosphere with normative color palettes and lighting types, with adaptable, durable, varied furnishings, so individuals can self-select seating configurations.

Resource centers

The recent literature on schizophrenia and related mental disorders and on emerging fields such as neuropsychiatry underscores the importance of the on-site resource center. A well-designed center houses educational resources in a supportive, attractive space while simultaneously embodying the care provider organization's community outreach mission. The asylum had a single, cramped room called the 'Medical Library', sometimes housed in the basement, housing the institution's collection of medical texts and scientific journals, a collection often off-limits to the patient. Contemporary health resource libraries encourage use by multiple constituencies. Where once only technical materials were housed, today a broad range of resources are accessible in hard copy and online. Preferably locate these functions within the social activity zone at the heart of the campus along a main circulation artery or near a central dining room. Design them as semi-open, with an age-appropriate zone for children and adolescents, with reading areas and comfortable seating and tables, and with the collection displayed on shelves and in stacks near computer stations. Create an inviting atmosphere. One or more full-time librarians staff these centers, with assistance provided by volunteers. Provide one or more offices, an adjacent conference room, with (in larger institutions) an auditorium; for patients, provide for confidentiality and personal security and safety. From the perspective of the public, also provide the option of privacy. Locate the resource center within a larger constellation constituting the social activity/community outreach resources of the campus, in proximity to the main entrance. Avoid noisy, highly trafficked areas or recreational activity zones (i.e., gymnasiums) and remote locations that are difficult to find (e.g., in the current CAMH library in downtown Toronto), while equally avoiding conditions that invite absconding. Alternatively, house the resource center in a commercial storefront, not unlike a small grocery or neighborhood branch library, again, without compromising personal safety or security (Figure 5.14).

Noise attenuation

Excessive noise directly impedes effective cognitive functioning, especially with respect to prefrontal cortical processes. In a recent experiment conducted in a psychiatric hospital, an overall mean sound level of 75.68 dB was recorded, with peak sound levels as high as 85–90 dB – a sonic range that can induce significant hearing loss. These noise levels, higher than comparable levels documented in general hospital medical, surgical, and intensive care units, call for greater attention to the deleterious effects of noise on hospitalized patients with acute psychiatric symptoms. Pagers and alarms are particularly intrusive in psychiatric treatment settings, and excessive noise levels are widely considered to have an adverse impact. For this reason, architects are well advised to devote sufficient attention to noise attenuation during the facility-planning process.[52] Hospital-generated noise has been studied for both its deleterious psychological and psychological impacts, including increased respiratory rates, heightened blood pressure, increased heart rates, and increased psycho-emotional stress levels. While music and ambient soundscapes can help to some degree to mask intrusive, potentially harmful sounds, this itself can dissolve into high distraction for the patient.[53] Uncontrollable noise can exert equally unhealthful outcomes in acute care hospitals, with their intrusive intercom code alerts and pager systems, alarms, bedrails, telephones, ice machines, pneumatic tubes, carts, and bedside medical alarms.[54] Designers need to be cognizant of recent design interventions to reduce adverse and disruptive impacts of such sudden, unexpected sounds.[55] Interfering, distracting sounds in mental health settings are proven contributors to occurrences of medical and nursing errors and in the United States, the Joint Commission for the Accreditation of Healthcare Organizations (JCAHO) cites noise as a chronic risk factor across a broad range of healthcare facilities, including psychiatric facilities.[56] Patients and families can help in their own way to control the unwanted consequences of excessive noise by informing the attending staff and the administration of any particular sources found to be especially annoying or grating or a source of agitation among patients.[57] As Florence Nightingale cautioned, 'Unnecessary noise is the cruelest absence of care.'[58]

Therapeutic colors

A residential or clinical facility with stark, monolithic, or drab spaces can adversely impact patient anxieties, with such conditions tantamount to a condition of sensory deprivation. Repetitiveness in the form of monotonous, undifferentiated surfaces was the norm in the modern psychiatric hospital and was clinically justified on the basis that such conditions' cleanliness and supposed 'purity' was of therapeutic amenity. Today, many care providers prefer a normative, naturalistic, or residential aesthetic in terms of color palettes. One replacement psychiatric hospital in Canada (2015) has been the subject of rather harsh critiques since opening day by the psychiatric staff for this very reason – its pervasive monolithic, all-white color palette is considered by some psychiatrists on staff to be a cause of numerous hostile outbursts among the patients.[59] Unsurprisingly, the topic of color palettes in psychiatric facilities continues to be a much-debated although still little-understood phenomenon. In 1931, Siegfried E. Katz, of the New York State Psychiatric Institute and Hospital, published a study in the *Journal of Applied Psychology* called 'Color Preference in the Insane'. In this early evidence-based investigation, 134 hospitalized patients were tested for their color preferences among six colors: red, orange, yellow, green, blue, and violet. No black, white, or shades of gray were found to be preferred and blue was found to be most popular. Men, in the aggregate, favored green, although female patients were divided between green, red, and violet as their most preferred color choice.[60] The literature on this remains far from conclusive today. That said, interpersonal differences among patients and staff representing different nationalities and cultures are to be taken into consideration, with the role of culture emerging as an influencer in design. A study in Nigeria conducted in five psychiatric hospitals over a 5-year period (1995–2000) examined the impact of inpatient ward colors on patients' behavioural outcomes. It was found that for 3,125 patients admitted across the five facilities, 73.3% recovered, of which 26.3% had occupied green residential units, 37.6% occupied blue, 5.1% occupied neutralized yellow, and the remaining 4.3% occupied an all-white-walled residential unit. When the units were then regrouped into two colors, namely dull (green and blue) and bright (neutralized yellow and white), out of the 73.3% that recovered, 63.9% were found to have resided and been treated in 'dull' wards and the remaining 9.4% were treated in 'bright' units. It was concluded that dull units had a more positive influence on 'recovery' rates.[61] James Ledbetter, a former psychiatric patient himself, recently launched the Madlove Project in the United Kingdom, where he solicited ideas from other former patients on designing 'an ideal', user-friendly mental health facility. And bright, psychedelic patterns on the walls was one of his foremost recommendations.[62]

Compositional inventiveness

Designers need the freedom to explore – freedom to translate innovative treatment theories and methods into an architecture that affords meaningful therapeutic amenity. This includes using new and interesting building massings and the freedom to incorporate skewing, pulling, pushing, slanting, folding, distorting, distending, and otherwise reinterpreting compositional form in new ways. The spatial distortion of wall and ceiling planes and curvilinear geometries are currently being brought to the forefront. These types of surfaces and volumes may on the surface appear counterintuitive – although they continue the ontogeny of rejecting the sterile orthogonality of the International Style psychiatric hospital. Inventiveness can allow for the unexpected to emerge – the unconventional, the ironic condition, to manifest – but only if implemented in a manner fully supportive of the physical and mental health needs and safety of all building occupants. Memorable imagery can be attained through inventive formal intervention, such as the sloped wall planes of the High Care Clinic in the Netherlands (CS 13), the curvilinear footprint of the Linn Dara residential treatment facility in Ireland (CS 18), and the sweeping geometries of the Lowry Unit in the United Kingdom (CS 14). Design strategies based in unconventional geometries and unanticipated spatial adjacencies can be furthered by means of the inventive application of color and material palettes, enlivening otherwise monotonous circulation zones, dayrooms, patient rooms, dining rooms, and therapy/treatment spaces. An unexpected column or a slanted, partially rotated, perforated wall or ceiling plane can be effective if viewed as a source of visual relief, as animated and novel, with such conditions becoming memorable in a positive way in psychiatric treatment settings and especially in facilities specifically geared toward children and adolescents.[63] The danger here, however, is that excessive use of such formal interventions to establish dynamic space can become disorienting or even overwhelming if taken too far in the other direction and may have a deleterious impact on directional (wayfinding) navigation – for example, staircases that progressively narrow in width; irregularly shaped, awkwardly positioned windows; wall surfaces that hover or appear suspended precariously or are too high or too wide; and distorted floor patterns. Excessive design experimentation may become countertherapeutic.

Spatial decompression

The modern psychiatric hospital was spatially compressive and dehumanizing, with its institutional, monolithic corridors, patient wards, and nurses' stations and lack of meaningful informal or in-between realms serving as places for informal social interaction. It was an architecture characterized by subtraction through subtraction: minimalism. Form followed function and function alone. On the other hand, spaces disconnected or far apart from one another can make movement between them difficult and time-consuming, and this can be equally countertherapeutic. Balance is attainable with the freedom currently existing to design a health-promoting built environment for psychiatric and substance addiction treatment that recognizes the limitation of a reductive architectural environment. It is about providing staff, patients, and visitors broader spatial experiences, opportunities, and freedom of choice in a far less compressive, minimalist environment. It is about the building simply *breathing*. 'Breathing' allows the building to become genuinely decompressed, in support of patients' desire for a perceived sense of relative unconfinement while in treatment. This is achievable through a process of pushing/pulling (disassemblage) of various constituent spaces – with such disconnection yielding entirely new types of space, in the process becoming meaningful (in-between) microspaces. This process can reveal spatial relationships otherwise likely to remain unrevealed. Disassembly/reassembly in this manner, in residential units in particular, can yield interesting in-between realms, both formal and informal, as in the case of Sou Fujimoto's Children's Centre for Psychiatric Rehabilitation in Hokkaido, Japan (CS 20). There, the aim was to establish an alternative paradigm, of not always having to use the same room in the same way, with the in-between spaces and zones just as important as the formal 'clinical' spaces.

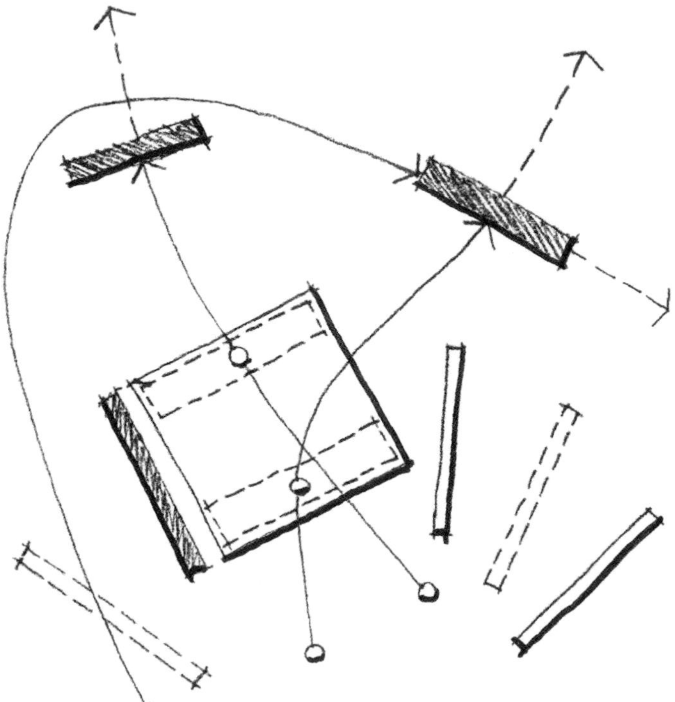

5.15 Achieve spatial decompression.

The provision of decompressed space can breathe life into facilities and their campuses, such as multifaceted courtyards and more informal options to be alone while remaining on the unit (i.e., a small private dining alcove on the unit vs. the main dining room, and small pockets of interior and exterior space nested within a larger space). Spaces that allow for cognitive decompression (refuge and personal choice) are preferred and more inviting compared to those that do not, a concept applicable to psychiatric hospitals and clinics (Figure 5.15).[64]

3 The inpatient care unit

Transitions, doors, and thresholds

The modern psychiatric hospital was about repetitiveness, regularity, and spatial compression. The doors and transitional spaces leading to and through various rooms and zones were often architecturally inconsequential, of relatively benign impact in terms of them having been consciously considered as 'designed' spaces. They often did symbolize, by contrast and often unequivocally, their critical role in establishing and reinforcing separation and confinement. There generally was little transitional space from the publicness of the main corridor to the semiprivacy of a patient's room or dormitory. The overt message was unwelcoming, intimidating, in the extreme. For its part, Hollywood historically depicted psychiatric treatment in precisely this type of setting, from the detox ward depicted at Bellevue Hospital in New York City in *The Lost Weekend* (1945), to the 1995 science fiction film *12 Monkeys*, to the 1999 film *Girl, Interrupted*. This representation of now-obsolescent imagery continues to persist in the public consciousness largely due to filmmakers' continuing obsession with the depiction of psychiatric treatment as a subnormalized human condition – as an altered or 'othered' form of human existence. The shopworn clichés – that is, featureless corridors, imposing staircases, foreboding doors – and associated negative reputation were once well deserved. Transitional zones – door thresholds, circulation elements, and the design of doors as aesthetic objects in their own right – are now receiving focused attention. Recently built facilities feature recessed thresholds color-coded to symbolize the individuality of that room's occupant (Figure 5.16). Single-leaf double-hinged doors, sliding pocket doors, and double-leaf (major-minor door) configurations allow for further design experimentation. In the latter, there exists a primary door and a secondary door, with the primary (major) door three feet in width and the secondary (minor) door approximately one half its width. This allows one door to be closed and controlled from the interior side of the room while the other is controlled on the outer (corridor) side (see Chapter 4). A further option, although less practical, is a door-within-a-door configuration, with the primary door containing a smaller (cutout) door within it. This smaller 'hatch' door is controllable from only the corridor side. The door and its threshold, regardless, still continue to harbor medieval connotations not unlike the small hatch doors of the panoptical asylums of the 18th century (e.g., the Glasgow, Scotland lunatic asylum [1810] with its small latch door in the prison cell-like doors through which food was pushed through to the hapless patient-inmate on the other side).[65]

Graduated territoriality

The concept of graduated territoriality is antithetical to the tradition of the restraint room, where the patient is closely monitored until he or she is deemed sufficiently calmed and able to exhibit a semblance of self-restraint. This does not mean that restraint rooms are no longer needed, because they still are in certain situations, but only in extreme circumstances. In programs

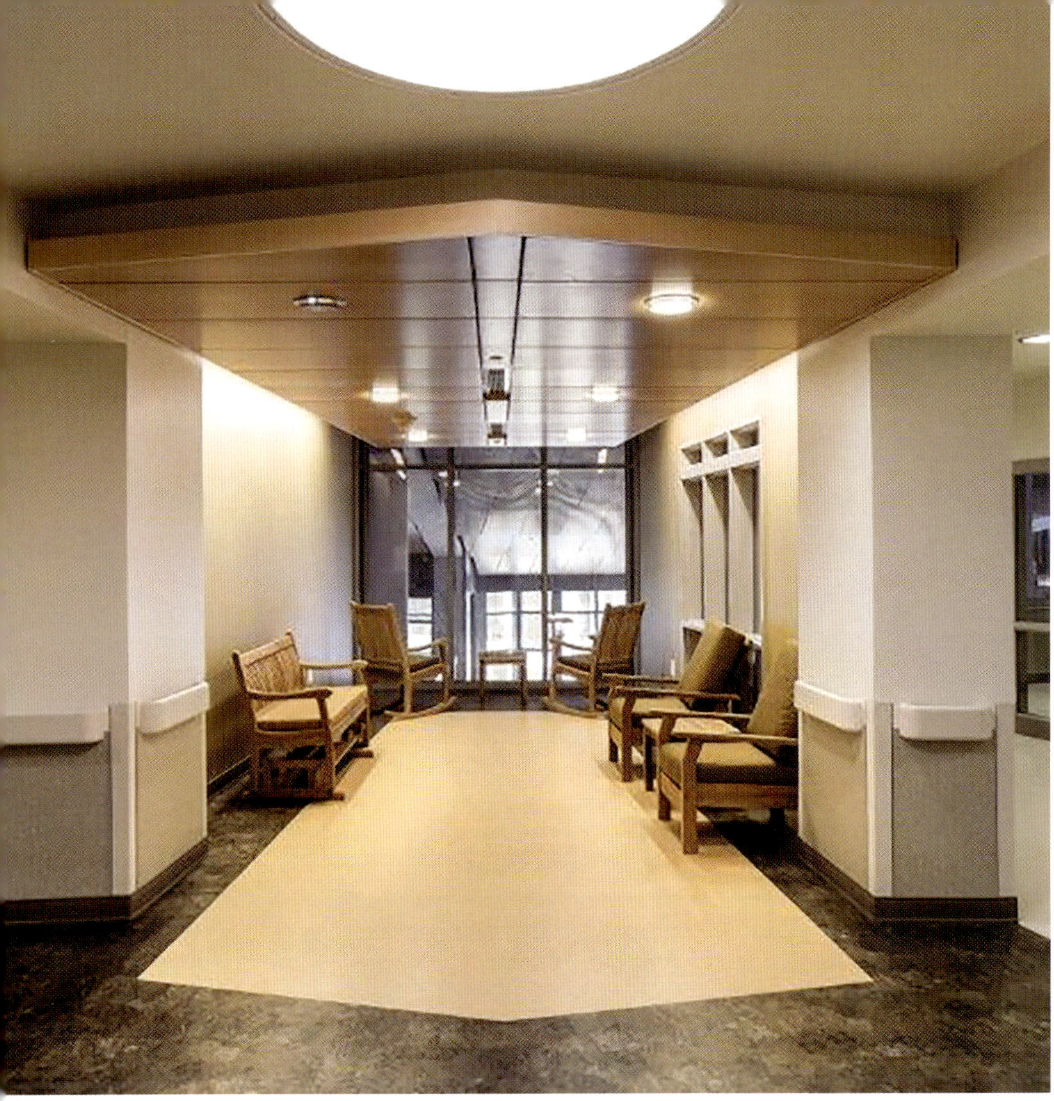

5.16 Transitional spaces near (and on) the unit.

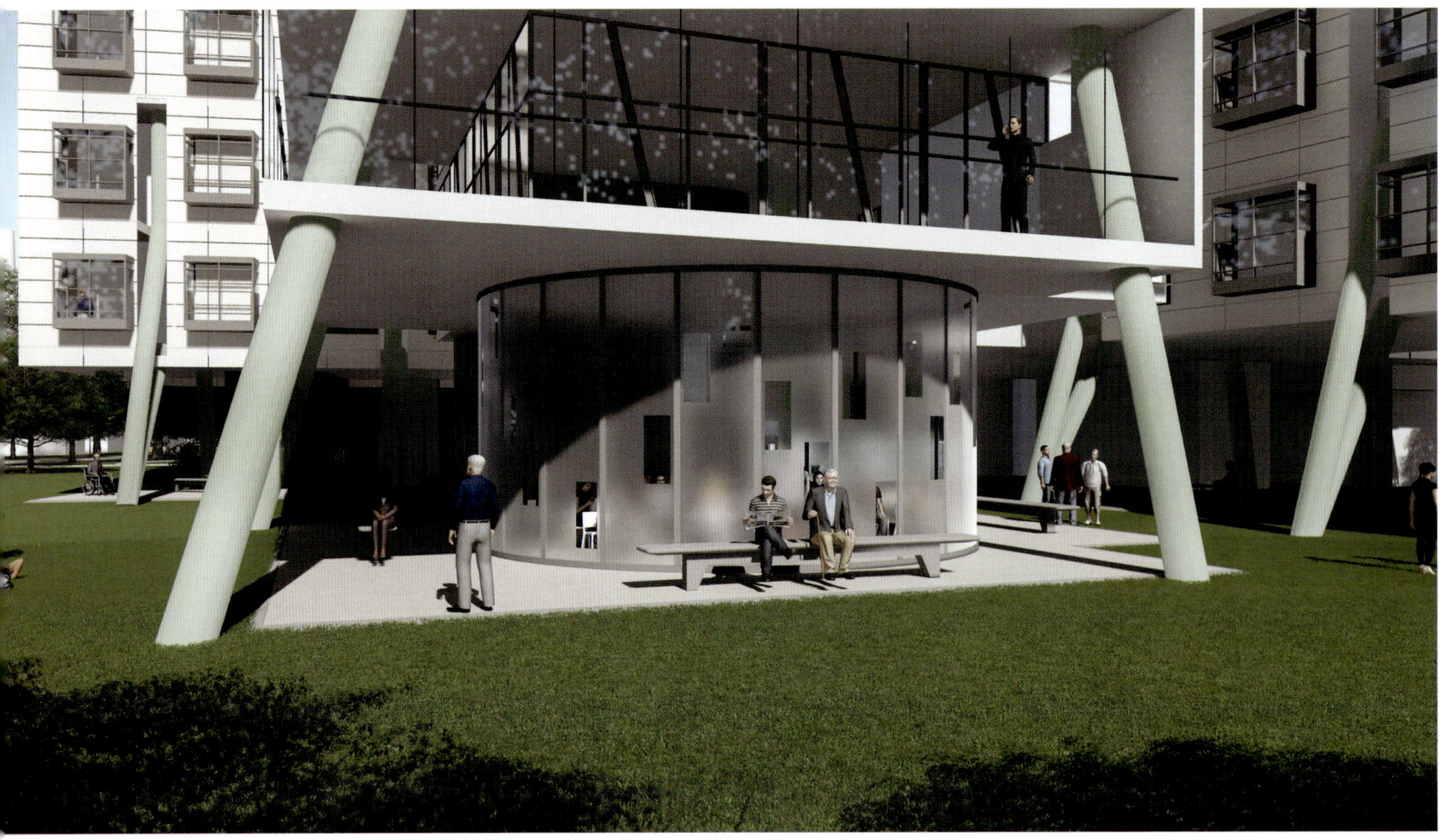

5.17 Provide multiple destinations points, such as a multipurpose gallery.

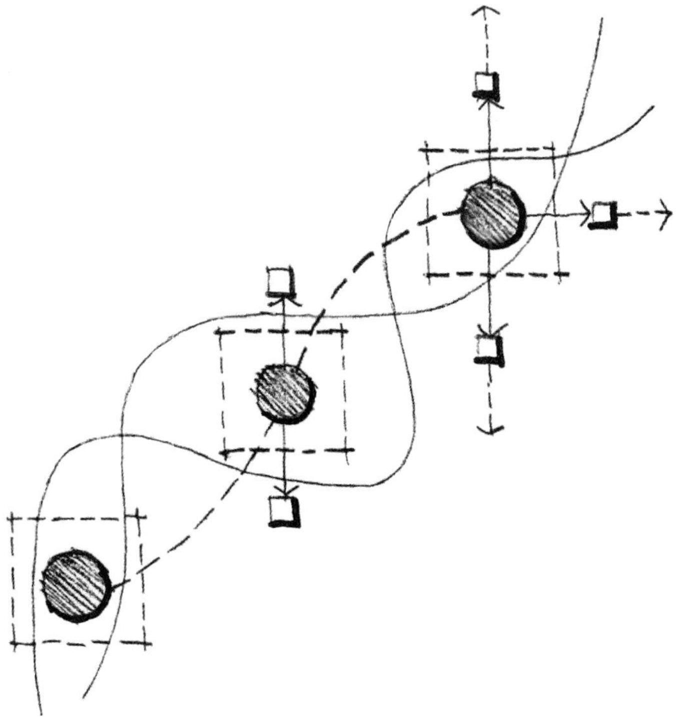

5.18 Graduated territoriality.

where a behavioural reward system exists, patient behaviour is far more often linked with a corresponding increase in the individual's personal rights and privileges. These additional rights and privileges are coordinated with an expanded range of spatial movement within the facility and grounds, as long as the individual demonstrates being capable of handling this added responsibility. Expanded freedoms are bestowed, therefore, as one *earns* additional privileges. The alternative CAMH proposal (see Chapter 4) features a ground-level rotunda in support of this graduated-territoriality concept (Figure 5.18). Recent evidence-based research on this issue suggests that policies resulting in extreme restriction on spatial movement continue to exacerbate increased levels of aggressive (and violent) incidents in psychiatric units. These findings further suggest that direct care providers should implement unobtrusive monitoring policies associated with graduated spatial freedoms through natural observation or other methods, without diminishing the patient's sense of control, independence, or self-dignity.[66] In stark contrast, the nurses' station in the modern psychiatric ward shielded the staff behind fixed-wire glass and locked doors, with the patient restricted to the outer confines of the ward. Movement was typically not permitted to off-ward therapy and observation rooms, or beyond, unless the patient was accompanied by a staff person. The philosophies of service providers have evolved to the point where, now, graduated ripples that symbolize the patient's unfolding freedom of movement within the facility and its grounds are to be encouraged by organizational policy. This can be aided by means of unobtrusive visual surveillance, with the patient moving about relatively freely.

Informal observation of this nature can occur within the parameters of a graduated sphere of increased patient spatial movement, in tandem with a rewards system. However, these policies will not always be possible, especially where a 24/7 high-security level is required, such as in forensic facilities (Figure 5.17).

Symbolic interactionism

Symbolic interactionism theory was developed by the social psychologist Herbert Blumer in the mid-20th century and retains currency in the context of mental health and addiction disorder treatment environments. This theory is premised on the centrality of how a patient actively shapes the narrative within her or his physical surroundings, rather than the patient existing as a mere passive participant, or observer, watching the unfolding flow of events. Blumer's mentor, George Herbert Mead, developed the origins of this theory some years earlier within the field of phenomenology.[67] He postulated a person's social construction and understanding of 'reality' occur through a process of continuously filtering multiple perspectives in an effort to articulate a unified synthesis. This implies that the patient exists not in the physical space composed solely of those constructed realities, but in a world composed of perceived 'objects', with these objects falling into one of three types: physical objects, social objects, and abstracted objects. Blumer distilled this into three fundamental tenets: first, humans act toward people, objects, and places on the basis of the meanings they ascribe to those things; second, the interpreted meaning of such things is derived from, or arises out of, the social interactions one has with others in one's immediate world and then with society at large; and third, these meanings are filtered through an interpretative process constructed by the individual as a means to cope with those sets of people, objects, and places encountered on a daily basis.[68] As such, virtually every physical feature of a physical setting, from the color of the walls, to the quality of the lighting, to the condition of the furnishings, is subject to its appraisal as 'good or bad', 'hostile or friendly', 'us versus them', and so on. By extension, an excessively institutional setting will likely elicit negative responses, whereas a salutogenic, compassionate, supportive setting will likely elicit a more positive appraisal. For instance, the patient will symbolically transact with the people, objects, and places in his or her immediate life while in treatment and will then, accordingly, make a determination as to whether these 'objects' are acting 'for' or 'against' him or her. Because of this, a worn-out, tired-looking facility with its torn, dilapidated sofas, chairs, and light fixtures and burned-out bulbs will likely be negatively appraised. This adverse verdict is extendable to apply equally to the people around oneself, with an adverse appraisal of the facility possibly tipping the balance toward an adverse behaviour taken out against others.[69]

Suicide prevention and materials, finishes, and equipment

Most suicide attempts occur within the first 3 days of admission, and approximately one quarter of all actual inpatient suicides occur within the first week of admission.[70] A determined individual will persist in finding a way unless the staff can intervene on a sustained basis, if need be the case. A core corresponding architectural issue is the degree to which the built environment is to look and feel 'normal'. This equally corresponds to the perceived openness of the facility and its surrounding grounds. It would be inadvisable to provide normative residential furnishings in a setting occupied by violent offenders because this would only provoke the furnishings' weaponization. Many caregivers assume such acts can and will occur, regardless. The normalization of the treatment setting, and the establishment of quasi-residential atmosphere, tends to result in fewer physical separations and requires a higher mutual trust factor, with the goal of the physical setting not having to replicate the old psychiatric hospital it replaced next door. The greater freedom of choice (control) in the new facility may result in a more positive (likeable) appraisal, with a greater probability for less aggressive acting-out behaviour ('Because there are no security windows at the nurses' station in this new building they seem to think I am not such a *bad* person after all'). Whether or not a progressive design strategy is adopted, every single item selected and every color choice carries direct consequences. Certain materials, finishes, and equipment items convey intrinsically positive messages, while others carry intrinsically negative messages: 'How far should the designer go, aesthetically and functionally, in creating a residential atmosphere?' 'Will the well-being of the occupants be placed in jeopardy if I swing the aesthetic pendulum too far away from the visibly secure conditions and regimentation of a *hospital*?' This requires an assessment index, or metric, perhaps something such as a *tempered materiality endurance factor*, or TMER, which would be an evidence-based score assigned to a given item's durability, resiliency, and aesthetic appearance quotient, reflecting the probability of its weaponization. A metric of this type might also take into consideration, during the design phase, the intended occupant's *perception* of the item (in its proposed application) within that item's total TMER score, which would represent, accordingly, a rating of its overall appropriateness relative to numerous other factors. Items subject to consideration can be pretested in a facility mock-up simulation context prior to actual construction.

Absconding

This is the act of running away, escaping, or of leaving the grounds unbeknownst to the administrative staff. It involves leaving under unpermitted conditions and often involves the individual running away and hiding or going somewhere where he or she is provided shelter or refuge. This behaviour dates from the earliest prisons and insane asylums. In England in the 17th century, patients who escaped from Bethlehem Asylum (Bedlam) in London were returned, if caught, and often harshly punished for their transgression.[71] Escaping the asylum became a pastime for some patients (and remains so), and sometimes these actions are aided and abetted by corrupt staff personnel. In the past, the formidable stone wall surrounding the asylum kept away the curious, mischievous, and those with harmful intent – while keeping inside those judged as incapable of safely living out in the community. Entrances to the grounds were strictly limited, controlled, and allowed only sanctioned persons to pass through. Similarly, only sanctioned equipment and supplies passed through the portals, although they often provided a clear way out for the absconding patient. Absconding continues in institutions around the world. A 51-year-old patient at Toronto's CAMH, diagnosed with paranoid schizophrenia, in 2001 walked out freely into the neighborhood for 14 hours before returning of his own cognizance, after having strangled a 41-year-old unit nurse to death; he was found not criminally responsible. It was the second such incident in a 3-month span at CAMH. That unit had supposedly been on 24/7 lockdown, with patients disallowed from leaving without a physician's note.[72] The judicious placement of open-air courtyards surrounded by protective residential units and support spaces is integral to numerous case studies presented in Chapter 6. These include the Vermont Psychiatric Care Hospital (CS 6), the Lowry Unit (CS 14), and Junction 17 (CS 17). Upper-level roof terraces can also function to inhibit absconding in this manner, with the building itself compositionally bracketing open exterior space while simultaneously functioning as a perimeter barrier. Other case studies employing this design strategy include the Marie Bashir Centre in Sydney (CS 4) and the psychiatric hospital under construction in Bispebjerg, Denmark (CS 25).

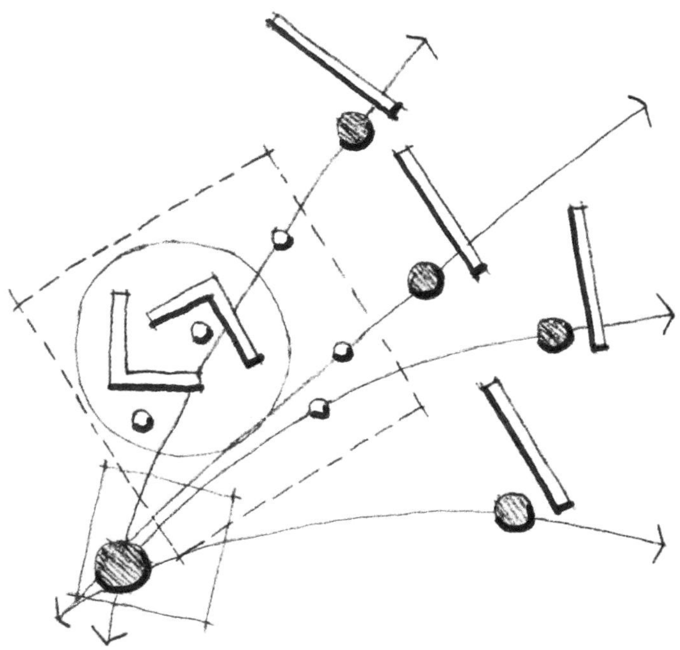

5.19 Workstation hybridity.

Workstation hybridity

The modern psychiatric hospital perpetuated policies that in some ways differed remarkably little from those governing the neoclassical open wards of a century earlier, including those that governed the design and construction of panoptical asylums.[73] The locked-in, fixed-wire glass, fortress-like nurses' station provoked patients' heightened levels of aggression, contributing to instigated acts of violence perpetuated against the staff and against other patients – with many a chair, table, or other weaponized object being smashed through the glass. The staff workstations at Ontario Shores in Canada (1996, Chapter 2) were originally completely open in plan, but later had to be closed in behind shatterproof glass. The preferred standard in many institutions now is to provide options – to provide more than one workstation, from a space nearly fully open in plan and appearance (nonsequestered), to a space least open in plan and appearance (highly sequestered). Residential units featuring multiple workstations within a decentralized hub-and-spoke network allow for staff to self-select their degree of contact with the patient, and vice versa. Being sequestered 24/7 behind shatterproof glass needlessly perpetuates the archaic *us versus them* status hierarchies of the old custodial institutions. Openness, with minimal physical barriers separating the direct caregiver from the patient, is preferable. However, when retreat becomes an absolute necessity, there must exist a safe zone that is readily accessible; this calls for workstation hybridity, which calls for design solutions that nest multiple interrelated workstations within one another, almost telescopically.[74] This can consist of a configuration of two (or three) types of workstations on the unit – the most open of which is simply a desk or counter, with the other(s) providing securable (locked) workspace. This strategy responds to the continued debate over the optimal degree of openness of nurses' workspaces on 24/7 residential units.[75] No longer will a one-size-fits-all approach suffice. The hybridity of the staff workstations at the Marie Bashir Centre in Sydney, Australia (CS 4), epitomize this. There, an open, unprotected desk is complimented by a second, fully securable workspace nearby. Recent digital technologies enable care functions to be decentralized and far less intrusive. With hybridity, staff functions are dispersible to interdependent workstations (Figure 5.19).

Medication administration

A psychiatric medication (PM) is a controlled psychopharmacological substance exerting an effect on the chemical makeup of the human brain and the central nervous system. Since the 1950s, these medications have been used in the treatment of a broad range of mental disorders, decreasing the necessity of long-term hospitalization in many cases (see Chapter 2). Broadly defined, there are six types of PMs: *antidepressants*, for the treatment of disparate disorders including clinical depression, dysthymia, anxiety disorders, eating disorders, and borderline personality disorders; *antipsychotics*, for psychotic disorders such as schizophrenia and mood disorders; *anxiolytics*, for anxiety disorders; *depressants*, including hypnotics, sedatives, and anesthetics; *mood stabilizers*, which treat bipolar disorder and schizoaffective disorder; and *stimulants*, which treat attention deficit hyperactivity disorder and narcolepsy. Medication administration (MA) is a central focus of the unit's designated medication nurse. The practice of MA involves directly interacting with most, if not all, patients on the unit, and this procedure is therefore highly interrelated with patient and staff safety. Nurse-patient interactions provide opportunities to develop rapport, resulting in a heightened level of mutual trust, and a well-designed MA station can have a positive impact in fostering mutual patient-staff trust.[76] In MA, there is involuntary and voluntary compliance. In the latter, a medication window or station is located at or directly adjacent to a staff workstation. The medication room is a secure space typically equipped with freestanding steel shelving racks, with rows of bins. The patient comes to the window to receive a dosage; the most highly trafficked dosage dispensing occurs right after breakfast, after lunch, before dinner, and after dinner. MA is time sensitive, providing the patient the opportunity to ask medication-related questions on a one-on-one basis. An abrupt attitude conveyed by the attending nurse can adversely impact patient behaviour, and in a recent study conducted in three inpatient psychiatric units, nurses who exhibited short-tempered behaviours with their patients or who did not fully explain why the patient's med type or dosage level was changed (while standing at the MA window station) resulted in a significantly higher occurrence of aggressive behaviours among patients, and subsequent higher levels of MA noncompliance.[77]

Code-alert responsiveness

The prevention of aggressive incidents, along with effective suicide-watch protocols, is essential.[78] To assist in this, hospital emergency codes are used in psychiatric hospitals worldwide to alert staff and others to various types of emergencies and incidents occurring on the premises.[79] Code alerts convey information quickly and with minimal interpretative misunderstanding among staff, while preventing stress or panic among visitors (and other patients). The institution's code lexicon is posted on walls and is often printed on employee identification badges for ready reference. In Ontario, Canada, the code-alert categories in 24/7 psychiatric facilities are as follows: black (a bomb threat or suspicious object), blue (cardiac arrest or medical emergency involving an adult), brown (in-facility hazardous spill), gray (evacuation or crisis), green (infrastructure loss or failure), orange (disaster), pink (cardiac arrest or medical emergency involving an infant or child), purple (hostage situation), red (fire), white (violent or highly aggressive person), and yellow/amber (missing person or child). When a patient becomes violent or otherwise out of control, staff personnel must lock down the unit or that larger portion of the facility occupied by the patient at the time of the incident. Staff must reach the scene of the event as expeditiously as possible and without undue obstruction attributable to any design or construction feature in the physical environment. This applies to routine daily operations as well as in the event of a renovation project that may shut down one wing or floor for a significant period of time. All such obstructions are unwarranted and bear life-and-death consequences. The various zones within the facility must be securable so staff can quickly deploy in code-alert scenarios. Therefore, being cognizant of the role of the built environment is indispensable, and simulation training is one effective tool as it exposes the staff to multiple possible scenarios. A 2012 report surveyed 519 psychiatry residents in 13 psychiatry medical residency programs across the United States to learn of their experiences in this regard. Of the 204 residents who responded, 175 (86%) indicated they had been threatened at least once, 145 (71%) reported being physically intimated, and 51 (25%) indicated they had been physically assaulted at least once, with the vast majority of these incidents occurring on locked inpatient units.[80] Often, it is a matter of the attending staff being alerted beforehand to the most probable (and improbable, for that matter) facility and campus-wide escape routes. Oculus Rift and similar recent simulation technologies hold promise in training staff personnel to more adroitly navigate their physical work setting to ensure their own personal safety, as well as that of the patient.[81]

Safe passage

The recent Star Wards project conducted within the National Health Service (NHS) network of psychiatric hospitals in the United Kingdom resulted in 74 findings, or tenets; these are centered on measures intended to establish a greater level of staff engagement in day-to-day work across the total work environment and to enhance patient and staff safety. A 2012 assessment of this multiyear program found numerous areas of improvement, particularly in patient satisfaction, staff morale, effective methods to decrease levels of boredom among patients, and successful methods to reduce the occurrence of incidents of aggression directed toward attending staff.[82] It was concluded, however, that it remains essential for staff to be able to readily obtain refuge in a 'safe zone' (on the unit) and, if

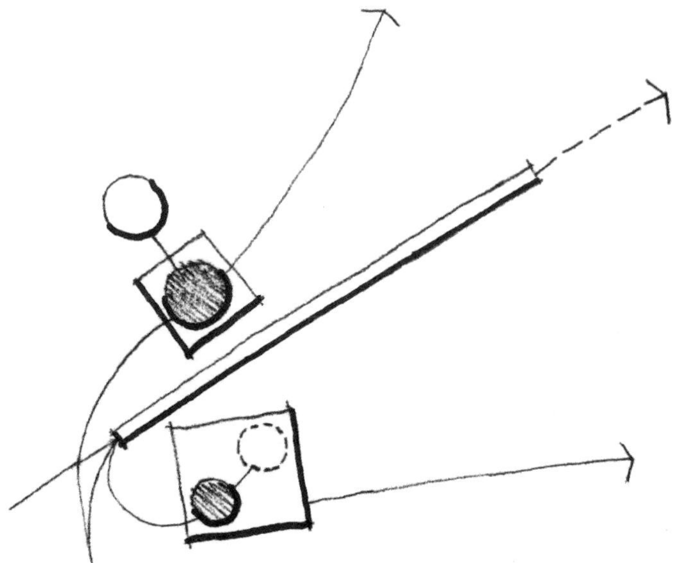

5.20 Provide multiple safe passage routes.

need be, to obtain safe passage elsewhere (off the unit).[83] Regarding implications for inpatient unit design, it is unacceptable for there to be no safe way out, and this holds for virtually every corridor and room in the facility. Accordingly, no one should be able to be 'cornered' anywhere at any time. An empirical study of psychiatric unit layout and amenities reported in 2011 underscores the importance of vigilance in door locking and properly adhering to exiting security protocols on acute psychiatric units.[84] The absence of safe passages off the unit (and conversely, safe passage *onto* the unit to aid imperiled staff) has resulted in many otherwise avoidable violent incidents being perpetrated against staff – and sadly, the legacy of tragic acts perpetrated against staff in mental health institutions has been a harsh reality since the construction of the earliest asylums. Statistics on the occurrence of such adverse events remain surprisingly incomplete even today and therefore inconclusive. Nevertheless, these incidents continue to be treated as nothing short of scandalous in the mainstream press and on social media.[85] The situation in many parts of the world does not appear to be improving either. Moreover, insufficient risk-assessment training of staff personnel occurs in many psychiatric diagnostic and treatment settings. Growing nursing staff shortages are a further contributor, as patients need and deserve the trust and structure provided by a properly staffed and trained professional team.[86] Neither the environmental design nor the health sciences evidence-based literature has drawn a definitive correlation between a unit's physical design and this issue. Regardless, in multilevel facilities, provide staff with a 24/7 dedicated or quickly convertible staff-only elevator, stairs, or bypass circulation arteries as needed in direct proximity for immediate access in lockdown conditions. When this occurs, ideally, adjacent inpatient units must still be able to continue functioning without interruption (Figure 5.20).

Seclusion protocols

Seclusion rooms no longer need adhere to the nearly bankrupt traditions associated with the old *restraint* or *isolation* room. The term 'restraint room' itself conjures negative images associated with suicide watch, self-harm, and violent acts carried out against others. Stereotypically, this space is poorly lit with padded walls surrounding a sole restraint bed at the center. It minimal function was to ostensibly deprive the patient from transforming any feature within the room into a weapon. This space was (and is) for removing the patient from the mainstream unit in order to preclude a violent or aggressive behaviour. A new wave of seclusion, isolation, chill, and time-out areas are being created in diagnostic and treatment settings as part of an international trend to deinstitutionalize the overall residential treatment environment.[87] These spaces do often typically continue to be housed in or near highly secure zones, near the staff workstation. Here, sequestering occurs for a prescribed length of time. The room may have an adjoining bathroom to preclude the patient from reentering the main unit. It may have a bed equipped with restraints, natural light, and soundproofed surfaces. Institutional policies in general discourage the use of these rooms for restraint purposes unless no viable alternative exists, where sequestering is necessitated due to a verbal or physical outburst or abusive incident – particularly when a patient becomes a threat to him- or herself or others. The patient may require seclusion for hours at a time without undermining his or her right to privacy or the opportunity to be in a quiet, still space. Chill spaces and time-out rooms are alternatives, and are increasingly common, without the comparatively high-security requirements of more traditional seclusion or restraint rooms. With the continued deemphasis on restraint usage, having a range of alternative spaces available on the unit or adjacent to the unit for sequestering the patient is important.[88] Besides a high level of soundproofing, wall, floor, and ceiling surfaces should be non-weaponizable without appearing austere. There remains some debate, however, as to the appropriateness of providing a 'residential-like' atmosphere. In a 2005 study of 56 inpatients on an acute care psychiatric unit, a residential-like, normative seclusion room was compared to an austere, hospital-like seclusion room.[89] It was found that residential-like space had a less-positive effect on behaviour than initially hypothesized. [90]

Restraint minimization

There is no need to review here the unfortunate history of inhumane, excessive, harsh restraint apparatus (isolation boxes, chains, clamps, etc.) historically applied to 'treat' those persons deemed insane. By the mid-1850s, proponents of moral treatment advocated for the total elimination of the practice of punitive restraint. Despite this, psychiatrists in Europe and in North America concluded at the time that restraints would never be completely eliminated.[91] Not until the 1990s would this practice once again be subject to reappraisal: 'Is physical restraint a necessary evil?' Media reports persist today of patient deaths and injuries sustained while held in restraints for prolonged periods, as well as of the occurrence of staff deaths caused by patients in association with restraining.[92] It remains a fact that since the nursing staff are held accountable for maintaining the safety of every patient, they often continue to view seclusion and restraint use as a necessary last-resort intervention. And of course the continued tragic, adverse impact of mental and physical assaults on staff must be taken into consideration and balanced with patient safety concerns in formulating an appropriate architectural strategy.[93] There is recent empirical evidence to suggest that changes in a unit's treatment philosophy can result in a positive modification of patient behaviour, resulting in the decreased use of seclusion rooms and restraints.[94] For the patient, injury is an ever-present risk, just as for the caregiver team. In 2014, the American Psychiatric Nurses Association (APNA) published a position statement, calling for effective oversight at all levels of government and private-sector organizations, evidence-based research and practice, and the minimal use of seclusion and restraints premised on the core assumption that every patient has the right to be treated with respect and dignity in a safe, humane, culturally sensitive, developmentally appropriate manner. The individual's self-choice and self-determination are to be maximized, and seclusion and restraints must never be used for staff convenience or purely for punitive or coercive aims. Rather, it must be used for the absolute minimal amount of time, and only to ensure the physical safety of all parties after other, less restrictive measures have already proven ineffective.[95] Individuals secluded or restrained must be allowed maximum freedoms while maintaining the safety of others, with the least number of restraint points (tie-downs) utilized, and under continuous observation. Policies to reduce or eliminate seclusion rooms and restraint usage must be coordinated with the organization's internal culture and implemented in such manner as to encourage preventative and alternative interventions in emergencies, as this will significantly aid in minimizing acts of aggression while promoting the safety of all.[96]

Continuum of comfort space

The patient room is where one can recharge and rest while gathering the wherewithal to reengage the next day's therapeutic regimen. But sometimes the patient may seek out other locations on the unit. One alternative is the comfort, or chill, room. The various options should represent a continuum of in-between places for the patient to relax or, as previously discussed, cognitively decompress. These places are essentially time-out zones, and the caregiver team can suggest them to a patient if an outburst is imminent or about to intensify if not immediately addressed. In a 2012 study on seclusion rooms, restraint use, and assaultive acts instigated by patients, 92.2% of patients who were placed in alternative rooms to conventional restraint rooms found them helpful when they experienced an increased level of distress. With the availability of this type of step-down room for the patient to voluntarily self-manage his or her distress *without being physically restrained*, the caregiver team can then engage in broader behavioural interventions.[97] It is one thing to provide an intermediate chill space, and another for the caregiver team to be trained to make the best use of it. A comfort or chill room is not to be misconstrued; a refuge space, by contrast, is generally a room indoors or an outdoor space where one *voluntarily* spends time, and its use may be 'suggested' but not required by the attending caregiver team. It is therefore recommended that staff caregivers receive appropriate training *a priori* on how to assess the multiple options to make the best use of less formal comfort and chill spaces, versus opting for a more physically intensive restraint room. The need may exist, here as well, to establish a new assessment scale, or metric, perhaps called the *Facility-Attuned Caregiver Engagement*, or FACE, scale. The FACE scale (and composite score) might consist of a continuing-education training module addressing the inner profundities of how to make best prescriptive use of a range of room/space options (Figure 5.21).

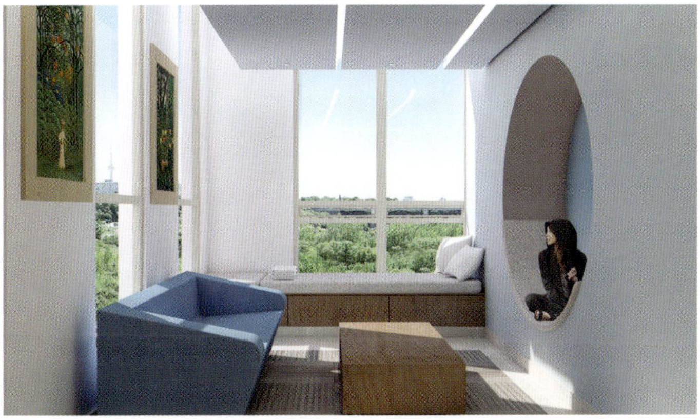

5.21 Continuum of seclusion and chill spaces on (and near) the unit.

Staff respite spaces

The caregiver team requires and deserves a getaway breakroom, and associated outdoor space. A psychiatric and addiction disorders hospital environment can be quite disruptive and unpredictable, depending on the type, age, and acuity of the patient cohort. The inability of staff to obtain privacy, and of always being 'on stage', is stressful in and of itself. The widely cited *prospect-refuge* theory of human involvement with the physical environment, as put forth by the British geographer Jay Appleton in the 1970s, remains applicable in this context, because individuals need a place to obtain periodic, if brief, periods of respite.[98] His theory, by extension, provides a framework for further distinguishing unwanted versus wanted interactions with others within the total treatment environment. Spaces supportive of socialization (prospect) differ from spaces that are territorially uncontrollable.[99] Spaces allowing for privacy and the feeling of getting away are preferred (refuge), and the provision of a range of spaces allows for prospect-refuge behaviours, with physical settings hierarchically nested as a mix of private, semiprivate, semipublic, and public spaces. A number of Chapter 6 case studies express this concept, including Hopewood Park in the United Kingdom (CS 3) with its patios, terraces, and informal getaway places. In Canada, the Southdown Institute's (CS 7) naturalistic central courtyard, and the 'pocket gardens' and roof terraces provided at De Hogeweyk (CS 10) in the Netherlands respond to this need for periodic respite. Prospect-refuge amenity is attainable in one of two ways: first, as embedded staff breakrooms (on unit), perhaps reconfigurable as user preferences change; and second, as autonomous spaces (off unit). In the first scenario, the ability to pull a curtain for visual privacy, rearrange furnishings, self-regulate lighting levels, and provide space for personal belongings can be effective. In the latter, a completely separate room elsewhere, away from the unit/workplace, perhaps with a different aesthetic, can be most effective. An empirical investigation reported in 2009 cited the importance of staff breakrooms with windows and interesting views, as this aids in alleviating stress. A study reported in 2013 called for providing connectivity with an outdoor garden or patio for staff-only use because these spaces are similarly linked to reduced workplace stress

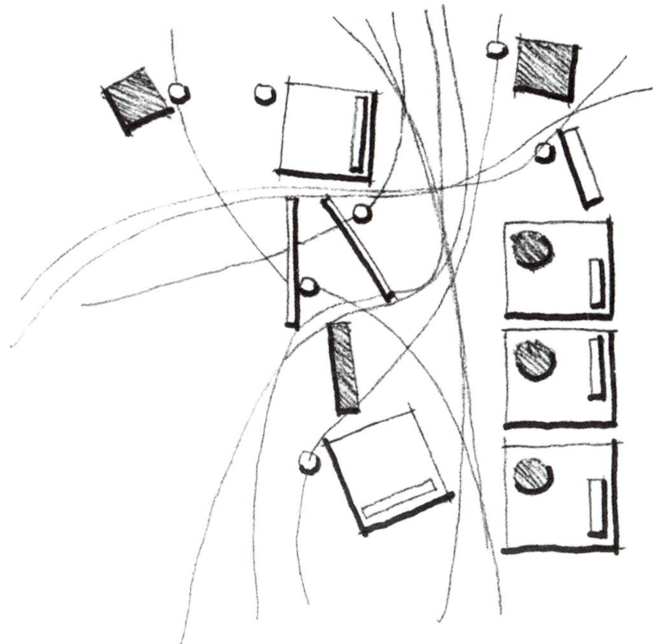

5.22 Examine viewing station typologies.

levels.[100] In a study reported in 2016, nurses deemed high-quality break spaces to be 'fairly' or 'very' important in terms of the potential to have a positive emotional impact on the staff and the patient (and in terms of carrying out facility management protocols).[101]

Viewing stations

Window seats and semiprivate alcoves strategically positioned along circulation arteries and at the end of corridors provide informal places to sit and engage in consultation, or simply function as *viewing stations*. When near the unit, yet not physically within it, they provide for short retreats without having to travel far. As places for social interaction when situated between more than one inpatient residential unit, they symbolize a transitional, in-between zone (Figure 5.22). In community hospitals, unfortunately, few places such as these exist. This is usually because the circulation realm is considered strictly utilitarian, transitory, and therefore a financially poor investment on a per-square-foot (or meter) basis compared to areas that 'directly' serve patient care needs. This bias is unwarranted. Occupants' exposure to interesting views of nature from within hospital circulation zones has been found to have a positive influence on spatial navigation and, by extension, helps ameliorate what might otherwise devolve into a stressful situation.[102] Semiprivate viewing stations are therefore ideally positioned along paths near (or within) the inpatient treatment unit. Insert them in between clusters of perhaps three to four patient rooms in either single-loaded or double-loaded unit plan configurations or at the end of a corridor; provide large windows – transparency – without compromising patient confidentiality. Alcoves need be no more than 5 feet deep to accommodate a built-in window seat and a wheelchair. When

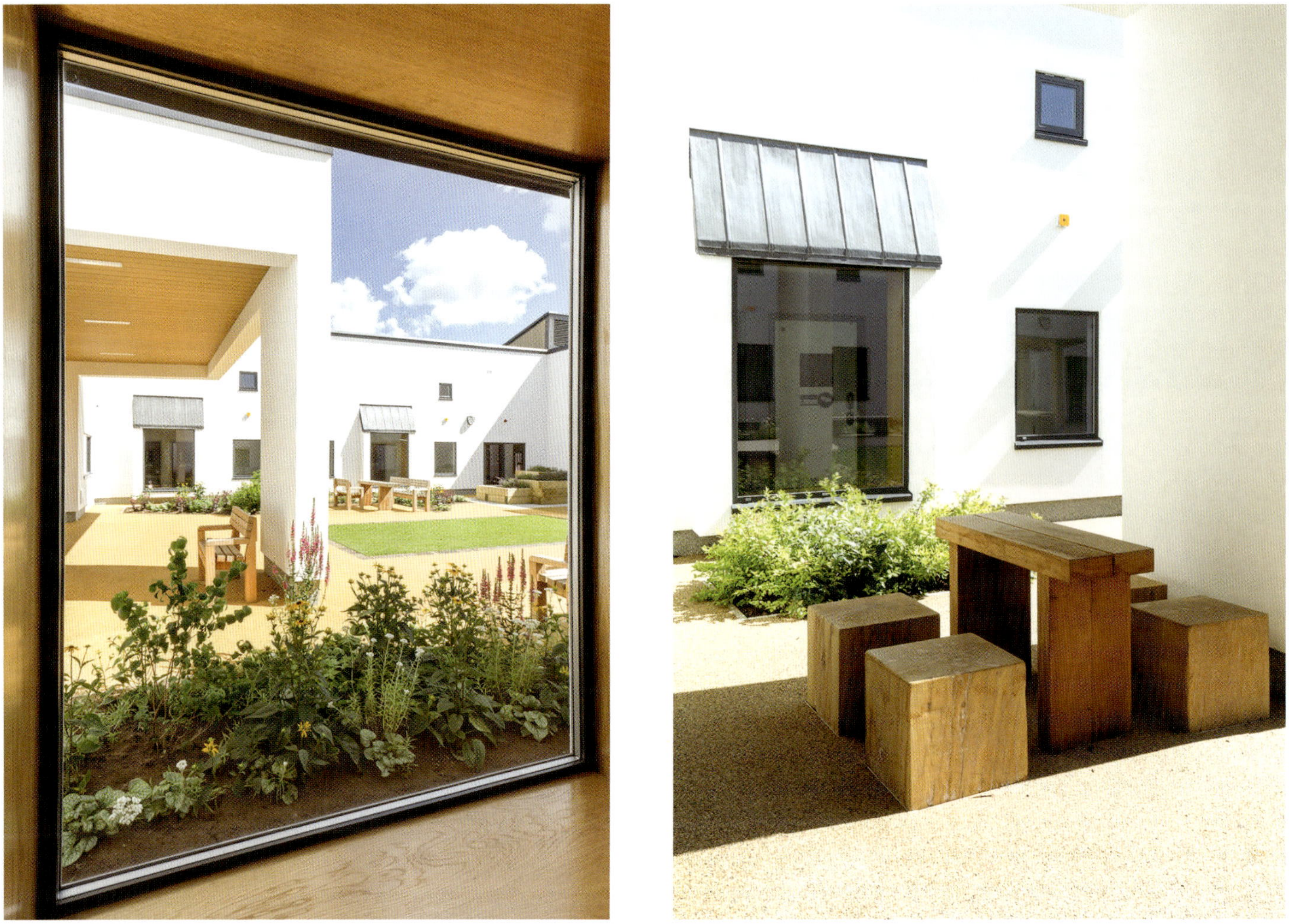

5.23a–b Windows overlooking interesting courtyards.

outdoors, the viewing station functions as an exterior 'room' extending the interior realm outward, a place for quiet contemplation and consults, perhaps sheltered and positioned between building wings, or on a rooftop garden terrace. Inventive landscaping enhances their function and memorability by means of vertical gardens, trellises, or plantings or by being located inside a winter garden. De Hogeweyk (CS 10) in the Netherlands features numerous indoor and exterior viewing stations of this type. Hopewood Park (CS 3) also stands out for its four exterior courtyards, each one with (interior-side) window seats positioned around the space – two such courtyards each feature six window seats stationed around the perimeter, thereby inviting year-round use as weather permits (Figure 5.23a–b).

Dayrooms

Dr. Thomas Kirkbride, in his 1854 book *On the Construction, Organization, and General Arrangements of Hospitals for the Insane*, considered prominently located dayrooms of fundamental importance.[103] Dayroom spaces have prevailed, providing a setting for diverse activities ranging from group therapy sessions to social events such as birthdays and anniversaries, dining, and a host of recreational activities. A wave of studies was conducted in the 1950s and 1960s on their optimal location and configuration in the modern psychiatric hospital. A main focus of this research was their amenity in encouraging social interactivity. These studies focused on furnishings, seating configuration, and the proxemic-visual relationship to the nurses' station.[104] Interestingly, some findings from this period remain relevant today. Regardless of the whether the facility is classified as high, medium, or low security, the dayroom symbolizes an important function and is essential in the daily life of the residential unit. These spaces are most often at the end of a corridor or situated between or across from clusters of patient bedrooms and staff supports. The nurses' station is often nearby, allowing for direct observation, 24/7, but the desire for direct adjacency is becoming noticeably less important in recently built facilities. The dayroom itself is therefore now relatively free to unrestrictively function as an attractive, autonomous space – to foster socialization and provide a change in scene. The dayroom/living area is no longer a boring

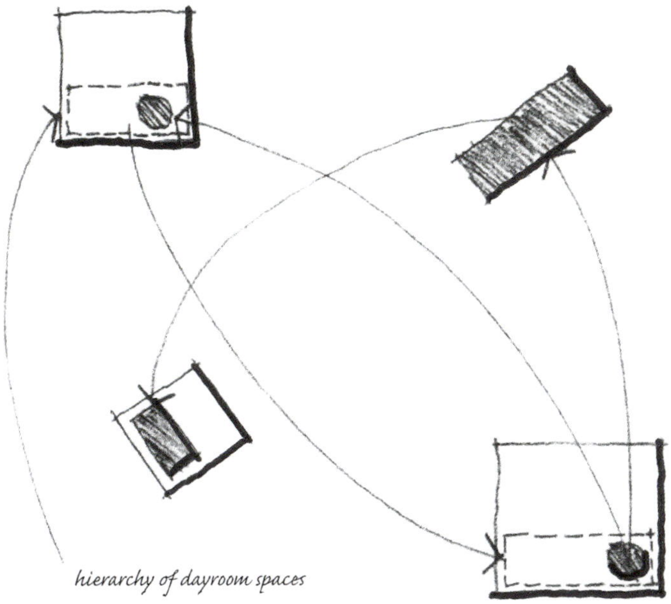

5.24 Day/activity rooms in and near the residential unit.

room down at the end of the hallway. It can function as the central activity hub – connecting private, semiprivate, and public realms, perhaps featuring multiple zones within a main room and ancillary rooms or zones serving specialized needs, for example, with one space (or room) serving as a media center, another as a small group space, and a third space connecting to the outdoors, such as a terrace or balcony (Figure 5.24). In one-level facilities, these zones may open directly onto courtyards. They function as protected, semisequestered space. In multilevel facilities, it is recommended that balconies and roof terraces are also fully explored for their feasibility in this regard. A hybrid dayroom/living space can function as the common ground between the unit and staff supports, such as at the Glenside Hospital, in Adelaide, Australia (2013), by Medical Architecture and Arts Projects, Ltd (MAAP) (Figure 5.25).

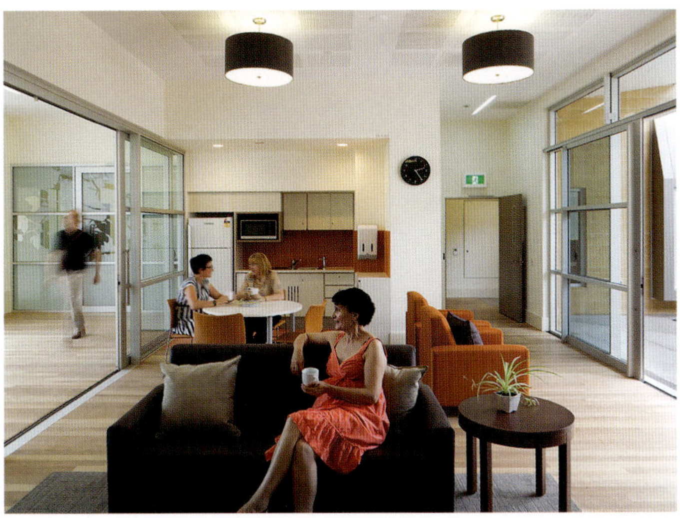

5.25 Explore day/activity room hybridity as common ground.

Geriatric psychiatry

This specialized area addresses the assessment, diagnosis, and treatment of complex mental health and addiction disorders that commence later in life, or those that originated earlier in life but persist into later life. Unfortunately, mental illness can appear in this stage of life, complicating psychiatric or substance abuse treatment. Aged patients are often treated for comorbidities, such as dementia, mood disorders, verbal and physical aggression, agitation, paranoia, wandering, persistent vocalizing, and depression. One or more of these symptoms are estimated to occur in 90% of patients during the course of dementia and are the most frequent reason for long-term care placement and chronic hospitalization. The focus of geriatric psychiatrists is to diagnose and treat individuals experiencing late-onset, complex, and severe depression with a suicide risk; late-onset psychotic disorders, delirium, and psychiatric complications from cerebrovascular accidents (CVAs); and Parkinson's and Huntington's diseases. Treatment is also provided for individuals with Alzheimer's, bipolar disorder, schizophrenia, substance abuse and complex disorders, combined with dementia. The treatment facility and its exterior environs should reinforce spatial orientation through the concept of *redundant cuing* – where spatial information is presented in multiple ways concurrently (i.e., sight and sound, or touch and sight). Such examples include the use of color, material change, room number, and a photo of the patient placed at the threshold to her or his bedroom, or choreographed surfaces (i.e., color-coordinated walls, flooring, and ceiling surfaces) and orientation through mutual reinforcement. A second design strategy is by means of *self-regulated environmental control systems*. This consists of mechanical heating, air conditioning, ventilation, and humidity control systems, allowing the building occupant to self-regulate and control the ambient room conditions. Ramifications include the ability to self-adjust temperature levels to suit the unique preferences of the aged individual, who often prefers interiors somewhat warmer than his or her younger counterparts. In a 2-year pilot project reported in 2014 in a geriatric mental health residential unit in Grand Rapids, Michigan, the incorporation of redundant cuing (navigational aids), together with larger room sizes, resulted in a reduced number of medical emergencies and use of restraints.[105] Design for normalization, personal choice, and personal control without sacrificing privacy, confidentiality, or safety. Aged patients with comorbidities (e.g., rheumatoid arthritis with a diagnosis of schizophrenia) can act out surprisingly quickly, without notice, and the result can be unpleasant, or worse.[106]

The patient bedroom

Patient room/bath unit

The patient bedroom and its embedded bath/shower unit (PR) occupies a central role in 24/7 mental health and substance addiction treatment facilities, and this role has evolved through the long history of psychiatry (Figure 5.26). If the dormitory ward was once about accommodating a large number of patients in a single space so their continuous observation could be maximized, today, privacy and autonomy is of far higher priority. These privatized spaces must neither pose a self-risk to the patient nor encourage any inherent physical attributes to become weaponized for use against others. The current emphasis in design is nonrestrictiveness, free from intrusive observation, physical isolation, or the incarcerating conditions of the past. The opportunity exists now to design a genuinely residential space that is inviting and properly supportive of therapeutic goals, including patient self-dignity, autonomy, and greater freedom of choice, with the most experimental architectural examples thoroughly rejecting the archetypal mid-20th-century modernist psychiatric institution. As in any period of reappraisal, there is no one sanctioned configuration above all others at this time, either in terms of size, layout, color, material palette, or aesthetic appearance. With the emphasis currently on projecting a normalized, quasi-residential atmosphere, however, patient- and staff-centered design is foundational to success and also the success of the larger unit, of which the bedroom and bath/shower unit are constituent components. The bath/shower unit is often, currently, positioned on the inboard (corridor) side of the bedroom opposite the perimeter (exterior) window wall. Numerous possibilities exist in overall unit configuration within this theme, from semicircular to rectangular layouts, with the footprint of the unit determining patient room shape, proportion, and size. New ideas are always emerging in professional practice, although a time-tested method for generating design innovation can be helpful here: the format of the two-stage architectural design competition

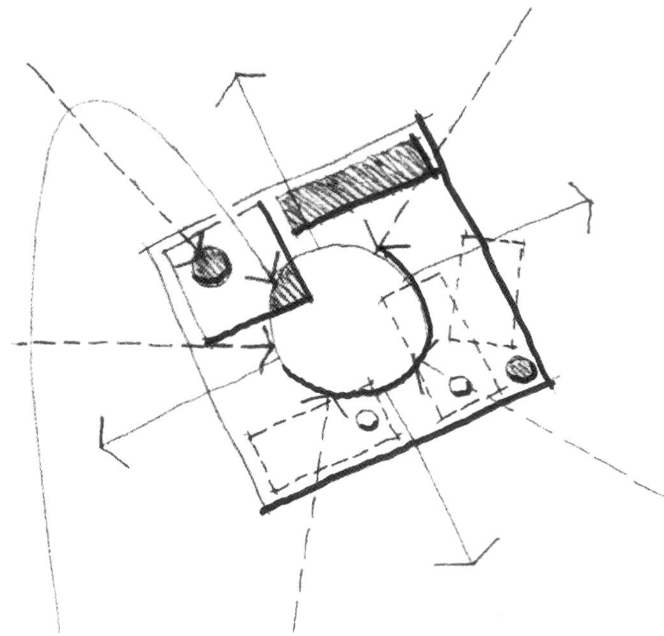

5.26 Explore patient room affordances.

is a vehicle for generating innovative new possibilities. This has proven useful to governmental agencies, private-sector clients, and philanthropic sponsoring organizations, as it enables the client-sponsor to comparatively examine the state of the art. One prominent recent example of the competition format as a vehicle for design innovation was the two-stage Kaiser Permanente Hospital of the Future competition held in 2012.[107]

Natural ventilation and daylight

The majority of case studies in the following chapter feature operable windows in the patient room. This is most often achieved by means of vertical or horizontal slatted windows, apertures narrow enough to not facilitate patient absconding. These apertures do, however, facilitate natural airflow, controllable by the patient and providing a degree of control over the physical environment previously impossible in the hermetically sealed megahospitals built in the post-World War II period. Then, the provision of natural ventilation was considered a contaminating element – polluting (or at the very least diluting) the quality of the indoor air within the building envelope. Omnipresent, ceiling-mounted fluorescent light grids became predominant. With widespread emphasis now on natural daylighting without compromising occupant comfort or safety, interiors are being reactivated in previously unattainable ways, influencing total building form, with narrower building footprints becoming mainstream (after 75 years of dismissal). Suffice it to say, dreary, poorly ventilated hospitals are harmful to one's psychological health. As for the therapeutic benefit of daylight, it influences human circadian rhythms, which maintain the body's sleep-wake cycles – a function housed in the suprachiasmatic nucleus in the hormone control center of the brain, the hypothalamus. The provision of a light box simulator in the patient bedroom is a valued amenity in this regard; this device can emit up to 10,000 lux of light, much brighter than a typical incandescent lamp, or a lower intensity of wavelength, such as the blue (470 nm) to the green (525 nm) areas of the visible spectrum, recommended in spaces receiving a moderate to low level of daily sunlight.[108] In addition, specify low-e glazing for exterior windows and a mixture of full-spectrum lighting, including ceiling-recessed incandescent light fixtures, cove lighting, and task ambient fixtures allowing the patient maximum freedom of choice, without compromising staff or patient safety. Beyond this, inventively incorporate skylights, clerestories, and bounced-lighting effects off interior surfaces, drawing light deeply into otherwise shadowed or windowless spaces. Finally, significantly minimize the overall carbon footprint through applied renewable energy systems. Configure the inpatient unit with single-loaded corridors to further maximize daylight and natural ventilation transmission, within sufficiently narrow building footprints.[109]

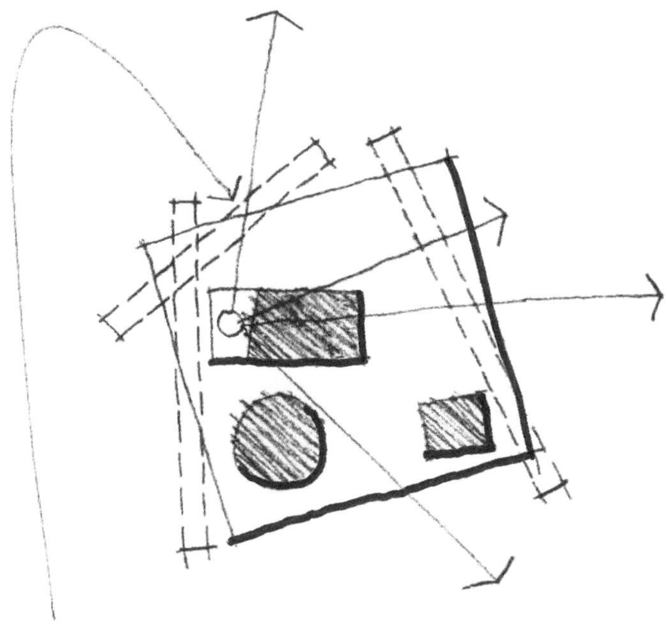

5.27 Reassess and reassemble prosaic room components.

Headwalls, footwalls, and window walls

The headwall need not house the technical apparatus required in an acute care hospital patient room (e.g., medical gases, elaborate electrical tie-ins for monitoring equipment for acuity-adaptable hospital beds, and so on). Regardless, design the headwall to be interesting, aesthetically and functionally. Create wall recesses and (color and material) accented walls, as well as built-in lighting, and provide space for a side table. The desk can be an autonomous element near the bed or along the opposite wall (or along the perimeter wall). As for the footwall, design for aesthetic and functional inventiveness with color and material changes, effective placement of the desk and the storage closet, and attentiveness to the bath/shower unit. Media connections, such as those for television and Internet viewing, is seldom allowed in the bedroom (although it may be feasible in some situations to provide a fixed-mount flat-screen monitor). As for the perimeter wall, this surface provides the opportunity to frame interesting views of the outdoors, while drawing in light and fresh air. The reimagining of all surface planes (including floor and ceiling planes) in the patient room envelope is an opportunity for positive (sensory) information (i.e., choreographed positive distractions) commensurate with the previously discussed tenets of attention restoration theory (ART) and the virtues of achieving automaticity in the architectural environment. The main challenge/opportunity of the patient room is to provide therapeutic affordance while it simultaneously functions as a reading, contemplation, and sleeping zone (Figure 5.27). Position the bed parallel (or perpendicular) to the perimeter wall, with a window seat or desk beside it with recessed incandescent lighting, safely mounted above. Provide a large 'picture window' with smaller inset operable windows to either side, above, or directly below, with open bookshelves or drawers built-in beneath the overnight bed along the window wall. In bedrooms where overnight accommodation is most appropriate, such as in pediatric units, a second sleeping space (e.g., a built-in or foldout bed) is helpful in some situations. The patient rooms at Seattle Children's (CS 19) feature a full-size bed for the patient plus a slightly narrower bed for overnight visitors' use. Strive to create a well-illuminated environment for the occupant(s) complete with a range of available options, without fostering self-risk.[110]

The patient bed

The patient bed, compared to its high-tech counterpart in an acute care hospital room, is low-tech, although it has an equally instrumental role in the patient's overall health status. The mental health and addiction disorder inpatient's bed is a relatively passive device, and its functional requirements can range from rudimentary to high restraint. In acute care, the bedroom is where the patient may spend the majority of his or her stay. In mental health care settings, on the other hand, the patient is encouraged to get out of the bedroom for the most part. Two predominant bed types currently are the nonmechanical *platform bed* and the mechanically operated *restraint bed*. Regardless of type, these devices must be highly durable, as they will receive more than their fair share of abuse over time. For restraint uses, commercially available products include the line of Medline beds and the line of Nemschoff Behavioral Health Beds, both of which feature underbed pullout drawers, while the CHG Platform Bed does not feature any underbed drawers. When full bodily restraint is called for, the bed must be able to severely limit the patient's sphere of physical movement. Here, commercially available products include Unique Care's Acute Mental Health Bed SWL 250KG and the Attenda Bed, by Norix. The Stryker Psych Bed provides a crank handle, central brake, and side rails, and is compatible with the Posey 8115 Restraint Net. In quasi-residential patient rooms, the bed selected will have a significant impact on the overall aesthetic, and it is important to attain a balance between functionality and a residential appearance. Many treatment centers now provide quilts and colorful bed sheets to soften the outward appearance of the bed; this policy has been adopted at Hopewood Park (CS 3), Roseberry Park (CS 5), Vermont Psychiatric Care Hospital (CS 6), and Ferndene Centre (CS 16). Ensure the attending staff team has consultative input in the bed selection process and is able to maintain unimpeded access to the patient bed from at least two sides within the room. It is highly inadvisable to specify an electric bed, as their relatively high rates of malfunction can cause accidents, and even death.[111]

Personalization and storage

Patients arrive at mental health and substance abuse treatment centers with relatively few personal belongings. Regardless of the length of hospitalization, adequate space is needed for proper and safe storage of personal items and artifacts. Patient dignity and self-awareness can be enhanced through the provision of multiple options and the freedom to self-personalize the bedroom to a degree. This can be achieved by providing bookshelves, a desk, and a full-height storage closet. These amenities should not provide hiding places, however, as this will invite their becoming a source of danger to the care provider, as well as invite self-harm. Consider a mix of freestanding and built-in furnishings and securable (locked) storage units, affixed to a wall surface, and not subject to weaponization. Personalization similarly denotes freedom to operate window blinds to block out unwanted light; to avoid being seen from the outside; and to control the transmission of fresh air, the room's lighting fixtures, and portable handheld devices (if allowed). Children and adolescents may desire to bring in items including clothing, shoes, books, and portable electronic devices (if allowed). The inpatient room in many case studies in the following chapter accommodates these aforementioned personalization measures, including bookshelves beneath window seats, along the footwall, beneath the bed, or along the headwall next to the bed. The Worcester Recovery Center and Hospital in the United States (CS 15) provides storage nooks and options for personal artifacts, as does the Östra Healthcare Centre for Psychiatry in Sweden (CS 2). As mentioned, it is inadvisable to provide locked storage shelves, drawers, and closets (unless they are able to be unlocked by staff). In some institutions, most personal belongings are by policy required to be stored visibly, always out in the open. As for other modes of personalization, provide a wall area for the display of art, produced by the patient during his or her stay.[112]

Bath/shower units

As recently as 1990, a private bath/shower unit embedded within the patient room was the exception, not the norm. Psychiatric hospitals previously featured communal bath/shower units for the majority of patients. These spaces were usually located at the end of a corridor and required the patient to always leave the bedroom, a practice now widely viewed as depersonalizing. Respect for the personal hygiene needs of the patient is of priority in recent facilities. Within the patient room, this space should be readily accessible and fully compliant with universal design standards (i.e., size, proportion, and equipment). But where should this space be located within the patient room envelope – inboard, outboard, or at midsection? An outboard location minimizes the remaining exterior window-wall area and is therefore less preferred compared to an inboard location. With the bath/shower unit positioned on the interior or corridor (inner side), the full width of the exterior perimeter wall can accommodate a built-in seat, desk, pullout second bed for overnight visitors, or below-window open shelves or pullout drawers. Attractive surfaces, flooring, ceilings, sinks, water closets, grab bars, roll-in shower zone, lighting options, and nonhospital color palettes are essential ingredients. In private rooms, the unit should be a single volume without compartmentalization; in the case of semiprivate bath/shower units (two private rooms sharing a single unit), there is justification for compartmentalization, as it allows two patients to use the space concurrently. Regardless, for patient and staff safety and self-risk reasons, do not provide a 'closed' water closet or shower compartment. Depending on its orientation, provide a clerestory above to transmit light. As for unit doors, the location and swing orientation of the bath/shower unit door remains problematic – if it is a continuously hinged swing-out device, it must not impede corridor-side sight lines into the patient room or invite its commandeering as a shield or weapon. The width and bulk of most bath/shower room doors unfortunately invite their misuse in potentially harmful ways; a prudent strategy is to specify a sliding pocket door, although these, too, have their disadvantages. Explore the use of vertically louvered doors, within a bifold C-curved or L-shaped pocket wall cavity.

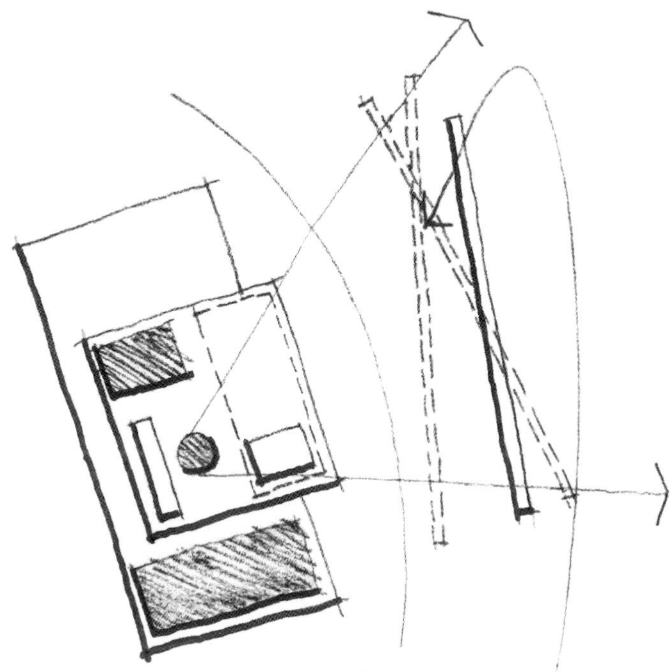

5.28 Explore digital view surrogation.

Surrogate view representations

Environmental sampling, not unlike digital music sampling, has opened up fascinating new design horizons, enabling the outside world to be drawn into the patient's immediate realm. Few patient bedrooms, dayrooms, dining rooms, staff break rooms, or therapy spaces can have that equally amazing view of a nearby mountain range. What about the rooms with the worst views on the unit? What of those rooms that remain in shadow even on sunny, cloudless afternoons? The challenge of enhancing window and window-wall view informational content through view surrogation (externally) can transform a less-than-ideal condition into a far more preferred condition. This requires harnessing the recent explosion in digital media technology, including handheld devices (Figure 5.28). Various media are to be weighed comparatively for their therapeutic value in the healing experience in this regard, and handheld devices (where allowed) can transform a patient or therapy counseling room. *Inboard surrogation* is defined as in-room equipment, such as wall-mounted flat-screen TV/Internet monitors, perhaps grouped into a grid (of four, or more) to allow concurrent or multi-view projection, with each monitor equivalent to an individual window aperture. *Outboard surrogates*, inventive adaptations of existing Mediamesh (micromesh, see Chapter 4) technology, can externally project vivid, evocative view informational content to patient bedrooms and other spaces otherwise experiencing restrictive view or daylight conditions. This sampling system consists of high-durability, high-brightness 'content profiles' projected onto a lightweight, stainless-steel mesh device installed on a facing wall plane. Interestingly, this technology is yet to be applied anywhere within a healthcare facility, at this writing. Mediamesh, its trade name, is capable of displaying complex images and can simulate, expressively, any view scene, and informational content is highly modifiable. The therapeutic amenity of this technology – simulated 'views' projected from an exterior source – can be synchronized with the passing of day to night, daily weather patterns, and the changing seasons. The Fort Worth-based Cook Children's Hospital recently opened a new parking structure featuring a 3,400-square-foot Mediamesh screen mounted on one corner of the structure's exterior façade, announcing its hours of operation.[113]

Semiprivate bedrooms

Semiprivate patient rooms and small wards remain the norm in many mental health care and substance addiction treatment centers around the world. Two-, three-, and four-bed inpatient configurations remain relatively functional in cases where more than one patient can demonstrably benefit from the social interaction and mutual support this arrangement can provide (although this is not to be construed as a universal endorsement). Suffice it to say, long gone (good riddance!) are the large, undifferentiated open dormitory wards filled with underattended

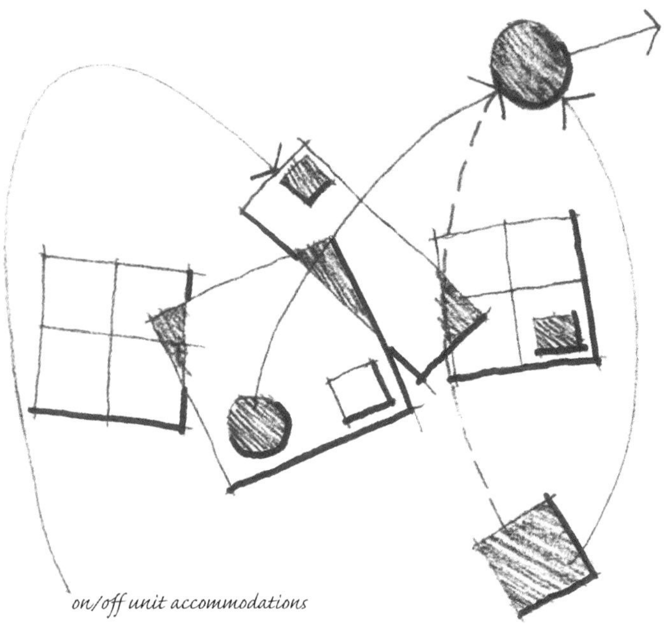

5.29 Provisions for overnight visitors.

patients, who are often undermedicated (or overmedicated). Certain patients can benefit from this type of semiprivacy, including patients in treatment for nutritional and other compulsive behavioural disorders. Each semiprivate (two-bed) bedroom should have its bath/shower unit shared, ideally, by no more than two patients. In wealthy, developed nations, the all-private-room psychiatric hospital has become the norm – although certain variations remain acceptable here as well, such as in the case of patients admitted for overnight observation and assessment. The case for the all-private-room acute care hospital has been forcefully made in North America based on the results of (rather inconclusive) evidence-based research – research premised on the argument that single-occupancy rooms are *always* safer than semiprivate rooms from the standpoints of both the caregiver team and the patient. Privacy advocates claim this also renders a healthcare facility more attractive from a marketing standpoint, as it will make the facility and campus look and feel more like a hotel.[114] Nonetheless, the case for the all-private-room acute care hospital remains just about as inconclusive as that for the all-private-room psychiatric hospital or substance addiction treatment center, in the sense that only a relatively small number of empirical investigations have been conducted in acute care psychiatric facilities on this issue, as mentioned previously. With so little corresponding empirical research reported, the question of who is assigned a private room should hinge on more than the ability to pay for privacy – because a private room may not always be in the patient's best interest. For this reason, an 80/20 mix of private to semiprivate room types is recommended.

Overnight accommodation

Recent thinking on patient room design calls for more opportunities for family and friends to be present on the unit, to a degree deemed mutually feasible in consultation with attending unit staff. It is a delicate balancing act because the presence of intrusive 'strangers' may trigger spontaneous aggression or acts of violence in other patients.[115] Since its founding in 2010, the Institute for Patient-Centered Design, Inc., in the United States has sponsored an annual competition on patient room design for mental health facilities. The core aim for entrants is to create an environment that maximizes patients' personal dignity, comfort, and control over their room settings without sacrificing staff, patient, or family member safety. Prior submissions have featured bedrooms with high-tech amenities and sustained person-nature connections in the form of wall murals, large windows, and full-spectrum lighting. Curiously lacking in these entries have been overnight bed accommodations for significant others. This can, however, be a positive therapeutic ingredient in pediatric psychiatry. At Seattle Children's (CS 19) 44-bed child and adolescent psychiatric unit, each bedroom has an 'exaggerated depth' window seat that doubles as an overnight sleeping space. Many families travel long distances from home to hospital, and in the case of pediatric psychiatric facilities, the family may wish to be as near as possible to allay the anxieties of the young patient. Having a sleeping berth provides a convenient option for parents (especially those traveling from afar). This is particularly valued among the parents of young patients undergoing overnight (preadmit) observational assessment. For these reasons, consider lift-up, pullout, or permanently fixed second-bed arrangements in the room. Alternatively, provide space for a second bed to be brought into the room. At the very least, a foldout chair or recliner can be provided. In cases where the family would have to travel a considerable distance nightly, consider providing a studio apartment unit on-site, or elsewhere nearby.[116] Two families can share a single overnight unit, each with a private bedroom, with communal living/kitchen and bath/shower units, not unlike a shared hotel suite with connecting doors (Figure 5.29).

4 The diagnostic and treatment realm

Trauma unit intake

The State of Arizona has a chronic shortage of psychiatric beds and the fewest mental health and addiction disorder service providers anywhere in the United States as of 2017. Its community-based outpatient clinics and hospital emergency departments (ED) have become overwhelmed by the sheer volume of unmet need. Lacking insurance and service providers locally, the mentally ill turn to community hospitals as the option of last resort, and as a result, ED wait times are skyrocketing. Some providers are at long last beginning to invest in building new inpatient facilities, and Banner Health, one of the main providers in Arizona, estimates 16,000 mental health patients are admitted to its ED annually, including suicidal patients and individuals suffering from severe schizophrenia and psychotic episodes. In response, Banner constructed a new behavioural health hospital, a US$36 million investment that houses 96 private-room beds.[117] Many community hospitals in the United States face a similar quandary: having inadequate beds for psychiatric admittances, forcing long waits, or only admitting a new patient when an insured (fully cost-reimbursed) patient is discharged. Third-party insurance providers in the United States provide scant coverage for psychiatric inpatient care, as discussed in Chapter 3. This is a main reason why so few new psychiatric hospitals have been built in the United States in the past quarter century. In countries with universal health coverage (i.e., single-payer systems), the situation is often different. Whether the context is a standalone psychiatric hospital or a community-based medical center, access to high-quality care is of utmost priority. The ED should therefore be easily identifiable with clearly discernable signage, day and night. Provide vehicular access, good lighting, and parking in proximity. Upon entry, intake and triage must occur expeditiously. Many psychiatric admittances are walk-up patients and a significant percentage are homeless who have simply been 'dumped' at the nearest ED. CAMH in Toronto operates a 24/7 ED independent from all other acute hospitals in that metro area. Its staff is trained to diagnose and treat a wide spectrum of mental illnesses and recommend whether an individual should be transferred for admittance to another local institution or to its own inpatient facility nearby (see Chapter 4).[118] Current thinking on ED unit design emphasizes multiple pod configurations whereby one or more pods can be dedicated for only mental health and substance-addicted patients. In hospitals lacking space for pods or similar dedicated treatment rooms or zones, it is recommended that 'convertible' space be provided with locked bins for storage of all equipment in the event a patient attempts to grasp an object from an open drawer and suddenly transform it into a weapon.[119]

Music therapy (MT)

Since ancient times, music has nurtured the human soul and continues to be an effective treatment modality in health promotion, including recovery from sickness and disease. In contemporary psychiatry, there is increasing interest in the use of MT in the treatment of a broad range of disorders.[120] Music can help an individual regain a sense of inner peace, and its socialization dimensions draw people together, and this has proven effective in the treatment of depression. Music was utilized to treat psychiatric illness in ancient Greek and Roman cultures. The Greek philosopher Pythagoras is considered the founder of MT. The oldest known documentation of medical practices, the *Kahum* papyrus, refers to the use of incantations for healing the sick.[121] Later, Florence Nightingale recognized the therapeutic affordances of music in hospital wards during the Crimean War in the 1850s, where she discovered the sounds of woodwind instruments to be particularly soothing to her patients. In the United States, in 1950, the National Association for Music Therapy (NAMT) was founded; Music Therapist-Board Certified (MT-BC) is the title currently ascribed to its practitioners, and there are generally three types of MT applied as an adjunctive treatment method in medical/psychiatric practice at this time: contemplative MT, combined MT, and executive MT. Contemplative MT involves listening to music for a prescribed time span on a scheduled basis and occurs either alone or in a group format. Combined MT involves engagement, often by means of the patient self-selecting the music he or she listens to, and executive MT manifests in many forms, including the writing and performing of music while in treatment, either individually or in a group therapy context. The pioneering jazz cornet player Buddy Bolden suffered from schizophrenia and from age 30 was committed to the Louisiana State Insane Asylum at Jackson, where he organized a jazz band that performed there regularly until his death at age 54 in 1931. Applied MT is effective for a range of psychotic and mood disorders, developmental and neurological disorders, and anxiety; in some applications it may be prescribed for up to 12 hours per day. It allows for diverse applications in diverse settings and is also administered in geriatric psychiatry with patients with Parkinson's disease, to improve cognitive motor skills. It is also proven effective with children and adolescents in treating agitation reduction and social phobias.[122] The portability of playback devices is what allows MT sessions to occur virtually anywhere, indoors or outdoors. By contrast, executive MT sessions require a group room environment to facilitate composing and performing music, including provisions for instrument storage, rehearsal and performance space, and perhaps access to an outdoor performance space.

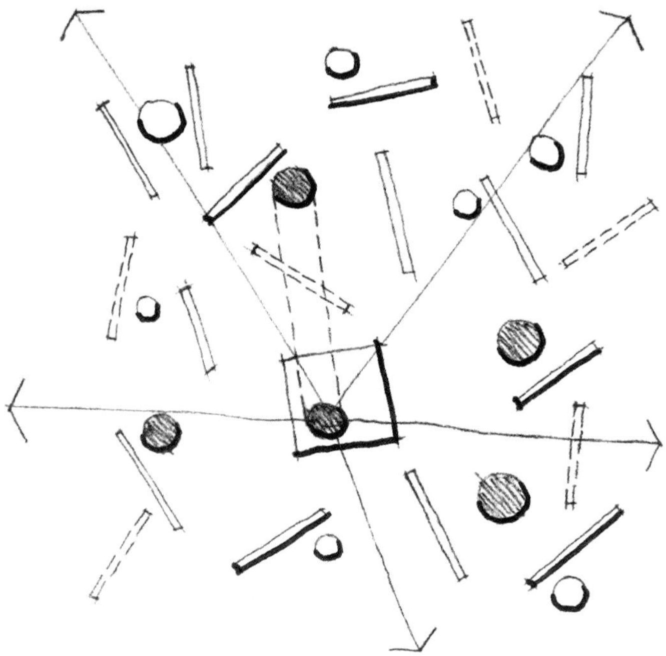

5.30 Art therapy.

Art therapy (AT)

Art has been a psychotherapeutic contributor in healing since the earliest institutions in the Far East, the *asclepia* of Ancient Greece, and the earliest mosque hospitals in the Middle East. In religious-affiliated insane asylums in Europe, Christian icons, including the Virgin Mary and Catholic saints, were displayed in public lobbies, chapels, courtyards, and in patient wards. By 2000, artworks in hospital environments had almost entirely turned away from religious iconography, with the notable exception of religious-affiliated care provider organizations. Even there, overtly religious themes in works of art have continued to be somewhat deemphasized.[123] In 1883, the superintendent of Bethlehem (Bedlam) Asylum in London, United Kingdom, began the practice of commissioning original murals in the wards, and female patients in one ward at the time painted a series of intricate panelized wall murals. Recent artworks produced by psychiatric patients were the subject of a museum exhibit in London in 2013 featuring the works of Richard Dodd, who created many of his most famous works while himself a psychiatric inpatient.[124] The American Art Therapy Association, founded in 1969, has grown to become an international association, and it recommends AT as a proven treatment method for borderline personality disorder, anxiety disorders, and phobias, by means of drawing, painting, sculpture, and active creative engagement with various allied art media.[125] For patients suffering from eating disorders, AT has similarly proven effective though a technique called *body image tracing*. Patients compare a self-drawn outline of their bodies to a true outline of their bodies. Patients suffering from PTSD, including young children, have benefitted as well, with AT proving effective in fostering mood enhancement and self-esteem.[126] It is recommended that spaces provided for AT are themselves interesting and psychologically uplifting because a stimulating space can stimulate creativity. Provide large windows facing north, with ample space for tables, easels, a ceramics area, storage, and the display of recently completed artworks by patients, and locate AT exhibit space in the public realm of the institution. Allow for freedom of choice, providing connections to the outdoors and in the local community for artmaking; these measures reinforce recent empirical research on the role of AT in the reduction of psychopathologies, particularly in schizophrenic patients (2011). In general, the literature on AT makes scant reference, quixotically, to the specific contributing function of the built environment in psychiatric and substance abuse treatment settings (Figure 5.30).[127]

Recreational, animal-assisted, and play therapy

These three treatment modalities address individuals' mental health with regards to physical, cognitive, emotional, social, and leisure time well-being. All are individualized to the patient's physical capabilities, emotional needs, and specific lifestyle. Recreational therapy is defined by the American Therapeutic Recreation Association (ATRA) as treatment for restoring, remediating, or rehabilitating persons suffering from injury, chronic illness, and disabling conditions. In the United States, the National Council for Therapeutic Recreation Certification (NCTRC) provides certification. The field's origins stem from the work of Florence Nightingale, who placed a high value on patient's outdoor leisure activity, with the term itself first formally coined by the Menninger brothers, who were keen on its inclusion in treating the mentally ill at the Menninger Foundation Hospital. Since the 1940s, it has been a prominent component in therapeutic intervention, with indoor spaces initially centered on the gymnasium and the swimming pool, with the gym serving as the nexus for team sport activities (e.g., basketball and volleyball), and indoor therapy pools facilitating both individualized or group activities (Figure 5.31a–b).[128] Many psychiatric institutions also included bowling alleys at this time, as it emerged as a popular sport in post-World War II North American society. Animal-assisted therapy consists of guided interactions between a specially trained animal and an individual or group, with sessions facilitated by a trained animal handler. Also known as pet therapy, these structured interactions are proven to improve patients' mental health status and emotional outlook. This type of therapy occurs indoors and also in outdoor settings, particularly with dogs,

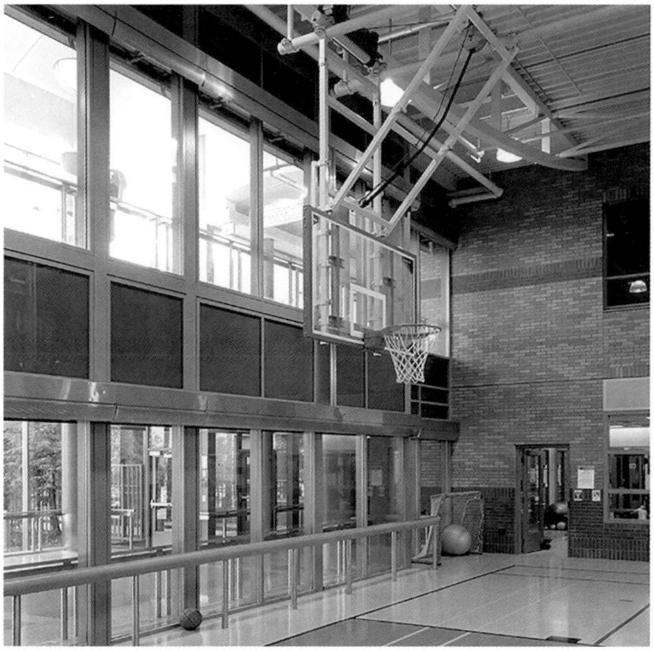

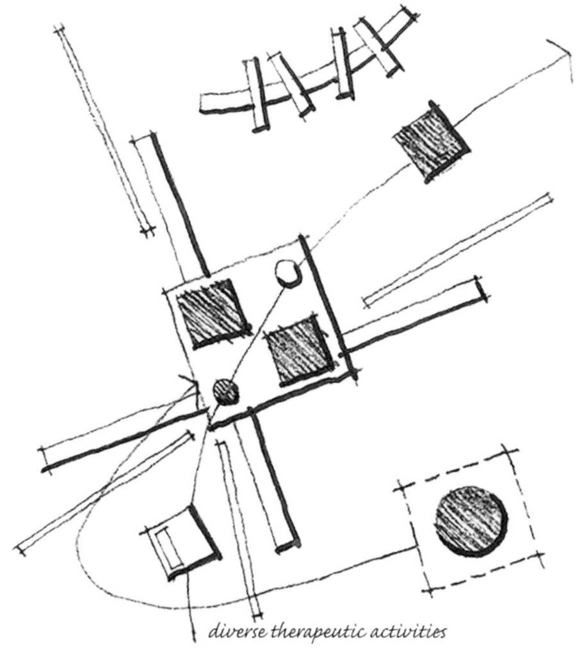

5.31a–b Provisions for recreational, animal-assisted, and play therapy.

birds, lambs, and horses.[129] Play therapy is typically administered to children aged 3–11, and is particularly useful as a diagnostic assessment tool with this age cohort. In 1982, the Association for Play Therapy (APT) was established in the United States and this organization is now international in scope. Play therapy/treatment is generally of two types: nondirective and directive. In the former, the child or adolescent is encouraged to work toward his or her own solutions to emotional problems through unstructured play, with relatively few boundaries imposed (psychodynamic therapy). A second scenario involves guidance and structure provided by a therapist vis-à-vis a group session or individualized activities (cognitive-behavioural therapy), with toy usage occurring as a fundamental method in either treatment regimen. Provide access to natural daylight and ventilation and seamless connectivity with the outdoors whenever feasible.[130]

Consultation/group rooms

In psychiatry and social work, the majority of patients receive mental health counseling in outpatient settings in private practitioners' offices and freestanding clinics.[131] From a sensory and aesthetic perspective, the physical space where counseling sessions occur is therefore of obvious importance. Dr. Jose Ribas, a psychiatry resident in the process of establishing a private professional practice, recently photographed 28 consult/group therapy offices and personally interviewed a subset of 12 care providers among all who created these spaces, in order to learn why the therapists appointed (personalized) their spaces as they did. He reported a typology ranging from the highly generic and minimalist to approaches reflecting the personal idiosyncrasies of each therapist. The trend of therapists to further personalize their therapy counseling spaces is gaining wider attention. These spaces no longer need remain resolutely minimalist, and this process of treatment-setting reappraisal (and enhancement) holds the potential to yield psychological and transactional benefits in therapist-patient interactions. These settings, whether a private consult room or a larger group session space, function, prosthetically, in support of the patient while in treatment. The trend to self-personalize psychotherapy spaces by the attending therapist, or by the parent service provider organization, currently spans a spectrum of approaches, from traditionally passive and minimalist, to intentionally active and visually stimulating.[132] On the minimalist end of this spectrum, counseling spaces are generally nondescript with respect to their lighting, furnishings, and color palette. On the other end, these spaces are de-institutionalized – that is, they use saturated colors, wood paneling and flooring, articulated ceilings, residential furnishings, plants, audio soundscapes, antiques, and artworks depicting nature and landscapes and equestrian themes. In one empirical study (2008), posters featuring nature scenes in outpatient therapy counseling settings were assessed as being significantly less stressful compared to comparable therapy settings lacking nature-themed posters.[133] K.L. Backhaus researched therapists' and patients' perspectives on the design of the physical[134] environment of private (individual) and group therapy settings among other reference sources.[135]

Virtual and augmented reality therapy

Environmental simulation technology is fostering inventive therapeutic applications in psychiatric and substance abuse treatment. Although more severe diagnoses typically require pharmacological intervention, techniques such as cognitive-behavioural therapy (CBT) and exposure therapy (ET) can be effective in the treatment of anxiety disorder, panic disorder, phobia, and obsessive compulsive disorder (OCD).[136] Anxiety disorders alone are estimated to affect upward of 40 million people in the United States currently, and treatment expenditures total approximately US$42 billion annually. Virtual reality (VR) technology has been applied in virtual reality exposure therapy (VRET); VRET has shown promise in military contexts in the treatment of ADHD, PTSD, depression, and numerous related mental health disorders. *Alternative realities* can be displayed on a flat-screen monitor or experienced by wearing headsets with viewfinders. This technique has proven successful in preparing combat soldiers for difficult hostage negotiations on the battlefield and in treatment of PTSD in veterans returning from the Iraq War.[137] Effective treatment interventions using VRET do not as a rule require pharmaceuticals. Other examples of simulation techniques include remote teletherapy between home and clinic. Some success is being achieved in using VRET in CBT. For example, if a person spends an inordinate amount of time obsessing about plane crashes and accidents, that individual will likely avoid air travel. VR is 'real' enough to simulate many anxiety-inducing stimuli and is safe and controllable; for certain childhood conditions, such as early onset developmental disorders and autism, VRET is anticipated to become widely used and of particular benefit in medically underserved communities, transcending geographical borders where the caregiver team is physically remote from the location of the patient. This decentralization of treatment through telemedicine and self-guided simulation technology/therapy holds much promise. Commercial providers of software and hardware include CleVR in the Netherlands, Psious in Spain, and Mimerse in Sweden. VirtualRet is a tool for psychologists and therapists to help evaluate and treat types of phobias. Unello Design produces meditation and relaxation therapy modules for Google Cardboard and for Oculus Rift. Eden River simulates nature experiences, and Zen Zone consists of a simulated, immersive, self-guided meditation 'journey'. In other contexts, patients are exploring the efficacy of therapeutic VR *sound sculptures* using three-dimensional music-based smartphone apps.[138]

5 Outpatient treatment environments

Inviting imagery

As mentioned earlier, the patient's and family's first impression of a treatment facility and its campus environs is critically important. The perceived/communicated image of the facility will be of enduring significance, and it will either induce a patient to enter into treatment or influence him or her otherwise. Whether the patient is in need of acute psychiatric care or outpatient services, the first impression matters, and this pattern has prevailed throughout history. In the Middle Ages, the image projected by the institution mattered no less in one's decision to seek out help, where the hospital's 'accident room' was specifically created for the treatment of injuries sustained in everyday life; it was also the place where persons with mental health disorders went (or were brought to) seeking help. In the case of those whose condition was considered non-life threatening – social outcasts, the abject poor, the melancholy, or those merely deemed a public nuisance – these individuals were turned out each night due to insufficient *inpatient* space in the hospital, hence they were referred to as the *outpatients*.[139] Outpatients with mental disorders typically experienced delusion, depression, delirium, and violent behavioural tendencies, considered untreatable as judged by conventional medical practices at the time, and as such they were disallowed from the hospital proper. By the 19th century, large urban hospitals, out of sheer necessity, established inpatient sections (units) for the insane with bed capacities dependent entirely upon the availability of residual or otherwise leftover space. This led, in time, to a freestanding custodial asylum being built far from the acute care hospital, providing specialized treatment on the assumption the patient was infinitely better off in a less chaotic, pastoral, tranquil atmosphere far from the city (see Chapters 2 and 4).[140] Today, as discussed previously, the psychiatric unit in most urban medical centers is chronically overcrowded, with little space or amenity for outpatient treatment of any type. Today's overcrowded facilities continue to be indicative of mainstream society's dismissal of the importance of mental health, a pattern no different from what has occurred for centuries. As for outpatient clinics, some are independently owned and operated as storefront clinics, others as part of a local for-profit or publicly operated healthcare network. Recent outpatient clinics include the Sowa Unit in Japan (CS 21), the CAMH Village Family Health Team Clinic in Toronto (CS 22), and Sydenham Gardens in London (CS 23). The Sowa Unit inventively reappropriated its fragmented site through the use of strategic views overlooking pocket courtyards, small spaces that inventively reflect inward. At the CAMH Village Family Health Team Clinic, the clinic is housed in a storefront directly abutting the street, in stark contrast to the spaciousness at Sydenham.

Adaptable spaces

In a recent study of 4,526 individuals with problematic addictions who sought out treatment at a rehabilitation center in Quebec, Canada, 61% were males, with a mean age of 39 years. Patients resided in neighborhoods where, on average, 21% of inhabitants were low income, and most lacked access to social services. Clients had a history of an average 11.4 consultations with social workers and 8.6 consultations with psychiatrists over a 2-year period, and 83.3% had availed themselves of only one type of treatment program while a patient at the clinic. The most frequently utilized programs were outpatient adult services (55.3%), followed by outpatient youth services (14.2%), addiction emergency and triage services (12.6%), and detoxification services (11.2%). Approximately 62.4% received a diagnosis of having a mental disorder, including a substance abuse disorder (SAD). The main diagnostic categories were anxiety disorders (41.8%), followed by SADs (38.2%) and mood disorders (21.5%), with 15.6% suffering from the combination of drug as well as alcohol abuse disorders. On average, many of the outpatient clinic clients suffered from chronic physical conditions, most commonly chronic pulmonary disease, liver disease, and uncomplicated hypertension conditions.[141] This study and its wide range of patients underscore the necessity of providing spaces adaptable to a broad range of treatment regimens in outpatient clinical settings. Individual and group therapy spaces should be flexible and reconfigurable, with multipurpose rooms for large group therapy sessions – equally adaptable to accommodate a variety of events, from poetry readings, concerts, 12-step meetings, and various types of individual and group therapy activities, to yoga and related mind-body treatment programs, to film screenings. Locate the most highly used spaces within these clinics nearest the main entrance so they are readily identifiable and immediately accessible to persons with physical or sensory mobility restrictions. Locate the outpatient clinic at street level whenever possible, with other services located on upper levels, as in the case at Marie Bashir Centre, in Sydney (CS 4). Provide clinical spaces that can double or triple function, as this will maximize the overall amenity of the facility regardless of whether it is an indoor- or outdoor-based treatment environment (Figure 5.32).

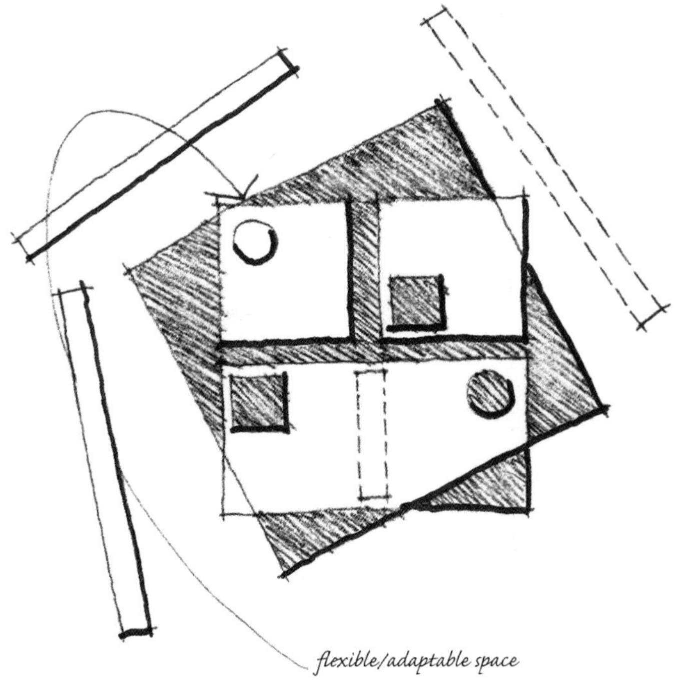

5.32 Explore spatial adaptability strategies.

Age-appropriate realms

It is not uncommon for children and adolescents at an outpatient mental health/addiction disorders clinic, especially if there for the first time, to experience heightened anxiety. Regardless of diagnosis (e.g., eating disorder, depression, or early signs of a more severe mental illness), the situation may be fragile, even volatile, with the probability of an aggressive or uncooperative behavioural occurrence.[142] Ideally, the design and appearance of the outpatient clinic environment communicates normative values that provide positive reinforcement. For example, a student who has been expelled from middle school involuntarily due to an inability to function successfully there in a 'normal' classroom environment may easily interpret the outpatient clinic as excessively authoritative and little more than an extension of the hated school setting. From the earliest planning stages, therefore, provide an age-appropriate environment that does not inadvertently trigger such adverse reaction to the outpatient clinic environment. Incorporate age-appropriate imagery in spaces frequented by children and adolescents from the first moment of arrival, beginning with the entrance and public circulation spaces. Forms, colors, materiality, and the careful orchestration of every space used for therapy sessions can help to establish an antiauthoritarian atmosphere.[143] The pediatric patient will benefit from the feeling that the physical environment is there to provide emotional reinforcement in a manner unavailable elsewhere to the same extent.[144] On the other hand, over-the-top supergraphics of cartoonish scenes and large animals can be off-putting as well. Eschew clichéd imagery in favor of subtle artworks and wall treatments and varied and interesting ceiling heights and fenestration, without their becoming caricatured, disorienting, or distracting. If an outdoor play-therapy space is provided, ensure it is equally age-appropriate, with safe play objects and surfaces allowing for staff observation to be effectively yet not obtrusively conducted. In larger clinics, provide multiple realms with each coordinated to a specific client age-group cohort, where practicable, such as separate waiting rooms for children apart from adolescents, and those apart from adult patients. In the United States, the design of outpatient mental health/addictive disorder clinics is governed in part by the Health Insurance Portability and Accountability Act (HIPAA), a set of federal regulations enacted to ensure that minimum patient privacy and confidentiality standards are met and maintained.

Nomadic vehicular clinics

Mobile vehicular clinics that provide mental health/addictive disorder services are an effective method in addressing the needs of medically underserved outpatient populations. These clinics on wheels function as important corollaries to fixed-site, brick-and-mortar clinics and are capable of reaching and serving a significantly wider geographic catchment area by reaching individuals without personal transportation or who have been unwilling or unable to seek out care in the past. Mobile units are premanufactured with thousands having been built over the past 50 years, ranging from the tuberculosis (TB) and polio screening units manufactured in the 1950s to the contemporary kidney dialysis units, primary care clinics, cancer screening units, and blood donor units deployed throughout the world today. Clinics on wheels are designed and manufactured for specific types of services, and a significant number of mobile units have been designed and deployed as mental health/addictive disorders outpatient clinics.[145] Regardless of the type of service provided onboard, they share common attributes, including uni-body compartmental configurations whereby the driver's compartment is located within the main cabin. Uni-modular mobile units have the advantage of diagnostic and treatment zones autonomous from the driver's area yet housed within a shared compartment. Relatively few psychiatric hospitals deploy mobile units of this type, In a recent study (2011) conducted in South Carolina in the United States, it was found that undocumented migrant farmworkers who suffer from depression and anxiety disorder greatly benefit from this type of mobile unit coming to their rural community.[146] Such service providers, whose units travel a set circuit on a weekly scheduled basis, cover a number of rural counties and fill an acute void left by the absence of fixed-site clinics in these places. Here, seeing the nomadic clinic arriving at its weekly deployment site in town is tantamount to a being thrown a life jacket.[147] A typical unit includes provisions for one-on-one counseling, as well as small group sessions. Provide a safe and secure medication dispensary on board, one or two private counseling/exam rooms, and a group space for up to eight persons. If funds allow, commission the design and manufacture of mobile units with pop-out side modules (bays), as these allow a virtual doubling in size of the unit footprint. Finally, ensure the unit is docked when not in service in a safe zone protected from vandalism or theft, and during supply replenishment.

6 Landscape therapeutics

Hierarchy of landscape realms (a) – As previously discussed, the spatial sequence leading to the typical post-World War II psychiatric hospital was seldom 'inviting', usually conveying a message of omnipotence and bureaucratic authority. Nature/landscape was held in abeyance as a passive element in the equation, often relegated to secondary status because the singular focus continued to be on the 'Institution'. From the moment of first arrival on campus and throughout the spatial sequences leading to the main entrance and within, this is no longer the case. The campus arrival sequence and entrance to Perkins + Will's Fleury Medicina e Saúde, Healthcare Ibirapuera Unit, in Sao Paulo, Brazil (2011), features natural daylight, trees, and abundant ground plantings. Landscape/nature is experienced hierarchically as green spaces encompassing public, semipublic, and semiprivate spaces. The three primary user constituencies of a psychiatric and substance abuse treatment center – staff, patients, and patients' visitors – are equally benefactors. At the Highcroft Psychiatric Hospital (2002) in Birmingham, United Kingdom, by Medical Architecture, Ltd., exterior landscaped space totals 54% of the overall campus footprint, resulting in a network of interconnected, nested outdoor activity spaces (Figure 5.33). The buildings surround central gardens, linked by exterior features and paths of varied configuration. Incorporate site and architectural design strategies allowing opportunities for the building(s) to therapeutically 'breathe', reaching outward/inward simultaneously. Eschew dark, dreary 'light wells' (often deceptively labeled on the site plan as 'courtyards). Employ horizontal and vertical cutouts as volumes for transmission of natural daylight and fresh air, and create view sight lines directionally coordinated with various visual and multisensory focal points (i.e., a fountain, sculpture,

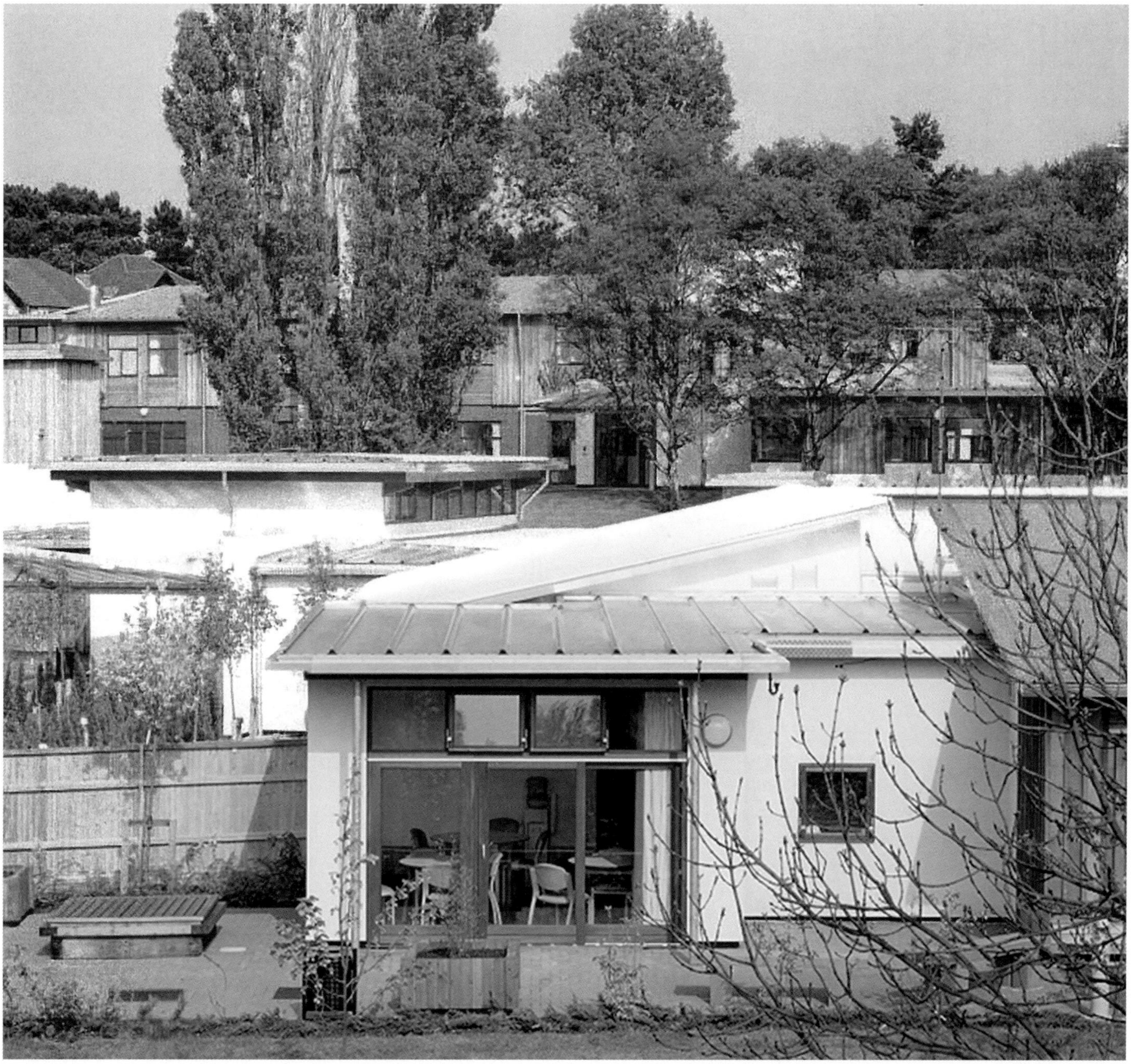

5.33 Hierarchy of landscape realms.

staircase, cluster of trees, a garden). Bisect these spaces with fluid circulation paths – natural extensions of adjoining interior realms. At Rehab Basil, in Switzerland, by Herzog and de Meuron (2002), the building envelope features nine 'breathing courtyards' within a large, articulated box, resulting in a highly theraserialized condition. Avoid residualized, off-the-beaten-path spaces with blind ends, as such conditions can be both unsafe and unhealthy. Weave outdoor-indoor 'rooms' together in a seamless tapestry, endeavoring to calibrate the proportions of therapeutic spaces/volumes with open green space relative to the size and volumetric scale of the total facility and its campus environs.[148]

Habitat conservation

Tragically, in the 21st century we have now arrived at the point of having destroyed nearly two thirds of all wildlife species on our planet in a mere 50-year time span. A recent, damning report released by the World Wildlife Fund (WWF) documents the dramatic decline in the world's animal populations as thousands of species now struggle to survive against an implacable and highly determined enemy: *Homo sapiens*. The 2016 iteration of the biennial *Living Planet Report* reported a 58% decline in vertebrate populations from 1972 to 2012, warning that if current trends continue unabated, the world will have already permanently lost a massive number of its wildlife species by 2020. Human populations deeply, adversely impact the spectrum of vertebrate life – fish, birds, mammals, reptiles, and amphibians. The global challenge at this point must shift to halting this precipitous decline in species. The rapid decline of wildlife species is a consequence of the 'five horsemen' of the coming environmental apocalypse: habitat loss, overexploitation, pollution, invasive species, and global climate change. Cumulatively, these forces have already deleteriously impacted 3,706 species documented by the WWF on land, in the world's oceans, and in inland freshwater habitats. Unbridled urbanization, the unabated clear-cutting of rainforests, senseless big-game poaching, and massive ocean overfishing now require the equivalent of 1.6 Earths in order to provide the goods and services humanity consumes *each year* as the expansion of the human ecological footprint results in rampant overconsumption of finite resources. It is well known that the wealthiest nations consume the largest footprints, and changes to this modus operandi must include the complete revamping of the Earth's food production systems to rebalance human consumption levels with planetary capacity limitations.[149] In a curious reprise of the past, the recent trend to build new on grounds (near an old asylum) may be prudent from an ecological perspective because ample land is already owned by care provider organizations in those places. In exurban and rural settings, it will be essential to rebalance habitat species-conservation initiatives with environmental ecosystem conservation. Often, the architect's brief will extoll the virtues of its new facility's bucolic site without any mention of its adverse environmental impacts on the local ecosystem or on local animal species (Figure 5.34). In response, four alternate designs for a 40-bed inpatient and outpatient treatment facility in a Toronto neighborhood, developed in a graduate design studio directed by this author in the fall of 2016 at the University of Toronto, illustrate a balancing strategy between these determinants (Figure 5.35a–b and Figure 5.36a–d). From clockwise, these site/building design concepts are the work of Jordon Wong (a), Rotem Yaniv (b), Kiwoung Cho and Gefei Pan (c), and Kelly Chin and Parham Karimi (d). Collectively, these diverse yet environmentally attuned site/building concepts illustrate the virtues of carefully examining *a priori* multiple, balanced site strategies as a means to avoid adverse environmental and animal species impacts.

Horticultural therapy

The benefits of horticultural therapy include opportunities to emotionally recharge and obtain respite by engaging in social interaction through gardening. Food grown and consumed on-site can be a source of sustenance for the patient; recent evidence-based research at a psychiatric hospital in Greece reinforces these benefits. Green spaces and gardens for this purpose can help patients experiencing mental disorders or seeking liberation from the shackles of addiction.[150] Nature itself holds the power to reignite the human inner spirit to provide the strength to take on the challenges that lie ahead.[151] Endeavor to provide trees, gardens, diverse ground plantings, and a continuum between exterior and interior realms (e.g., a dining room connected to an outdoor terrace followed by an open lawn). The relationship of these to inpatient housing and recreational therapy spaces is of importance. They should be inviting and not too difficult to master, functioning as an antidote to the intensity of conventional therapy counseling. More and more service providers are gearing these spaces, originally intended primarily for patients, for use by staff as well. A therapeutic garden is far more than a visual device, and this was achieved at Sydenham in London (CS 23), where a typology of spaces on-site is provided, each zoned for a particular type of horticultural therapy session. These zones consist of vegetable gardening, flower gardening, a greenhouse for year-round gardening sessions, multiple platform-gardening bays for individuals who are wheelchair bound, and multiple storage spaces for equipment and supplies (Figure 5.37).[152] Pockets of seating dispersed throughout these spaces support the need for personal contemplation, informal socialization, small group sessions, and certain leisure activities, and when these amenities are able to function as a source of food consumed on-site, they further symbolize patient empowerment. This is not entirely dissimilar from policies perpetuated in the asylums of the 19th century – where the asylum farm was the site of 'work activity therapy' for the patient, as well as a food source for the institution. In British Columbia, Canada, the 'Colony Farm' psychiatric hospital operated a farm continuously on-site from 1909 to 1983.[153] Provide more than just a single outdoor space for these functions, and wherever feasible, create virtual outdoor rooms and associated exterior spaces orchestrated in support of patients of all ages.

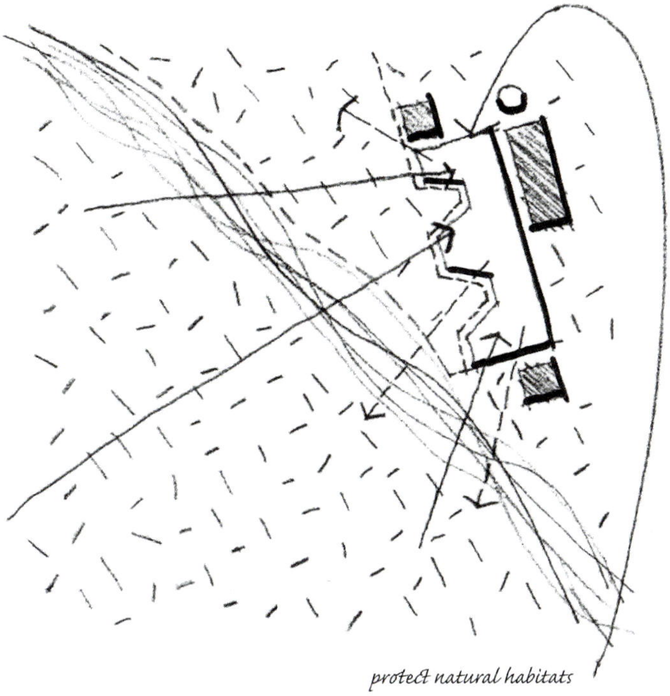

Figure 5.34 Habitat conservation advocacy.

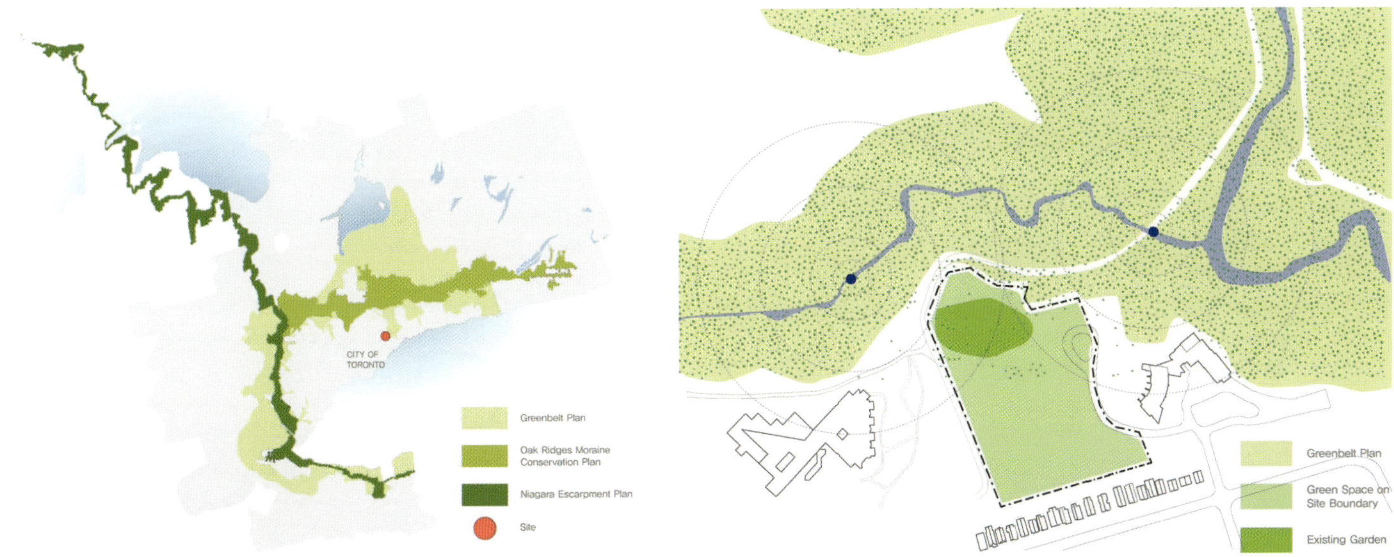

5.35a–b Tread lightly on natural ecosystems.

Microlandscapes along narrow spines

Narrow vertical and horizontal circulation passages and residual spaces, such as in-shadow light wells, typically problematic, are transformable through thoughtful landscape design strategies. Cutouts, open volumes, slices, and perforations examined in plan, elevation, and in section during schematic and design development phases can inventively draw light downward into spaces otherwise devoid of daylight or nature (Figure 5.38). These strategies can be effective in activating the interiors of midrise healthcare facilities on dense urban sites. The Centre for Cancer and Health in Copenhagen, Denmark, by NORD Architects (2012), features a prominent cutout, demarcating the main arrival and principal interior arrival axis. The Lady Children's Hospital, in Brisbane, Australia, by Lyons Architects with Conrad Gargett Architecture (2014), features bright colors and striking exterior materials; this hospital has garnered numerous awards, including the F.D.G. Stanley Award for Public Architecture, the Karl Langer Award for Urban Design, and a design

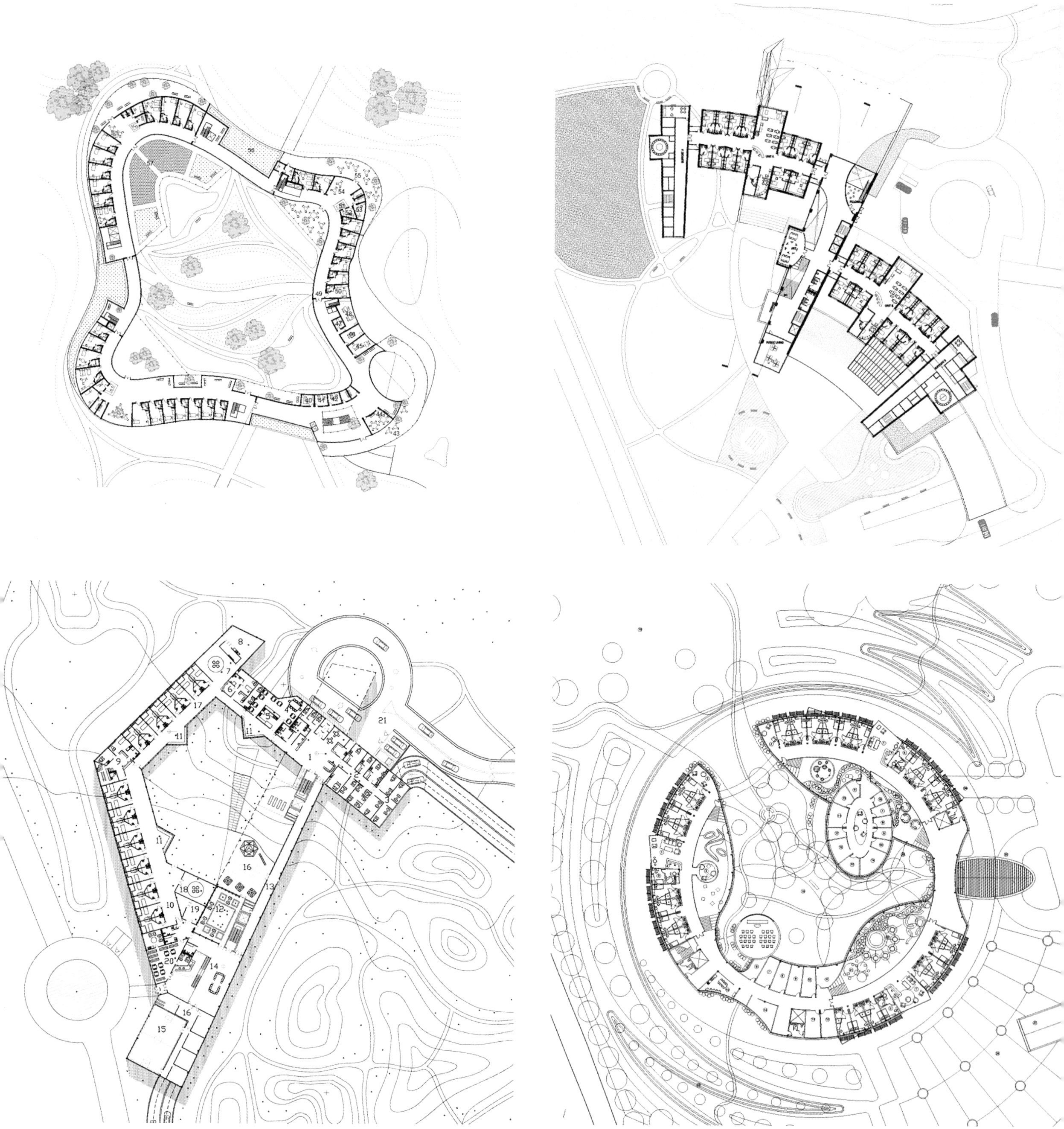

5.36a–d Explore multiple site and building typologies.

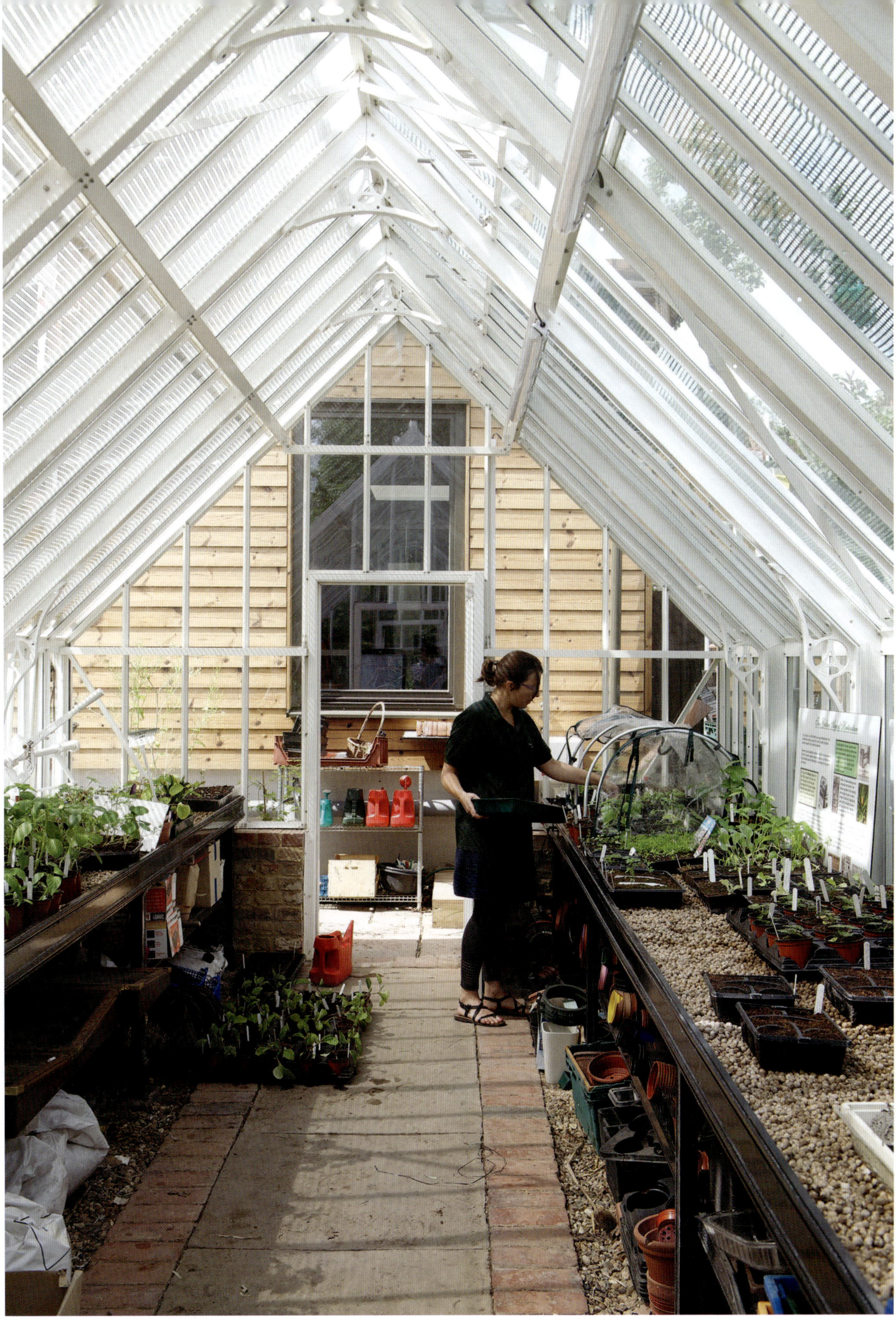

5.37 Horticultural therapy greenhouse.

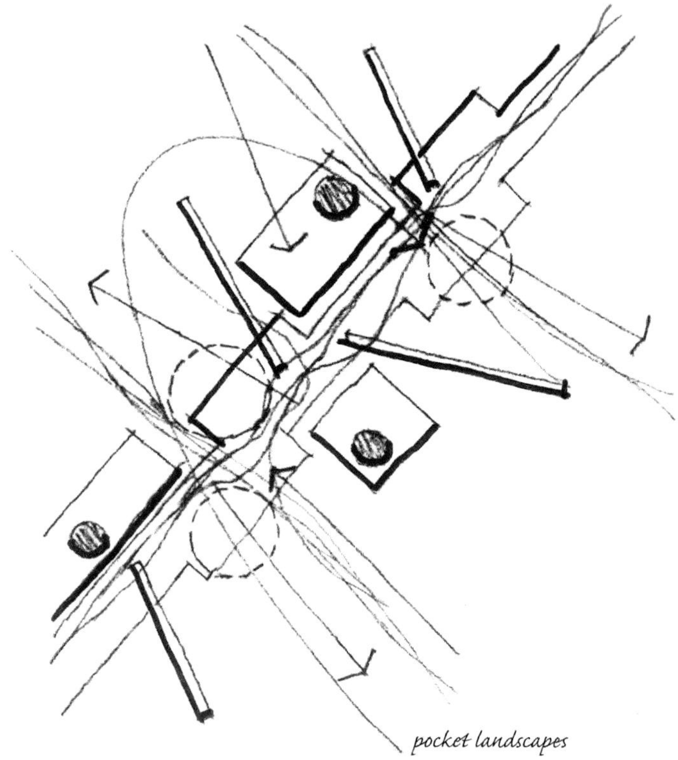

5.38 Incorporate microlandscapes along narrow spines.

award from the International Academy of Design and Health. Lady Children's Hospital also features large cutouts visible from the exterior, each configured as a cantilevered box/tray protruding outward, symbolically engaging in dialogue with its urban surroundings, and these examples simultaneously serve as exterior balconies.[154] Oblique or unusual vistas, created through the interjection of vertical and horizontal gardens and through the slicing and perforation of the compositional massing, create vegetated 'oases'. An inventive way to achieve these vertical and horizontal microlandscapes occurs at the Polyclinic, in Split, Croatia, designed by 3LHD Architects (2012). This medical institute is sited near a seashore, and multiple cutouts are visible from afar on the upper levels of this 10-level building. These elements draw in breezes and natural light while providing dramatic views outward, yet appear as random holes in a slice of cheese, and semipublic terraces and hanging gardens are interspersed. The linear rock garden at the Dandenong Mental Health Hospital (2011) in Melbourne, Australia, by the Bates/Smart Group with Irvin Alsop Architects, transforms an otherwise residual space into something much more interesting (Figure 5.39). In a third variant, the nearly dozen exterior courtyards, situated in between projecting alternating A/B A/B patient housing and medical wings at the Rikshospitalet in Oslo, Norway, by Medplan Arkitekter (2008), feature various types of gardens combined with open lawns.[155]

Roof terraces

Memorable buildings of the 20th century for designed health, notably the historic Paimio Sanatorium in Finland by Alvar Aalto (1929), feature roof terraces and linear gardens situated high above the ground level.[156] A viable strategy is to create one or more open-air terraces, with each autonomous from the others, protected by a perimeter security buffer. A second strategy is to provide cascading open-air terraces, interconnected, stepped downward in a serialized manner from uppermost to ground level, such as the Marie Bashir Centre, in Sydney (Figure 5.40). Alder Hey Children's Hospital, in the suburb of West Derby, in Liverpool, United Kingdom (2016), by BDP, features multiple salutogenic design concepts, including multiple undulating stepped roofs with inset balconies (Figure 5.41). This institution, founded in 1914, thoroughly reinvented itself from a staid Edwardian institution to one clearly embracing its immediate landscape. A terrace on the second level overlooks a large courtyard, gardens, and walking paths; other green, sloping roof surfaces are inaccessible to patients and yet appear otherwise.[157] The winning entry in the design competition for the psychiatric hospital at Bispebjerg Hospital, in Denmark (2018), by Friis & Moltke Architects, features landscaped roof terraces for patient, staff, and visitor use, where terraces are accessed via staircases connected to exterior courtyards on lower level(s) with pockets of seating, garden plots, low plantings, trees, and views of the surroundings beyond (see Chapter 6). The alternate design proposed by this author for CAMH in Toronto (see Chapter 4) features roof terraces on the uppermost level of two new inpatient pavilions, with multiple garden plots, seating, a winter garden, and a workshop for horticultural therapy (with a perimeter security buffer of clear-vision Plexiglas 10 feet high with fold-over mesh panel). These roof terraces afford views of the neighborhood and Toronto skyline (Figure 5.42). In general, provide a blend of interior and exterior spaces in response to organizational policies, patient needs, and staff goals, and balance visual privacy with safety; avoid 'fishbowl' effects where others can peer in on patients, as this will cause agitation. Use planting materials durable and virtually impossible to transform into weapons; provide a mixture of amply sunlit areas and shaded places, without too much of one or the other extreme, and plant species aesthetically pleasing to the senses (sight

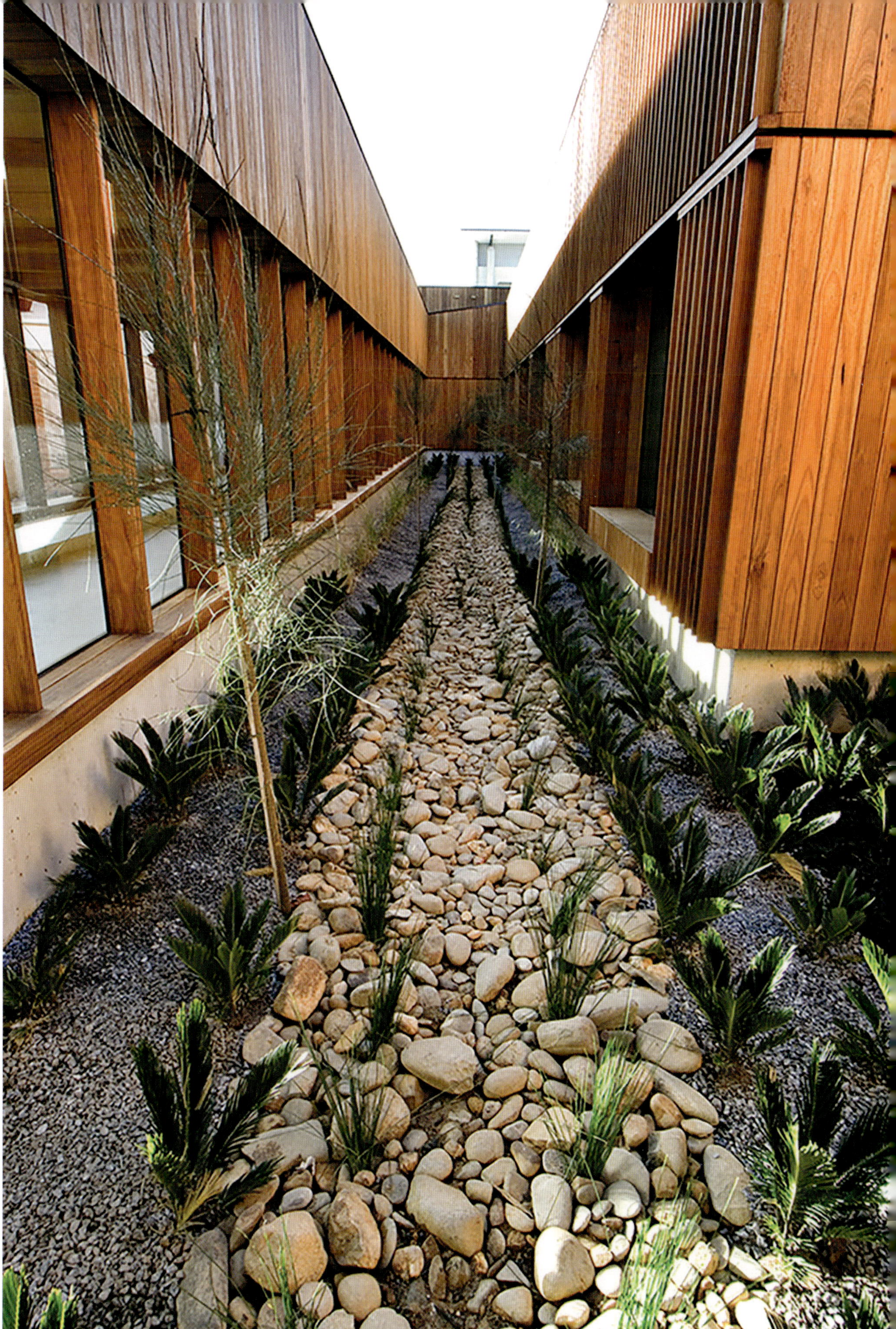

5.39 Pocket gardens (in residualized spaces).

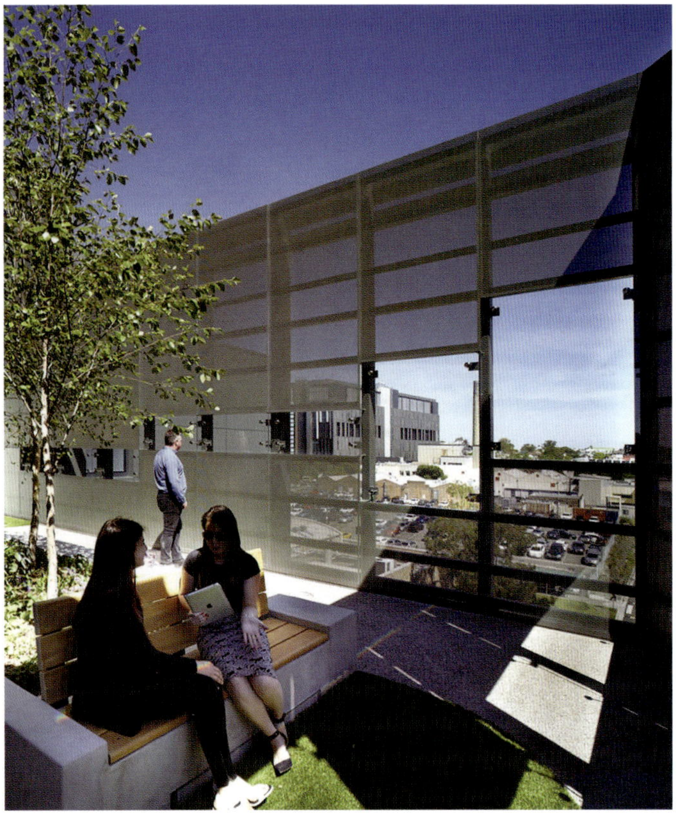

5.40 Roofscapes as therapeutic gardens.

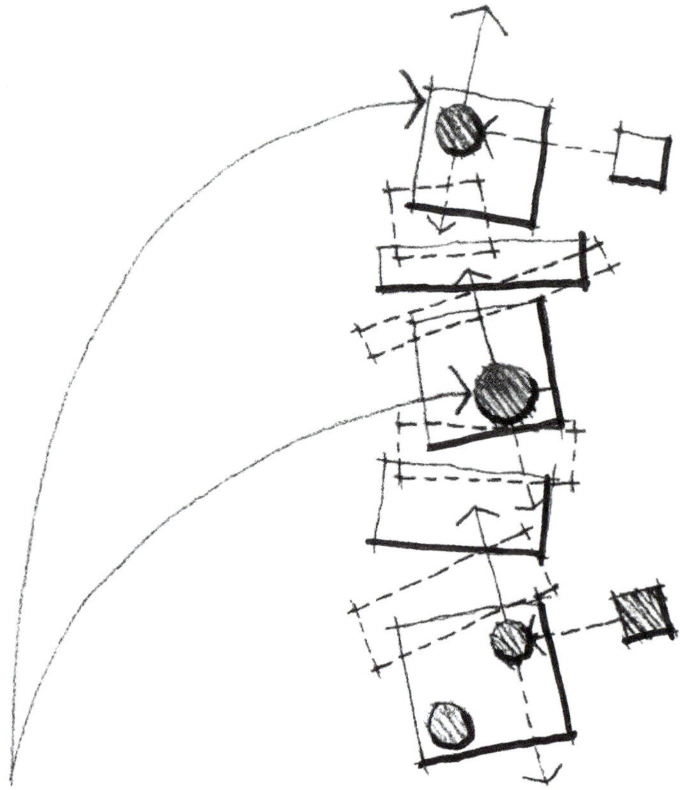

5.41 Cascading green roofscapes.

and smell) while assiduously avoiding plantings irritating to the human touch.[158]

Ecological stewardship

Psychiatric hospitals and addiction disorder treatment centers are environmental polluters, with their toxic materials often improperly stored on-site, only to end up in solid waste landfills outside the city limit. It will no longer suffice for any service provider organization to hide behind facile public relations efforts, attempting to whitewash its environmentally harmful actions. The US Environmental Protection Agency (EPA) provides an online Energy Impact Calculator to determine the carbon footprint profile for any given ZIP code in the nation. It is no longer acceptable to be an institutional laggard in terms of implementing ecological/environmental best practices. The means to do the right thing exist, from the retrofitting of heritage buildings (i.e., repurposing heritage buildings; see Chapter 4) and pilot demonstration projects in campus-wide waste recycling and solar and wind energy, to sustainable land uses and water retention practices, to successful on-site microfarming demonstration projects. Healthcare organizations need to lead in helping to eradicate toxic lead levels from the local water supply and the food chain.[159] In North America, the LEED-affiliated *Green Guide for Healthcare* began in 2003 and is a joint effort between Health Care Without Harm and the Center for Maximum Potential Building Systems.[160] It consists of a point-based metrics system that closely parallels the mainstream LEED (Leadership in Energy Efficient Environmental Design) certification rating program. These metrics are geared toward assessing the environmental stewardship level of hospitals and other healthcare facility types. In the United Kingdom, the National Health Service (NHS) some years back initiated an assessment tool called NEAT for its new construction and renovation projects, and it has helped to foster ecologically sustainable best practices. The need exists to launch similar efforts in medically underserved regions. In the United States, Catawba Hospital, a state-run psychiatric facility in Virginia, recently completed an extensive retrofitting of its campus that yielded significant energy savings though reduced overall power consumption and a decrease in facility operational costs resulting from retrofitted heating, ventilation, and air conditioning (HVAC) systems. All of the campus's 21 buildings were retrofitted and the central chilled-water plant was replaced. On-demand lighting systems were installed, and this effort has since been extended to include conserving the agricultural character of its immediate surroundings, a project known as the Landcare Initiative. This consists of grassland habitat conservation (to restore local quail species)

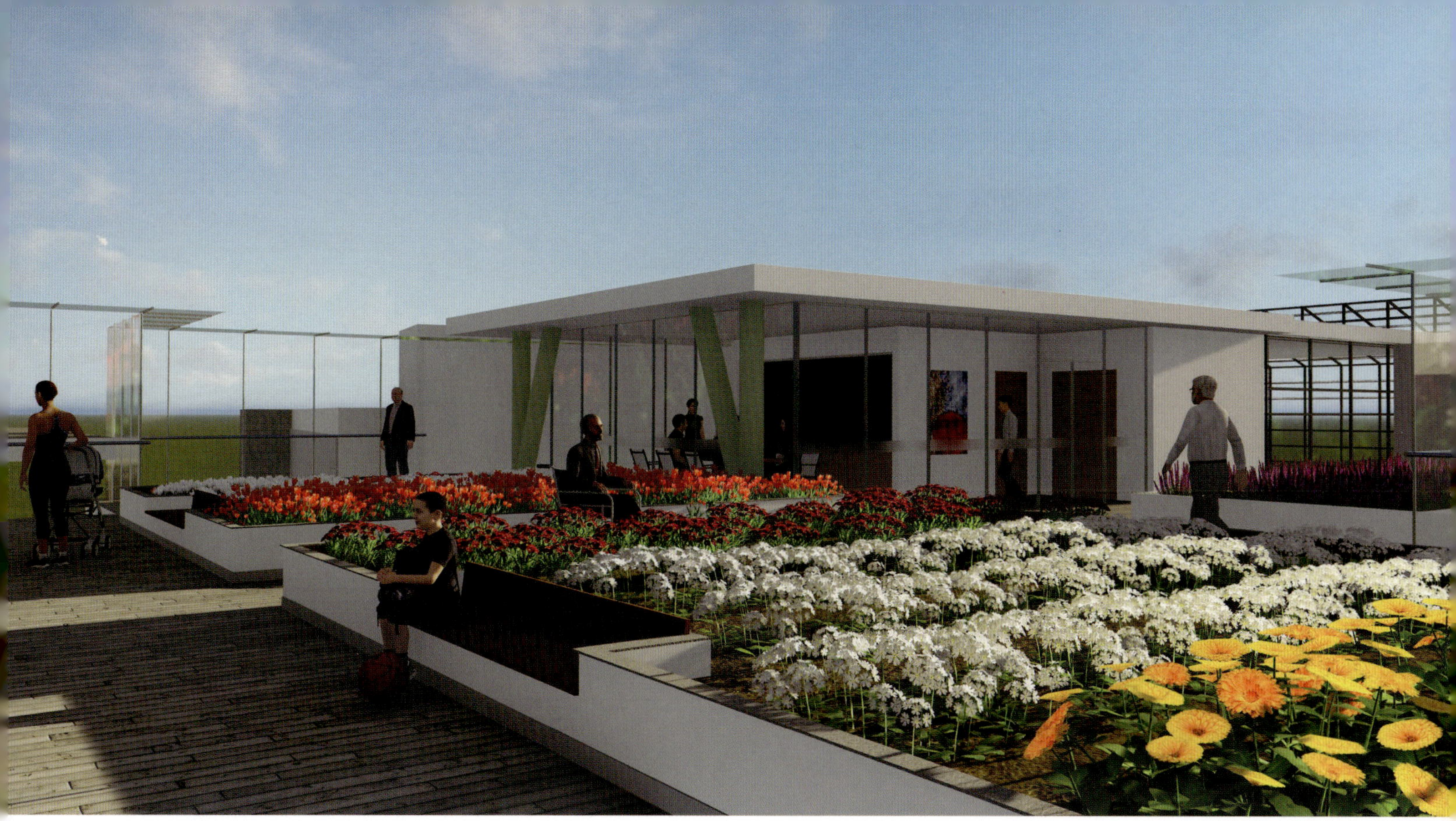

5.42 Roofscape horticultural gardening.

with the recultivation of warm-season grasses grown locally, judiciously harvested to help power the hospital's central heating infrastructure.[161]

7 Administration and total environment

Health-promoting policies

Noncommunicable diseases (NCDs) have reached epidemic levels in poor and wealthy nations alike, according to recent data released by the World Health Organization (WHO).[162] The unhealthful consequences of sedentary lifestyles and poor diets (i.e., obesity, hypertension, and diabetes) are increasing globally as standards of living rise and more people migrate to urban areas. The intersection between unhealthy lifestyles, physical inactivity, mental illness, and substance addiction has been studied extensively, and arguably, global strategies are required from here on out to combat this dangerous trend (see Chapter 1).[163] Comorbidities are on the rise, such as obesity crossed with depression.[164] In the United States, post-World War II urban sprawl fostered unhealthy lifestyles for three generations. Driving everywhere caused one to sit excessively, and the absence of sidewalks and associated amenities rendered it nearly impossible to travel anywhere without a car, giving rise to deleterious mental health consequences. While it remains a challenge for transportation planners to get people out of their beloved private autos, it remains equally challenging to improve transit access so patients can reach the nearest mental health clinic. Building a new mental health/addictive disorders residential campus on a greenfield or brownfield site far from the urban core does little to alleviate this. The challenge boils down to how to improve access to services while simultaneously promoting healthier lifestyles. The auto becomes the first (and perhaps only) option when services are located remotely from transit routes connecting to and from nearby towns and cities. Service provider organizations can benefit from working in partnership with other local agencies toward providing healthier transit alternatives. Provide families with a loved one in outpatient and in 24/7 programs with viable, commodious, and economical transit options, as this will accrue multiple affordances, including increased care utilization levels. Health-promoting transit linkages between home and treatment center will foster numerous spin-off benefits. Of equal importance is the provision of accessible, commodious, and healthier network options for transiting between home and workplace for staff persons.[165]

Grassroots outreach

Healthcare provider organizations, acting in their own perceived self-interest, do not always do what is in the best interest of the communities they serve. This has been happening for centuries. Supposed administrative (misguided) 'leadership' with respect to the built environment takes on myriad manifestations, including insensitive initiatives that an institution may attempt to foist upon its unsuspecting local neighborhood in the name of 'improving care'. A proven method for engendering genuine mutual trust from an institutional perspective and community-based constituency perspective is by simply making a genuine effort to listen to what is being said – listening to the public's feedback. Listen to various grassroots stakeholder constituencies about what they care most about; their vocalized concerns can be translated into more responsive community relations and into more responsive build-environment capital-improvement initiatives/outcomes to improve the quality and delivery of services (Figure 5.43). Address any lingering communication disconnects between the institution and its community stakeholders explicitly and early on. The status quo will often not suffice, and it requires hard work by all stakeholders to overcome the status quo. And sometimes an institution may feel blindsided by local mental health advocacy groups' concerns and demands. For example, the United States is currently plagued by a seeming unending wave of mass shootings by deranged perpetrators who, in the vast majority of cases, had previously been diagnosed with a mental disorder but somehow fell through the cracks of the 'system'. Fragmented care supports have been cited repeatedly as a main reason for this worsening national epidemic.[166] In response, a community grassroots group may demand better early warning detection of these tendencies in adolescents and teens as a leveraging point in negotiations over a proposed facility expansion. The unprecedented flow of information is further empowering grassroots groups' efforts, such as an editorial in a special issue of the *Lancet* in 2007 titled 'Scale Up Services for Mental Disorders: A Call for Action', calling for immediate action to improve and intensify the scope and quality of programs for the early detection of mental illness, in poorer and in wealthy countries alike.[167] This is but one example of the negotiated interdependency between psychiatric care and the built environment in the era we live in.

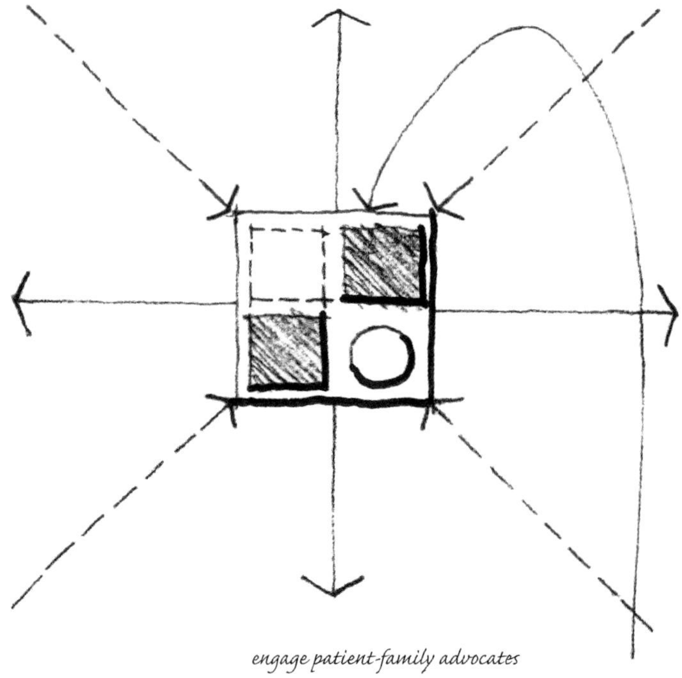

5.43 Engage in grassroots community outreach.

Patient, visitor, and caregiver team safety

The physical safety of patients, visitors, and direct caregiver teams must remain a top priority for those who administer mental health and substance addiction treatment facilities. Many effective organizational policies for reducing and eliminating acts of patient aggression have been reported in the literature.[168] A recent study in the United Kingdom focused on improving staff and patient safety in psychiatric wards based on data collected in 31 wards at 15 hospitals; each institution was subjected to a detailed pre- and postperformance assessment. Employing a data collection method known as the Safewards Model, 10 interventions were each assessed to learn new ways to improve staff-patient interpersonal communication protocols. It was found that aggression, self-harm, and related threatening behaviours could be decreased by 15% and coercive control of patients (restraint use) could be decreased by 24% using this method. The findings in this report centered on the importance of innovative and empathic methods for engendering positive patient-caregiver team communications and proven methods to eliminate internecine conflict.[169] As it is, psychiatrists, psychologists, social workers, and other direct caregivers whose clients commit suicide may experience, in the aftermath of these occurrences, a subtle yet corrosive stigma directed toward them. This can take the form of subliminal disapproval emanating from their non-mental-health professional colleagues. Worse, this can manifest in the form of lawsuits, with such actions taking a significant toll on the psyche the mental health specialist – rendering one perhaps less willing to take on suicidal patients critically in of need of emergency counseling in the future.[170] On the matter of facility-acquired infection, the research literature in the health sciences has long acknowledged the function of the physical facility as a contributing transmission path for sickness and possibly death (i.e., airborne infection, infection acquired through human contact, and infection via potable groundwater supplies). According to the US Centers for Disease Control and Prevention (CDC), each year an estimated 648,000 people in the United States develop a hospital-acquired infection and nearly 75,000 of these victims die.[171] Psychiatric patients, for their part, can be uncooperative, even intransigent, in terms of maintaining proper personal hygiene, in their adhering to their prescribed daily medication requirements, and with respect to many related sickness-prevention issues. These patients also tend to have higher rates of chronic infection due to histories of substance addiction – for example, human immunodeficiency virus (HIV) infection, hepatitis B or C, or tuberculosis.[172]

Patient and family empowerment

A century ago, individuals judged to suffer from a mental illness lacked collective voice, and this dismissive attitude on the part of psychiatric institutions extended to patients' families.[173] By extension, in the age of the insane asylum, patients and their families were rarely if ever consulted on matters related to capital improvements, such as a renovated or expanded facility. In psychiatric diagnosis and treatment, the patient's personal stories are documented in the medical case history, and patient empowerment/reempowerment rests in being able to recount and confront past issues and difficulties. Rehabilitation consists of reclaiming one's sense of personal worth, dignity, competence, and control and recognizing the hidden powers in positive, mutually supportive, life-affirming interpersonal relationships. Similarly, being consulted in matters related to the built environment, of feeling that one's opinions are valued, can yield positive outcomes. Compassion need not be limited to the treatment regimen per se. Meaningful consultation in the case of a capital improvement initiative can be about involvement in public meetings and predesign meetings with the architects and staff, as well as the organization's representatives genuinely listening to what is being said by patients and their families. Hidden agendas or superficial 'lip service' are corrosive. In the United Kingdom, the Bradford City Clinical Commissioning Group initiated a program it dubbed Grass Roots, a process of that drew together diverse local stakeholders in consultation sessions to review specific projects and proposed therapy/counseling resources, and how to best establish effective communications for the solicitation of grassroots mental health advocacy groups' input. More than 1,949 online posts consisting of patient/family feedback were received from 3,987 individuals, with 209 of these coming directly from former mental health patients and their families.[174] Similarly, patients were consulted in a design installation called 'Madlove: A Designer Asylum' by the British artist-activist James Leadbitter. Leadbitter, a former psychiatric inpatient himself, has exhibited at prestigious art venues, recently exhibiting his prototype psychiatric unit design in Liverpool, United Kingdom.[175]

Life-cycle performance metrics

Life-cycle assessment (LCA), also known as eco-balancing or cradle-to-grave building assessment, takes a long view of the operational performance of a healthcare facility with the goal of regenerative sustainability. This begins at the earliest stages of the capital improvement planning process, involving key stakeholders and encompassing a predetermined occupancy life span (e.g., 20 or 30 years). It encompasses all major building materials and assemblies, structural and environmental control systems, type of construction, maintenance and upkeep determinants, growth and retrofit options likely to play out over the predetermined time frame, periodic human health status, satisfaction and performance assessment, biohazard and solid waste disposal factors, and anticipated campus-facility resilience in the face of external threats to daily operations such as the impacts of climate change (Figure 5.44).[176] The success of LCA depends on interdependent internal and external data streams, and its mainstream acceptance remains somewhat hindered by biases against prefabricated, off-site built healthcare construction techniques. As for master planning, LCA assessment tools exist to demonstrate to an owner/client the likely environmental sustainability consequences that can occur relative to various site-planning and building-design options. Specific issues comparatively analyzed may include climate change variables such as the effects of atmospheric acidification, eutrophication, fossil fuel depletion, smog formation, ozone depletion, ecological toxicity, and on-site water retention and recycling system options. Multiple data inputs and outputs are analyzed and assessed for their predicted performance, and environmental programs for LCA applications include ISO 14000 – the most generally applicable and flexible program – developed by the International Standards Organization (ISO), the British Research Establishment Environmental Assessment Methodology (BREEAM) launched in

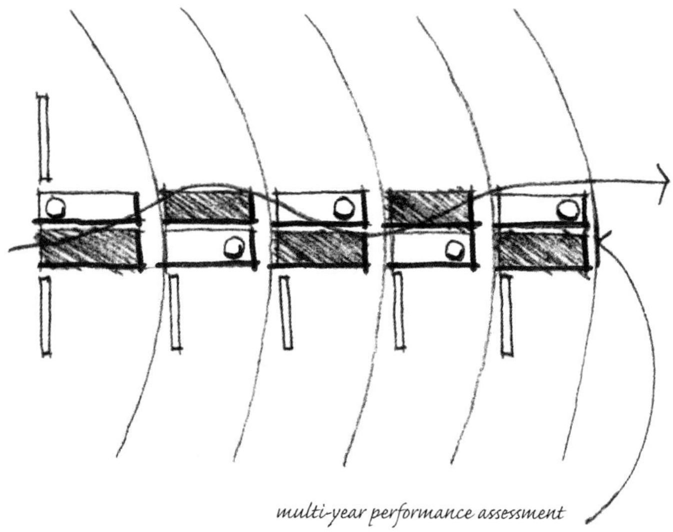

5.44 Adopt life-cycle performance metrics.

1990, BREEAM Canada, and BREEAM/Green Leaf. In 1996, this program was introduced to Canada and is now known as the CSA Plus 1132 Standard. The Green Building Challenge (GBC) is an international building assessment tool and is in many ways equivalent to the well-known LEED (Leadership in Energy Efficient Environment Design) program in North America. In Australia, NABERS (the National Australian Building Environmental Rating System) project is gaining considerable momentum at this time. Recently, *embodied energy* has come to the forefront, generally defined as the sum of all energy required to extract raw materials and then to produce, transport, and assemble the elements of a building at its site destination.[177]

Valuing evidence-based design research

As discussed in Chapter 2, the inpatient psychiatric ward was the subject of considerable evidence-based research conducted in the 1960s and 1970s.[178] Whether then or now, the facility CEO is a vital link in providing leadership to ensure administrative oversight translates into staff-, patient-, and family-centered policies, which in turn will yield positive outcomes with respect to the scope and quality of care. Zimring et al. (2008) conceptualized a systematic evidence-based facility-procurement process consisting of the importance of due attention accorded (in this order) to strategic business planning; facility and campus master planning; transitional planning to ensure smooth operations in relocating from an existing to a new facility; and in the programming, design, and construction phases, with continuing oversight occurring through to the commissioning and postoccupancy retrofit phases following a period of initial occupancy.[179] This process is driven by focusing on the end users – the daily occupants.[180] Initiated by the Washington, D.C.–based Institute of Medicine, the 'To Err Is Human' patient-staff safety report and subsequent patients' rights movement, as it pertains to the elimination of medical errors in mental health and addiction disorders centers, are noteworthy as the report's recommendations can ultimately dictate a facility's success or failure. The goals of mental health care provider organizations differ little from the broader patient-staff safety movement in acute care hospitals in this regard.[181] It behooves psychiatric and substance addiction service providers to incorporate evidence-based perspectives into the planning and design of new and renovated treatment facilities. Practices or policies perceived as nontransparent may boomerang and come back to haunt the organization. Instead, from the outset, foster a rigorous evidence-based protocol grounded in measurable outcome metrics subject to continuous reappraisal by the organization and its internal and external stakeholders. Then translate these outcomes into policy and built form, such as the demonstrated cost benefits of evidence-based design interventions that began as a series of one-off interventions and in time evolved into the policy implications associated with the Fable Hospital 2.0 Project (2011).[182]

Valuing therapeutic design interventions

The opportunity exists for mental health and addictive disorder service provider organizations to employ salutogenic (therapeutic) design as part of the organizational mission statement, and one example of this is partial hospitalization. Partial hospitalization programs encourage the patient to transition from a 24/7 facility as he or she progresses through his or her treatment, as complimented by a network of neighborhood-based outpatient mental health clinics. Salutogenic design strategies can aid this transition, because they can facilitate the coordination of 24/7 residential centers and outpatient-only facilities as a single continuum, each building type with specific architectural amenities, person/nature/landscape amenities, functional supports, and formal aesthetic language, achievable through such measures as redundant cuing, layering/collage, superimposition, and interpretive deconstruction/reassembly. The aim is for all program sites within the care network to become architecturally interdependent and yet diverse.[183] Explore administrative paradigms to leverage and harness synergies between management strategies, human resources, and the built environment. Attention restoration theory (ART) is but one theoretical perspective that can guide this process, as ART places priority on emphasizing the affordances of therapeutic design.[184] Care settings perceived as inherently interesting and that repeatedly draw us back to them possess restorative qualities and accordingly can be of positive psychological impact. Strive to match organizational transparency with architectural and landscape transparency because service provider organizations that fail to capitalize on this opportunity in their coordinated inpatient and outpatient facilities are subject to eventual sclerosis.[185]

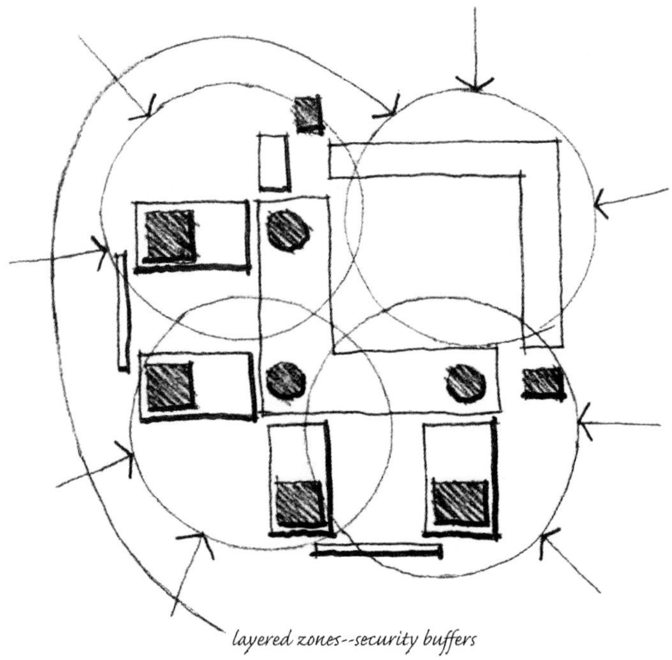

5.45 Choreographed security systems.

Security affordances

Individuals with mental and addictive disorders are fundamentally entitled to receive treatment in a care setting neither threatening nor disempowering. Recent advancements in campus security and surveillance technology make it possible to establish layered, overlapping zones of security beginning at the campus perimeter and penetrating into the heart of the campus/facility, not unlike concentric rings. These rings culminate in the inpatient residential unit.[186] Provide secure buffer zones beginning at the site perimeter, including all parking areas, the main arrival sequence and building entry, public spaces, and semiprivate and private zones throughout (Figure 5.45). Unobtrusive security measures – infrared imagery, lasers, miniature video cameras, and card reader sensors at access points – are effective in many situations. Achieve a balance between campus/building security measures and equipment with a humane philosophy of care – distinguishing between static security and dynamic security measures – combined with honor-code policies whereby patients are rewarded with additional spatial freedoms in accord with their behaviour.[187] Case study precedents in Chapter 6 incorporate a variety of such balanced security interventions, from strictly physical security measures, to behaviour modification policies, such as at Hopewood Park (CS 3), the Vermont Psychiatric Care Hospital (CS 6), the High Care Clinic (CS 13), the Ferndene Centre (CS 16), and the Hokkaido Children's Centre in Japan (CS 20). In each of these examples, fences and walls are minimized or avoided altogether in favor of the building complex itself functioning as primary security device (the physical footprint and its composition) together with progressive behaviour modification policies. The more transparent the intervention, the better, as illustrated in the alternative CAMH proposal (see Chapter 4), where the exterior balcony's 'walls' are transparent without compromising safety and security (Figure 5.46). The total security system should be a primary consideration from the earliest phases in design in order to avoid unsightly interventions having to be installed later. Most importantly, avoid security barriers/systems that may be perceived by the patient as restrictive, overbearing, or prosecutorial.

Health facilities and informatics

The electronic health record (EHR) movement in the United States has been endorsed by the American Psychiatric Association (APA) and was a tenet of the American Recovery and Reinvestment Act of 2009 (ARRA). This legislation included an unprecedented US$19 billion earmarked for application throughout the United States vis-à-vis the Health Information Technology for Economic and Clinical Health (HITECH) Act, and associated Health Information Technology (HIT) legislation.[188] The APA's Committee on Mental Health Information Technology (CMHIT) subsequently developed a tutorial to help service providers select an EHR implementation strategy and to assist commercial vendors in constructing useful EHR systems for use in psychiatry and behavioural health field applications. The APA Internet home page includes a section on key questions to ask before entering

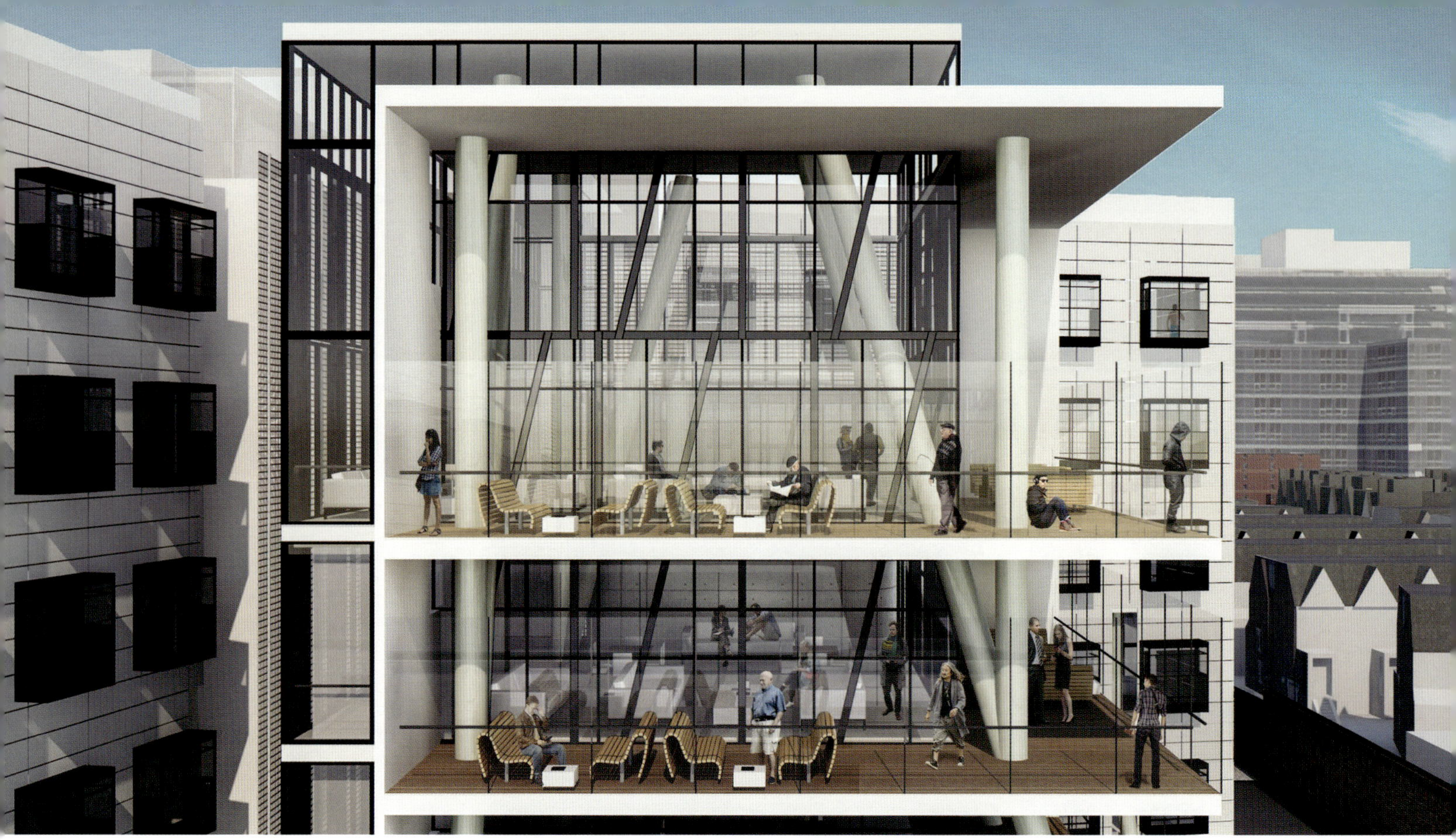

5.46 Safe, secure (upper-level) terraces and balconies.

an EHR agreement. A parallel organization, the Behavioral Health Information Technology (BHIT) Coalition, was established in 2010 and is composed of allied organizations dedicated to advancing public policy initiatives and advocates for the adoption of the full potential of EHR technology.[189] In 2014, an industry commercial vendor, Capterra, reported that 21% of all US mental health and addictive disorders service providers used some form of EHR at their program sites. IT spending by these providers represented only 1.8% of their total operating budgets, however, and 30% of providers cited high upfront investment costs as a leading barrier to further EHR implementation.[190] A parallel development has been the emergence of personal health records (PHRs). Patient's EHRs are particularly valuable in the aftermath of disaster events, where the individual patient may be suddenly uprooted, dislocated to another community, and in urgent need of medications or emergency counseling (see Chapter 3). One implication of advanced e-health informatics has been the obsolescence of bulky medical records storerooms, although there sometimes still remains a need to maintain a backup paper version of the PHR.[191]

Disaster preparedness and resiliency

Every healthcare organization needs a well-rehearsed emergency preparedness plan. A prescripted plan of action is of tremendous benefit, particularly in anticipation of climate change impacts such as rising sea levels, intense rainstorms, hurricanes and typhoons, periods of drought and associated water shortages, and related events likely to impact sudden population migrations and the immediate quality of life. In the case of St. Rita's nursing home in St. Bernard Parish, in suburban New Orleans, United States, the floodwaters from Hurricane Katrina filled this one-level facility nearly to the ceiling within 20 minutes. The owners were put on trial on 35 counts of negligent homicide and 24 counts of cruelty to the elderly and infirm patients who died within. Patients drowned in their beds and wheelchairs. The owners maintained that keeping these frail patients in place was safer than subjecting them to the trauma of forced evacuation.[192] Eight years later, the owners of the nursing home were acquitted of guilt in the deaths, although this tragedy is a cautionary tale for mental health and addiction disorder service providers.[193] While an extreme example, the fact remains that every inpatient and outpatient treatment center should have a strategic plan in the event that staff and patients must be evacuated offsite (or relocated to safe quarters elsewhere on-site). More broadly, entire communities should have coordinated, well-rehearsed emergency preparedness plans in place.[194] A small number (between 22 and 42) of psychiatrists returned to New Orleans in the fall and winter of 2005, in the immediate months following Katrina. Prior, there were between 196 and 208 psychiatrists practicing in the New Orleans area (for a population of 480,000). Most local hospitals shut down their psychiatric wards afterward, and the number of chronically mentally ill incarcerated in Orleans Parish Prison increased exponentially, and remains quite high today.[195] Additionally, extra security measures must be in place to anticipate possible acts of violence or attempts to abscond when a facility is in pre- or postdisaster lockdown or in the process of being evacuated. In high-risk zones, it is advisable to hold preparatory evacuation drills

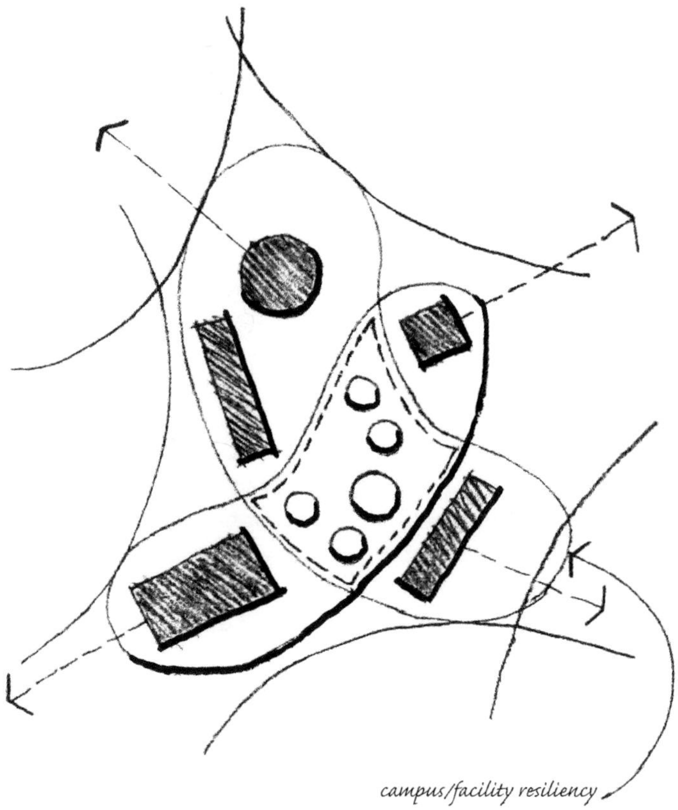

5.47 Design for disaster preparedness.

bimonthly. Rapid response can mean the difference between life and death. (Figure 5.47).

Eco-humanism and capital resource management

An eco-humanist perspective in design, as it applies to the built environment for healthcare, involves placing equal priority on both human and ecological well-being. As such, 10 territories for engagement were recently delineated by Peters and Verderber (2017), consisting of the need for (1) the minimization of the facility/campus carbon footprint, (2) resilient and sustainable/regenerative facilities for healthcare, (3) the use of functional deconstruction (scaled-down) strategies to reduce the sheer size and complexity of healthcare institutions and more carefully attune them to their local communities, (4) highlighting the role of landscape therapeutics and nature in treatment and healing, (5) emphasizing on the value of residential design strategies as opposed anachronistic design traditions associated with postwar institutionalism and custodialism (see Chapter 2), (6) emphasizing stakeholder advocacy and social inclusiveness throughout the planning and design process, (7) placing high value on the provision of salutogenic (therapeutic) design in the interiors of healthcare environments, (8) incorporating tectonic innovations in the healthcare environment, (9) inventively repurposing existing healthcare (and other) adaptive/adaptable resources to new healthcare purposes (versus thoughtless demolition), and (10) adopting strategies to ensure that any new interdisciplinary knowledge acquired is mobilized and disseminated so future similar initiatives can benefit.[196] Building information modeling (BIM) applications in healthcare facility planning and design can be effective in minimizing construction waste materials and can significantly improve the eco-humanist quotient.[197] LEAN can also be of aid in this regard, as a systematic method for waste minimization ('*muda*' in Japanese) within a manufacturing system, with the aim of not sacrificing productivity. It makes obvious that which adds value by reducing everything extraneous (which is not adding value), a management philosophy derived from the Toyota Production System (TPS) and identified as 'lean' in the 1990s. LEAN, when combined with BIM, synthesizes functional space-planning efficiencies during design and also in postoccupancy performance assessment, streamlining the total supply chain of materials, reducing overall waste and project delivery cost, and maximizing time efficiencies, and carbon neutral materials and building assemblies.[198]

Salutogenic partnerships

Salutogenic design and the public-private partnership (PPP) process for the procurement of healthcare facilities are not naturally compatible with one another. The former focuses on the promotion of human health and well-being; quality of life; environmental sustainability; and inspired, eco-humanist, and life-affirming aspects of the built environment. The latter consists of strictly defined business protocols to reach the highest 'feasible' design standard in the most cost-effective way. They are increasingly interconnected in further developing the world's healthcare infrastructure (Figure 5.48). PPP can be highly problematic to manage, and examples of unqualified success remain relatively few. Ken Schwarz, writing in *World Health Design* in 2015, summarized the pros and cons of PPP:

> Fortunately, there is a broad range of experience to learn from. For nearly twenty years PPP has been applied to healthcare projects and its use continues to evolve around

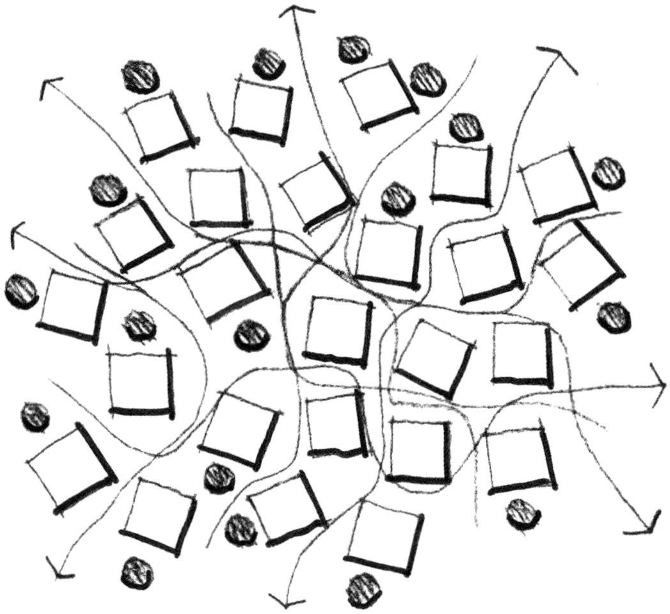

5.48 Establish sustainable, salutogenic partnerships.

> the world . . . the UK, Canada, and Australia are in the uppermost tier (where) literally hundreds have been completed. This reflects the largely nationalized healthcare systems of these countries, strong private-sector capability, and political will. On the other hand, the more fragmented and privatized healthcare systems, such as that of the United States, have been far slower to take up PPP.

He then summarized some of the hard lessons learned, citing recent case studies. The 'pros' of PPP include providing access to private capital markets, integrating total building delivery from project start to daily operation, and imposing a strict discipline resulting in on-time and on-budget building delivery (citing the fact that many high-quality facilities have resulted from this process). PPP spreads out the risk over many years relative to the upfront initial financial investment, establishes long-term contractual relationships for building delivery and maintenance (up to 30 years), and allows projects to be built that would otherwise have remained entirely unbuilt. The potential pitfalls of PPP, on the other hand, include it being slow and tedious to procure, with many legal disputes arising between the private-sector landlord and the public-sector tenant; this can hamper both design quality and long-term building performance. A PPP can incur higher upfront borrowing costs, and undue pressures to maximize shareholders' return on investment can diminish the quality of the final built outcome. Promises made up front during the project's bidding phase often can end up being ignored later on when the preferred (winning) bidder takes over, with the tone and structure of the entire enterprise often souring quickly for all parties. PPPs are, by fundamental contractual design, composed of rival individuals, firms, and corporations, and this alone can overcomplicate and greatly dilute the final built outcome. Finally, the salutogenic design aspects of a project can be totally overwhelmed, even obliterated, by the competing objectives of various stakeholders. Regardless, Schwarz cited successful case studies, including hospitals recently built in the United Kingdom, Northern Ireland, Canada, and Australia.[199] To date, the United States has not been a significant player on the PPP field in the realm of healthcare facilities.

PART 3

Case studies

CHAPTER 6

Case studies 1–25

The projects

Comprehensive treatment: medical campus/district

Kingfisher Court, Radlett, Hertfordshire, Greater London, England, UK
P+HS Architects, Leeds, UK
Östra Healthcare Centre for Psychiatry, Göteborg, Sweden
White Arkitekter AB, Göteborg, Sweden
Hopewood Park, Sunderland, England, UK
MAAP (Medical Architecture and Arts Projects, Ltd.), London, UK
Professor Marie Bashir Centre at the Royal Prince Alfred Hospital, Sydney, Australia
Peckvonhartel (pvh), Sydney, Australia/Silver Thomas Hanley (STH), Sydney, Australia
Roseberry Park, Middlesbrough, England, UK
MAAP (Medical Architecture and Arts Projects, Ltd.), London, UK
Vermont Psychiatric Care Hospital, Berlin, Vermont, USA
architecture+ (Prime Architect), Troy, New York, USA, with Black River Design (Associated Architects), Montpelier, Vermont, USA

Comprehensive treatment: autonomous

The Southdown Institute, Holland Landing, Newmarket, Ontario, Canada
Montgomery Sisam Architects, Toronto, Ontario, Canada
Helsingor Psychiatric Hospital and Clinic, Helsingor, Denmark
JDS/BIG Architects, Copenhagen, Denmark
Residence and Day Centre for the Mentally Handicapped, Barcelona, Spain
Aldayjover Arquitectura Y Paisaje, Barcelona, Spain
De Hogeweyk (Dementia Village), Weesp, the Netherlands
mbvda (Molenaar & Bol & Van Dillen), Vught, the Netherlands
Centre for the Mentally Handicapped in Alcolea, Cordoba, Spain
Taller de Arquitectura/Rico+Roa, Cordoba, Spain
Margaret and Charles Juravinski Centre for Integrated Healthcare, Hamilton, Ontario, Canada
Cannon Design, Buffalo, New York, USA/architecture+, Troy, New York, USA
High Care Clinic, Oegstgeest, the Netherlands
de Jong Gortemaker Algra (dJGA), Rotterdam, the Netherlands

Forensic treatment centers

The Lowry Unit, Prestwich, Manchester, UK
Gilling Dod Architects, Lancashire, UK
Worcester Recovery Center and Hospital, Worcester, Massachusetts, USA
Ellenzweig, Boston, Massachusetts, USA/architecture+, Troy, New York, USA

Child and adolescent treatment centers

Ferndene Children and Young People's Centre, Northumberland, Prudhoe, Newcastle-upon-Tyne, UK
MAAP (Medical Architecture and Arts Projects, Ltd.), London, UK
Junction 17, Prestwich, Greater Manchester, England, UK
Gilling Dod Architects, Lancashire, UK
Linn Dara Child and Adolescent Centre at Cherry Hill Hospital, Dublin, Ireland
Reddy Architecture + Urbanism, London, UK
Seattle Children's Hospital Psychiatry and Behavioral Medicine Unit, Seattle, Washington, USA
ZGF Architects, Seattle, Washington, USA/Medical Planning: architecture+, Troy, New York, USA
Children's Centre for Psychiatric Rehabilitation, Hokkaido, Japan
Sou Fujimoto, Architect, Tokyo, Japan

Ambulatory treatment centers

Sowa Unit, Saitama, Japan
Kensuke Watanabe Architecture Studio, Tokyo, Japan
Village Family Health Team Clinic, Centre for Addiction and Mental Health, Toronto, Ontario, Canada
ARK Architects, Toronto, Ontario, Canada
Sydenham Garden Resource Centre, London, UK
Architype, London, UK

Prognostications

Leaside Behavioural Health Centre, Toronto, Ontario, Canada
Gabriel Valdivieso, Quito, Ecuador
New psychiatric hospital, Bispebjerg, Denmark
Friis & Moltke Architects, Aarhus, Denmark/PLH Arkitekter, Copenhagen, Denmark

Twenty-five case studies are presented in this chapter, organized according to a six-part architectural typology. They represent a cross-section of public- and private-sector medically based programs with the exception of one (Sydenham Garden Resource Centre in London, United Kingdom). All facilities opened no earlier than 2006 (except for the two unbuilt case studies, 24 and 25); each expresses innovative principles of sustainable site planning and architectural design and each a progressive treatment philosophy with respect to residentially based or outpatient-based care (or both). A number of case studies represent a new approach, some radical. The more experimental firmly challenge the status quo in terms of expressing inventive solutions to nettlesome issues, whether related to site context, program imperatives, or architectural and landscape design strategies. The six types are:

Comprehensive treatment: medical campus/district – These six case studies are urban institutions providing comprehensive inpatient care, situated in proximity to (or immersed within) an existing medical center. The parent medical center typically houses acute care and specialized services, including a children's hospital, hospice center, outpatient clinics, and related supports, such as car parks and landscaped exterior space. All are publicly owned and operated, with some administered by local healthcare authorities and others by a parent, countrywide ministry of health.

Comprehensive treatment: autonomous – These seven are autonomous institutions, independent of a medical center campus context. They are campuses onto themselves (Helsingor Psychiatric Hospital and Clinic, in Denmark; and De Hogeweyk, in the Netherlands). Some are in quasi-rural settings (Centre for the Mentally Handicapped in Alcolea, Spain, and the Southdown Institute, in Newmarket, Ontario, Canada). They are freestanding, and range in size from 20 beds to upwards a of 300. Site environs facilitate patients' and others' immersion in nature as part of treatment. Many are rural, including some on the grounds of former insane asylums.

Forensic treatment centers – These case studies are innovative in rejecting custodial institutionalism and conscious and thorough dismissal of past traditional forensic architecture. Albeit, it remains a challenge to fully break from the past for these facilities house many patients who would otherwise be incarcerated, some for life. One case study is small in scale and quasi-residential, while the other is a large state-run institution where a genuine effort was made to create a quasi-normative 'village'.

Child and adolescent treatment centers – These case studies were planned and constructed for persons' aged 6–18 for specialized treatment, including eating disorders, depression, bipolar disorder, and personality disorders. One is part of a large urban medical center (Seattle Children's) while others are housed on freestanding campuses (Children's Centre for Psychiatric Rehabilitation, in Japan, and the Linn Dara Child and Adolescent Centre on the campus of Cherry Hill Hospital, in Dublin, Ireland).

Ambulatory treatment centers – Outpatient mental health and substance addiction clinics constitute, in many places, the largest percentage and fastest growing building type. The need for accessible, community-based services is considerable and particularly acute in chronically medically underserved communities. Unfortunately, few such clinics attain a high level of design excellence. The three represented here are in Japan, Canada, and the United Kingdom, and represent three quite different strategies.

Prognostications – Two unbuilt projects are included for their innovative design qualities and for questioning the current state of the art. The first is an unbuilt proposal for a neighborhood-based inpatient/outpatient residential treatment satellite campus for the Centre for Addiction and Mental Health (CAMH) in Toronto, and the second is the winning design competition entry for the replacement psychiatric hospital being constructed in Bispebjerg, Denmark. The latter opens in 2018.

Sixteen case studies have earned, at this writing, architectural recognition for design excellence in local, national, or international awards programs. These projects were deemed by panels of peer judges as representative of current thinking in architecture for health as pertaining to psychiatric and addiction disorder building types. Individual projects express interesting idiosyncratic aims and philosophical orientations of owner-clients and also the preferences and functional needs of patients and direct caregivers who inhabit the facility.

At the campus-wide scale of inquiry:

Case studies include facilities built in urban districts, in suburban neighborhoods, and in exurban contexts. With land valuations typically highest in dense urban contexts, the tendency is for those to have a somewhat restrictive footprint and a greater number of floor levels. If the campus consists of more than one building in this context, they will be in closer physical proximity to one another, often with parking provided in a deck below street level. In suburban contexts, the campus will tend to have a significantly larger physical footprint with parking provided at grade. In the case of exurban campuses, some new or replacement facilities are being built on, or next to, the grounds of former insane asylums, with the new facility occuping a portion of the grounds.

At the building-scale level of inquiry:

Many case studies involve the repurposing of an existing structure, and in other cases a new facility built in proximity to an existing heritage building. Some are housed in a one-level structure whereas others in midrise structures. Many feature courtyards of varying size and amenity, including green roof terraces functioning as outdoor rooms, many of which envelope the immediate building context on two or more sides. These spaces house therapeutic gardens and recreational therapy amenities such as a ball field, track, or basketball court. Every case study is examined in relative to its own aesthetic vocabulary, particularly from the standpoint of its *residentialist* qualities, including wayfinding, connectivity to nature vis-à-vis natural daylight, ventilation, and window-view amenity.

At the unit or patient room level of inquiry:

Individual rooms and the relationship between interior and exterior space are examined with regards to habitability, aesthetics, materiality, size, proportion, and the degree to which a given space supports larger diagnostic and treatment program priorities. Similarly, amenities for families and visitors are of importance, as are the functional and emotional support needs of direct caregiver staff. This pertains to staff travel and walking distances, personal safety, places for respite for staff, and the ability of occupants to maintain perceived control of their immediate environment to a reasonable degree – influencing one's overall psycho-emotional well-being, attitudinal disposition, and resulting physical behaviour. Specific attention is devoted to nurses' stations and associated workspaces in the residential unit, whether *shielded* (entirely enclosed), *hybrid* (partially enclosed), or *unshielded* (open) in configuration, and appearance, and security amenity.

In terms of sustainability and ecological inquiry:

The concept of net-zero (*zeroality*) or net-plus (regenerative) building and campus poses unique challenges for any hospital or related residential care facility; for they are among the highest and most energy-consumptive of all building types because they must be operational 24/7. The movement to transform these types in this regard continues to proceed at a less rapid rate compared to, say, educational, housing, and museum building types. Nonetheless, case studies are examined here from this standpoint with regards to daily and life-cycle operational costs, and measures taken to minimize the carbon footprint. Materials of construction, retrofitting measures, building envelope efficiency, and environmental control systems are addressed. Innovative landscape design and site maintenance strategies are examined, including xeriscaping and green roofscapes, rainwater harvesting, geothermal systems, and the sourcing of locally available materials and methods of construction. Public transit and cycling amenities are similarly examined.

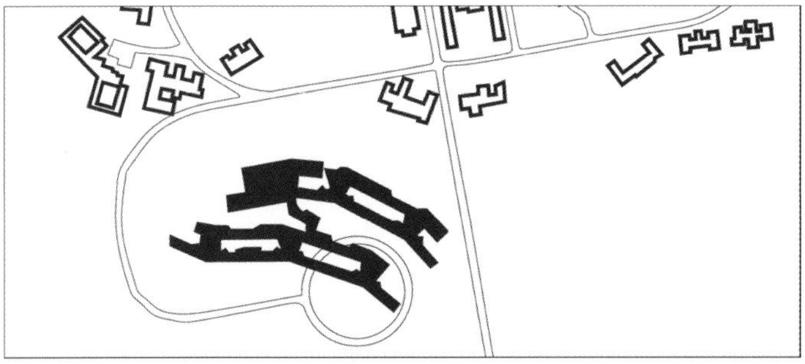

1 Kingfisher Court, Radlett, Hertfordshire, Greater London, England, UK

ARCHITECT: P+HS Architects, Leeds, UK
LANDSCAPE ARCHITECT: P+HS Architects, Leeds, UK
CLIENT: Hertfordshire Partnership University NHS Foundation Trust
FEATURED MATERIALS: Timber
COMPLETED: 2014
INPATIENT BEDS: 86
SITE/PARKING: 5.5 acres/150
HOSPITAL/TREATMENT CENTER SIZE: 38,000 square feet
NURSES' WORKSTATION: Shielded

Context/site

This campus was built at Hertfordshire Partnership Foundations Trust's (HPFT) Kingsley Green site near Radlett, in conjunction with the University NHS Foundation Trust. Kingfisher Court is a £42 million investment and its planning and design occurred over a 4-year period. It was built near the Kingsley Green Hospital, formerly the Harperbury Hospital (1928–1973), and the Middlesex Colony Institution (1936–1973), in a rural district northwest of London. It is an example of the 'recovery model' the NHS is promoting in its new buildings, with an emphasis on lifestyle normalization. The recovery model of psychiatric care centers on rehabilitation for success in everyday life in the community and views mental health treatment as constituting a continuum of care. The design process was participatory, with extensive meetings and workshops involving key stakeholder constituencies, including patients and their families. This pertained to site planning, building design, and building-campus usage. P+HS won this commission in a design competition, and nearly 2,000 hours were subsequently devoted to extensive rounds of consultation. The facility's 86 private bedrooms were deployed in five residential units: acute adult care, frail and self-vulnerable adults, and behavioural learning illness and disability.

At the outset, the design team walked and documented the site in order to take in its somewhat peculiar yet beautiful topography; the design response was a one-level facility, informal in its imagery, arranged as a collection of smaller-scale buildings. Because of its informality, the overall appearance of the campus is inviting and welcoming versus the typically harsh institutionalism of the asylums of the past (Figure 6.1.1). Absent are imposing, institutional façades or monolithic elevations with few windows. The facility is set in 11.5 acres of woodland and natural landscape; extra effort was made to avoid views directly overlooking walls or fences. The palette of colors and design of the courtyard spaces echo their broader surroundings. Campus directional signage reinforces a pervasive sense of informality. The parking area is centralized at the front (arrival side) of the campus. The various buildings' exteriors are sheathed in vertical wood siding, with brightly colored walls in courtyards and elsewhere. The entrances to the buildings are modest in scale to not appear imposing or authoritarian; the campus design strategy emphasized visual diversity and this is perceivable as one walks the grounds. The low-rise silhouette of the buildings is punctuated by many spaces where some buildings appear to wrap around them, giving them a unique identity and further contributing to visual diversity. The compositional massing yields interesting roofscapes that are consciously residential in materiality and form (Figures 6.1.2 to 6.1.4).

Building/unit

The public arrival zone connects to a reception/living room featuring a large fireplace that projects the ambiance of a rural retreat or manor. The image of this space establishes the tone of the campus and its horizontal connectivity with its landscape. The lobby features a café, and interior 'streets' radiate from this point to the five various residential units; the sports therapy, art therapy, and physical therapy rooms; individual and group consultation area; and a horticultural therapy area. The circulation paths connecting these core functions are interspersed with window seats for informal social interaction, not entirely unlike the experience of sitting on a bench along the main street in a village. The primary circulation routes, with their natural light and ventilation, differ from the dreary, double-loaded corridors of prior generations of mental health institutions. Seating is provided outdoors and is protected by extended eaves (Figures 6.1.5 to 6.1.7a–b). Exterior courts are

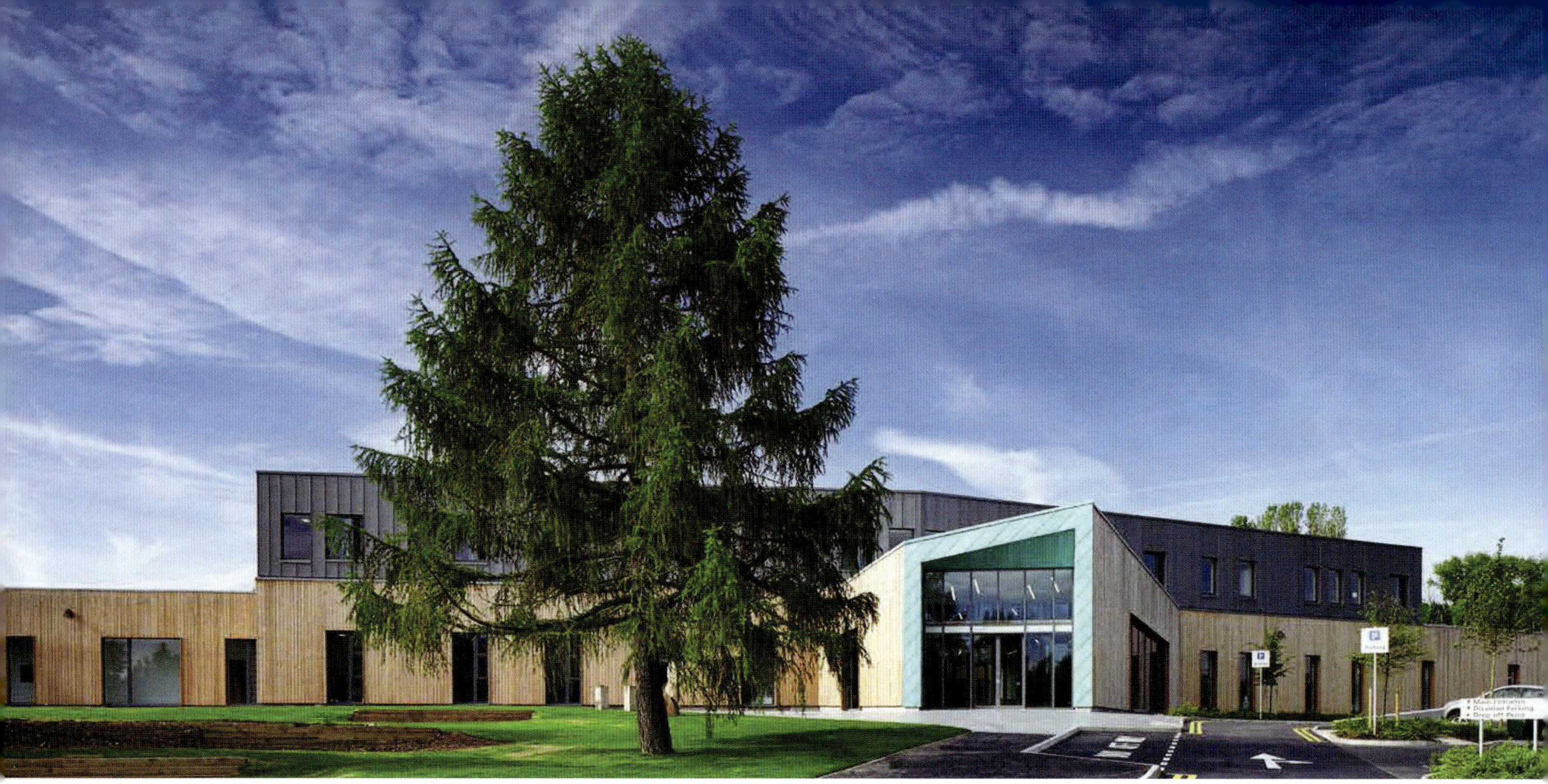

6.1.1 The main approach to Kingfisher Court.

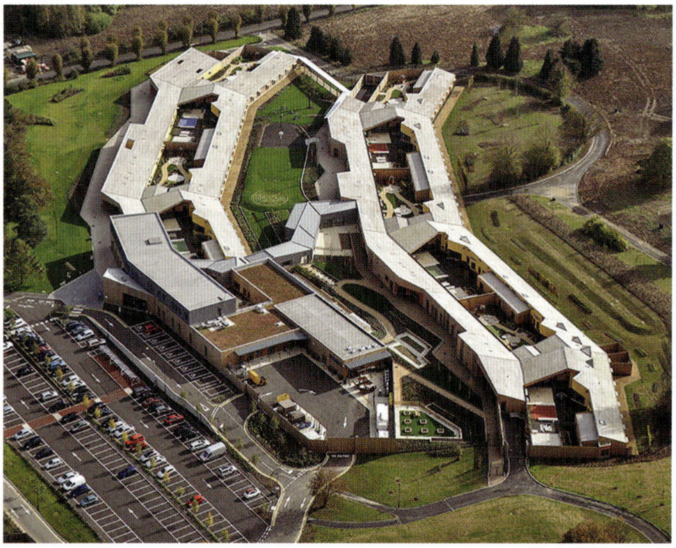

6.1.2 Footprint zigzags with various types of open spaces and the principal building bands interspersed.

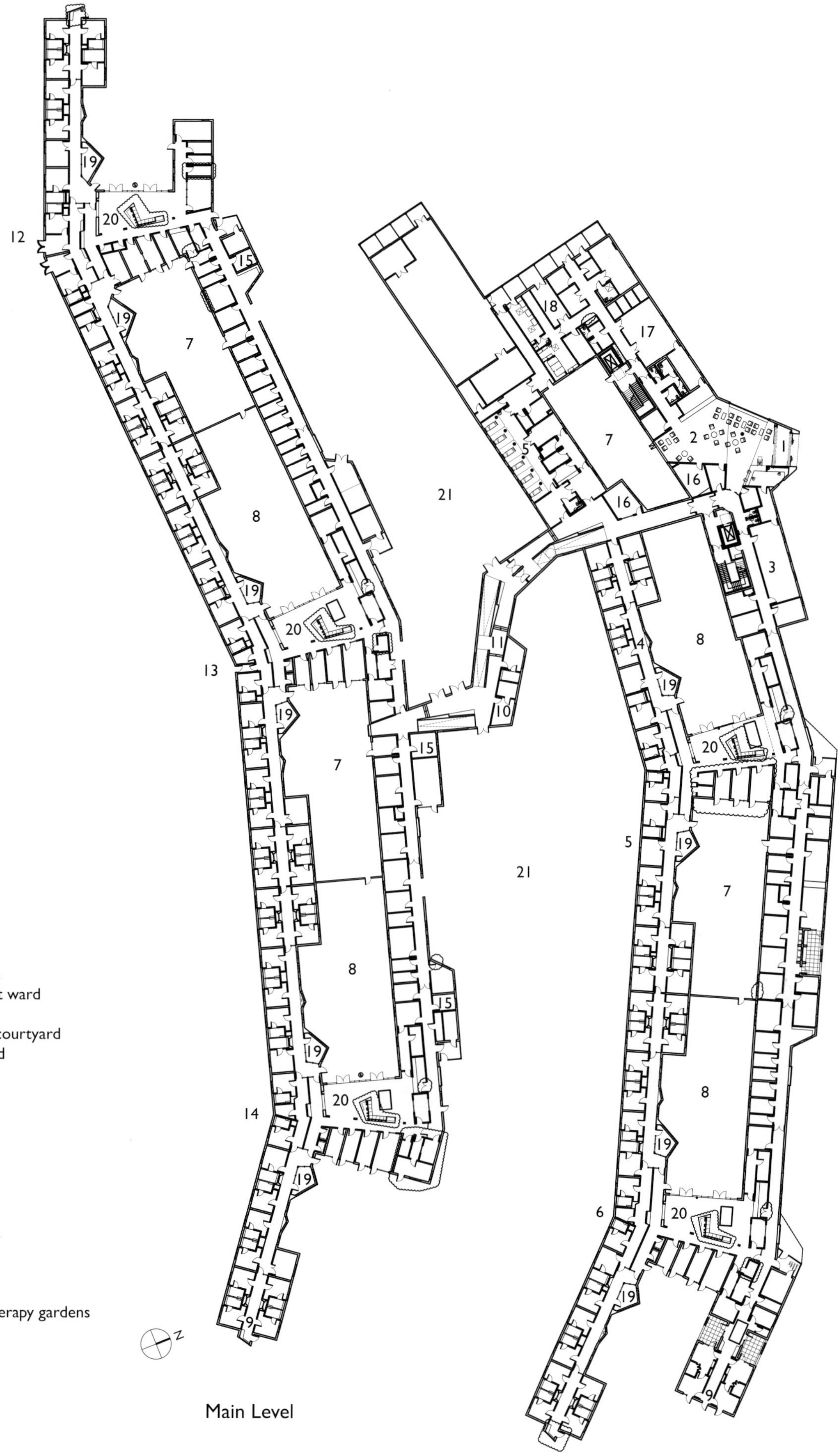

Key:
1 main arrival
2 reception
3 administration
4 central support
5 vulnerable adult ward
6 acute ward 1
7 contemplative courtyard
8 active courtyard
9 seclusion unit
10 guest suites
11 circulation link
12 LD ward
13 acute ward 3
14 acute ward 2
15 staff support
16 staff training
17 dietary support
18 central support
19 quiet room
20 dining/dayroom
21 horticultural/therapy gardens

6.1.3 Residential units at Kingfisher Court are linearly configured, resulting in single-loaded circulation arteries that draw natural night into interiors.

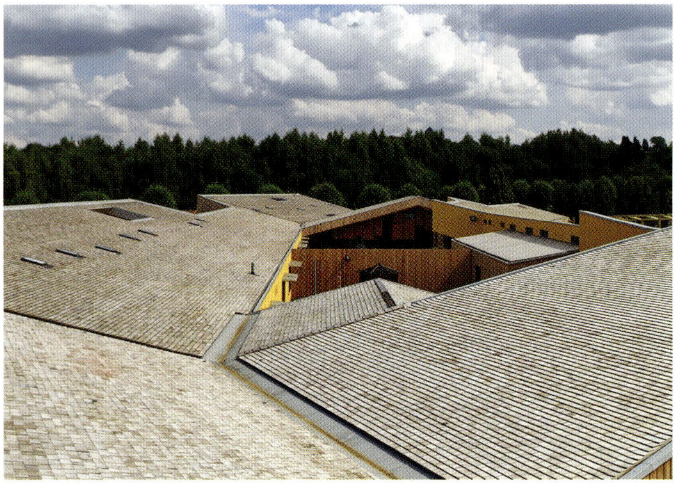

6.1.4 Intersecting roofs create an informal pattern, avoiding the rigid institutionalism of anachronistic asylums.

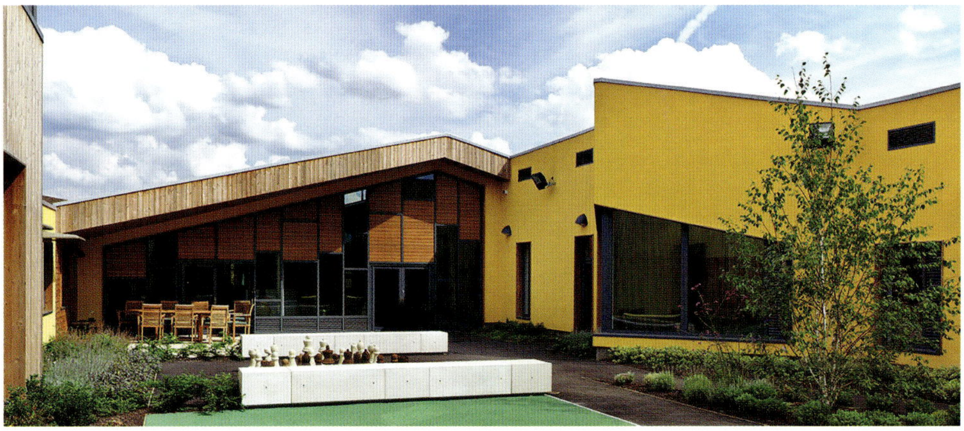

6.1.5 Courtyards are residentially scaled and feature varied materials and geometries.

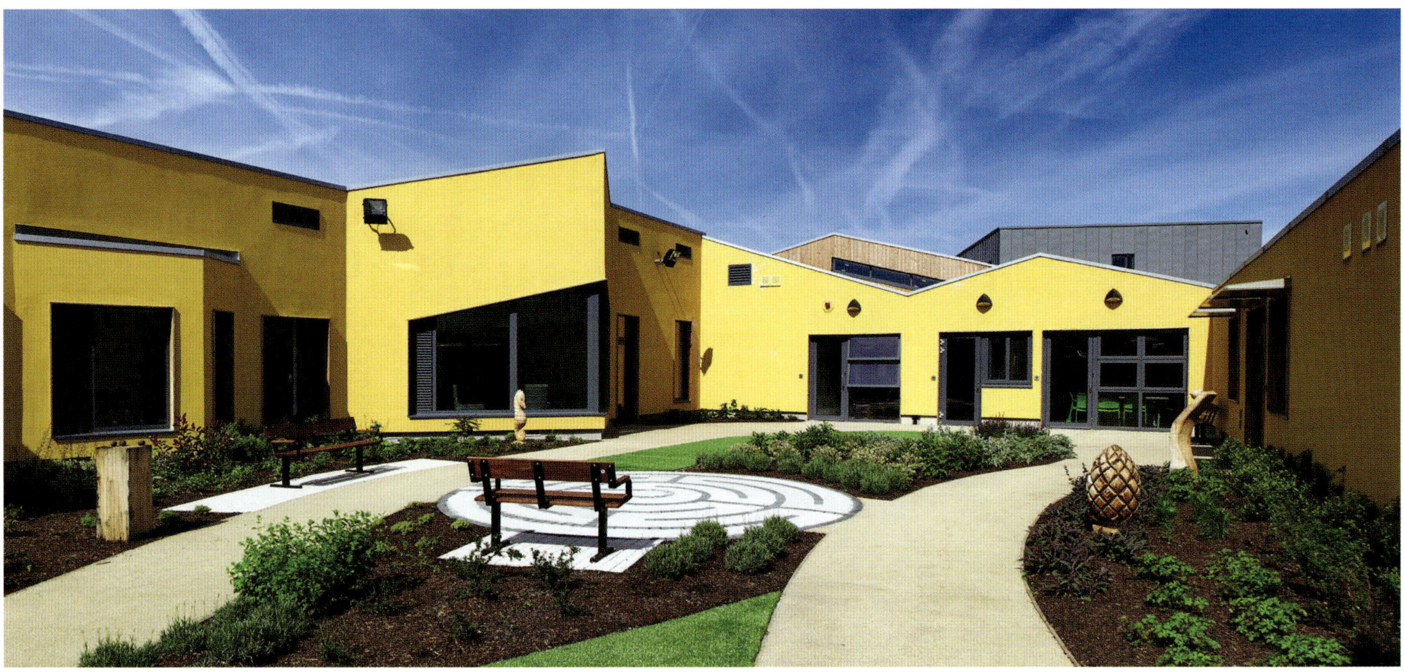

6.1.6 Walking paths, seating areas, and ground plantings in a garden court at Kingfisher Court.

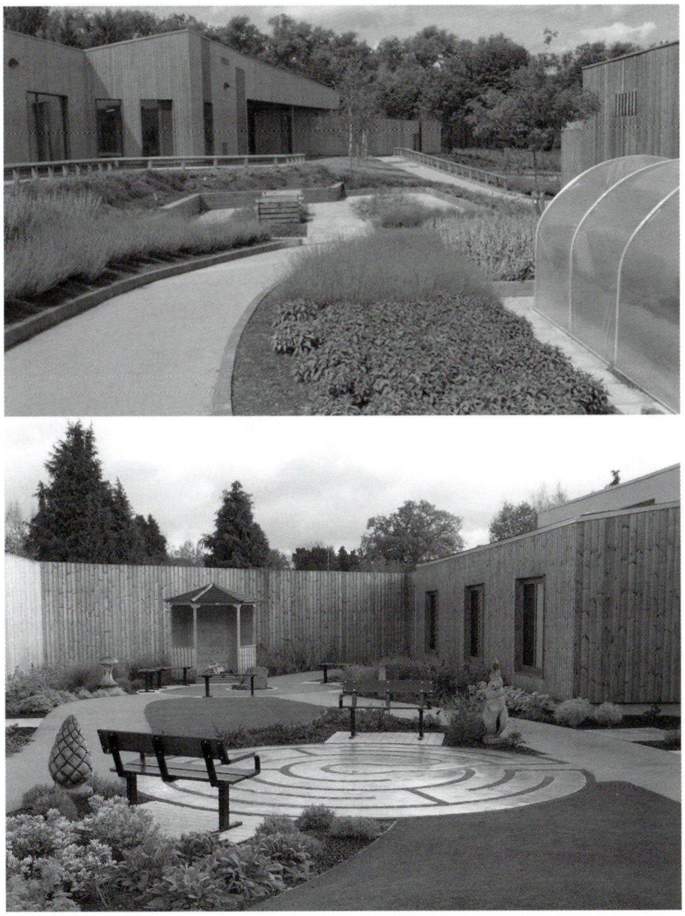

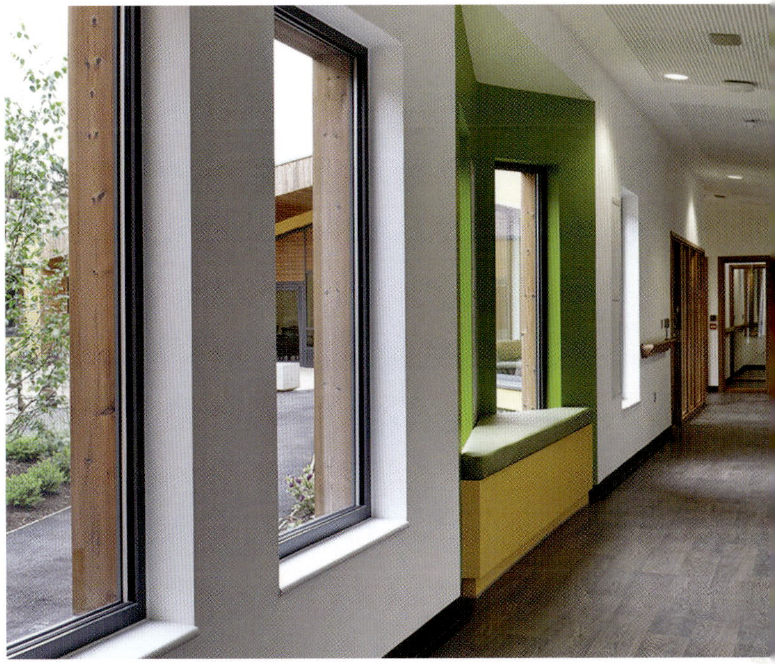

6.1.7a–b No two exterior courtyards are identical, as these exterior 'rooms' provide varied seating, paths, and related amenities, including a labyrinth.

6.1.8 Numerous windowsills along corridors on the residential units double as seating alcoves.

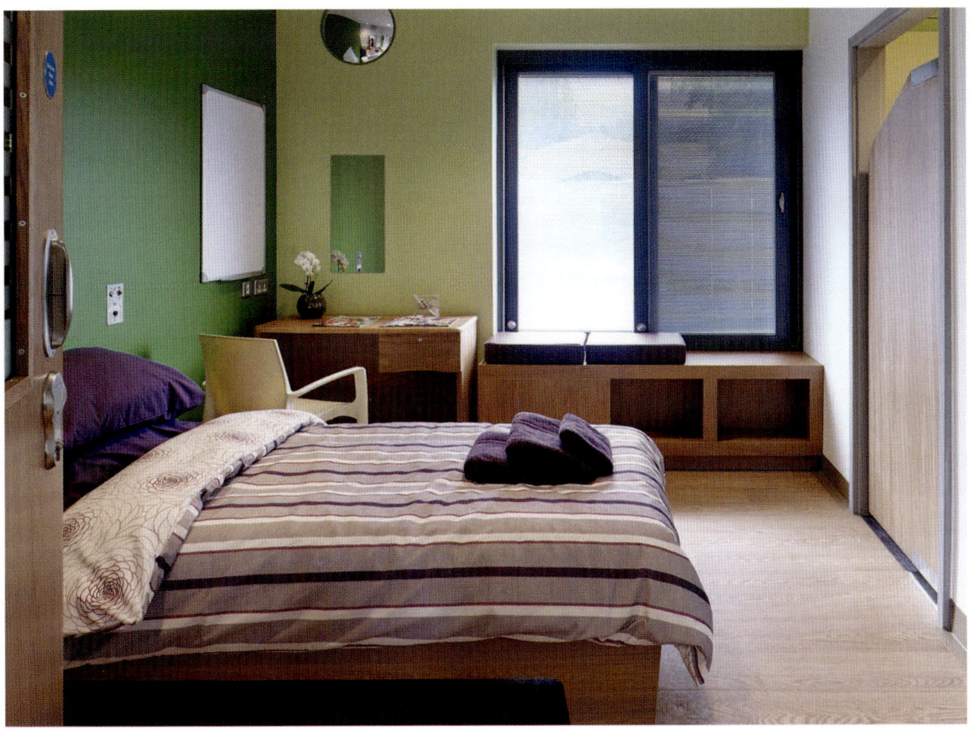

6.1.9 Patient room furnishings and aesthetics are similar to a college dormitory.

designed as 'rooms', with some more generously landscaped than others. The interior furnishings are residential throughout, reinforced by simulated natural wood flooring and natural wood–sheathed doors, door frames, and sloping ceilings of variable heights. This condition extends throughout the residential units and in most therapy and consultation spaces, including 51 such rooms available for therapy and consultation uses. The metaphor of an informal village street extends to the provision of places for chance encounters or simply as places for quiet contemplation. The aforementioned window seats are provided for this purpose and are positioned in proximity to the residential units (Figure 6.1.8). As the patient progresses through one's treatment program, she or he is gradually able to move about more freely on the campus, spending more time, for instance, in the pocket courtyards at the center of the residential units, as expressive of the graduated territoriality concept (see Chapter 5). A 'High Street' connects the two main buildings on the campus.

The local Contemporary Arts Society served as the fine arts consultant for this project. It suggested 10 artists but eventually reduced this number to two (Nicky Hirst and James Ireland). Various artworks are displayed in public circulation spaces, works both large and small in scale, including a series of bronze cast pillars, with each depicting a bark sample indicative of a local tree species. At the end of one corridor, a glass-like film overlay appears, as if depicting a bright sunrise. Hirst contributed a series of nature-themed and private residence–themed wall photomurals. A series of immovable 'collectibles', including pinecones, seashells, an eaten apple core, and large pebbles are displayed along the corridor windowsills and in the outdoor courts. The residential units also feature natural light, and patient rooms are equipped with dormitory beds, desks, chairs, and a built-in window seat. The windows are operable, drawing in natural ventilation, and a storage closet is provided. Flooring is of simulated natural grain, and walls are accented in natural hues inspired by the surrounding open landscape (Figure 6.1.9). Kingfisher Court is a psychiatric facility self-consciously different from most others of its type, rejecting the minimalist aesthetic commonly associated with places for incarceration, and in so doing providing a welcoming alternative.[1]

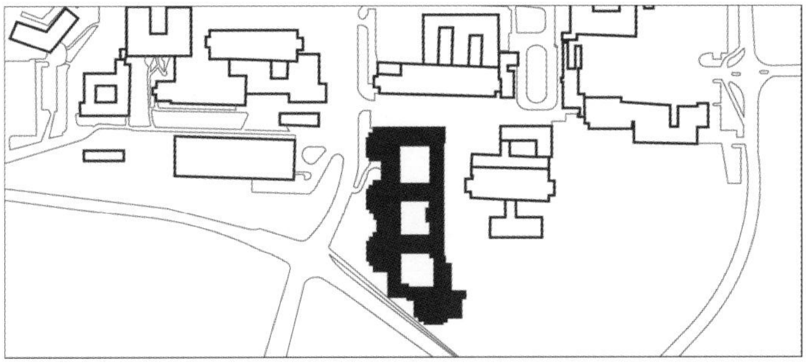

2 Östra Healthcare Centre for Psychiatry, Göteborg, Sweden

ARCHITECT: White Arkitekter AB, Göteborg, Sweden
LANDSCAPE ARCHITECT: White Arkitekter AB, Göteborg, Sweden
CLIENT: Västfastigheter
FEATURED MATERIALS: Glass panels, birch timber
COMPLETED: 2009
INPATIENT BEDS: 120
SITE/PARKING: 12 acres/175
HOSPITAL/TREATMENT CENTER SIZE: 154,000 square feet
NURSES' WORKSTATION: Hybrid

Context/site

This psychiatric replacement hospital is located in a suburban district of Göteborg and is part of an acute care and rehabilitation services medical center. It replaced an outmoded post-World War II psychiatric hospital in Lillhagen. The design team was charged with creating a normative treatment environment and from the exterior, the residential units at Östra recall Herman Hertzberger's social housing in the Netherlands in the 1980s, with their white stucco façades and De Stijl-inspired fenestration. The sloping topography, combined with compositional massing, contributes to the appearance of a hospital that is fitted, or slotted, into its site. The hospital's parti is organized around multiple courtyards; outdoor spaces allow patients' contact with nature in a secure setting, surrounded by residential, therapy/treatment, administrative, and staff supports. The main entrance, lobby, and reception area are three levels in height. Each of the courtyards is themed, one primarily for recreational activity, a second primarily for contemplation, and a third essentially for gardening and social interaction (Figure 6.2.1 and 6.2.2).

The three pavilions, located on the south edge of the site, are all three levels in height and in proximity to specialized treatment zones for one-on-one therapy, group therapy, art therapy, physical therapy, and recreational therapy. Each unit has a solarium and a small exterior light court in proximity to the three large courtyards. The circulation network is hierarchical, with major-scale (double-loaded spaces) and minor-scale (single-loaded spaces) relationships in evidence. The residential units on each floor are organized around a central core that houses a nurses' workstation, unit living room, kitchen, dining room, and social activity area, all grouped around the aforementioned exterior light court; this space provides spatial orientation and draws natural light to the heart of the unit and associated semiprivate spaces. A dayroom is located to one side in the corner of the unit, and its adjacent solarium serves as a screened-in porch not unlike in a private residence, with its bright yellow awnings visible on the exterior and its operable windows. Circulation paths on each unit are appointed with indoor plantings and artworks (Figures 6.2.3 to 6.2.5).

Building/unit

The residential units are spacious, configured to allow for freedom of movement with (reasonably) minimal restriction, as per the earned degree of freedom of movement of each patient (Figure 6.2.6). Patient rooms are provided with a private bath/shower and storage unit and are equipped with residential furnishings. A storage unit is situated between two exaggerated-in-depth windowsills, with these sills functioning as seating nooks. The L-shaped grouping of the patient rooms on each unit minimizes staff walking distances, and furnishings allow for multiple arrangements as needs change. Wood-grain flooring surfaces complement a palette of muted wall and ceiling colors (Figure 6.2.7). The patient rooms afford respite and privacy, without the patient feeling disassociated from the main social activity hub of the unit, surrounding the exterior garden court. When privacy is desired, options for this exist as well. The hospital's treatment philosophy allows the patient maximum, reasonable, freedom to self-determine how one uses the various spaces both on and off the unit, a policy at the core of the institution's rehabilitation programs.

Östra was the site of an evidence-based design research investigation led by Roger Ulrich a few years ago, as discussed in Chapter 1. The main building and its immediate environs were found to embody 10 evidence-based architectural and interior attributes Ulrich et al. identified at that time as associated with

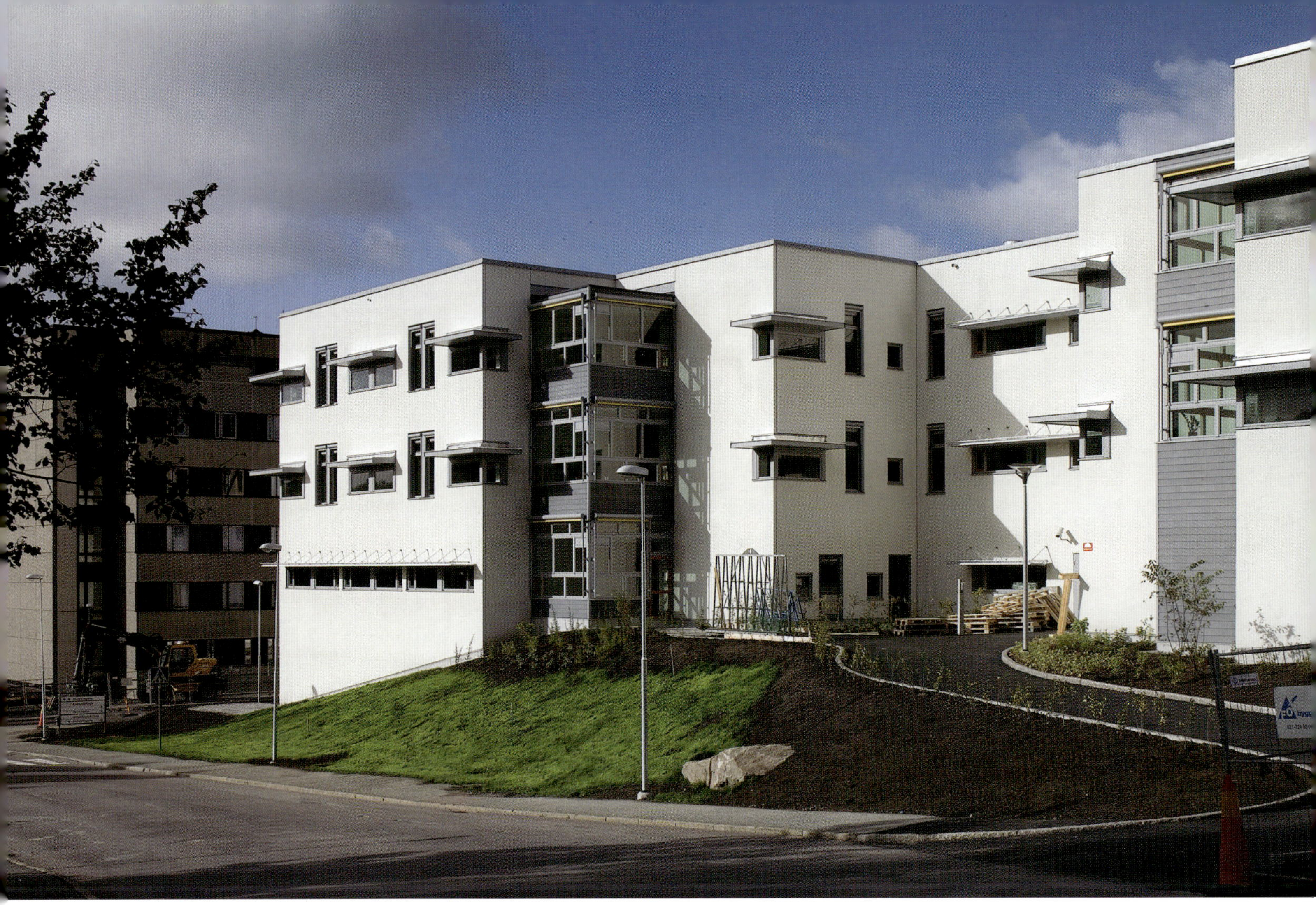

6.2.1 Exterior view of the Östra Healthcare Centre for Psychiatry.

a reduced need for the use of physical restraints with patients during treatment. These 10 design attributes, all in evidence on this psychiatric care campus, included single-patient rooms, small-scale residential units of 12–18 beds each, moveable furnishings (seating in particular) in sufficiently spacious dayrooms, measures to reduce noise levels throughout the facility, windows that afford views of nature, therapeutic garden spaces accessible to patients on a regular basis, works of art that are perceived as inspiring and therapeutic in their own right, the presence of natural daylight and natural ventilation, and nursing staff workstations in sufficient proximity to the inpatient residential core and its related supports. Ulrich contrasted the supportive architectural conditions found at Östra with their antithesis – the oppressive institutional conditions characteristic of post-World War II psychiatric hospitals – and compared those (in the outdated hospital that Östra replaced) to Östra's progressiveness (see Chapter 1).

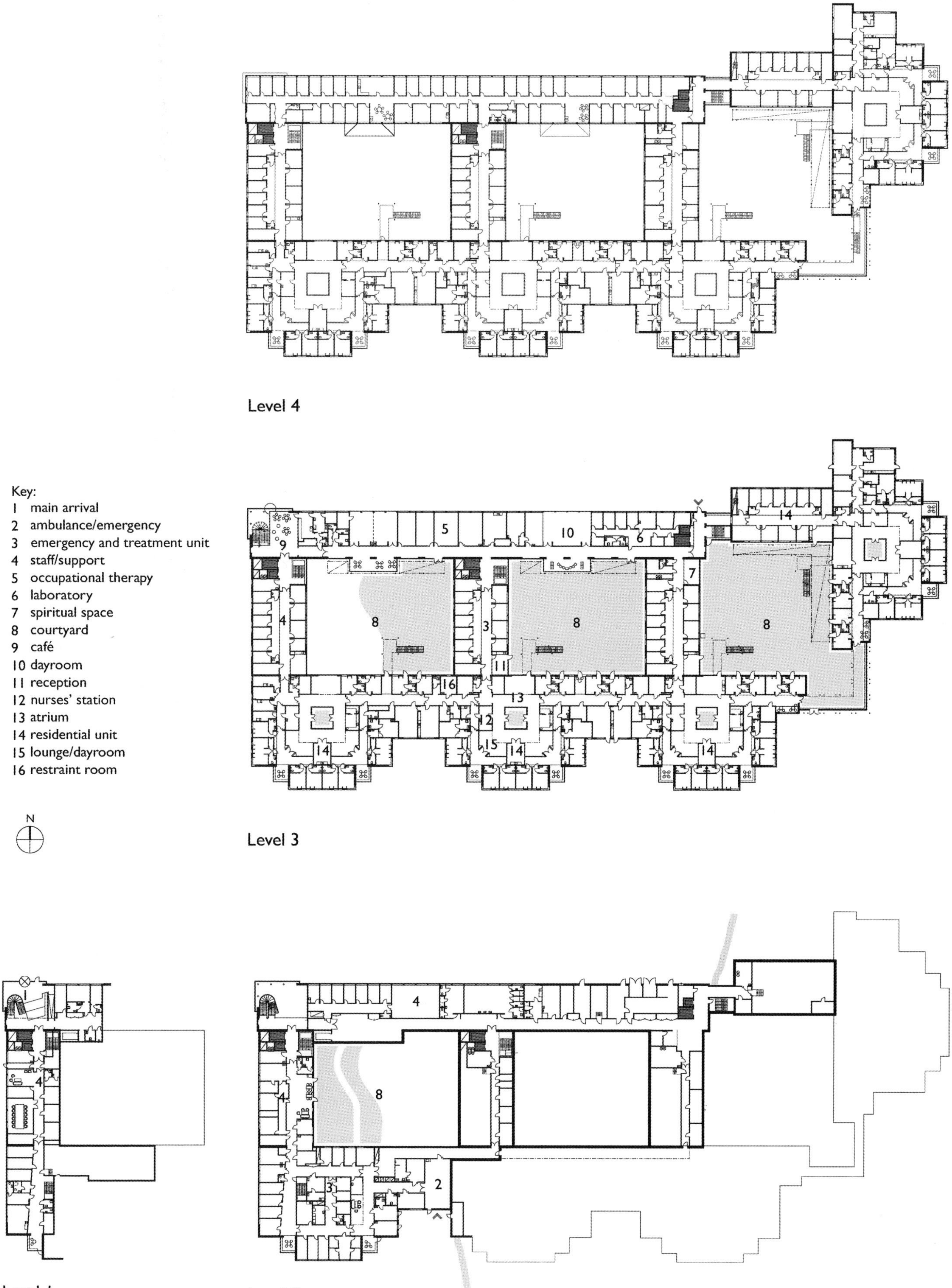

6.2.2 The centrality of the Östra campuses' three courtyards, with residential units located along the southernmost perimeter.

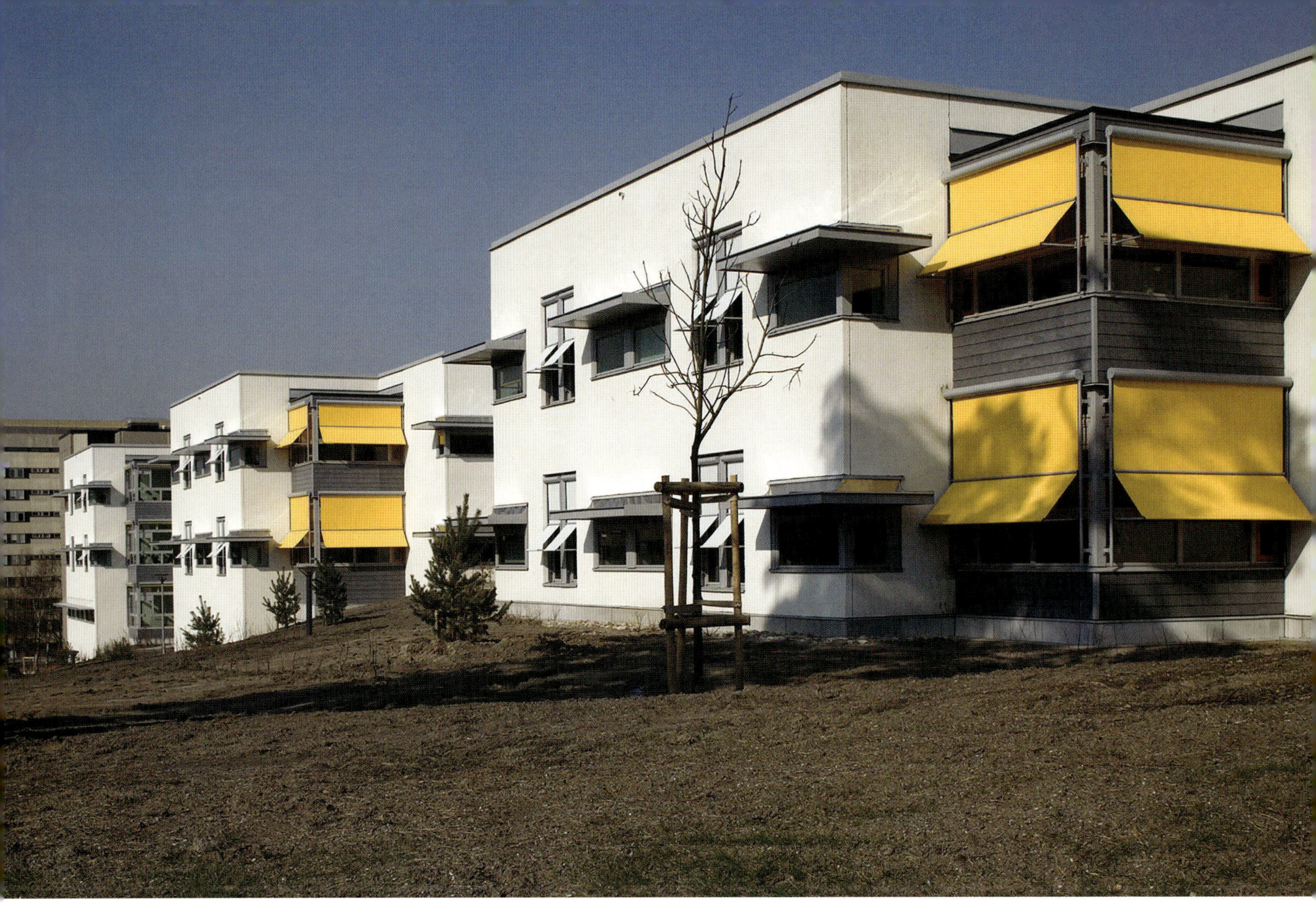

6.2.3 Living/dayrooms are positioned on the outer edge of each residential unit, activated by brightly colored awnings and projections.

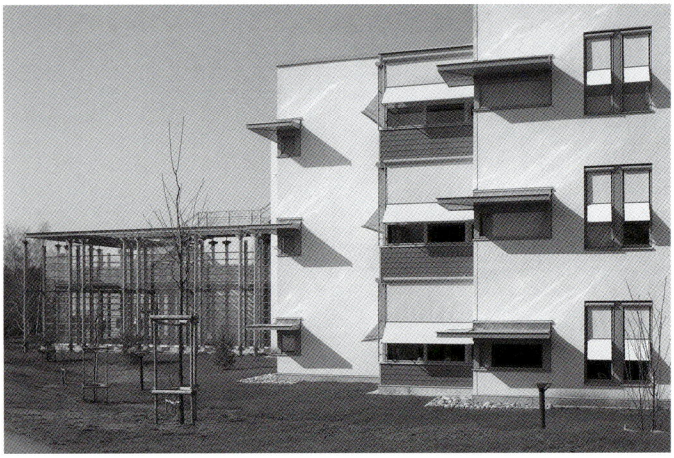

6.2.4 Fenestration patternsexpress internal functionality, not unlike a private residence.

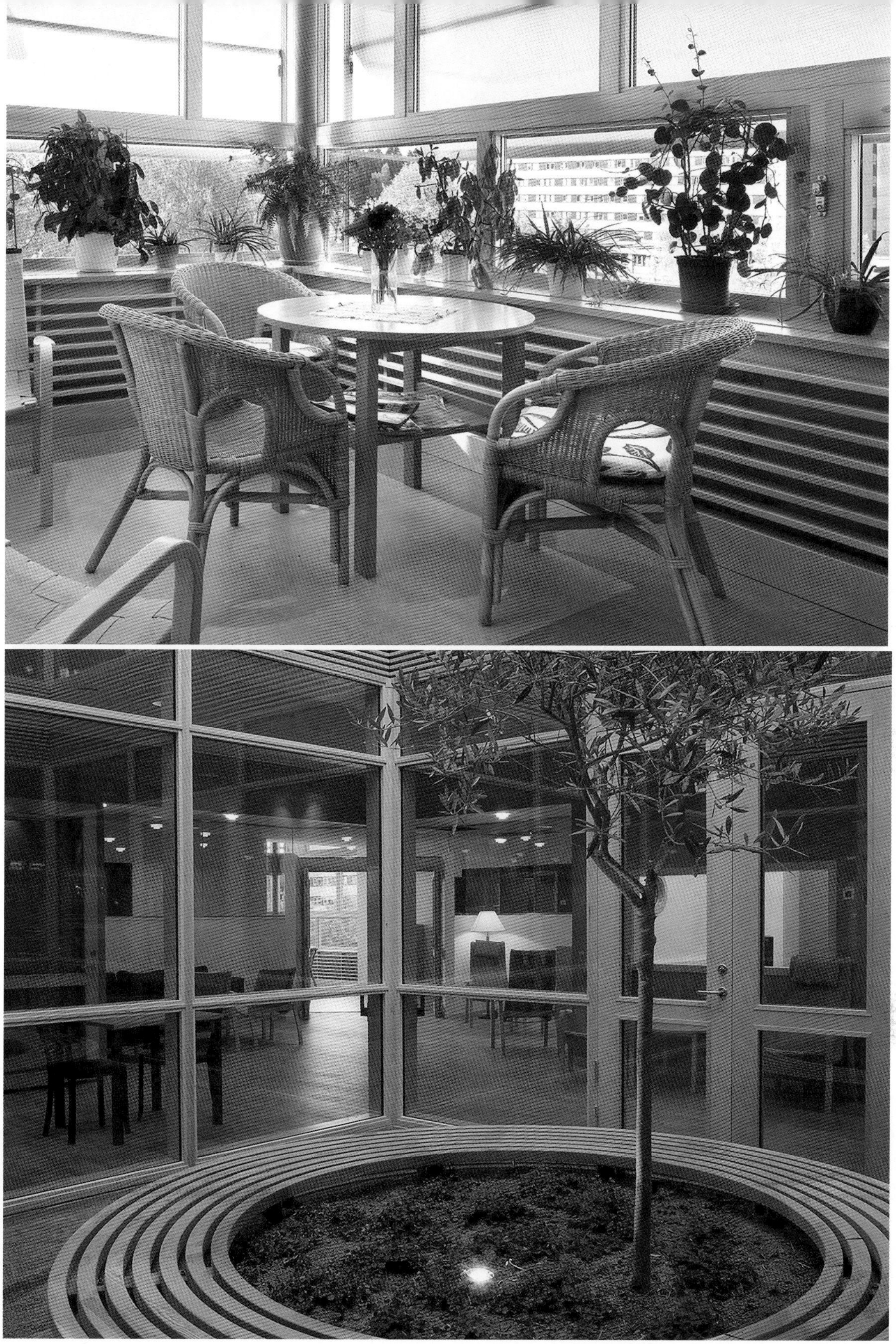

6.2.5 a–b The perimeter dayroom/living room is, in effect, a screened-in porch (top) with light court at center of the unit providing contact with the outdoors.

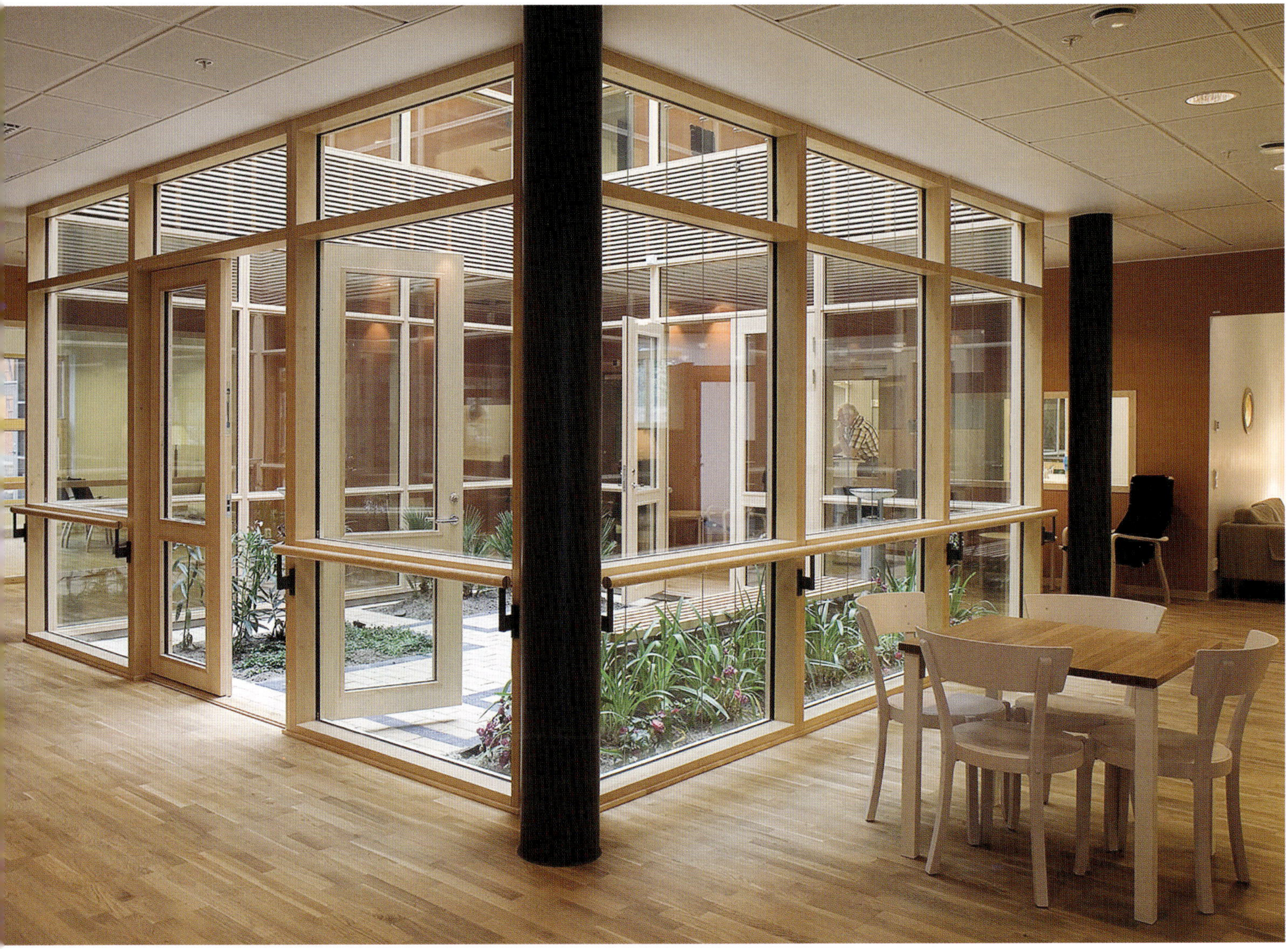

6.2.6 The light court features ground plantings, functioning as an 'outdoor room'.

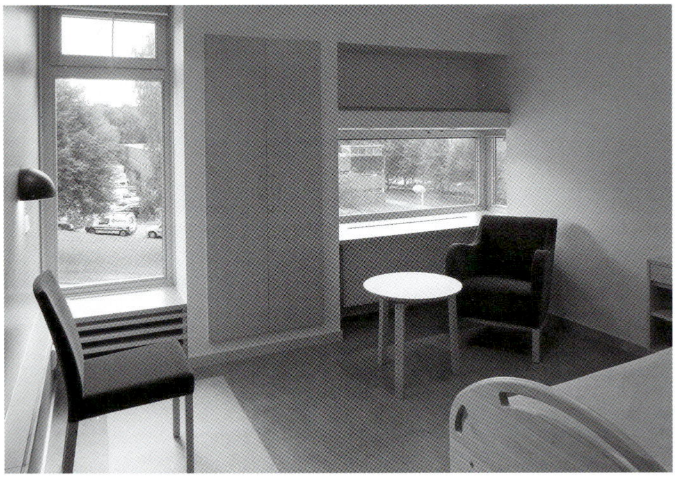

6.2.7 The patient rooms are all private, with reconfigurable furnishings and a built-in closet along the window wall.

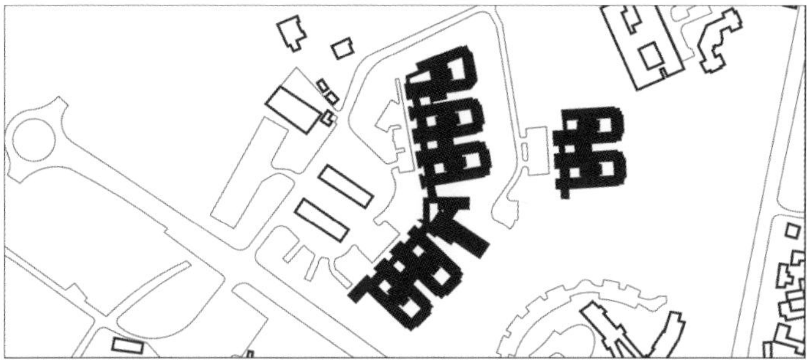

3 Hopewood Park, Sunderland, England, UK

ARCHITECT: MAAP (Medical Architecture and Arts Projects, Ltd.), London, UK
LANDSCAPE ARCHITECT: MAAP, London, UK
CLIENT: Northumberland, Tyne and Wear NHS Foundation Trust
FEATURED MATERIALS: Composite timber cladding
COMPLETED: 2014
INPATIENT BEDS: 137
SITE/PARKING: 40 acres/55
HOSPITAL/TREATMENT CENTER SIZE: 132,000 square feet
NURSES' WORKSTATION: Hybrid

Context/site

Hopewood Park was built to replace the old Cherry Knowle Hospital (located next door). The new campus sits atop a small ridge near the village of Ryhope, 16 kilometers from Newcastle, near the North Sea. It is primarily a rural district, and farmland surrounds the campus on three sides; to the north lies the town center. Hopewood Park's slightly elevated site provides broad, uninterrupted views of the North Sea, and also the southern district. The campus plan was inspired by the river and ravine that cuts through the site as it flows out to the sea. This inspired the designers to create a watercourse; this water feature flows through the site, originating at the main entrance and then 'flowing' from northeast to southwest on-site. The Barton Centre functions as the main building and principal social activity center. This arrival zone is inviting in appearance, with the facility's overall size not readily apparent to the visitor upon first encounter.

This building, rather narrow and oblong, houses the central administration, and it functions as a datum line of sorts in terms of establishing a relationship to the eight residential units and their various supports. The inpatient residential units are each themed by name – that is, Longview Unit, Bridgewell Unit, Beckfield Unit, and so on. The network of single-loaded corridors and circulation spaces, most of which feature large windows and views to the outdoors, collectively add to the facility's navigational amenity. This heightened level of indoor-outdoor connectivity expresses, in many places, theraserialization. Options for future expansion of this facility exist along the southern edge of the campus. Additionally, St. Benedict's Hospice, the Wellfield Day Unit, and the Meadow View Manor are all in relative close proximity (Figures 6.3.1 to 6.3.5), and the landscape design incorporate local plant species seamlessly connecting immediate environs with the surrounding broader landscape.

Building/unit

The eight residential units, and much of the entire facility and campus, is one level in height. Early on it was decided to organize the eight units around large courtyards, with the various buildings' wings buffering and sheltering these spaces. This resulted in a series of high-security gardens, while concurrently avoiding imposing, punitive-appearing walls and fences. Each unit is accessed through a landscaped front court and arrival foyer, a space shared by two inpatient units. Corridors that wrap around on three sides are bright and airy and look onto varied green spaces. The fourth side of most courtyards houses adjacent dayrooms, treatment rooms, and staff support. Large windows allow for visual connectivity in an open, quasi-informal atmosphere. The unit nurses' workstation is in proximity to the principal circulation spine used for transport of materials and supplies between and within units. Various staff supports are located within this core, a zone made more efficient by the back-to-back placement of the residential units in four pairs of two units. These various buildings step down in a terraced manner, in keeping with the site's rolling topography (Figure 6.3.6). This irregularity, moreover, makes possible the concealment of parking areas from direct open view. Pockets of parking are provided near the units and central support functions. The site's rolling topography allows for numerous semiprivate pockets of outdoor seating located in proximity to the residential units (Figure 6.3.7a–b). Public interior spaces feature wood paneling, with their surfaces embellished with hand carvings that provide a running narrative of the local area's history and folklore traditions and speak to the power of the human spirit to overcome mental illness through rehabilitation (Figure 6.3.8a–b).

At the center of each residential unit, two dayrooms and an adjoining quiet room overlook an outdoor courtyard. The

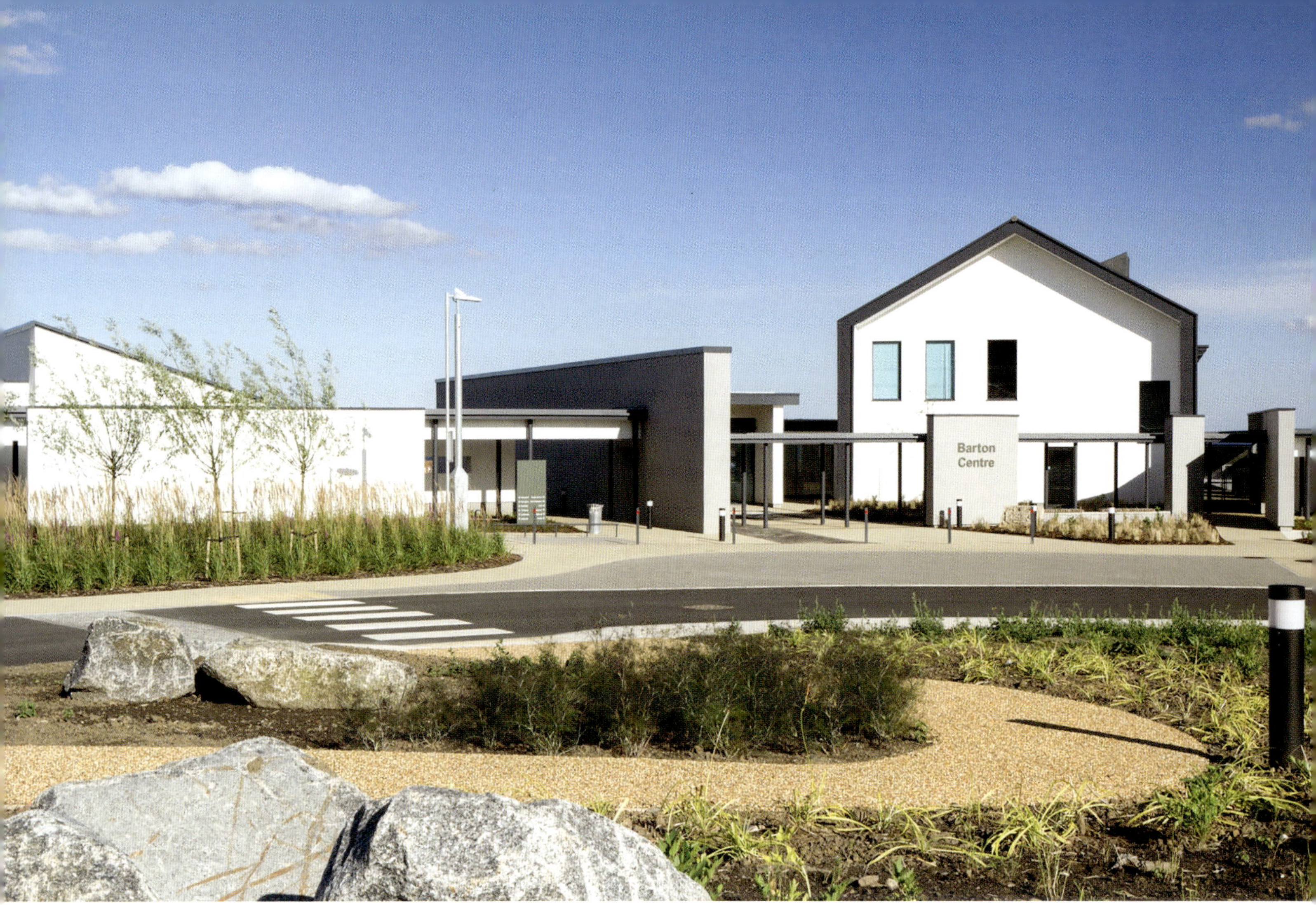

6.3.1 The arrival front court at Hopewood Park, in Sunderland.

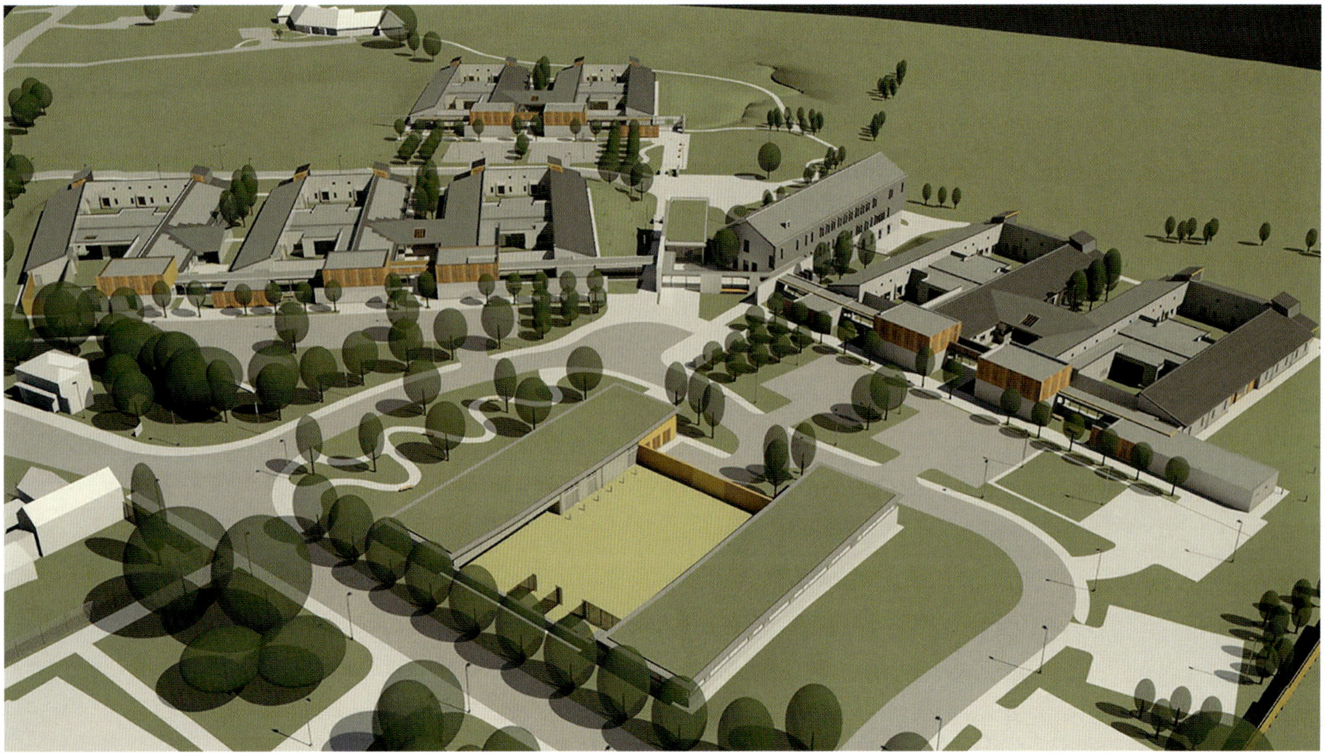

6.3.2 Inpatient units and treatment areas are configured as four one-level elements flanking a main building at the center.

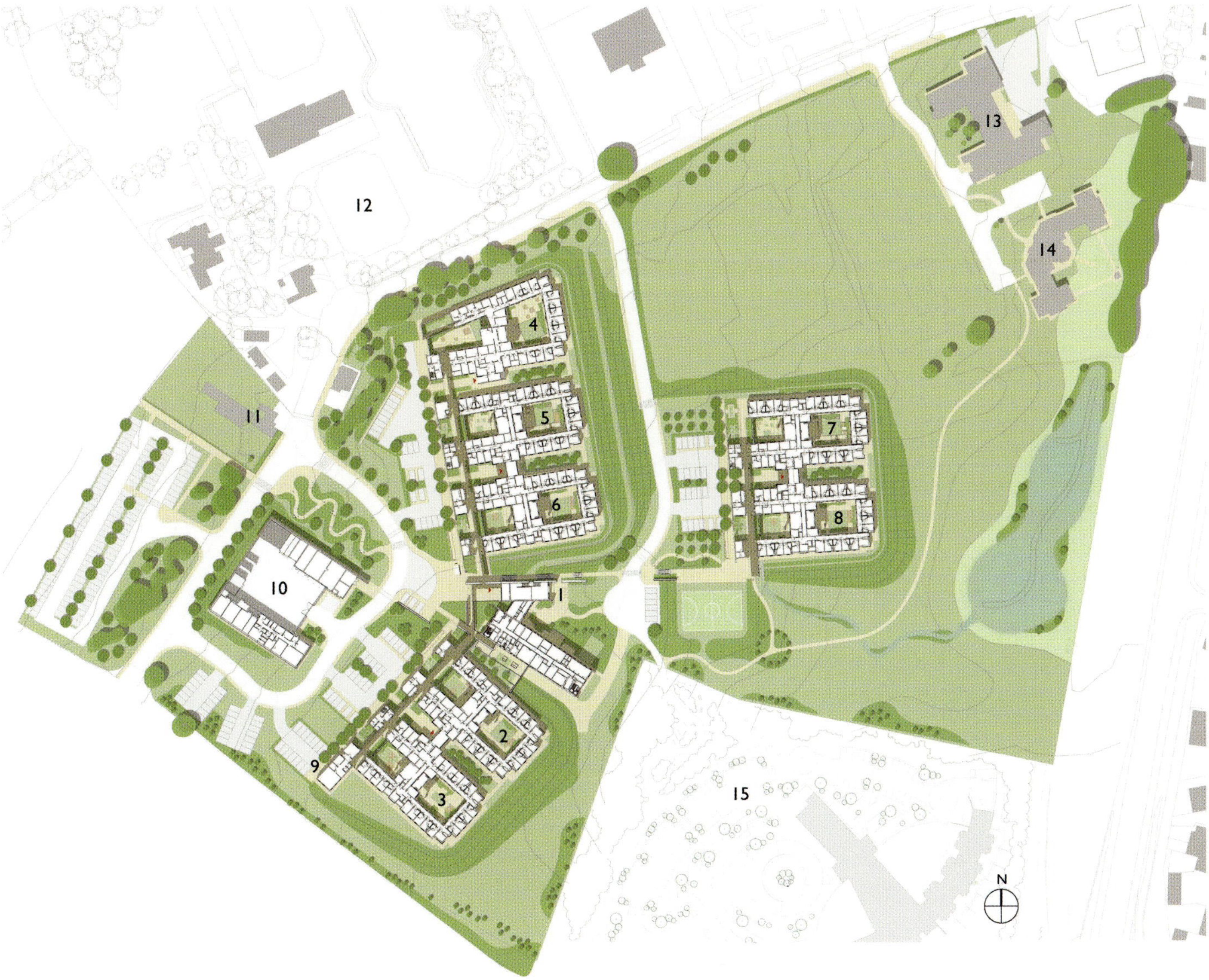

Site Plan

Key:
1 Barton Centre
2 Longview Unit
3 Bridgewell Unit
4 Beckfield Unit
5 Springrise Unit
6 Shoredrift Unit
7 Aldervale Unit
8 Clearbrook Unit
9 PMVA
10 FM Hub
11 Garden Lodge
12 Ryhope Engine Museum
13 Wellfield Day Unit
14 Meadow View
15 St. Benedict's Hospice

6.3.3 The campus houses seven inpatient residential units, each configured around a pair of courtyards.

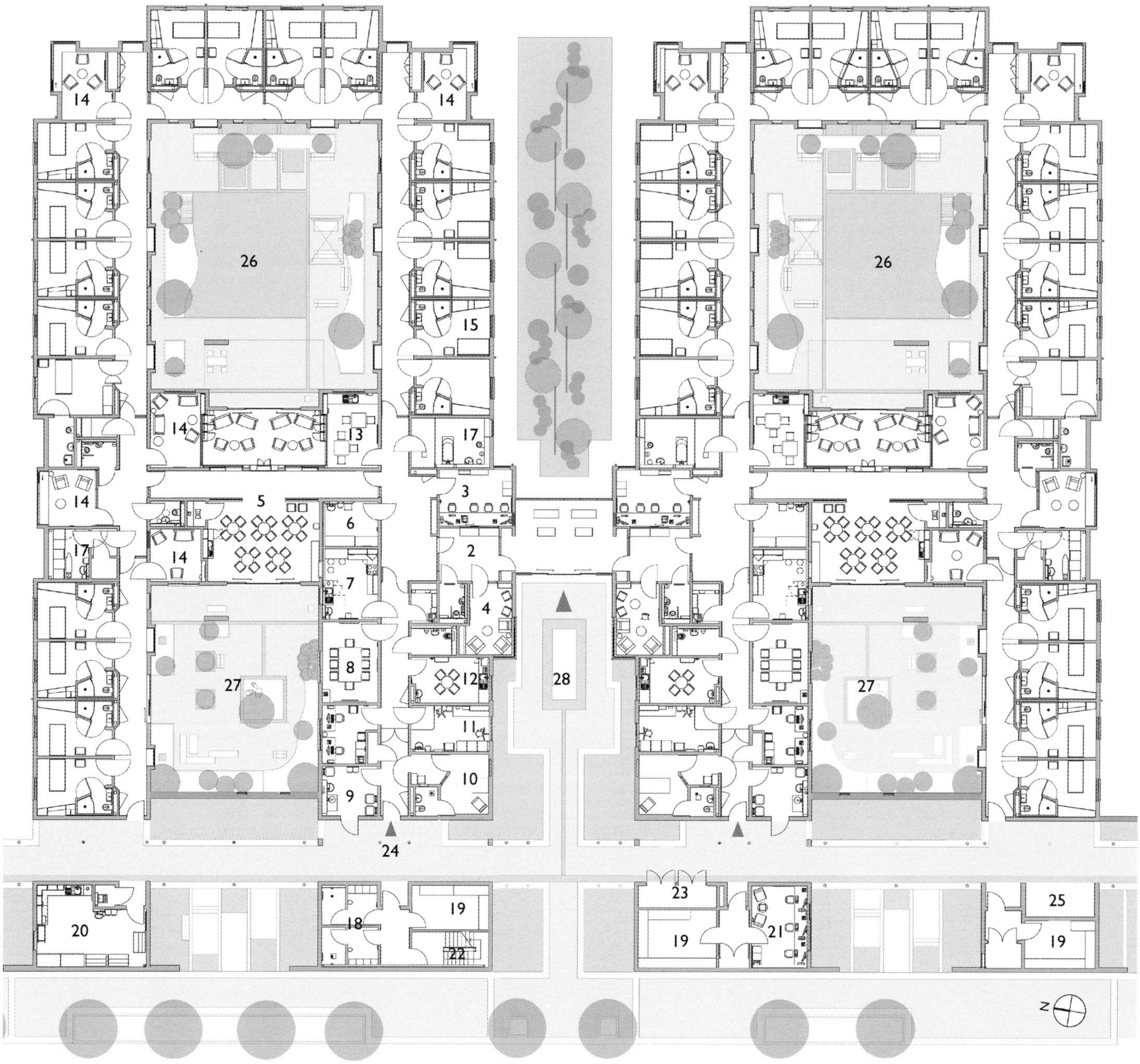

Level 1

Key:

1 entrance lobby	15 patient bedroom
2 controlled lobby	16 wheelchair accessible bedroom
3 ward office	17 assisted bathroom
4 visitor's room	18 staff change
5 lounge and dining area	19 general store
6 clinic/drug dispensary	20 regeneration kitchen
7 ward kitchen	21 ward manager's office
8 multidisciplinary team	22 access to 1st floor plant
9 dirty utility/disposal	23 FM store
10 seclusion	24 FM & discreet entry/exit
11 treatment room	25 bicycle rack
12 staff rest	26 passive courtyard
13 activity room	27 active courtyard
14 quiet lounge	28 arrival courtyard

6.3.4 The residential units' arrival forecourts and interior vestibules overlook a courtyard, and 'internalized' exteriors provide a mixture of active and passive space.

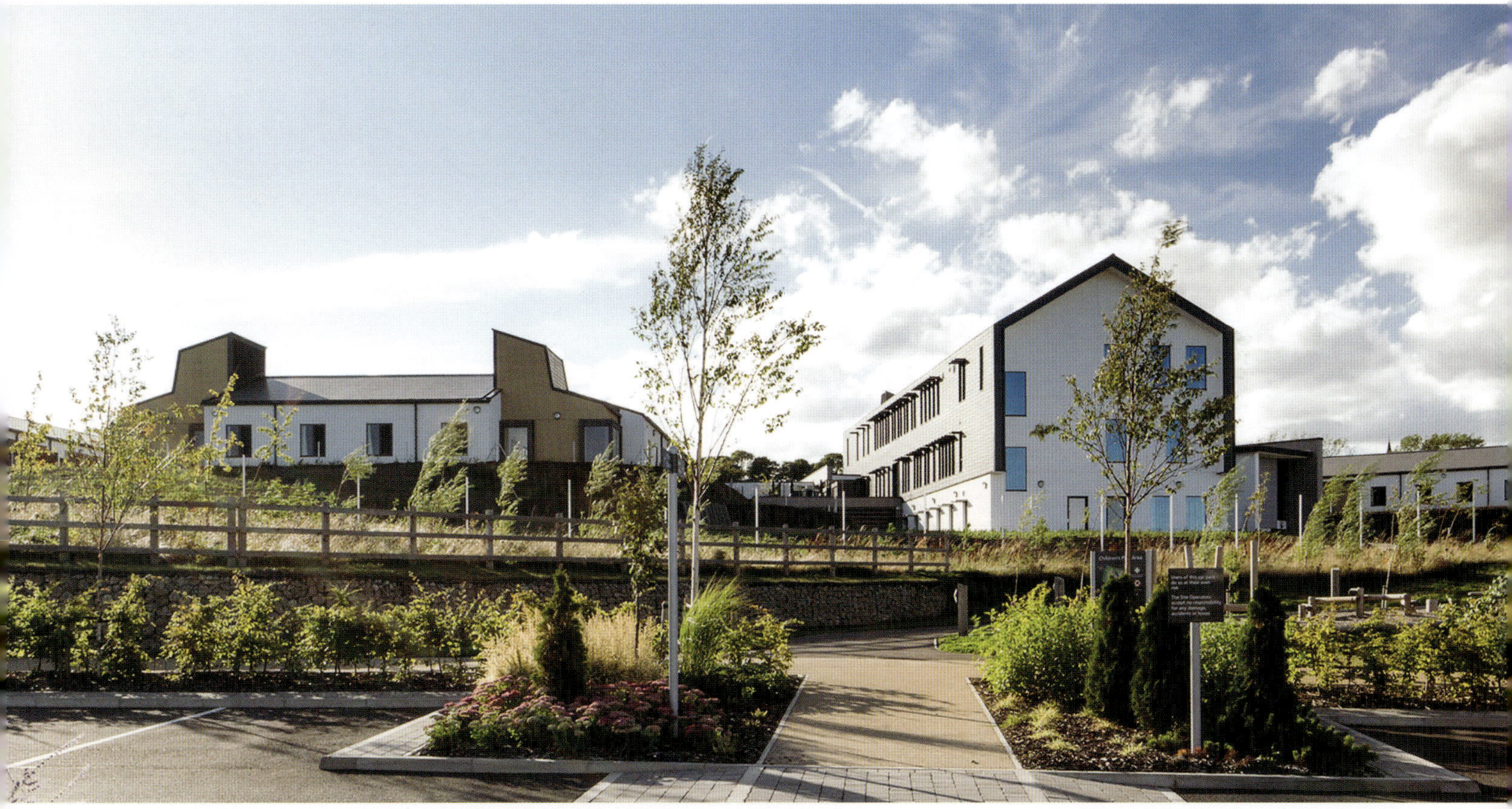

6.3.5 The terraced topography facilitats diverse compositional massings and exterior spaces.

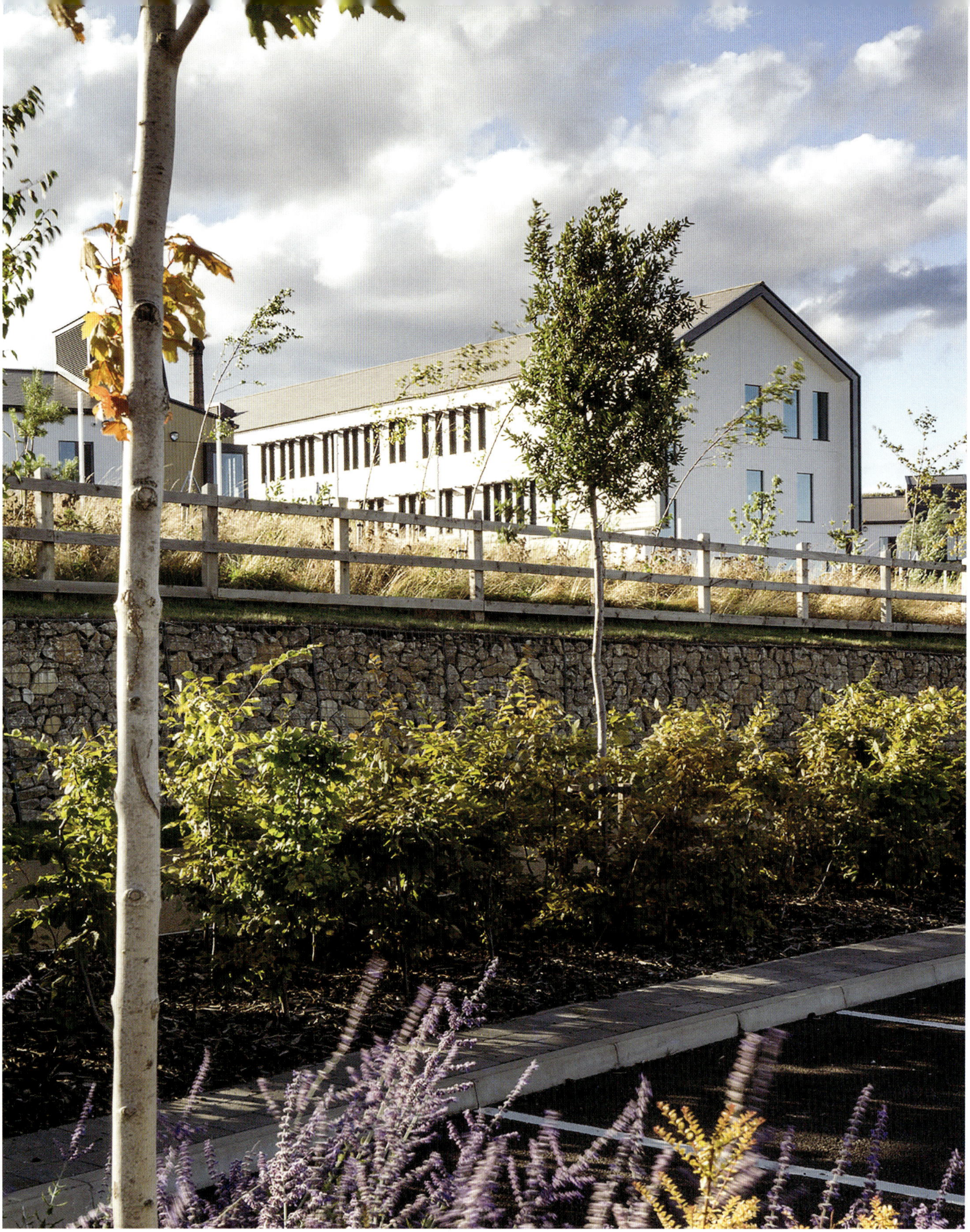

6.3.6 Semiconcealed parking areas are located in proximity to residential units at Hopewood Park.

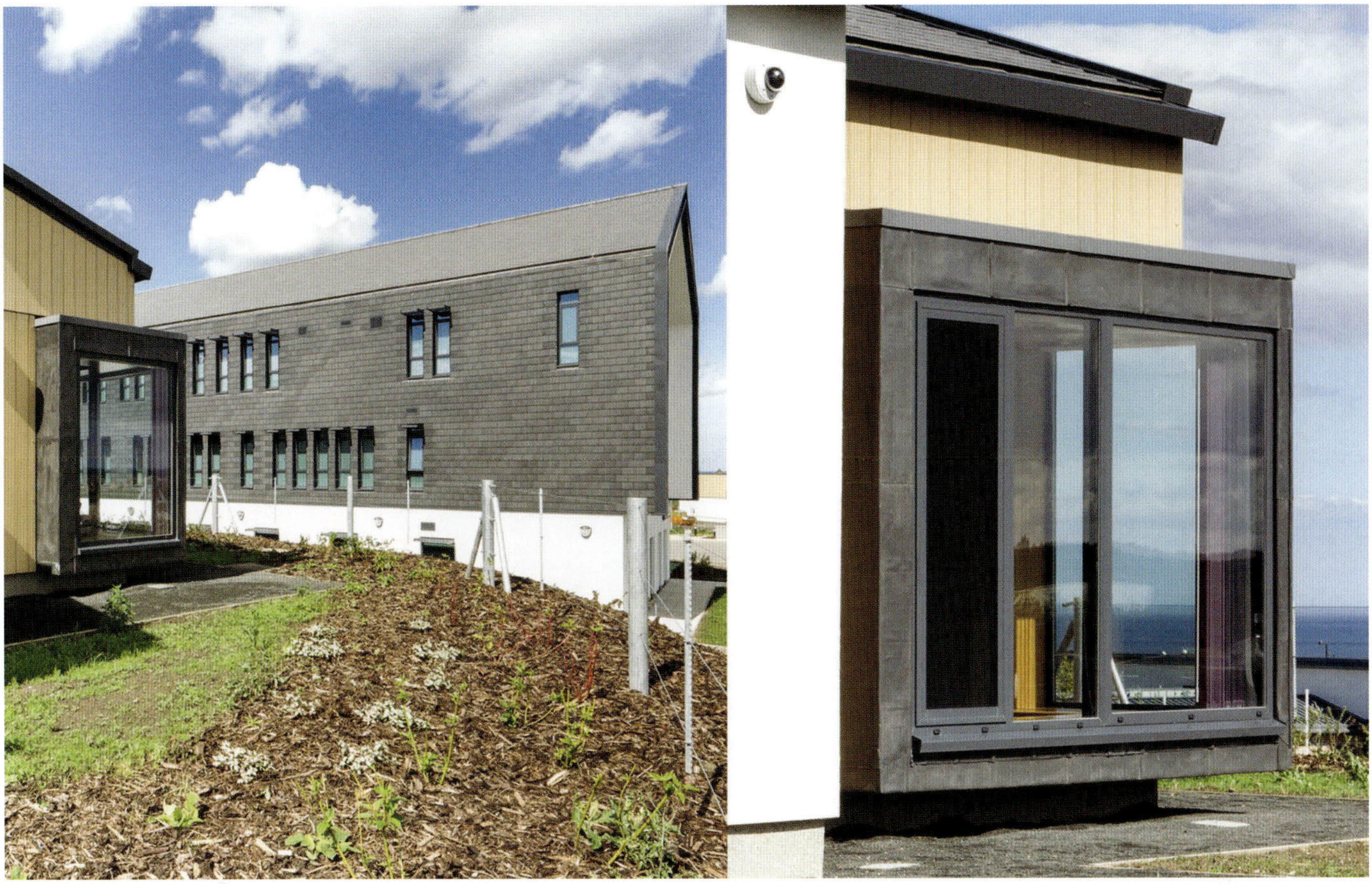

6.3.7a–b Exterior materials reflect local vernacular building traditions (left), and extended window bays are located at ends of circulation arteries (right).

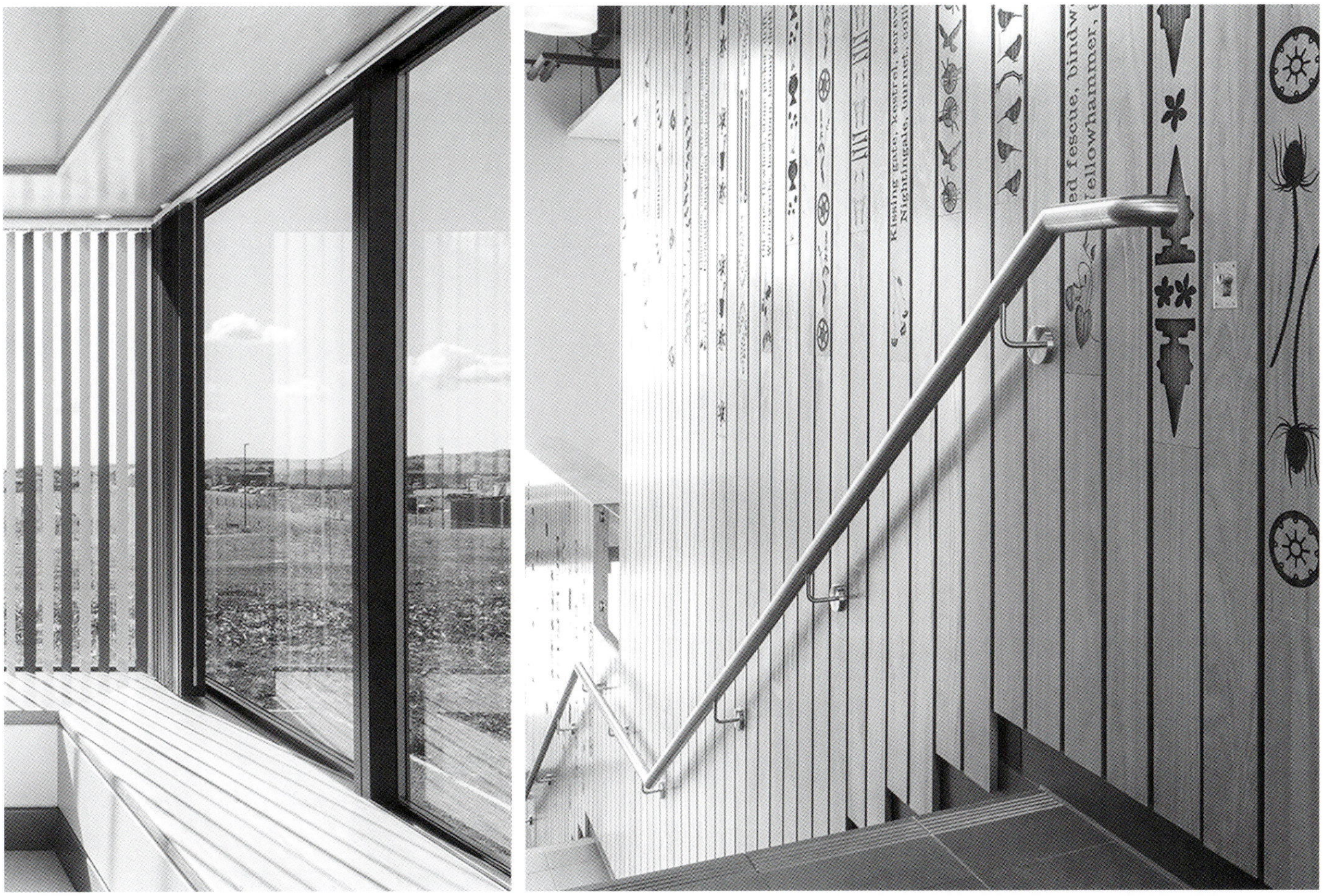

6.3.8a–b Circulation spaces feature large windows (left), with many wall surfaces inscribed with local literary narratives and iconic symbols (right).

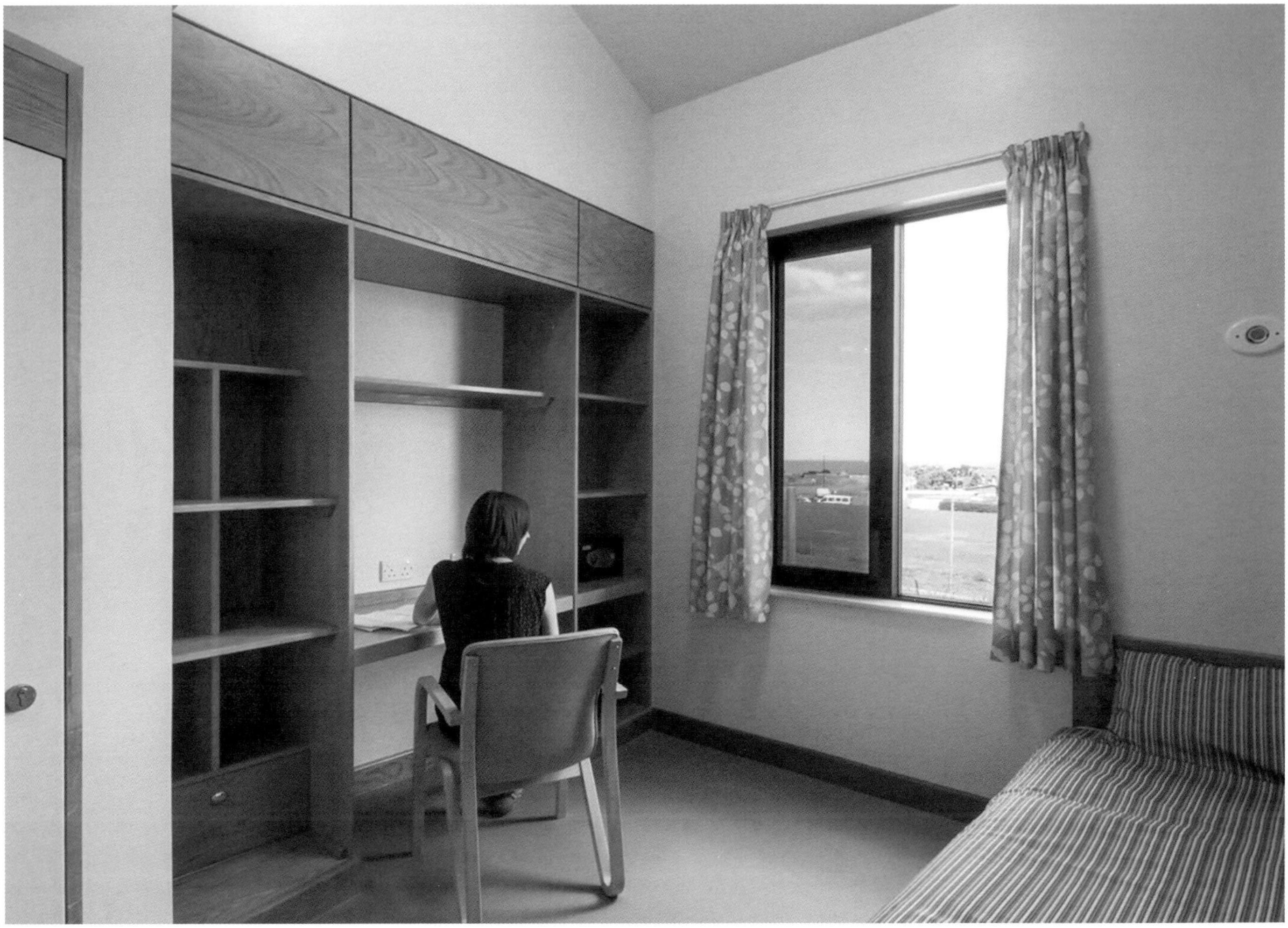

6.3.9 Patient rooms are all private, with dormitory furnishings and a built-in desk/shelving unit.

windows on the unit (and elsewhere in the facility) are operable; corridor lengths are minimalized despite being single loaded, with an interior window seat provided at the end of each circulation artery. Seclusion and quiet rooms are situated directly across from the nurses' workstation. Every patient room is private (single occupancy), with a private bath/shower unit and a large, operable window. Patient rooms are equipped with dormitory furnishings (i.e., a built-in desk and shelving wall unit for personal items). The architects' intent was for the inpatient unit to be residential in scale and appearance and relatively autonomous, thereby establishing for the patient a normative atmosphere. Potential reminders of institutionalism were carefully eschewed throughout, and to further underscore this strategy, natural materials are incorporated throughout both exterior and interior spaces. The ceilings in the patient rooms are vaulted, and their floor surfaces are of low-maintenance vinyl tiles. A network of video cameras facilitates unobtrusive observation of public and semiprivate spaces on this campus (Figure 6.3.9).

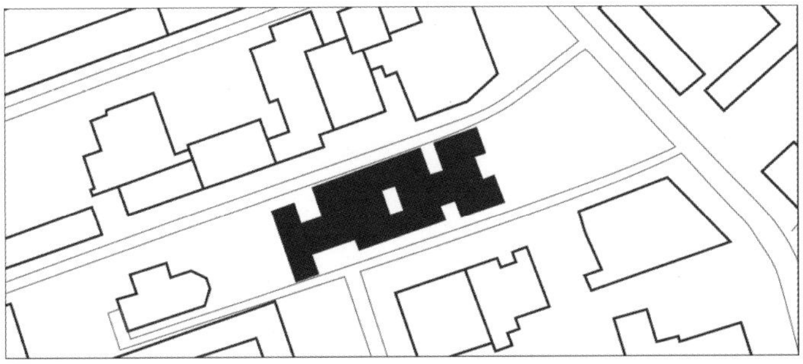

4 Professor Marie Bashir Centre at the Royal Prince Alfred Hospital, Sydney, Australia

ARCHITECT: Peckvonhartel (pvh), Sydney, Australia/Silver Thomas Hanley (STH), Sydney, Australia
LANDSCAPE ARCHITECT: Silver Thomas Hanley (STH), Sydney, Australia
CLIENT: New South Wales Department of Health Infrastructure
FEATURED MATERIALS: Unknown
COMPLETED: 2014
INPATIENT BEDS: 73
SITE/PARKING: 4 acres/155
HOSPITAL/TREATMENT CENTER SIZE: 122,000 square feet
NURSES' WORKSTATION: Hybrid

Context/site

Professor Marie Bashir Centre was initiated by the New South Wales (NSW) Department of Health Infrastructure, the Sydney Local Health District, the Royal Prince Alfred Hospital, and the University of Sydney. This six-level hospital was built within a medical district in the center of Sydney, near King George V General Hospital, Royal Prince Alfred Hospital, and the Brain and Mind Research Institute. It was named in honor of a former NSW governor in recognition of her significant contributions to the field of mental health. Services previously scattered at multiple sites were integrated in this new hospital. The functional brief called for its future expansion in the form of a second building to be built at a later time (directly to the east). For this reason, the first-phase building features precast concrete panels (on the facing elevation), removable for the purpose of connecting to any future addition. The anticipated future addition will at that time double the hospital's bed capacity (Figure 6.4.1).

Traditionally, psychiatric hospitals were built on large, open, remote sites far from the bustle and cacophony of urban life. The administration here opted, instead, to remain near its sister institutions versus relocating to a larger site on the urban perimeter, a decision that would have likely made possible a one- or two-level facility, versus the considerably taller structure that was built. The challenge therefore for the architectural/engineering (A/E) team became one of designing a midrise, relatively dense building encompassing the atmosphere and openness of a low-rise hospital built on a larger site. The design strategy was to create roof terraces, landscaped with outdoor amenities in direct adjacency to residences, therapy/treatment rooms, and various supports. These would allow inhabitants' direct immersion in nature, while providing dramatic views of the city. The resulting 'sky terraces' (architects' words) occur on the fourth, fifth, and sixth levels (Figure 6.4.2).

Building/unit

Compositionally, this facility is essentially a cube, with voids carved out at various intervals. This yields relative transparency and openness. Roof terraces are surrounded by interior spaces with full-height windows; varied colors; and residential-like wall treatments, materials, and finishes (Figure 6.4.3a–c). The patient experiences the freedom of choice to experience the regulated use of these spaces, within certain earned limits. The hospital's main level houses an emergency assessment/triage unit, the short-stay unit, and the central administration. The second level houses a satellite renal dialysis unit; the third level houses various clinics, including those for eating disorders and sexual health; the fourth level houses a 22-bed acute inpatient care unit; the fifth level houses a 22-bed, high-dependency inpatient unit; and the sixth level houses a 20-bed observational unit plus hospital-wide staff and family supports. On the fourth through sixth levels, inpatient units feature living and social activity rooms, therapy and recreational spaces, with window seating areas to encourage informal social interaction. Public and semipublic spaces on the residential units are generally spacious and noninstitutional in appearance. Green roof terraces feature semisheltered seating and the perimeter security screening device is noninstitutional in appearance yet secure, without impeding views of the city; high-performance exterior glazing was used throughout (Figures 6.4.4 and 6.4.5).

The 'outer' staff workstation on each unit does not have a security element to separate it from the surrounding spaces occupied by patients. However, a securable staff workstation is close by, if and when lockdown conditions become necessary. A main living/activity room opens onto a roof terrace on the third level (Figure 6.4.6). Wall murals were installed along many of the corridors, and these reference local residential streetscapes and gardens; scenes functioning

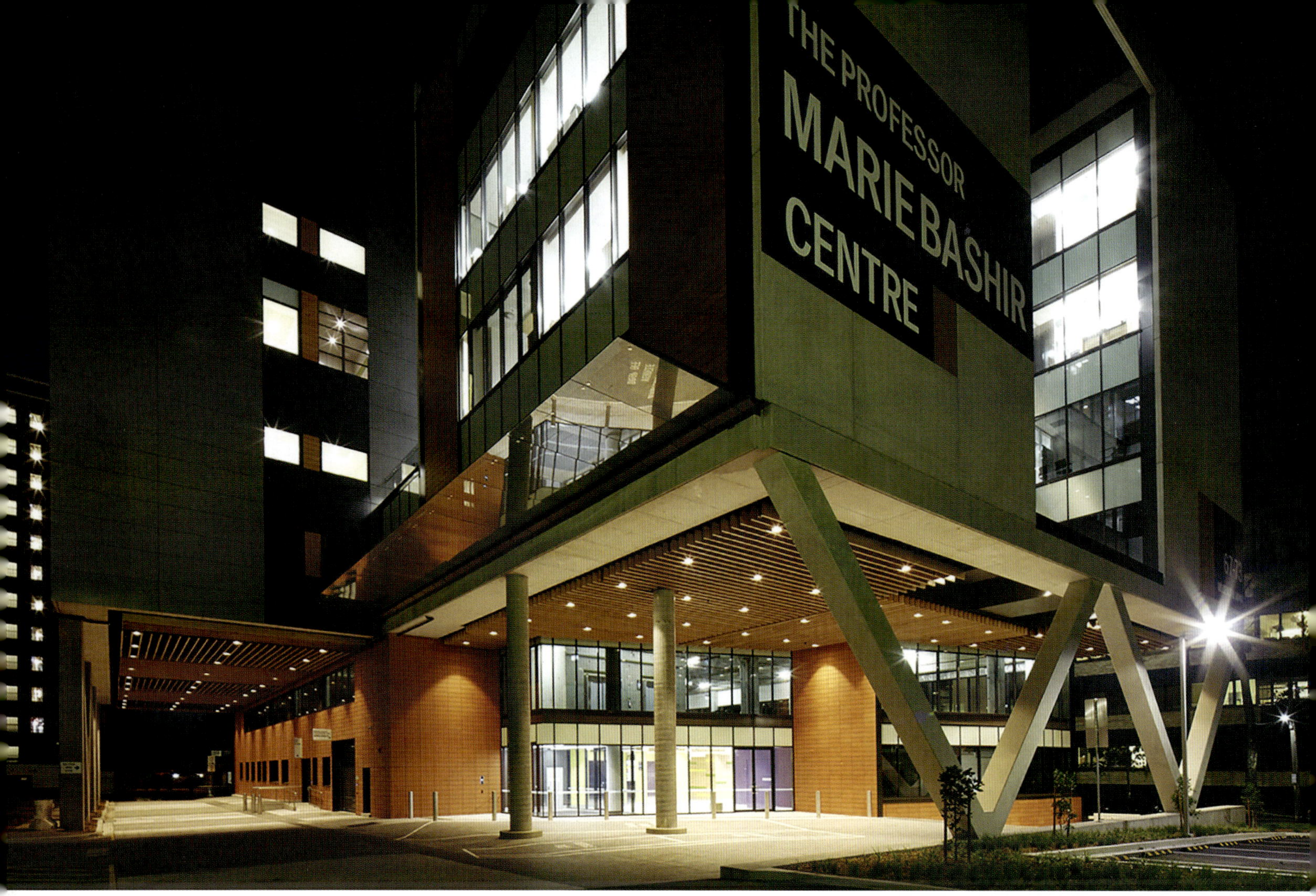

6.4.1 The Marie Bashir Centre main arrival court in Sydney, Australia.

to connect patients, cognitively, with everyday life in the surrounding city (Figure 6.4.7). All patient rooms are private, each with private bath/shower unit, built-in desk, seating area, headwall with storage bins, and simulated natural wood-grain flooring (Figure 6.4.8). The headwall is slotted, with variously shaped small nooks. Staff clinical supports are organized in a racetrack circulation loop; additional staff supports are housed at the ends of each floor. Because this hospital was procured through the public-private partnership (PPP) process, prototyping and spatial mock-ups were produced early on as part of a fast-track design and construction sequence that resulted in significant cost and time savings (see Chapter 5). With respect to the hospital's eco-sustainability, a key benchmarking tool used throughout the design and construction process was the Green Star for Healthcare V1; the outcome of this process was a bright, noticeably airy facility with natural ventilation and the ability to self-monitor and regulate its carbon dioxide and volatile organic compound (VOC) consumption levels.

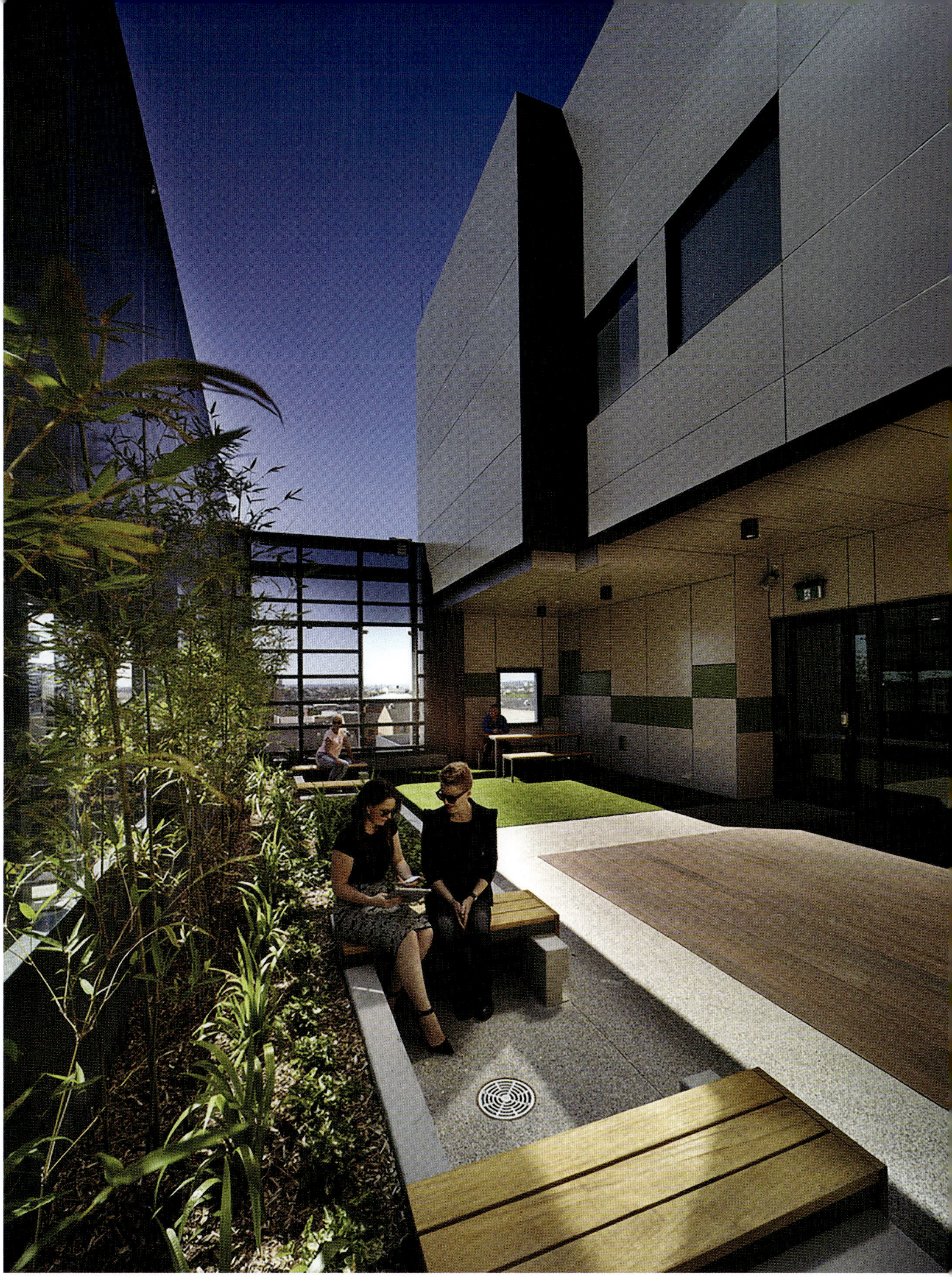

6.4.2 Roof terraces are landscaped, therapeutic extensions of adjacent interior space.

Key:
1 main arrival
2 lobby
3 conference/suite
4 outpatient clinics/
eating disorders
5 physical therapy
6 short-stay observation unit
7 MHAU
8 mechanical/energy
9 central services
10 loading dock
11 education/research
12 acute treatment unit
13 vertical circulation
14 nurses' station
15 group rooom
16 occupational therapy/
gym/music/sensory rooms
17 staff terrace
18 lobby
19 exterior courtyard
20 adminstration/staff
21 high-risk unit
22 servery (kitchen)
23 dining
24 quiet lounge
25 dayroom

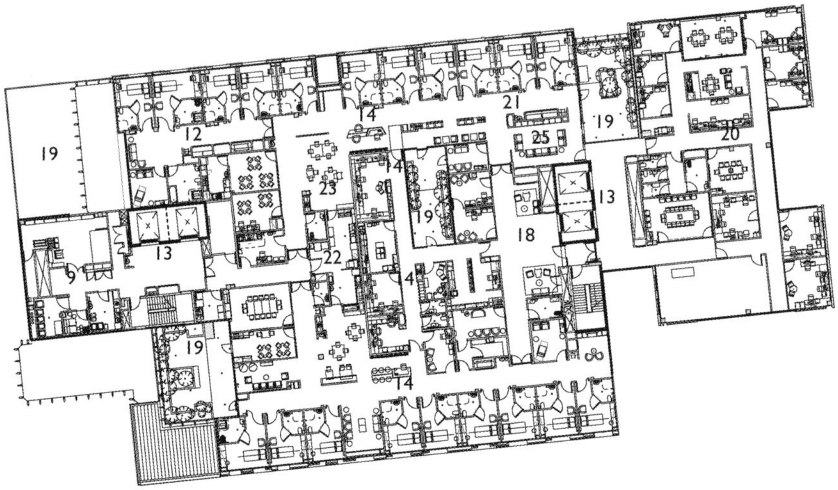

Level 5

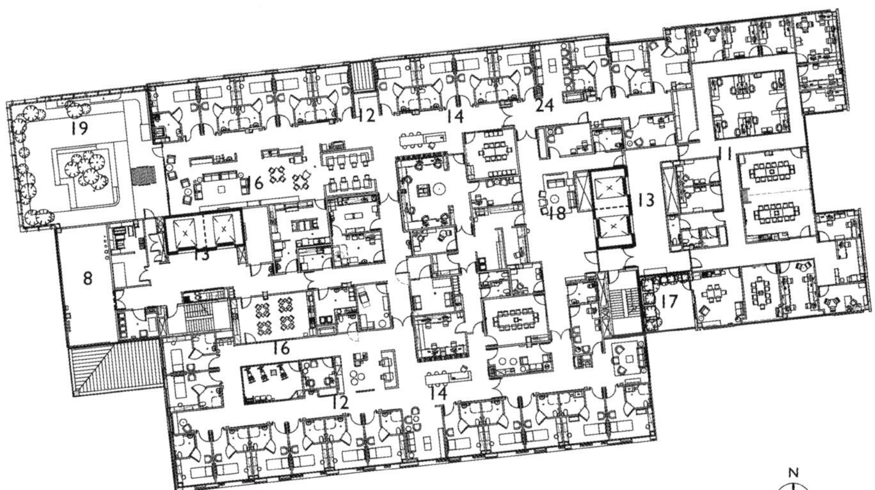

Level 3

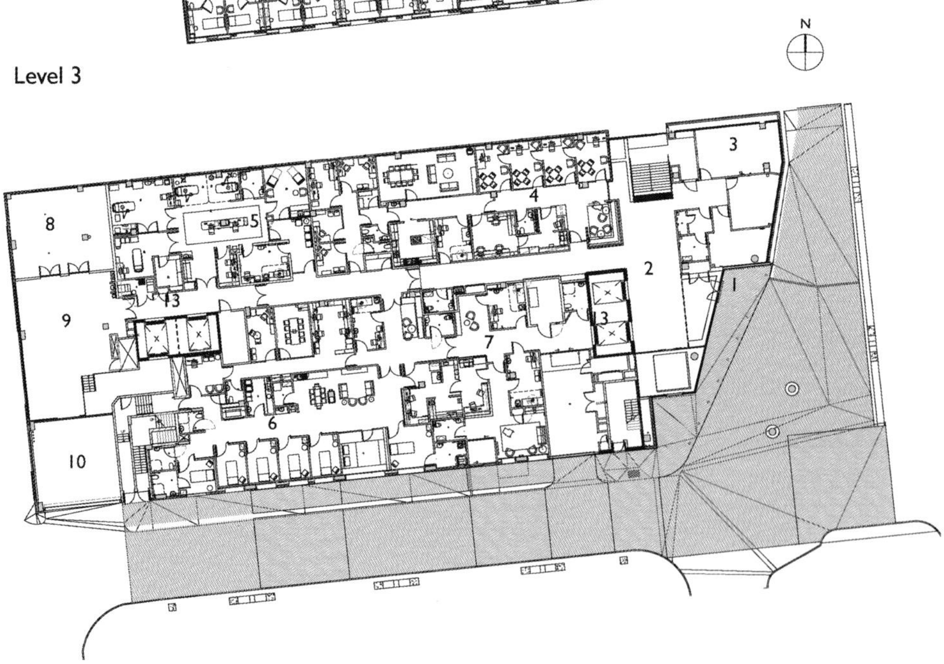

Ground Level

Figure 6.4.3a–c The hospital footprint is centralized, with patient rooms located along the perimeter of the units on upper levels.

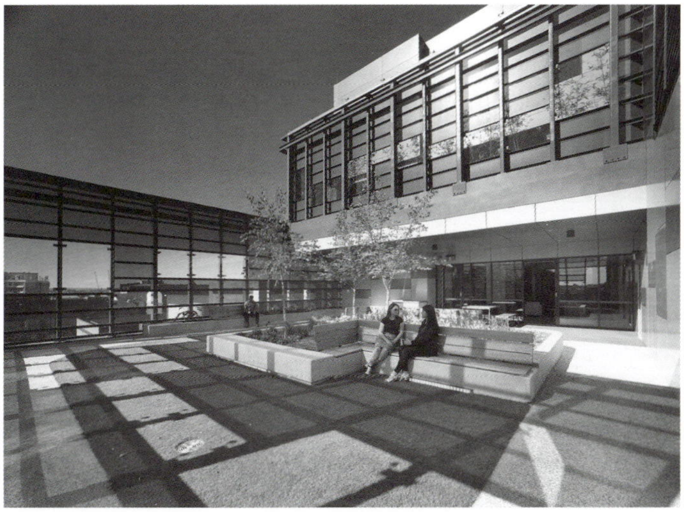

6.4.4 The roof terrace perimeter security (screen) device affords views of the city, and cantilevered floors provide protection from the elements.

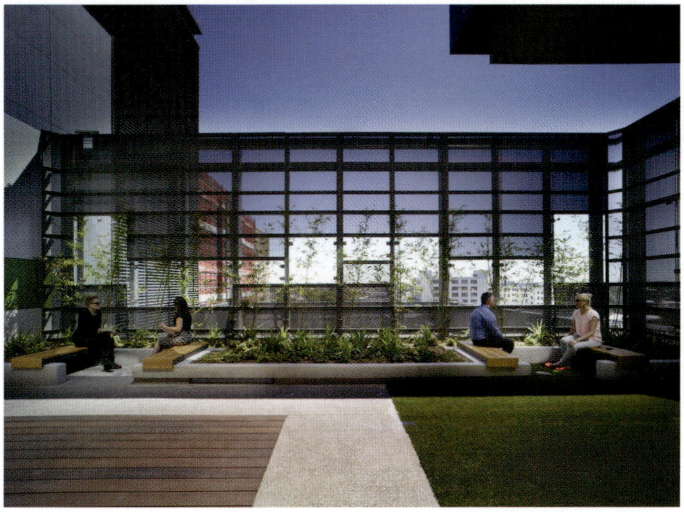

6.4.5 A perimeter security screen/wall contains a mixture of transparent and translucent panels, adjacent to seating areas and plantings.

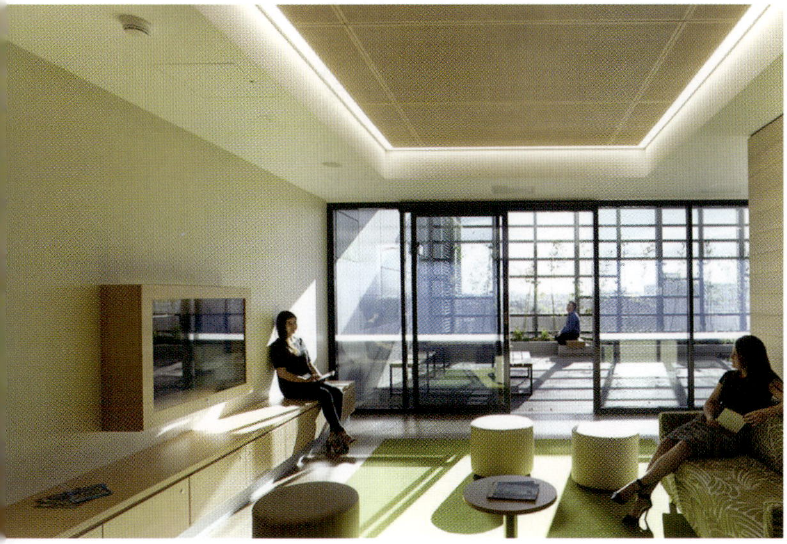

6.4.6 Activity/dayrooms open directly onto exterior roof terraces and transitional spaces.

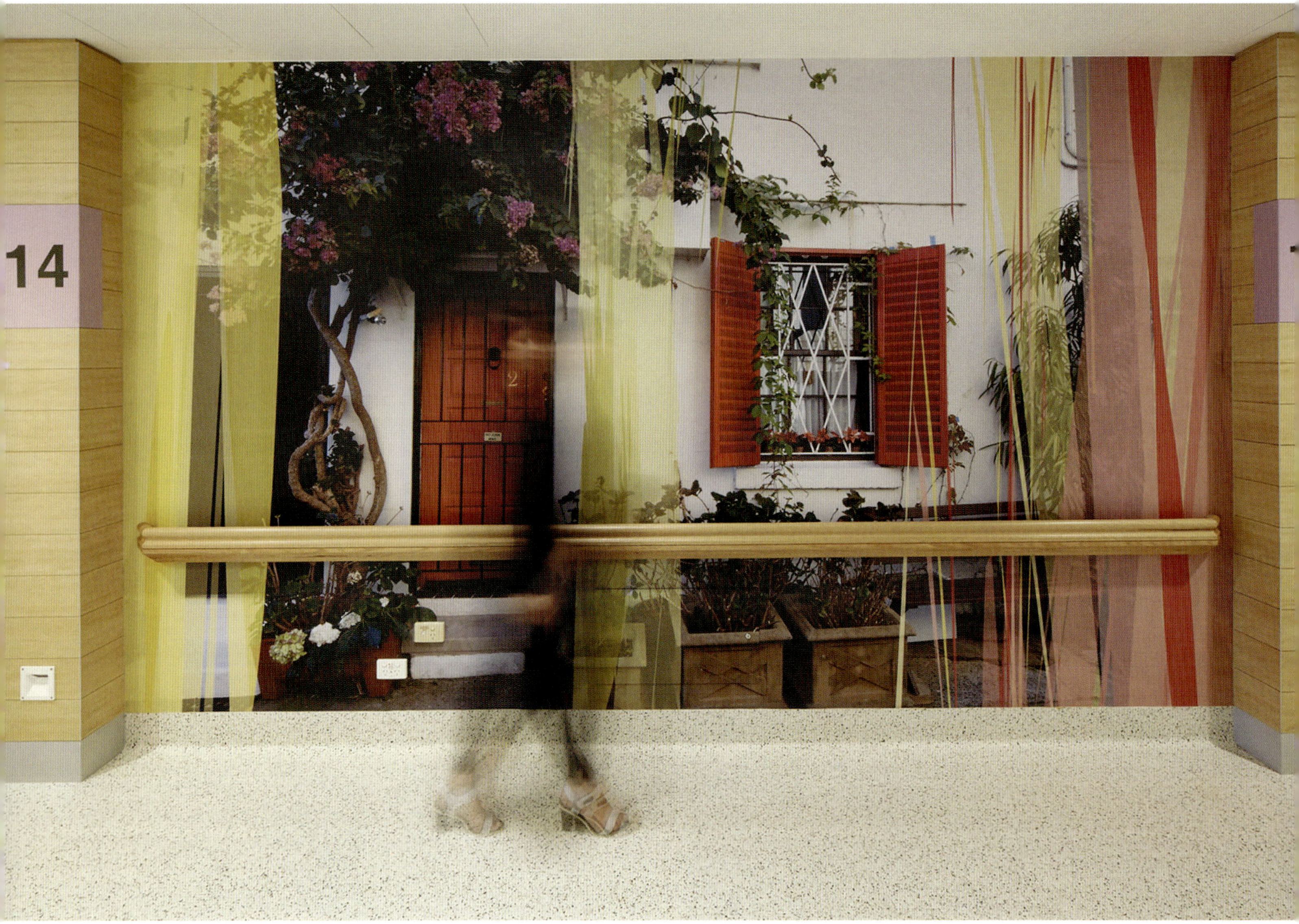

6.4.7 Murals depict local street scenes, reinforcing the hospital's relationship with its surrounding urban milieu.

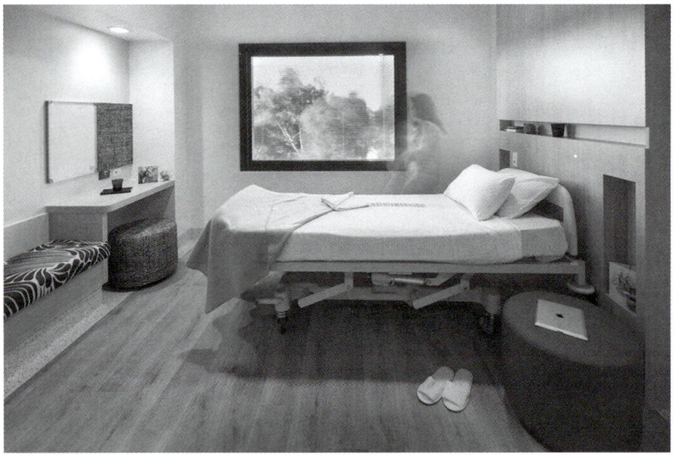

6.4.8 Patient rooms feature articulated headwalls, footwalls, and storage options.

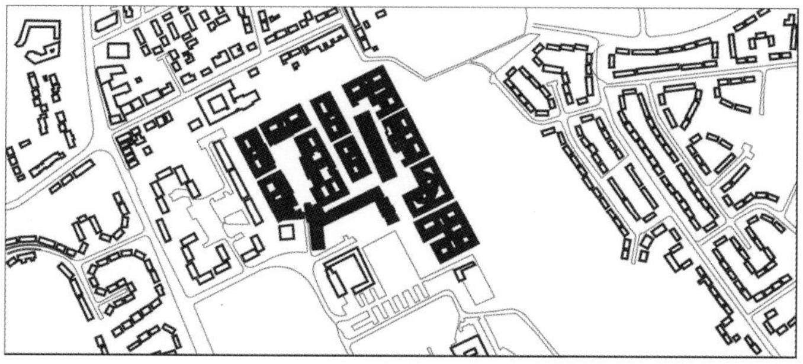

5 Roseberry Park, Middlesbrough, England, UK

ARCHITECT: MAAP (Medical Architecture and Arts Projects, Ltd.), London, UK
LANDSCAPE ARCHITECT: MAAP, London, UK
CLIENT: Tees, Esk and Wear Valleys NHS Foundation Trust
FEATURED MATERIALS: Prefabricated panels, timber
COMPLETED: 2010
INPATIENT BEDS: 312
SITE/PARKING: 15 acres/65
HOSPITAL/TREATMENT CENTER SIZE: 181,000 square feet
NURSES' WORKSTATION: Hybrid

Context/site

Roseberry Park psychiatric hospital was the largest replacement facility of its kind in the United Kingdom when it opened in 2010. The site, adjacent to the James Cook University Hospital, is located approximately eight miles from the North Sea. Residential neighborhoods lie beyond a rail line, just to the east. This facility was built on the grounds of the now-demolished Victorian-era St. Luke's Asylum, outside the town of Middlesbrough. The new campus provides inpatient acute mental health services; a learning disabilities unit; forensic services; and services for older adults with anxiety disorders, depression, and psychosis. The aim was to draw together on one site several services previously scattered across the broader region. This campus was seen as a key component in the NHS goal of delivering comprehensive psychiatric treatment in a noninstitutional, nonthreatening environment with a focus on rehabilitation. Its naturalistic site encourages engagement with the outdoors and for this reason it is horizontally oriented, as a one-level facility, a decision reached through an extensive, interactive consultation process with myriad stakeholders and NHS representatives (Figures 6.5.1 and 6.5.2).

The open courtyards at Roseberry Park allow for immersion in nature to an extent not possible at the psychiatric hospital it replaced. Adult inpatient and forensic units are physically semi-autonomous; this spatial separation was a requirement in the architects' functional brief. However, a number of 'swing beds' are provided in acute, adult, and forensic units in support of varied population types, as patient census levels fluctuate. A single-loaded corridor wraps around the courtyards, a fundamental decision made early on in the campus planning process. Small clusters of inpatient rooms and associated patient and staff supports are located close by. The administration building is three levels in height, located at the center of campus, functioning as a visual landmark. The decision to decentralize the various residential units, treatment rooms, and supports resulted in a human-scaled architectural and campus, obsolete environment – the antithesis to the now-closed hospital it replaced.

Building/unit

The campus is integrated into its immediate site context. Its aesthetic vocabulary is residentialist and generally normative. This was achieved in compositional massing, exterior wood sheathing, stucco, banded floor levels, full-height windows, and transitional zones at the residential 24/7 unit level, not unlike in a multifamily residence (Figure 6.5.3). The adult mental health treatment unit features an 'easy street' consisting of a fitness room, bank, activity/therapy suite, and a public café that adjoins the entrance plaza. This space serves as a nexus for family, staff, and patient social activity. The forensic unit is able to be expanded in the future by up to 64 additional beds. The residential units are situated directly next to a courtyard and the patient is encouraged to spend time outdoors (Figures 6.5.4 and 6.5.5a–b). The design and detailing of the courtyards (nearly 30 in all) is coordinated to the type and intensity of the patient population housed in the adjoining residential units. The various specialized buildings and their wings surround, as enveloping open spaces, precluding the need for obtrusive, punitive-appearing freestanding security fences or walls (Figure 6.5.6). Natural daylight activates many public and semi-public spaces, with window seats positioned at key intervals to allow for informal consults, and most dayrooms and activity areas open directly onto patios with low-scale plantings and benches (Figure 6.5.7).

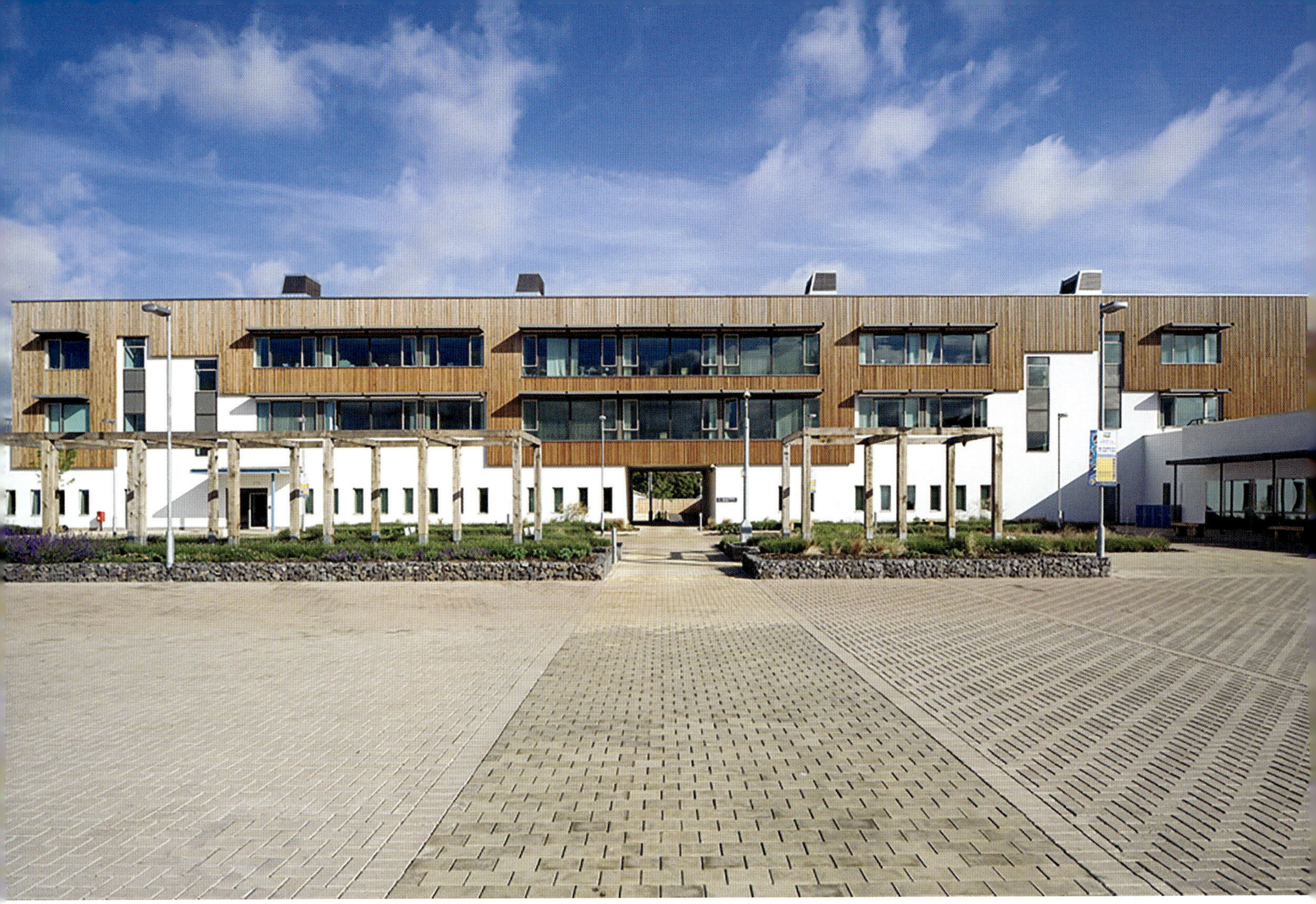

6.5.1 View of the main front court at Roseberry Park, in Middlesbrough.

The semipublic (social) and private realms are independent of one another, and each patient room (all single occupancy) on the unit is provided with a private bath/shower unit. Patient rooms are arranged in small groupings, with dormitory furnishings, including a bed, built-in desk, shelving, and closet (Figure 6.5.8a–b). With regards to eco-sustainability, building orientation maximizes natural light and ventilation transmission, and its structural frame was prefabricated off-site, manufactured exclusively from locally sourced timber. Many building materials are recycled from the demolished St. Luke's Asylum. A postoccupancy assessment of Roseberry Park was conducted (by the architects) 1 year after full occupancy, and findings were presented at the European Health Property Network (EuHPN) Workshop, held in Copenhagen, Denmark, in 2012. This campus, in general, through follow-up consultations, was found to have attained the general design intent and aims of the client agency (NHS), as well as those of the planning and design team from the predesign consultation phase.

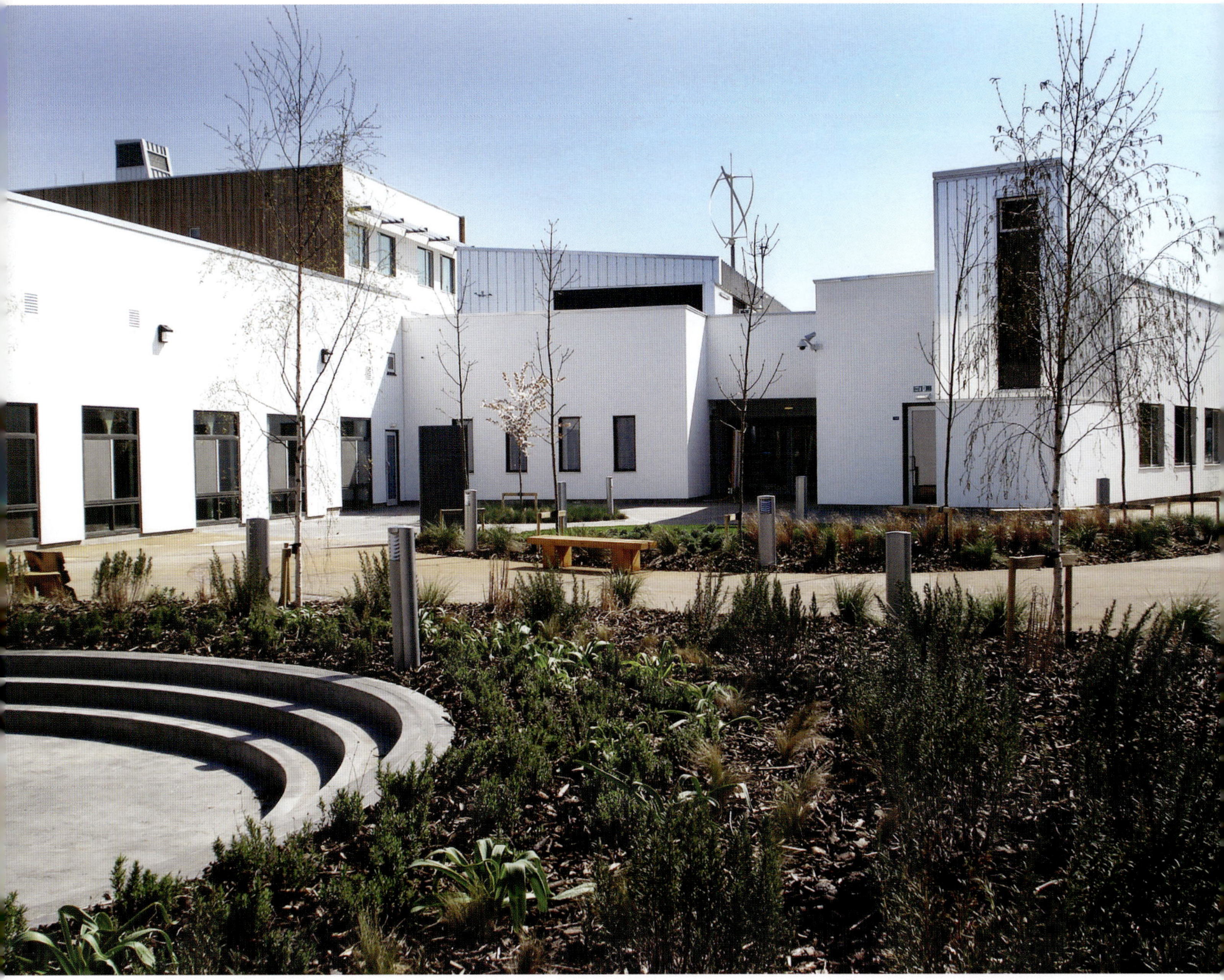

6.5.2 Courtyards feature varied geometries and coordinated landscape elements throughout.

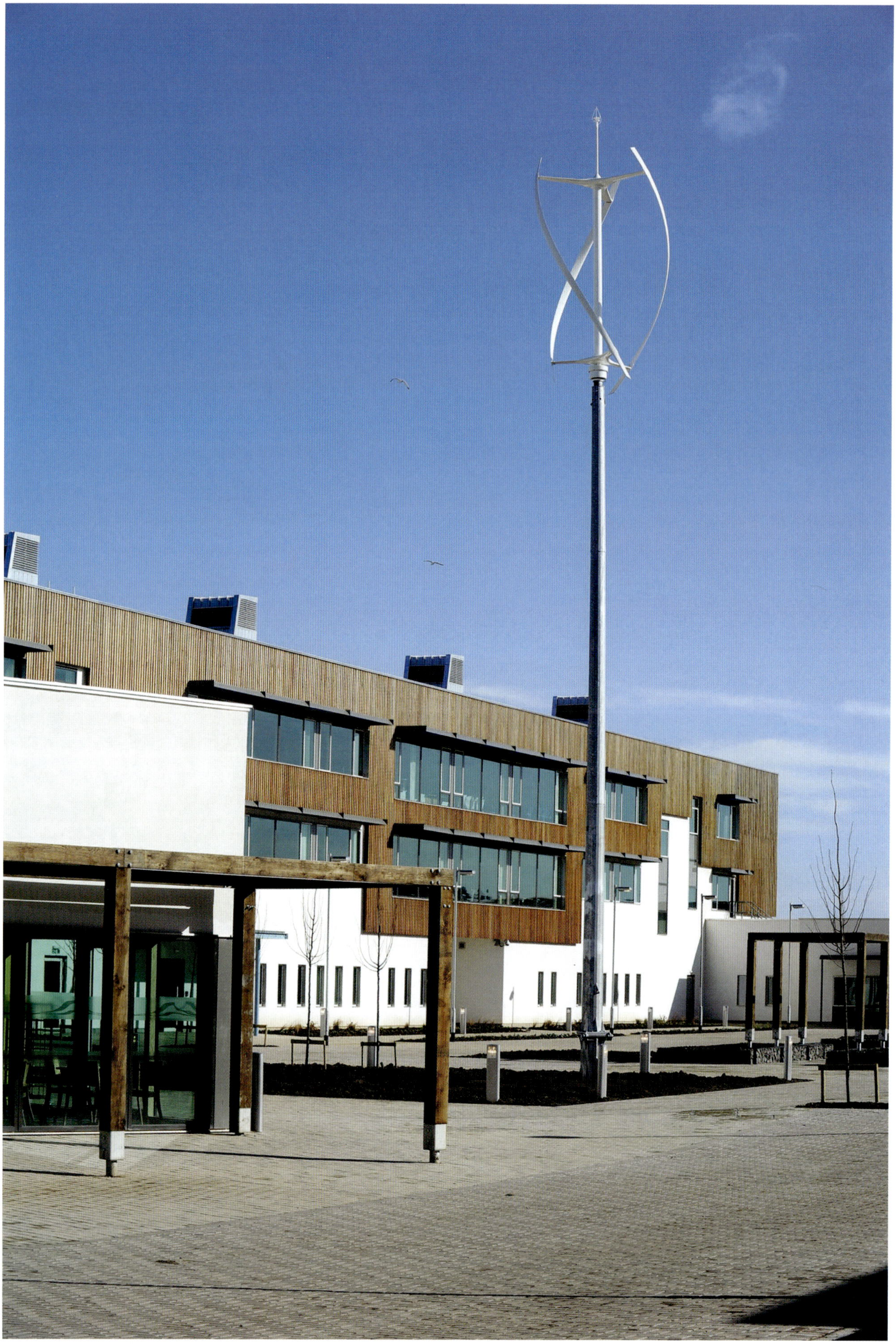

6.5.3 Landmarks (such as the totem) can foster spatial navigation.

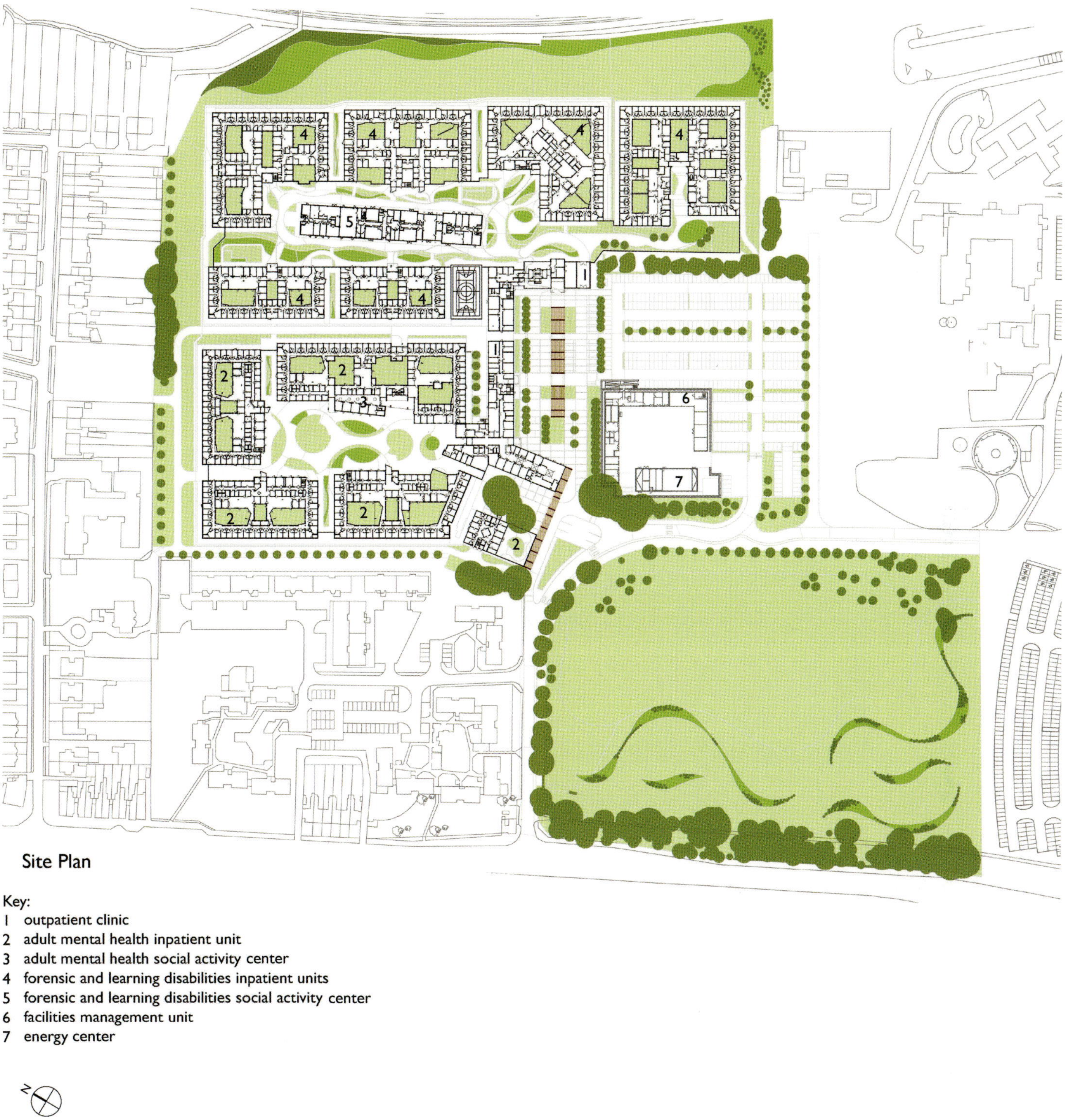

6.5.4 This architect's brief for this campus was decentralized into 12 realms, allowing hierarchical architectural and landscape amenity.

Key:
1 main arrival
2 exterior courtyard
3 dining room
4 day/group activity
5 staff/administration
6 inpatient treatment unit
7 communal hygiene
8 special accommodations bedroom
9 secluded dining
10 kitchen/servery
11 seclusion room
12 staff work area
13 nurses' workstation

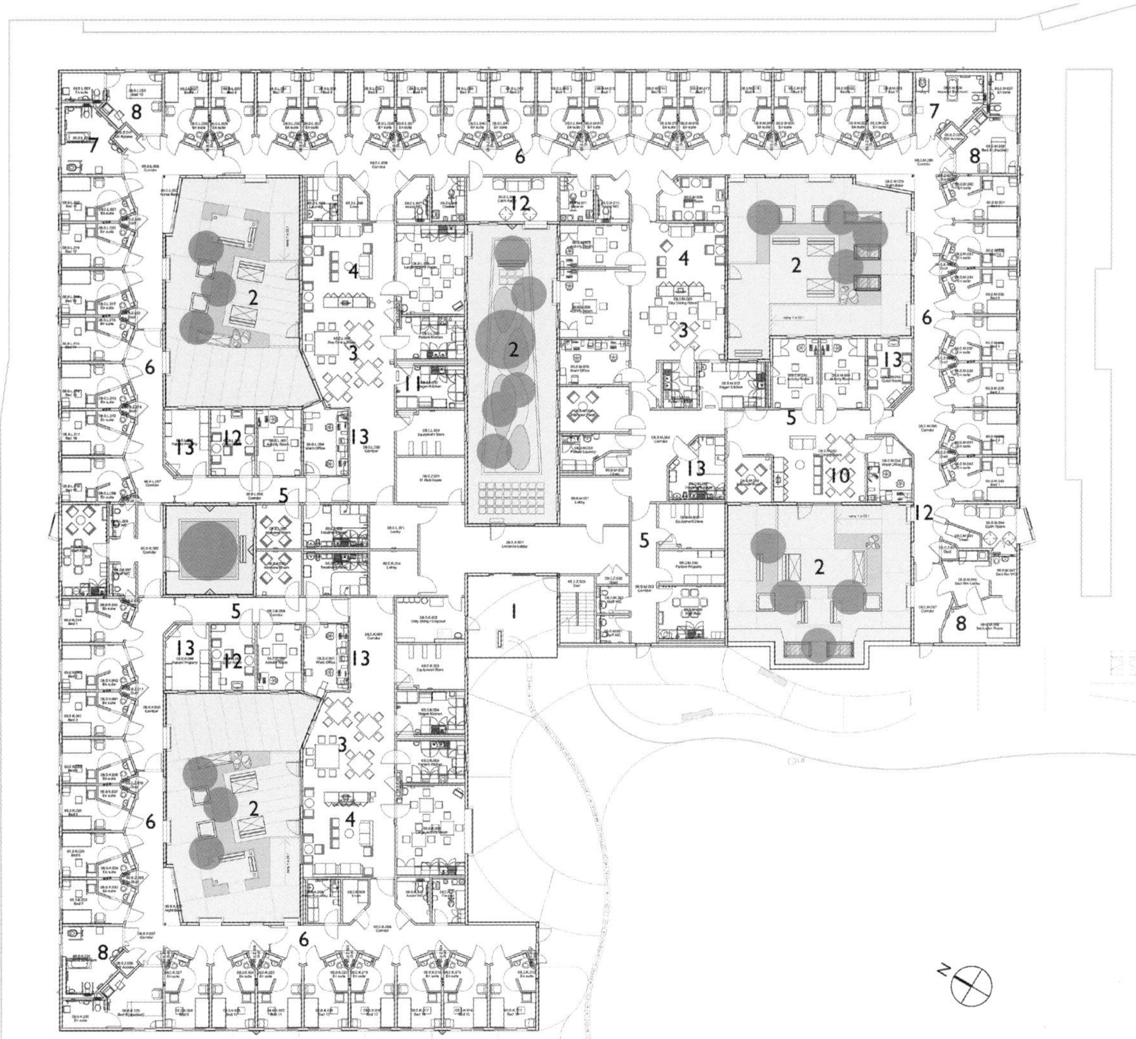

Level 1: Forensic/Learning Disabilities Mental Health Unit

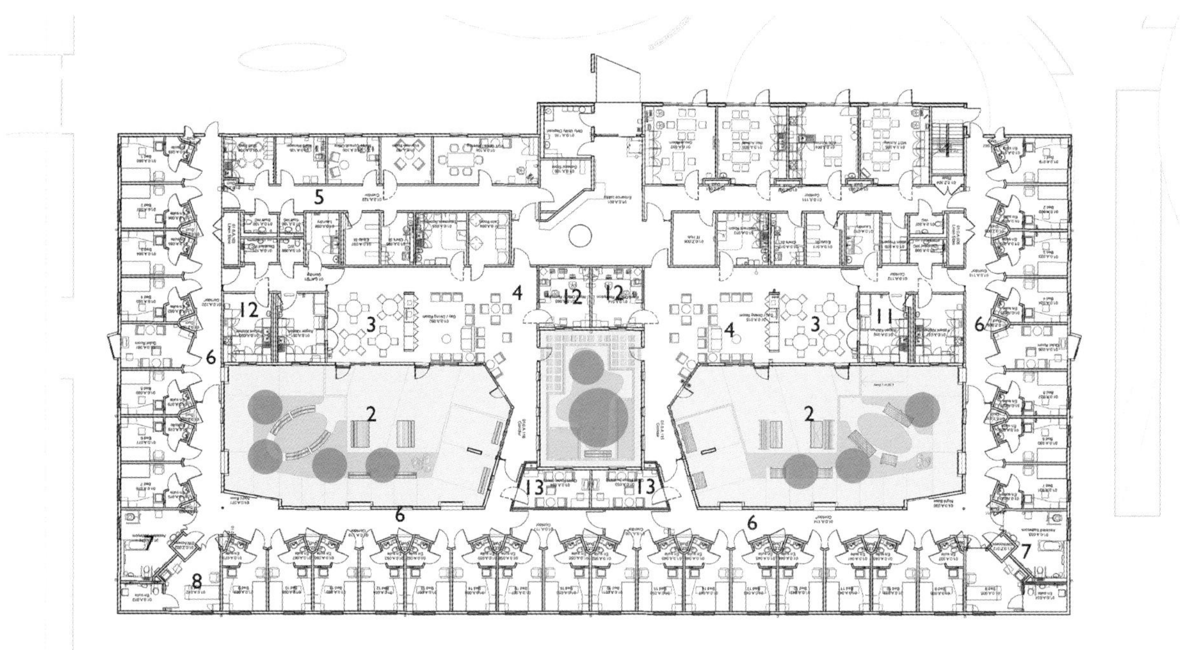

Level 1: Adult Mental Health Unit

6.5.5a–b The various residential units at Roseberry Park feature courtyards of varied size and shape, therapeutically supportive of those patients in nearest proximity, with all patient rooms located along the unit periphery.

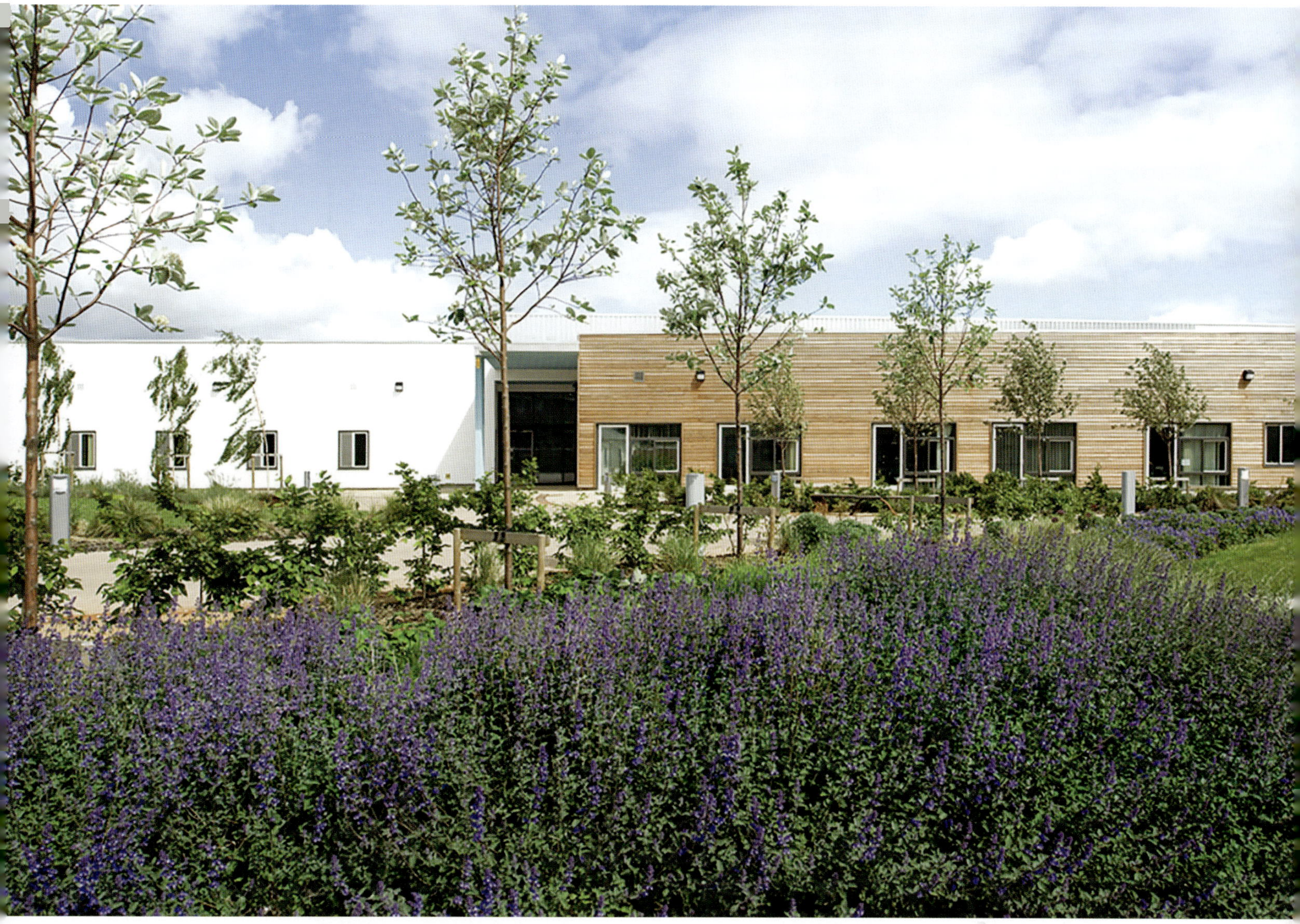

6.5.6 Plant species vary throughout the campus, strategically drawing in the broader surrounding landscape.

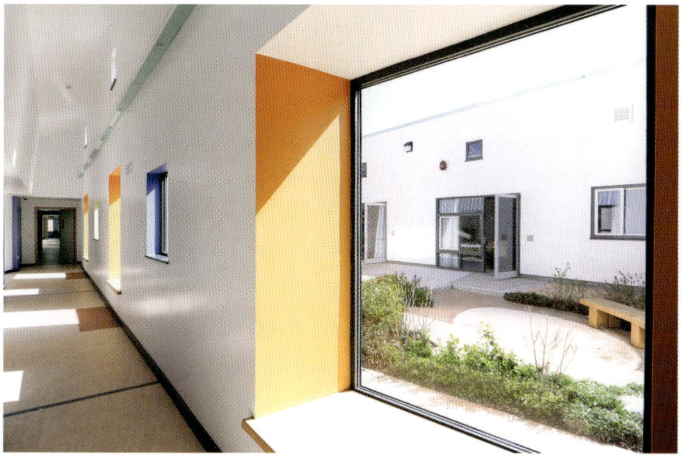

6.5.7 Windowsills along circulation paths in and near the inpatient units function as places for respite and informal consults.

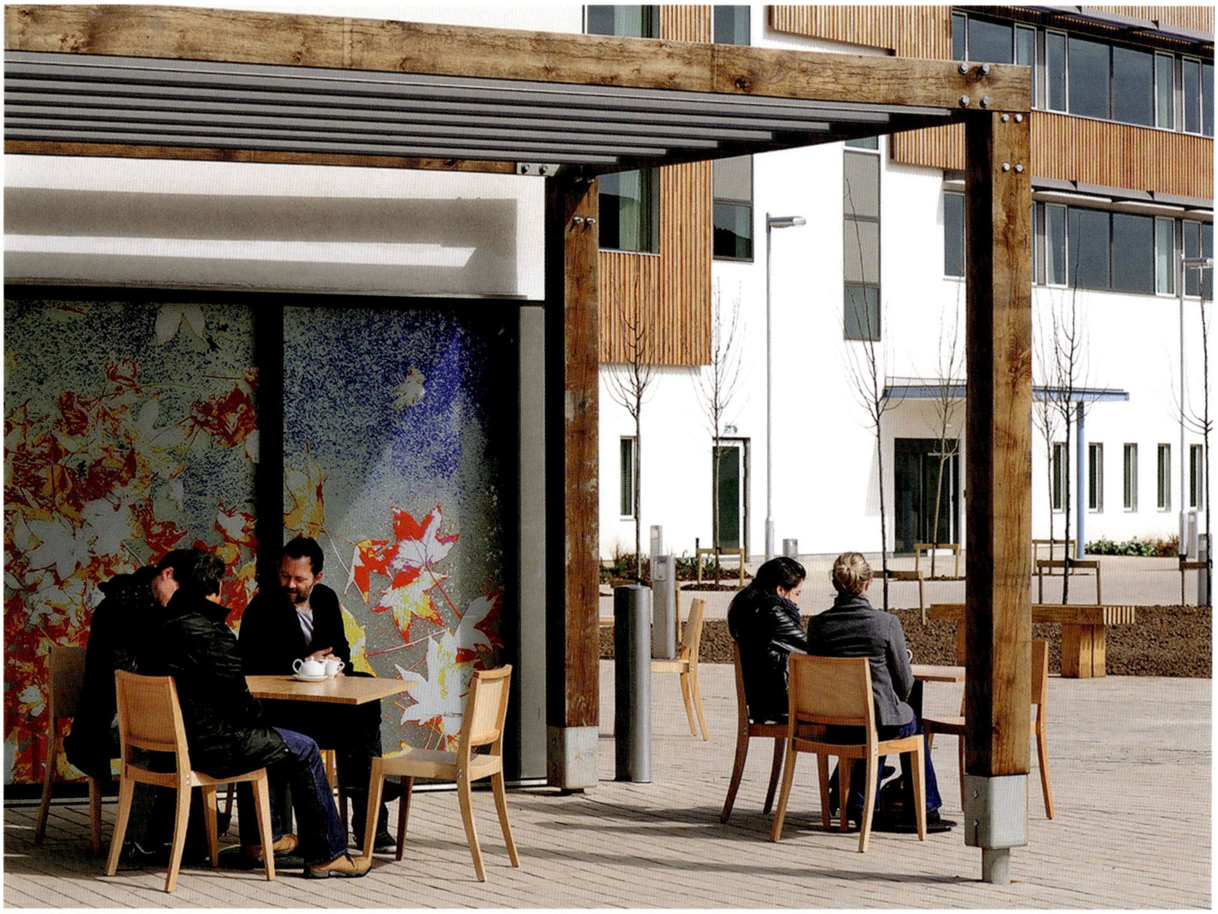

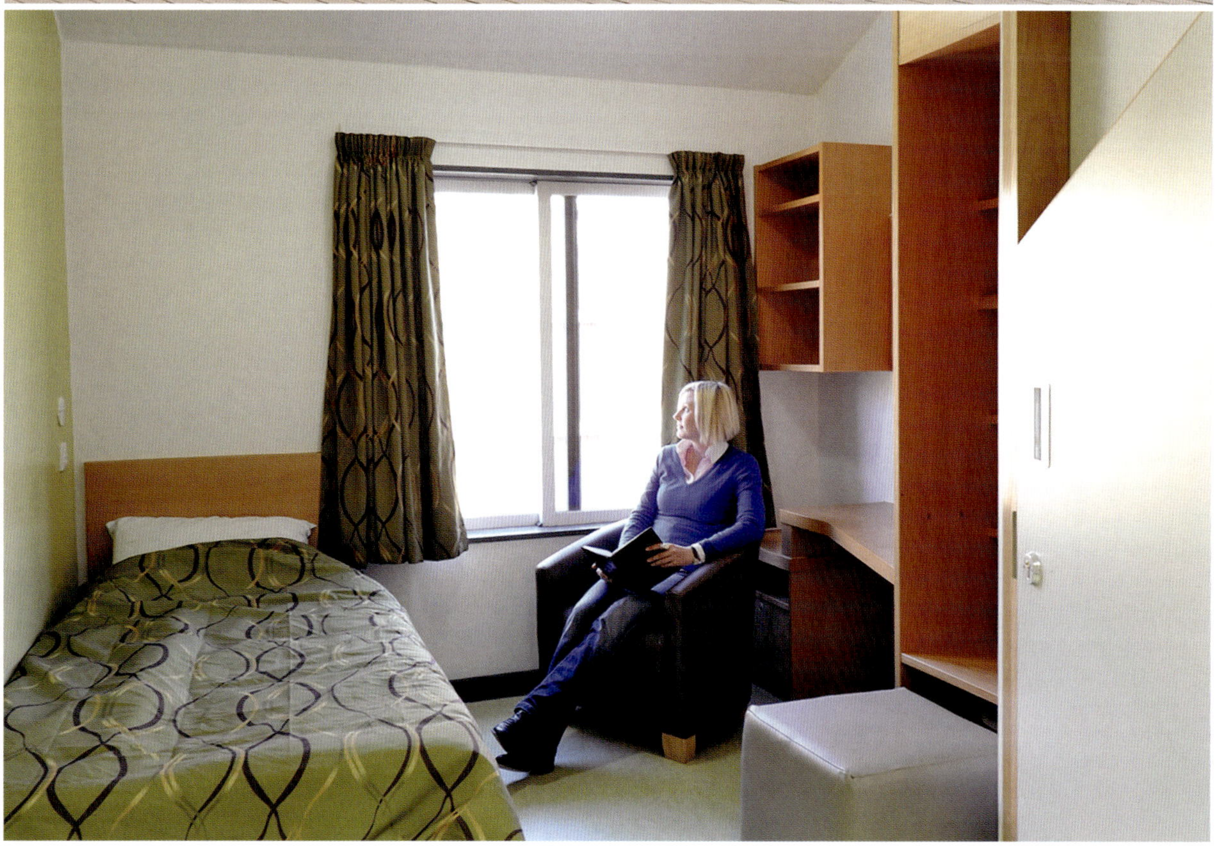

6.5.8a–b Semi-enclosed spaces such as a café in the central court (top) and the patient room (bottom) contribute to a noninstitutional aesthetic.

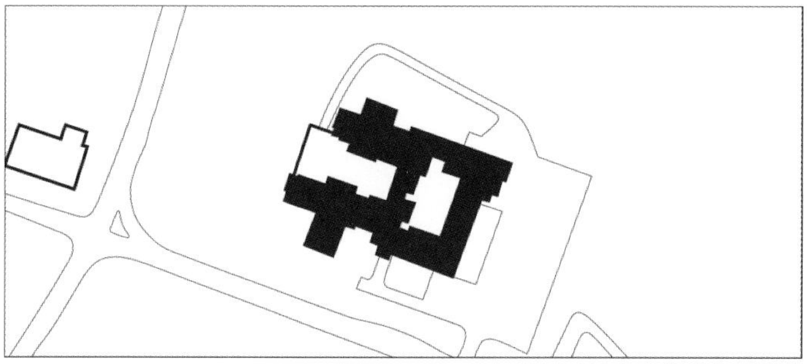

6 Vermont Psychiatric Care Hospital, Berlin, Vermont, USA

ARCHITECT: architecture+ (Prime Architect), Troy, New York, USA, with Black River Design (Associated Architects), Montpelier, Vermont, USA
LANDSCAPE ARCHITECT: Wagner Hodgson, Burlington, Vermont, USA
CLIENT: State of Vermont
FEATURED MATERIALS: Vermont bluestone and slate, locally harvested white ash
COMPLETED: 2014
INPATIENT BEDS: 25
SITE/PARKING: 12 acres/45
HOSPITAL/TREATMENT CENTER SIZE: 74,000 square feet
NURSES' WORKSTATION: Shielded

Context/site

In 2011, Hurricane Irene devastated much of Vermont and flooded the nearby state psychiatric hospital in Waterbury, Vermont, making it imperative that a replacement facility be built as quickly as possible. Psychiatric beds were reallocated on an emergency basis from the destroyed hospital to other, nonpsychiatric hospitals in the region, as the state proceeded with planning this 25-bed state-operated replacement hospital. The aging Vermont State Hospital had served the state's most acutely mentally ill patients, but its 19th-century facility was now obsolete and in a state of disrepair. In fact, the Centers for Medicaid and Medicaid Services (CMS) in the United States had decertified the old asylum hospital nearly a decade earlier (in 2003), and the state had slated it for eventual closure. With reconstruction funding provided by the US Federal Emergency Management Agency (FEMA), the State of Vermont was able to finance this long-overdue replacement facility to serve its most severely mentally ill. In response, a fast-track schedule was adopted and multiple groups of stakeholders worked closely and consistently within a tight time frame and construction schedule to see it to completion.[2]

This one-level facility was inspired by the recent wave of European psychiatric hospitals, the vast majority of which sought to proactively destigmatize, architecturally, the physical setting through the application of layered transparency, informal campus plans and building composition, and sustained connectivity with nature, with nature as a more consciously active therapeutic aspect in psychiatric treatment than in past generations. First, it was decided early on to create two prominent courtyards at the center. These courtyards are visible from virtually all adjoining indoor spaces and are for recreational therapy and help in establishing a normative, residential aesthetic. The various adjoining wings and support elements are variously coded by means of differentiated exterior materiality with, for instance, the administration unit in red masonry with Vermont slate panels, while other structures are sheathed in horizontal and vertical siding of varied patterns and colors. The residential units are situated to the rear of the campus; these elements are sheathed in this aforementioned board and batten siding, materials made from recycled fly ash, sourced locally. The courtyards are enclosed by fences relatively noninstitutional in appearance, with a semitransparent perimeter security element fabricated in wood and polycarbonate screening, appearing not unlike a high garden wall; stones are placed as landscape elements throughout the courtyards. The larger of the two courtyards features seating areas with a butterfly-shaped canopy near the center and an elliptical track and ball court. The entry portals are transparent, allowing views directly into the courtyards (i.e., to the canopy and its seating area) (Figures 6.6.1 to 6.6.3), with a circular labyrinth in proximity (Figure 6.6.4).

Building/unit

The admission unit was designed for patients that typically arrive in the custody of law enforcement. This necessitated a funnel-like sally port, remaining fully usable in inclement weather conditions. Vehicles arrive on-site at this midsection point on the campus, allowing for direct transference of patients from vehicle to the high-security entry vestibule/admit unit. The living rooms, quiet rooms, comfort rooms, and dining areas are located adjacent to the patient housing wings. A library, fitness room, a greenhouse, art therapy room, and dayrooms are nearby. A sensory immersion room is provided for contemplative therapy and respite. This facility consists of all private patient rooms, each with a bath/shower unit. Residential zones are clustered in groupings of four to eight beds. Patient rooms, treatment spaces, and many staff supports feature operable windows. The residential units are designed for flexibility. A prominent rotunda at the campus center is equipped with moveable screens for use for films and related media and doubles as a chapel, an *ad hoc* legal hearing room, and multipurpose/social activity space. Throughout the interior spaces, local vernacular building traditions are in evidence – that is, vertically slatted-wood paneling and rough-hewn shingles and masonry, with the overall vocabulary a far cry from the antiquated facility it replaced (Figures 6.6.5 to 6.6.7). This reinterpretation of the past and emphasis on the contemporary locality was extended to a 'creek' that runs, symbolically, throughout the interior, with various 'docks' stationed at patient room doors, and wood window seats positioned along corridors.

Each residential zone is themed to one of the four seasons, with corresponding color palettes, establishing a unique identity for each. This is underscored by a directional signage system that connects the various parts of a facility consciously configured to feel and look decentralized. The residential zones afford views of the surrounding woods (Figure 6.6.8). The inpatient room features built-in furnishings and individualized nodes to create the feeling of spaces larger than they actually are. Furnishings are dormitory-like, safe, and durable, and shelving is provided for personal belongings. Every patient room has two windows, a sloping ceiling above a built-in bed, accented walls in subtle earthen tones, and recessed incandescent lighting (Figure 6.6.9). According to Frank Pitts, the lead designer with architecture+,

> The bedrooms are designed on a model I had seen in Scandinavia where the bed is positioned such that one sits within a smaller enclosure, right next to a window, with the desk in a separate nook with its own window, each functioning as an independent, intimately-scaled space.[3]

This campus stands out as exemplary among recent North American 24/7 psychiatric facilities – specifically in a nation urgently in need of a new generation of progressively designed mental health and substance abuse treatment facilities.

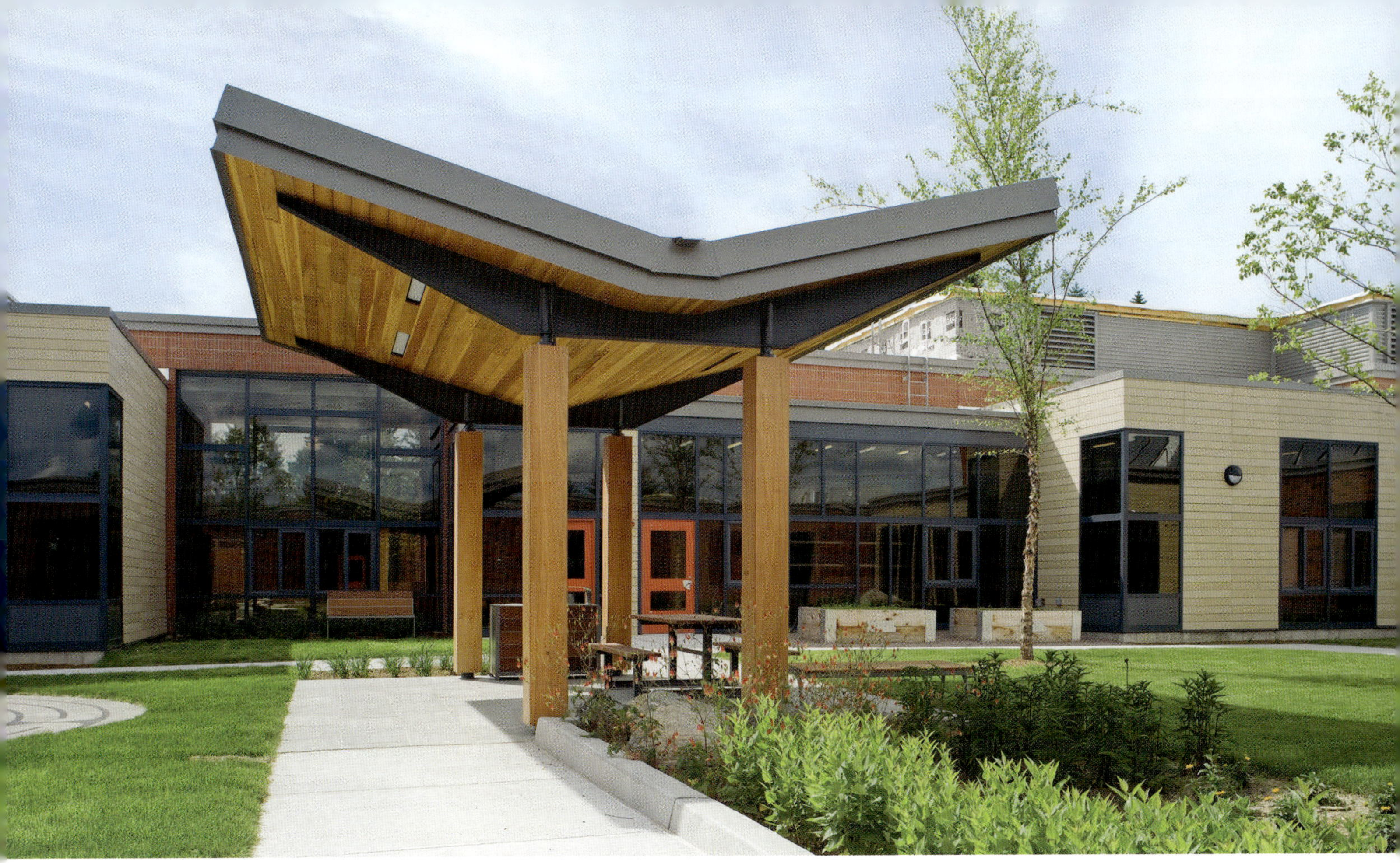

6.6.1 The butterfly canopy at the Vermont Psychiatric Care Hospital.

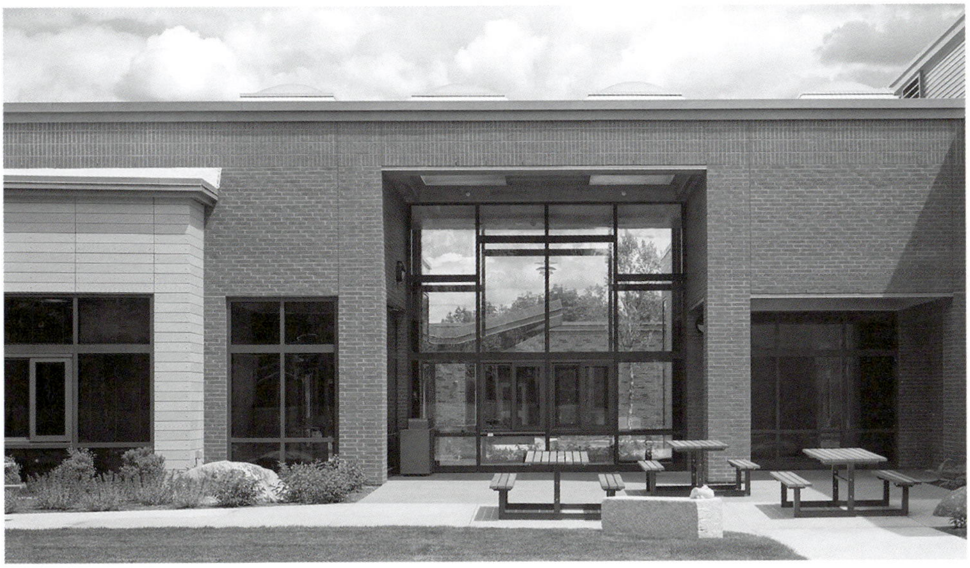

6.6.2 View portals function to de-mass the total composition and foster a sense of openness and transparency.

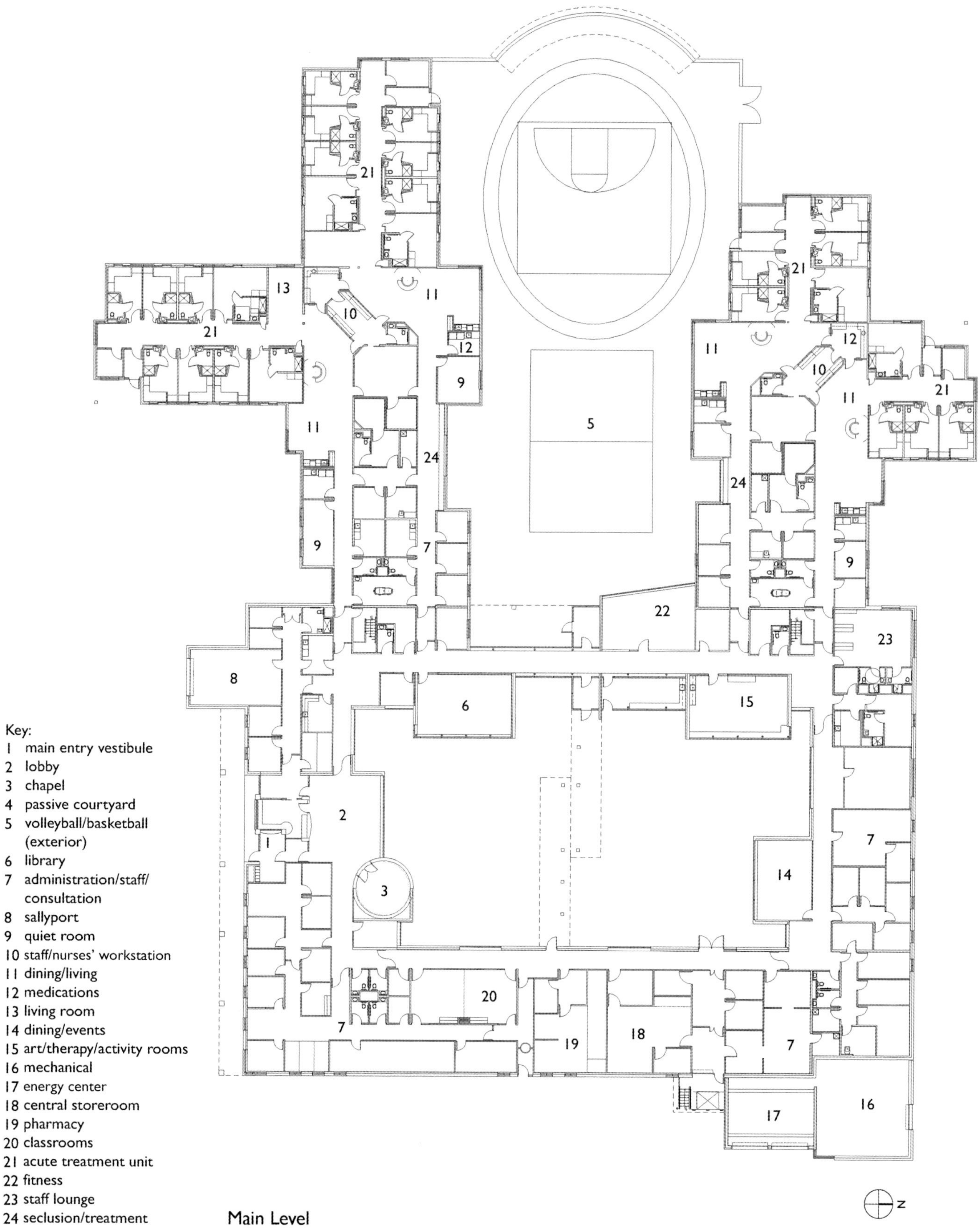

6.6.3 The facility is U configured, with a connector element at midsection linking two principal residential realms and various supports.

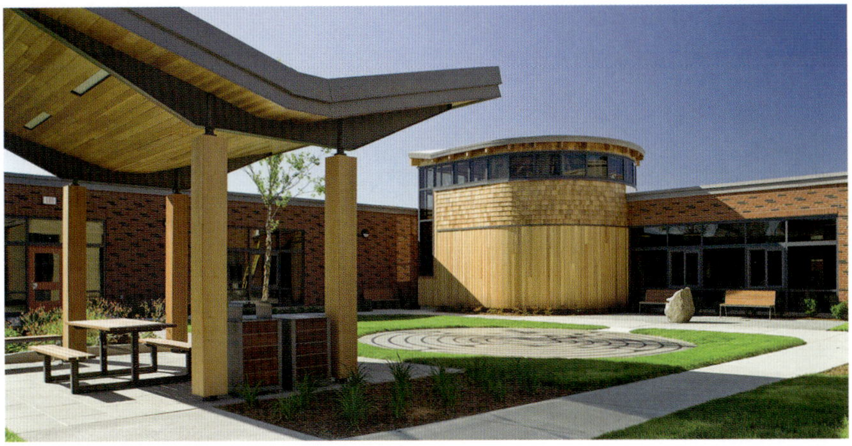

6.6.4 Multiple interior and exterior spaces are articulated as semiautonomous elements, providing compositional hierarchy.

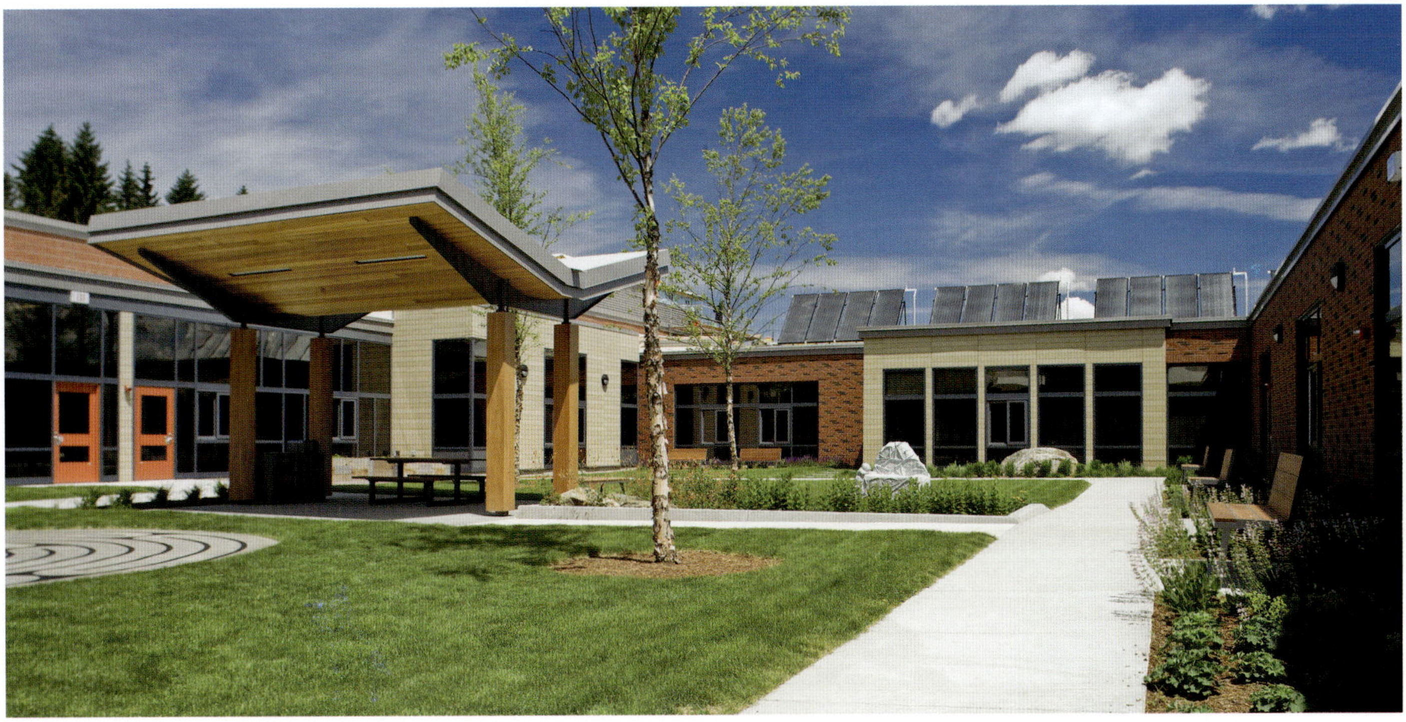

6.6.5 Courtyards feature active and passive spaces, including paths, covered seating areas, varied ground plantings, and recreational therapy area.

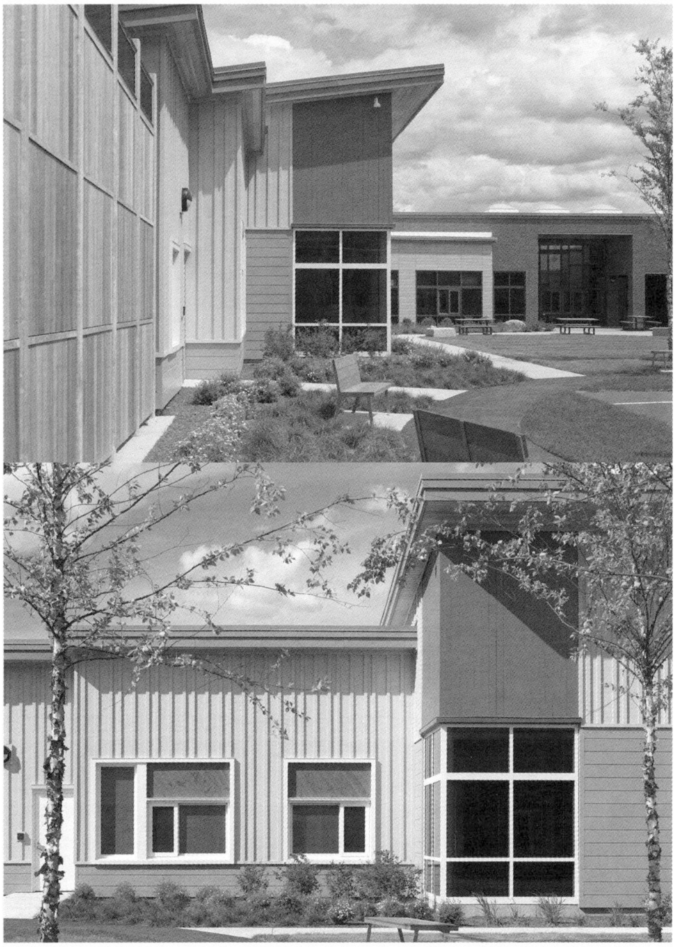

6.6.6a-b Compositional setbacks and varied roof forms allow for expression of smaller-scaled yet contiguous 'buildings', with varied exterior material palettes and fenestration.

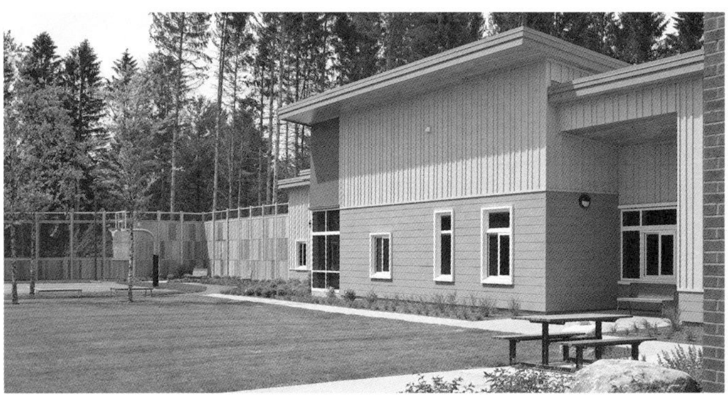

6.6.7 The perimeter barrier is a gridwall fabricated of steel and wood panel insets, visually extending buildings into the adjacent wooded site environs.

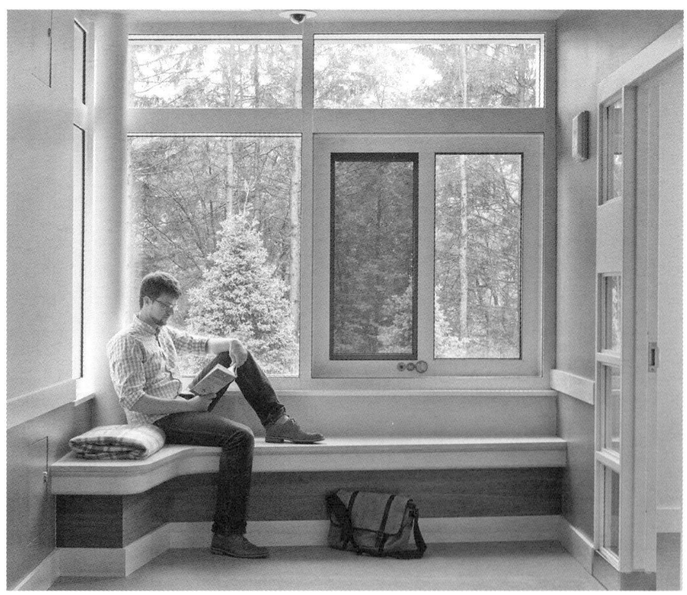

6.6.8 Residential units feature built-in seating, operable windows, and direct views of nature.

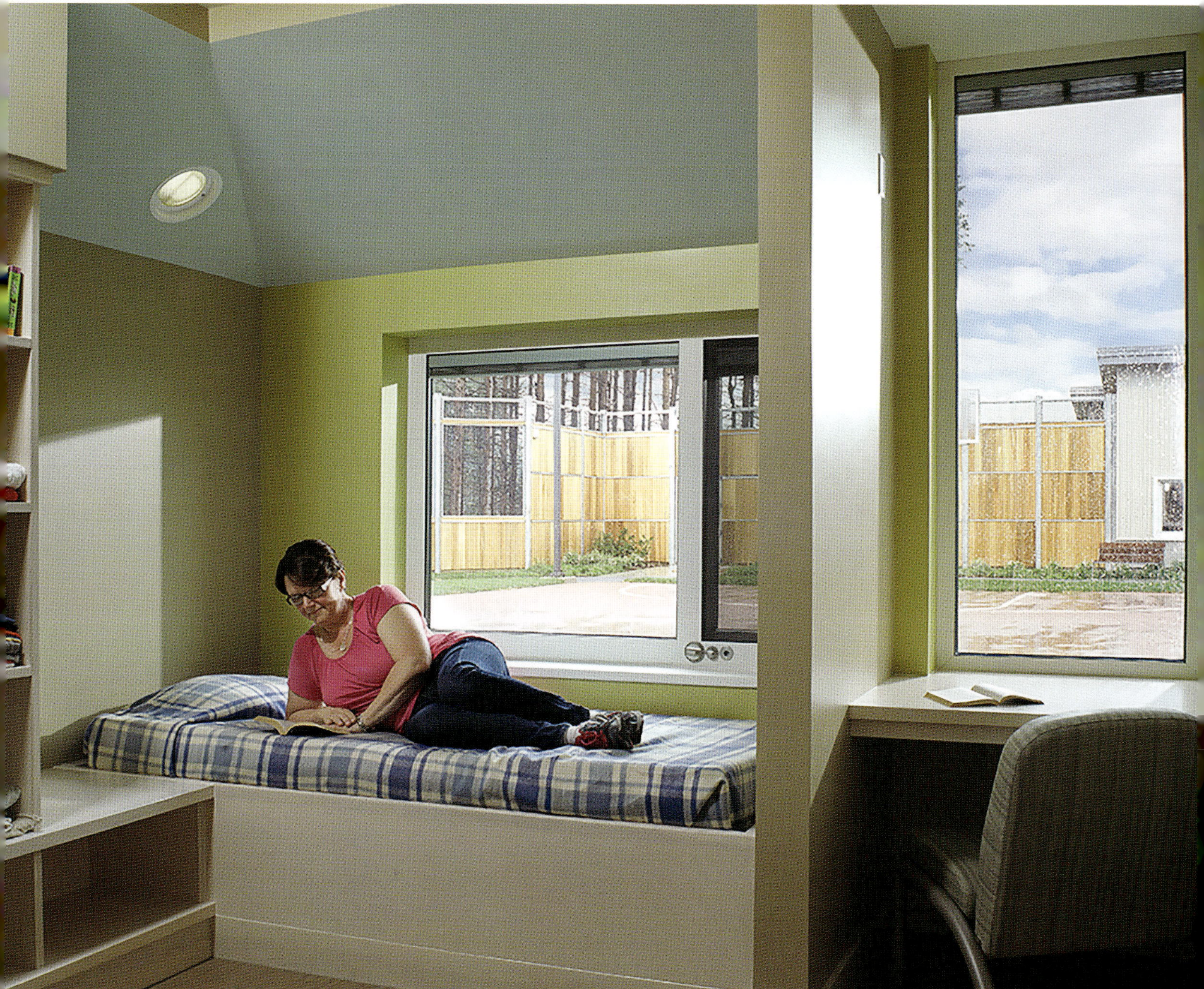

6.6.9 A color-accented patient room perimeter wall is divided into two built-ins (sleeping alcove and built-in desk) with sloping ceilings.

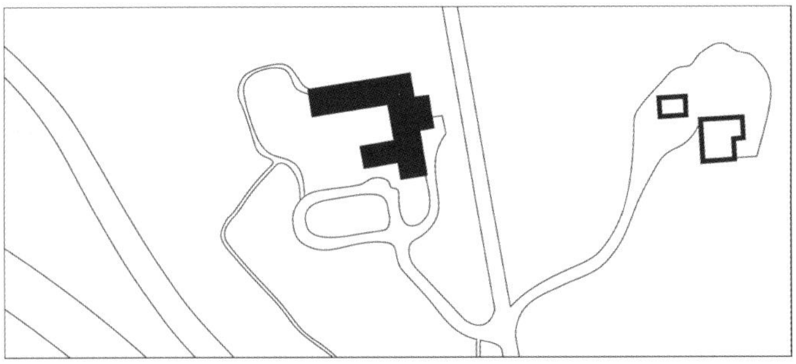

7 The Southdown Institute, Holland Landing, Newmarket, Ontario, Canada

ARCHITECT: Montgomery Sisam Architects, Toronto, Ontario, Canada
LANDSCAPE ARCHITECT: PMA Landscape Architects, Toronto, Ontario, Canada
CLIENT: The Southdown Institute
FEATURED MATERIALS: Timber and glass panels, masonry
COMPLETED: 2014
INPATIENT BEDS: 22
SITE/PARKING: 37 acres/36
HOSPITAL/TREATMENT CENTER SIZE: 12,200 square feet
NURSES' WORKSTATION: Open

Context/site

This rural retreat, located 40 miles north of Toronto, provides residential and outpatient mental health, chemical dependency treatment, and spiritual guidance to Catholic clergy and other vowed members of religious orders. Its education and consultation services promote health and wellness support care for church ministers so they can better serve their congregations out in the community. An interdisciplinary team of professionals combines advanced theories and best practices in the behavioural health sciences, within the Catholic spiritual tradition. The physical setting provides a contemplative environment conductive to healing while immersing the 'patient' in nature and landscape, with the treatment focus on rehabilitation. The program is centered on meditation, group counseling, and individual counseling. The institute is sponsored by the Canadian Conference of Catholic Bishops and the Canadian Religious Conference and is funded through private donations with financial assistance provided, as necessary, to ensure that no one is turned away. The Institute is unique within Canada; its clinical care team consists of registered nurses, social workers, and psychologists.

The Southdown Institute is located in a rapidly developing area on the northern fringe of Toronto, near a freeway and farmland currently under pressure for conversion to suburban development. At present however the site remains relatively remote and serene. In this regard, it is a bit reminiscent of Frank Lloyd Wright's Taliesin West, in Scottsdale, Arizona, a once-rural retreat, built in the 1930s that in time found itself surrounded by urbanity. The structure at Southdown is a modified U configuration, in plan, with a parking area and circular arrival drive at front, leading to the main entrance. From the vantage point of the main entrance only a small percentage of the total facility is visible at once, and this resulted from the designers' intent for the Southdown Institute to appear as a manor house retreat versus a formal 'hospital' or 'treatment facility'. The intent to achieve a human-scaled retreat ambience and aesthetic has been reinforced throughout the campus, with a strong physical and visual connection achieved with the immediate natural environment, on both its inward- and outward-facing sides (Figure 6.7.1 to 6.7.3).

Building/unit

The exterior is sheathed in natural-stained horizontal cedar siding, and its operable windows are scaled to appear non-institutional. Upon entering, one looks onto a wooded courtyard. This space has tall white pine trees and invites its use (Figure 6.7.4). It serves as the visual focal point, and the interior spaces are arranged around it on two sides. These include a chapel that doubles as a multipurpose space, prominently located and visible as one approaches. To the immediate right is the administration unit. The space features a large stained-glass mural along one wall and a vaulted ceiling. Theraserialization is employed in the form of strong indoor-outdoor connectivity. This pertains to principal circulation spaces with rooms situated alongside, and seating alcoves provide support for informal social interaction ad consults. A great room, located at the intersection of the two circulation arteries, contains a fireplace and expansive views with access to two outdoor terraces, one on the courtyard side, and another next to the great room and to the facility's 'back side' (Figures 6.7.5 and 6.7.6). The courtyard functions as a catalyst and the adjoining corridors are activated by its presence and its scale. Adjoining interior spaces feature wood floors and ceilings, and the dining area has a vaulted ceiling and clerestory windows, drawing light in while offering a view of the tree line and sky above.

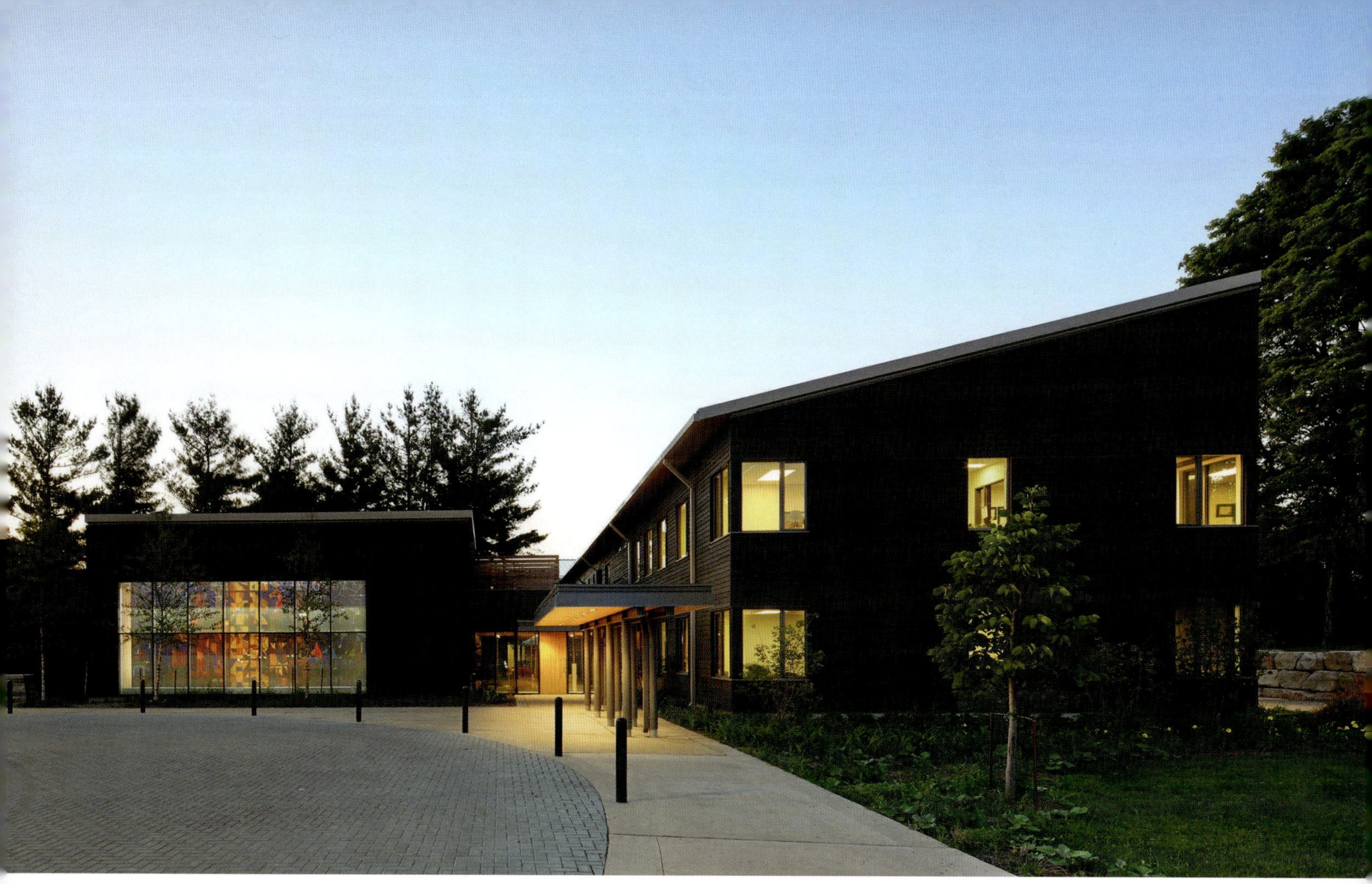

6.7.1 The main vehicular arrival zone at the Southdown Institute counseling center and retreat.

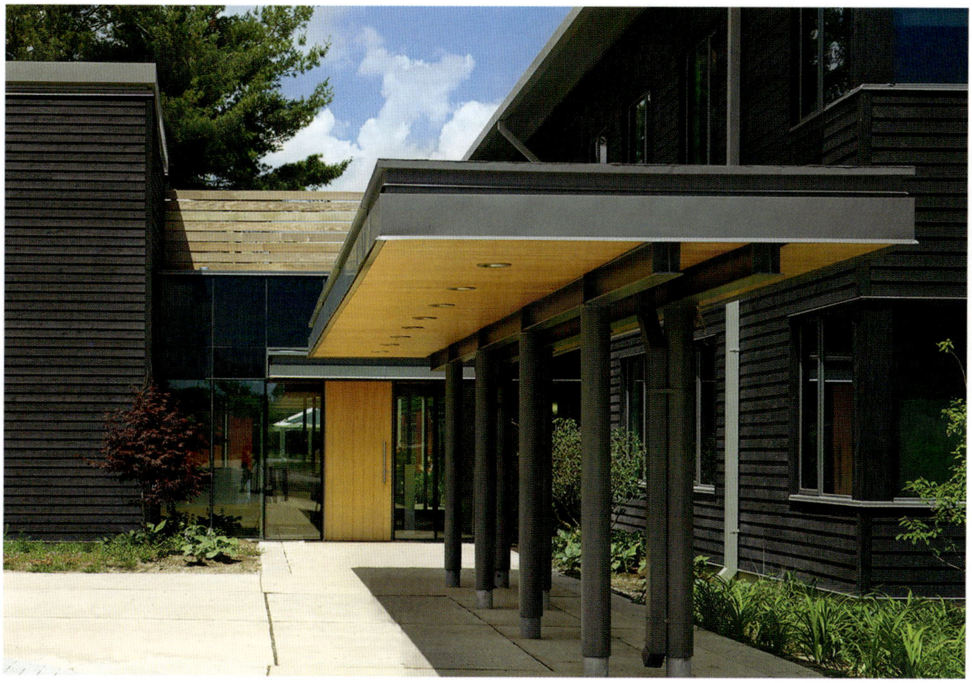

6.7.2 The arrival canopy is on axis with the semi public realm.

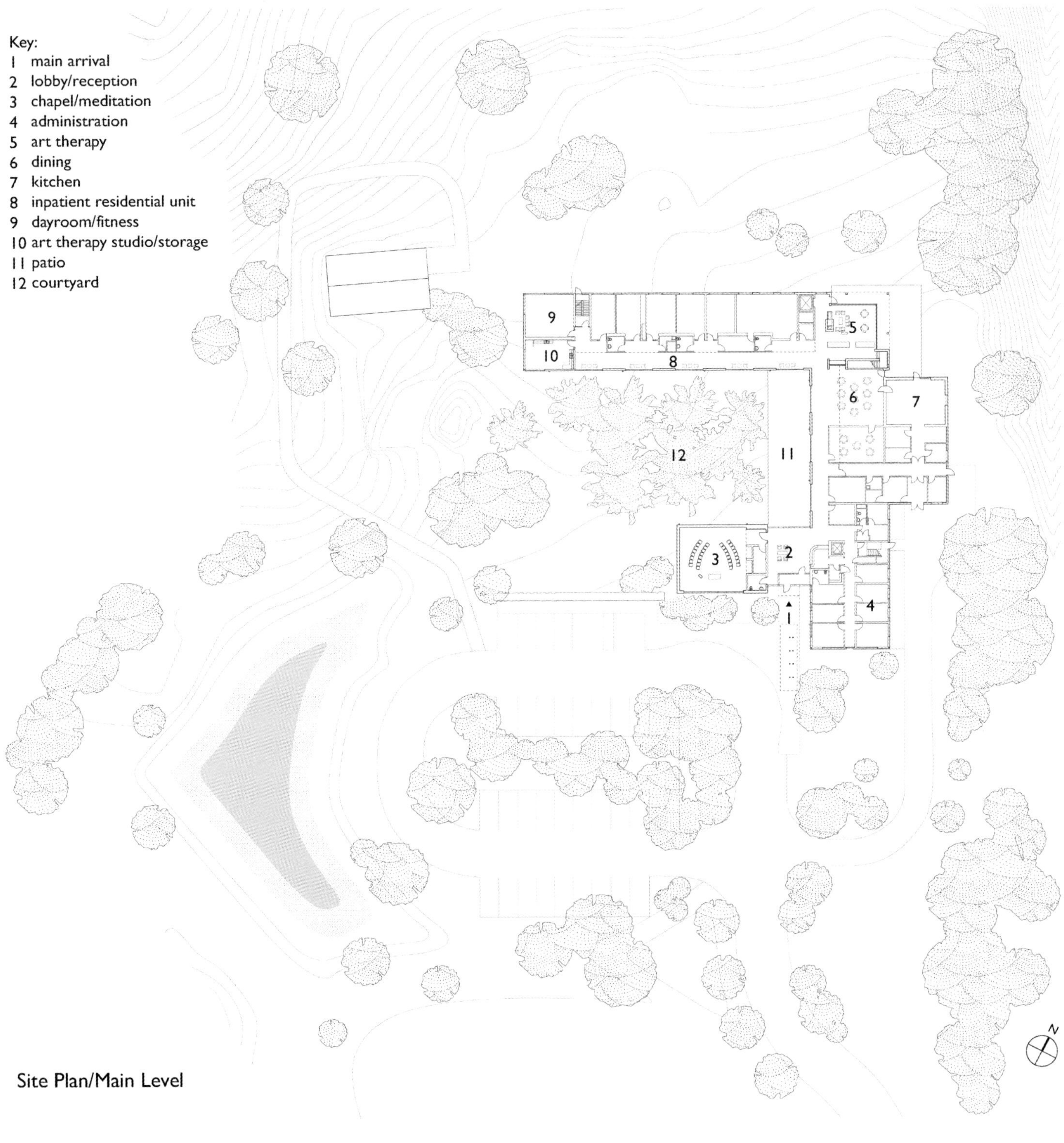

6.7.3 The building wraps around a stand of mature trees.

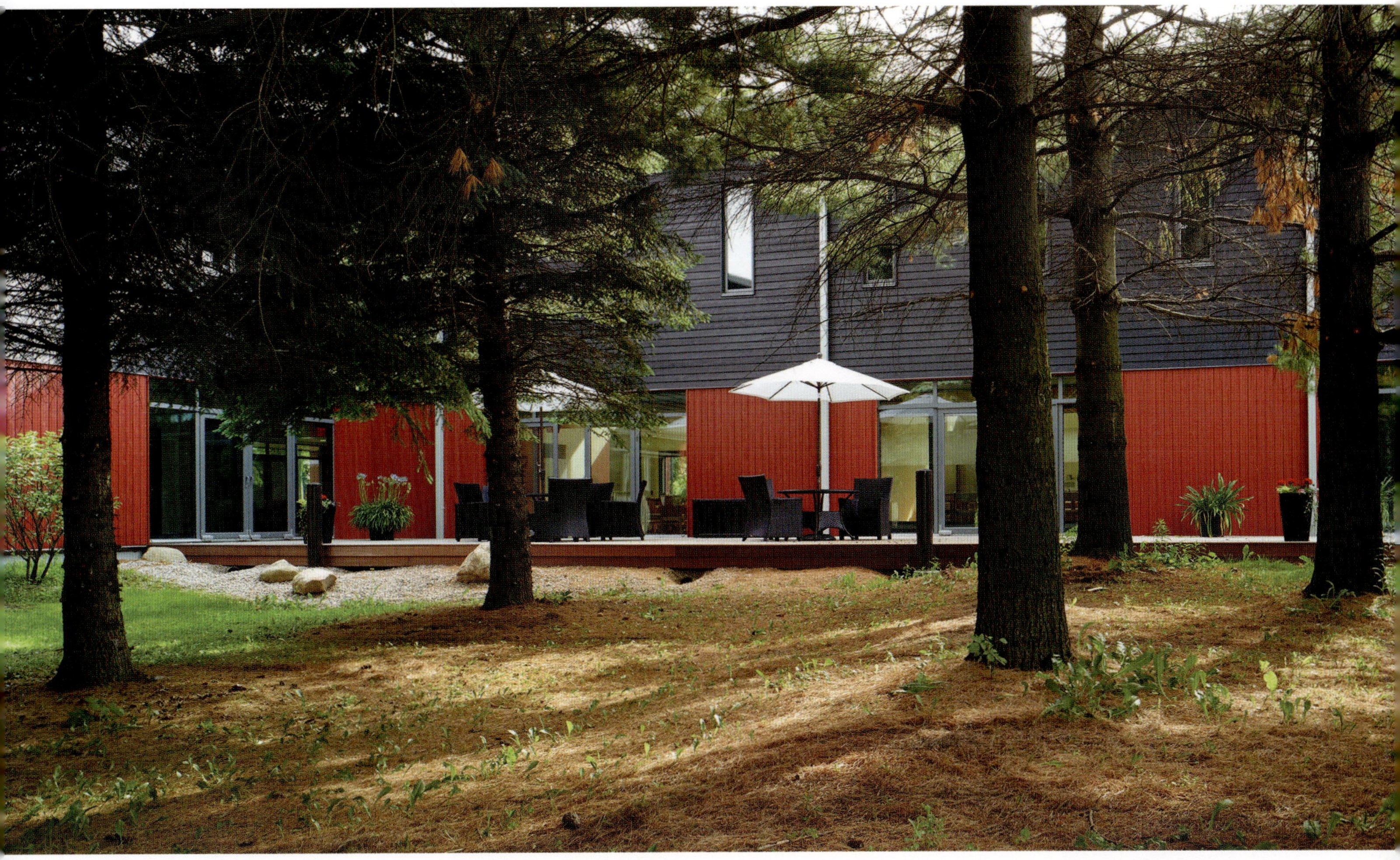

6.7.4 Spaces along two circulation arteries open onto wooded courtyard.

An indoor-outdoor continuum informs the orientation of the patient rooms, as these were set back from the corridor in order to feel more private; the bath/shower units are situated on the side nearest the corridor, and this allows for larger windows on the outer-facing wall. Some bathrooms are private, others semiprivate. Art therapy and group counseling/activity rooms are at the far end of the corridor, providing access to the outdoors (Figure 6.7.7). Residents' rooms are generally hotel-like in their furnishings, size, proportion, color palette, and ambiance (Figure 6.7.8). A second level houses additional counseling spaces and patient-resident bedrooms. Southdown Institute represents the small-scale, residentialist end point of a continuum of inpatient mental health treatment facilities perhaps best represented within this compendium of case studies at the other end point by the Marie Bashir Centre in Sydney, Australia (2014), and the Juravinski Centre for Integrated Healthcare, in Hamilton, Ontario, Canada (2013). These examples were, by contrast, built on dense urban sites and are more comprehensive care facilities. By contrast, the Southdown Institute shares perhaps its closest affinities with the Sydenham Garden Resource Centre in London, as both settings emphasize a decidedly low-tech approach in the provision of psychiatric and substance addiction counseling, emphasizing intrinsic therapeutic affordances of nature; both are small in scale, architecturally, while providing a multifaceted, deinstitutionalized experience.

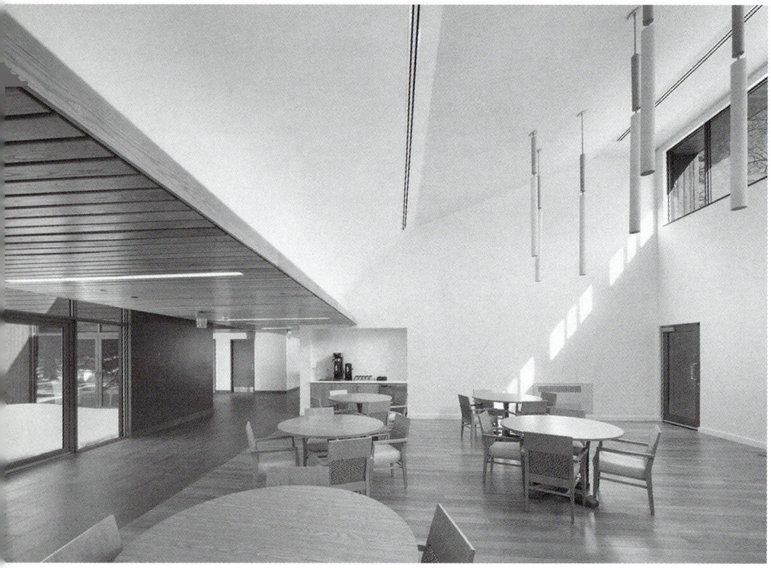

6.7.5 Varied ceiling geometries articulate semipublic spaces, including a communal dining room.

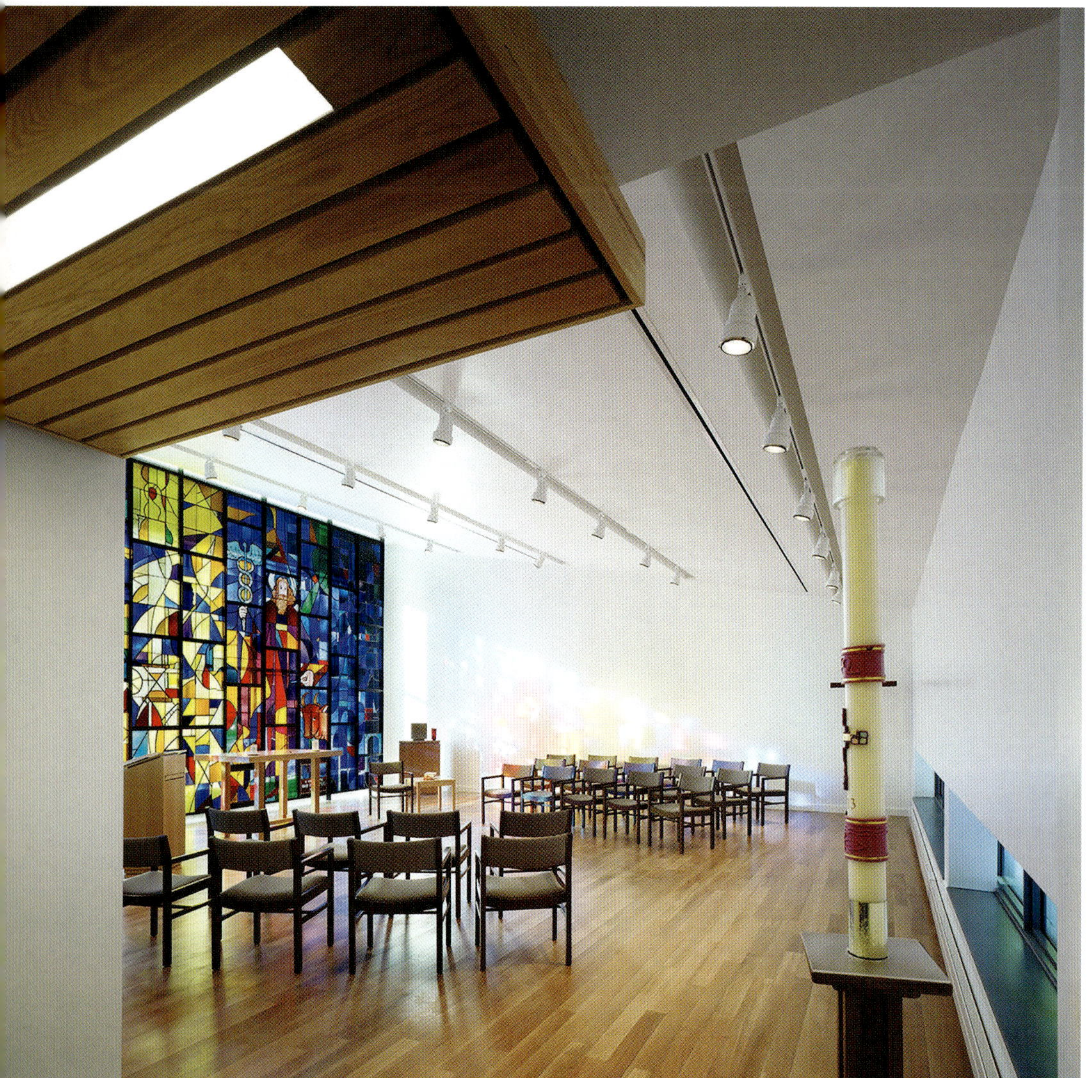

6.7.6 A large stained-glass installation is the focal point of the chapel.

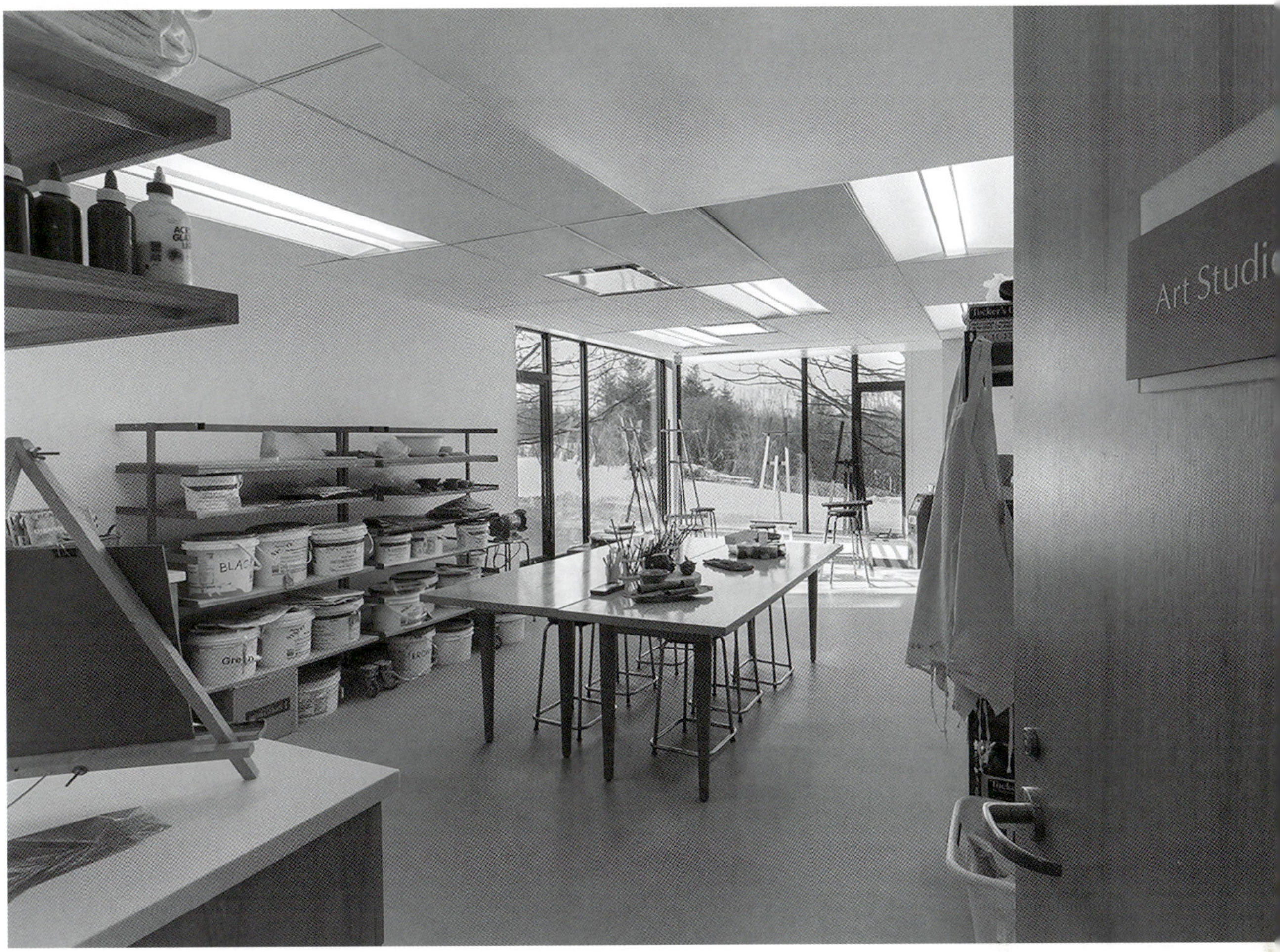

6.7.7 Therapy/treatment rooms open onto the back side of the campus.

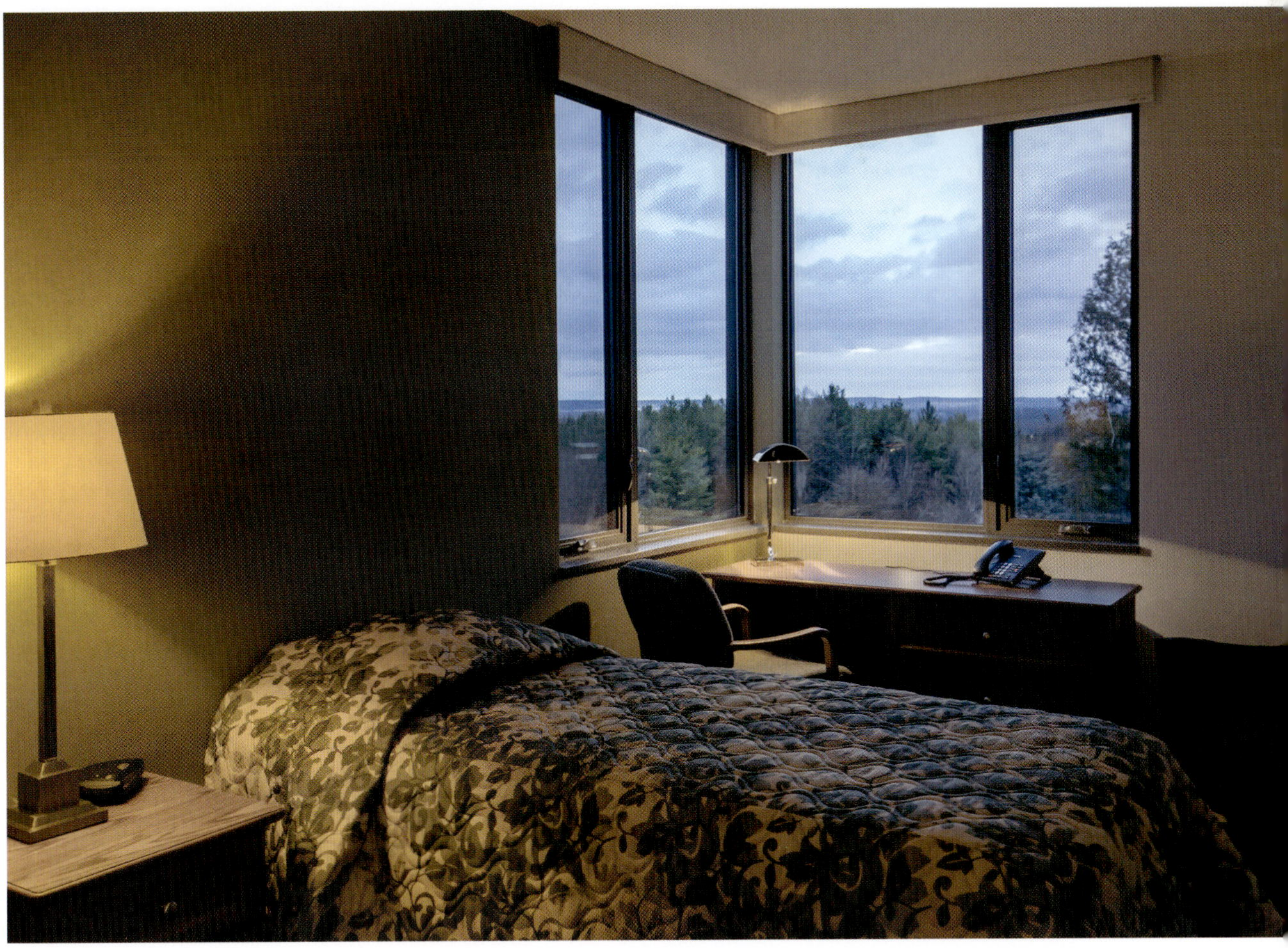

6.7.8 Bedrooms are hotel-like, with freestanding furnishings.

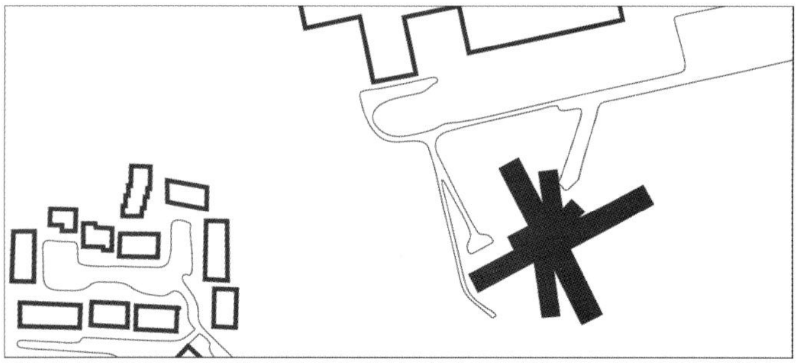

8 Helsingor Psychiatric Hospital and Clinic, Helsingor, Denmark

ARCHITECT: JDS/BIG Architects, Copenhagen, Denmark
LANDSCAPE ARCHITECT: BIG Architects, Copenhagen, Denmark
CLIENT: Ministry of Health
FEATURED MATERIALS: glass and steel panels, masonry
COMPLETED: 2006
INPATIENT BEDS: 75
SITE/PARKING: 22 acres/60
HOSPITAL/TREATMENT CENTER SIZE: 68,200 square feet
NURSES' WORKSTATION: Shielded

Context/site

This psychiatric hospital is located near the Danish-Swedish border and the old city center of Helsingor. The setting is essentially rural, with an International Red Cross hospital nearby, a supply distribution warehouse, and the administration center (across the road to the north). To the immediate east are residential subdivisions, with an elementary school located to the south of this residential area, near in proximity to the psychiatric hospital. The western edge of its site is farmland, extending far beyond in the landscape. As is the case with many recently built European psychiatric hospitals, the setting is rural, located at the edge of a city or town. The preference for a somewhat sequestered, even remote site is little different in this regard from that in the 18th and 19th centuries, with the ideal site for an asylum being remote from any major population center. The intent then, as now, was in some ways to remove the patient from the countertherapeutic aspects in his or her everyday life, a process essential to 'restoring' the individual by means of the latest treatment methods. This modus operandi allowed (then, as now) relative freedom for administrators and direct caregivers to experiment, although in the past this too frequently led to unfortunate mental health outcomes (see Chapters 2 and 4).

The architects, BIG Architects and JDS, in the case of the new hospital in Helsingor, sought, however, and in stark contrast to the dark past of European psychiatry, to eschew clichés and harsh stereotypes of neoclassical asylums, as well as mid-20th-century mental hospitals. This residential and outpatient treatment center is dramatically inserted *into* its sloping site in a manner that allows building and landscape to engage in a dialogue, and in some ways becoming one and the same – a symbiosis. The structure's formal compositional elements are deployed by means of a series of rotations and incisions; the resulting interior wings and exterior spaces simultaneously yield exterior cross-connections and varied landscaped roof planes. Overall, the plan is biaxial, with a pair of axes splayed as an X configuration; this results as a central commons/atrium nexus and adjoining outdoor space at the center of the X. From here, four narrow wings variously radiate outward as fingers reaching, in a way, with a central atrium functions as the core, or catalyst, from a spatial navigation wayfinding standpoint (Figures 6.8.1 and 6.8.2).

Building/unit

This hospital and clinic is, according to the architects' narrative, a *snowflake* in composition, with inpatient units and associated support functions articulated autonomously from therapeutic, clinical, recreational, and administrative zones (Figure 6.8.3a–d). Crossing a pair of axes is somewhat reminiscent of the panoptical asylums of the past, yet ironically, here, the intent was to *open up* the intersection of the axes by means of attaining covariances with landscape – whereas traditionally, the central atrium would have been used strictly for the purpose of staff surveillance of the patient-inmates – and in this respect, the central core is antithetical to its panoptical precursors. Taken further, every patient room is private and provided with a private bath/shower unit. Residential units are housed on the upper level of a two-level facility, oriented outward to maximize views of open landscape. The unfortunate, double-loaded, windowless, and dreary corridors of the past are avoided here as the result of the aforementioned splaying of the two principal axes. The decision early on to open up the central staff work zone, by carving out numerous small courtyards, allows light into adjacent occupied zones, otherwise devoid of natural daylight and views (Figures 6.8.4 and 6.8.5).

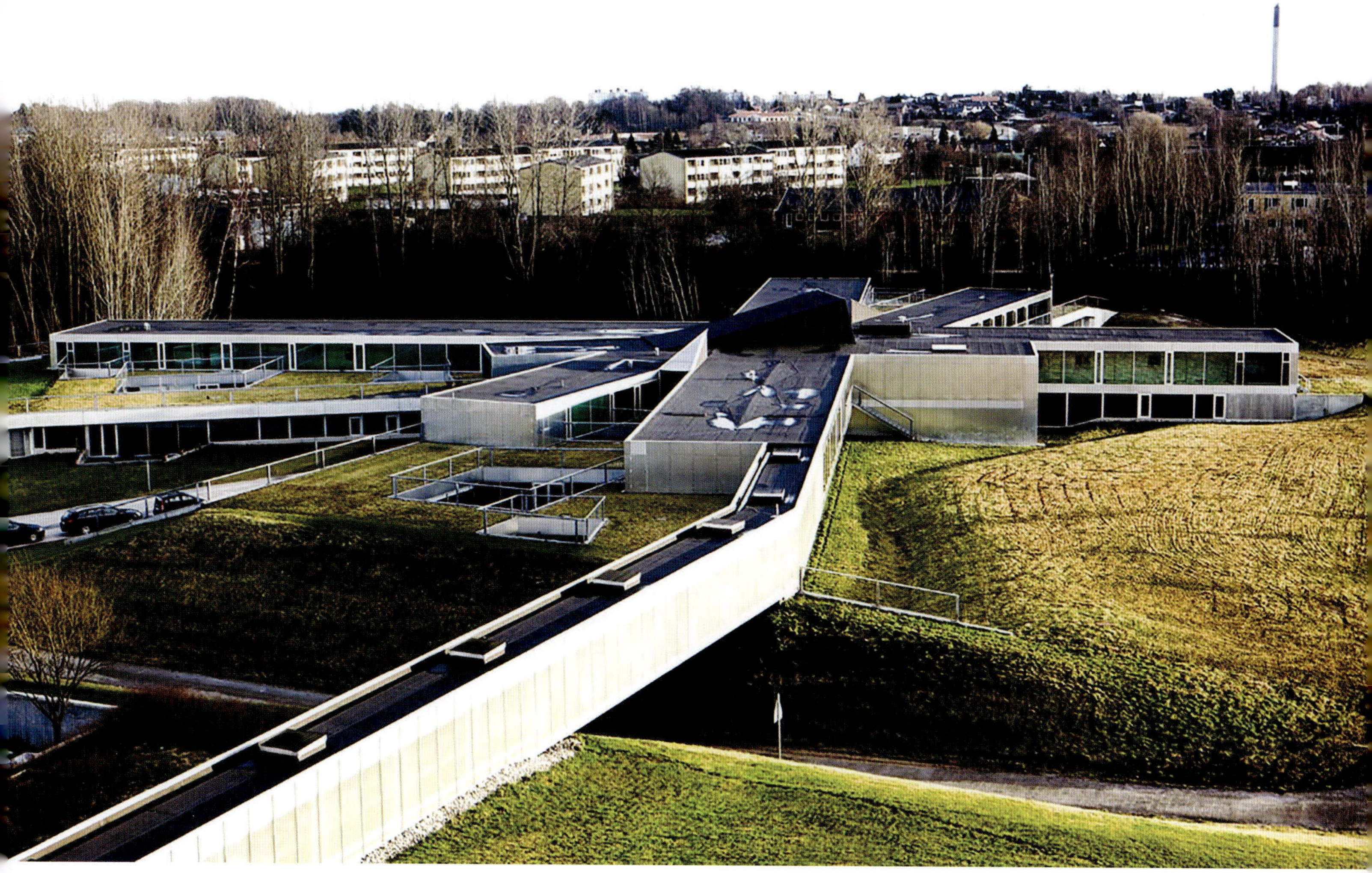

6.8.1 An umbilical link connects Helsingor Psychiatric Hospital and Clinic to an adjacent existing hospital.

The exterior space on both inboard and outboard sides of the inpatient room is rare, a condition seldom achieved in hospital architecture. On the outboard side, two inpatient units overlook a human-made retention pond, with a third inpatient unit overlooking the surrounding rolling landscape. Patient rooms have full-height glass windows and doors on both levels. The upper level features a continuous balcony spanning the length of the unit. Nurses' stations and unit staff offices are located in a work zone at the center, in proximity to centralized public space – that is, nearest the apex in each V-shaped inpatient unit, in plan. The outpatient treatment program is located on the lower level, and this unit is organized into five distinct visual elements by means of color-coded walls and floors, with corridors similarly radiating outward from the main atrium nexus at the center. This unit contains staff offices and related supports on one side and waiting areas on the other. A sloping skylight sitting atop the commons (atrium) functions concurrently as external visual landmark and spatial orientation device from within, drawing natural light into the atrium below.[4] A glass and steel pedestrian-supply bridge connects the psychiatric hospital with the aforementioned existing hospital (Figures 6.8.6 to 6.8.8).

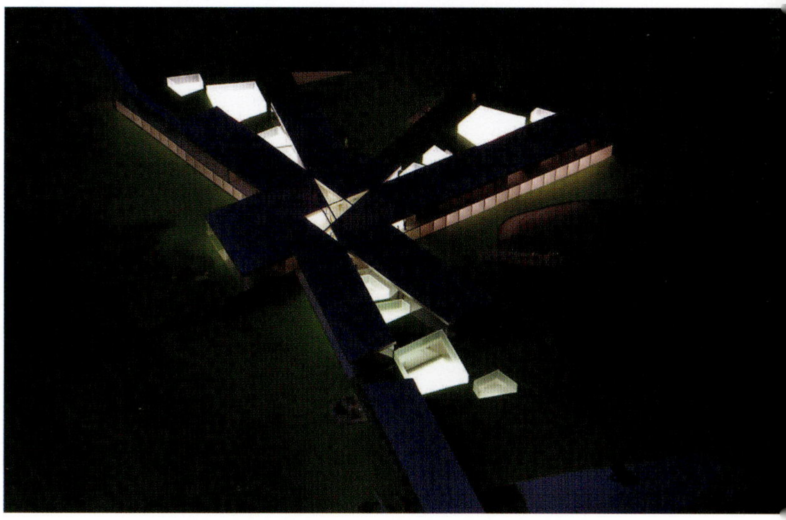

6.8.2 Viewed at night, semipublic interior and exterior spaces function as lanterns.

Key:
1 activity area
2 staff/nursing
3 living/activity
4 seclusion
5 nurses' station
6 staff support
7 inpatient residential unit
8 main arrival axis
9 lobby/reception
10 courtyard
11 living room
12 administration
13 commons area
14 dayroom/activity
15 treatment/counseling
16 art/music/sensory therapy
17 dining
18 multipurpose
19 fitness/gymnasium
20 roof terrace

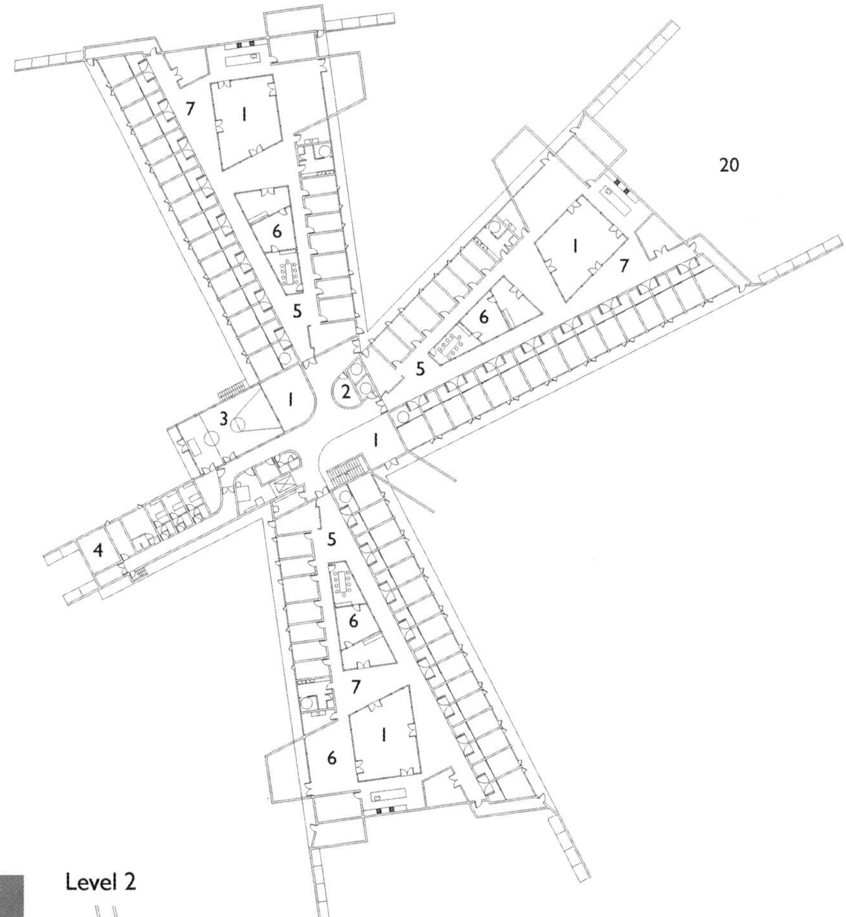

Level 2

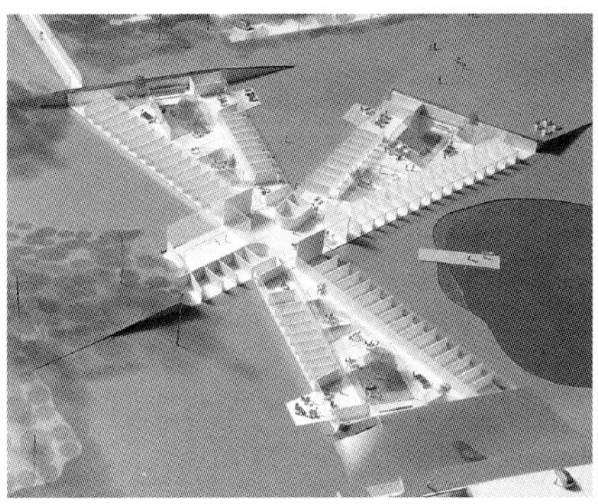

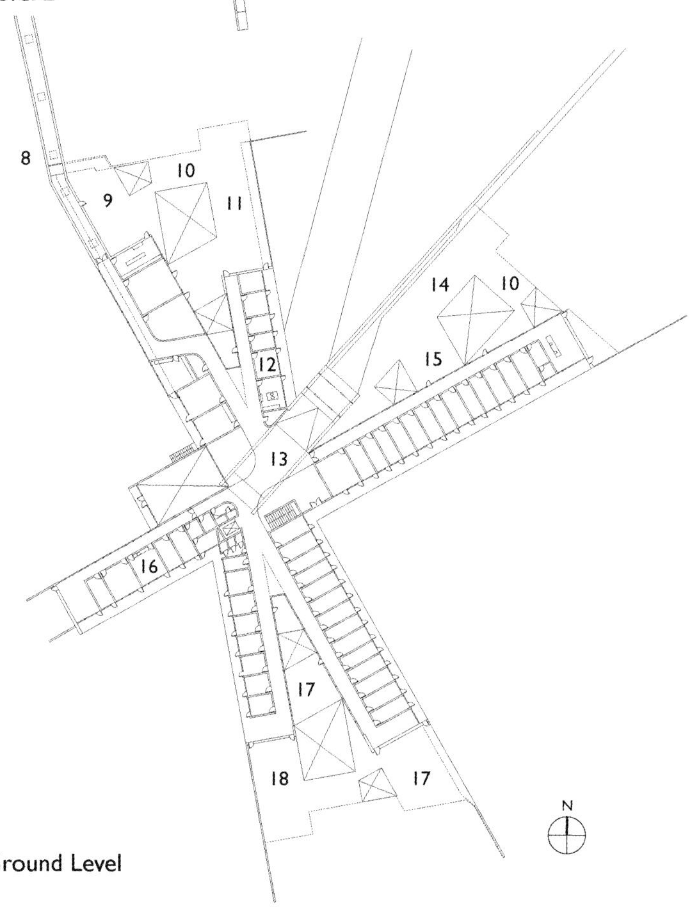

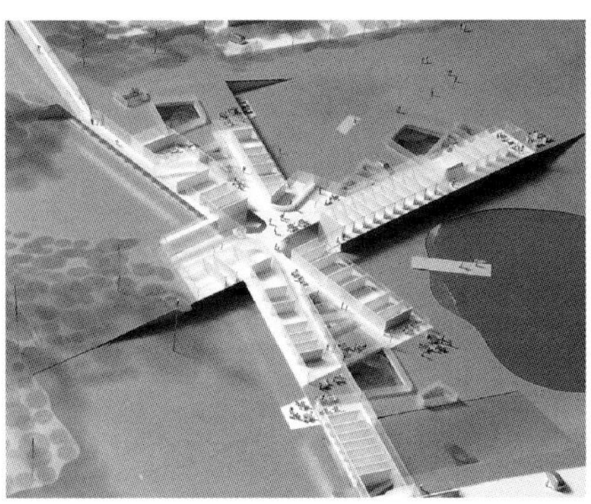

Ground Level

6.8.3a–d The splayed residential unit axes yield in-between zones, providing adjunctive therapeutic support.

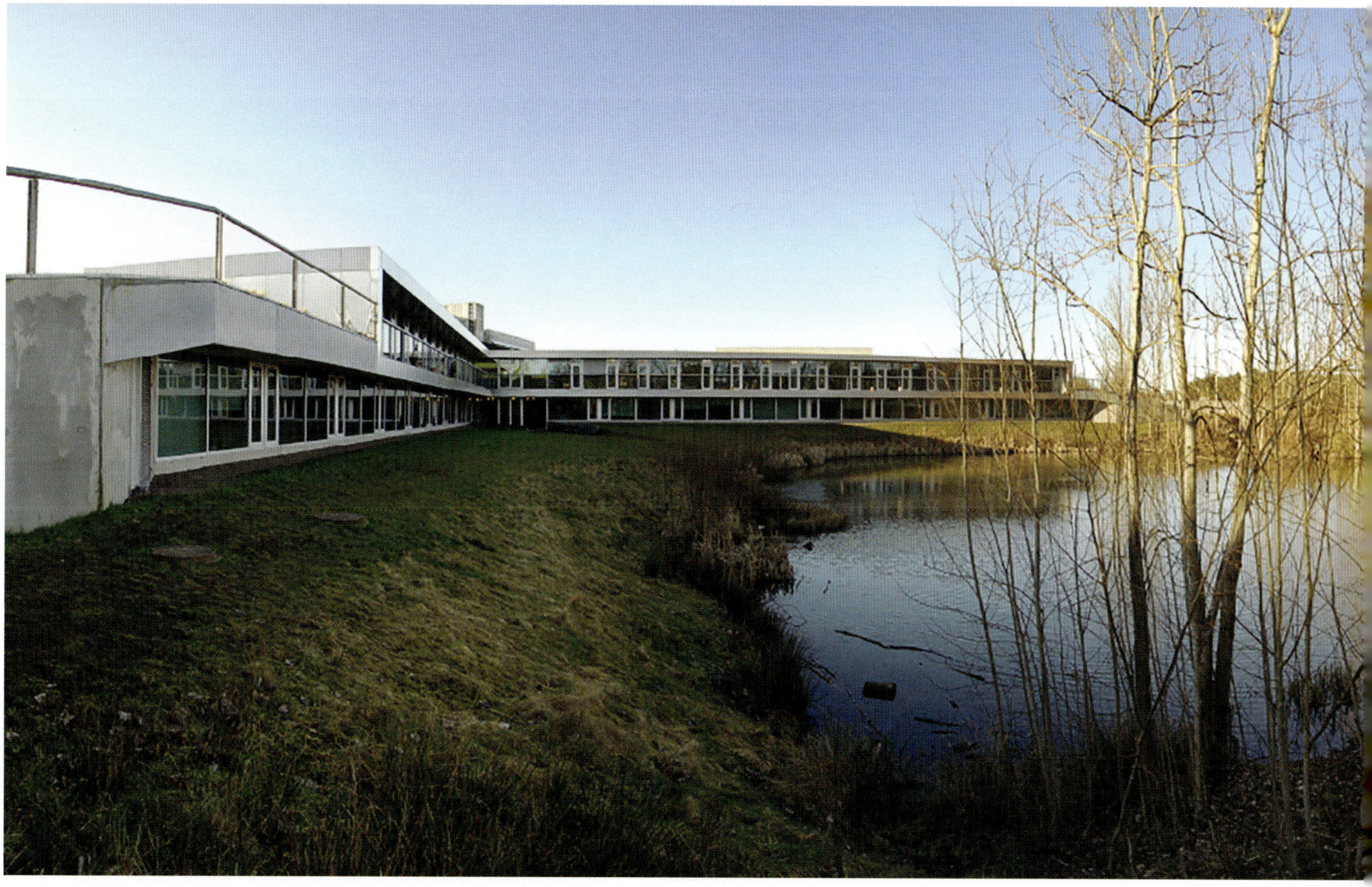

6.8.4 Residential units overlook a human-made retention pond.

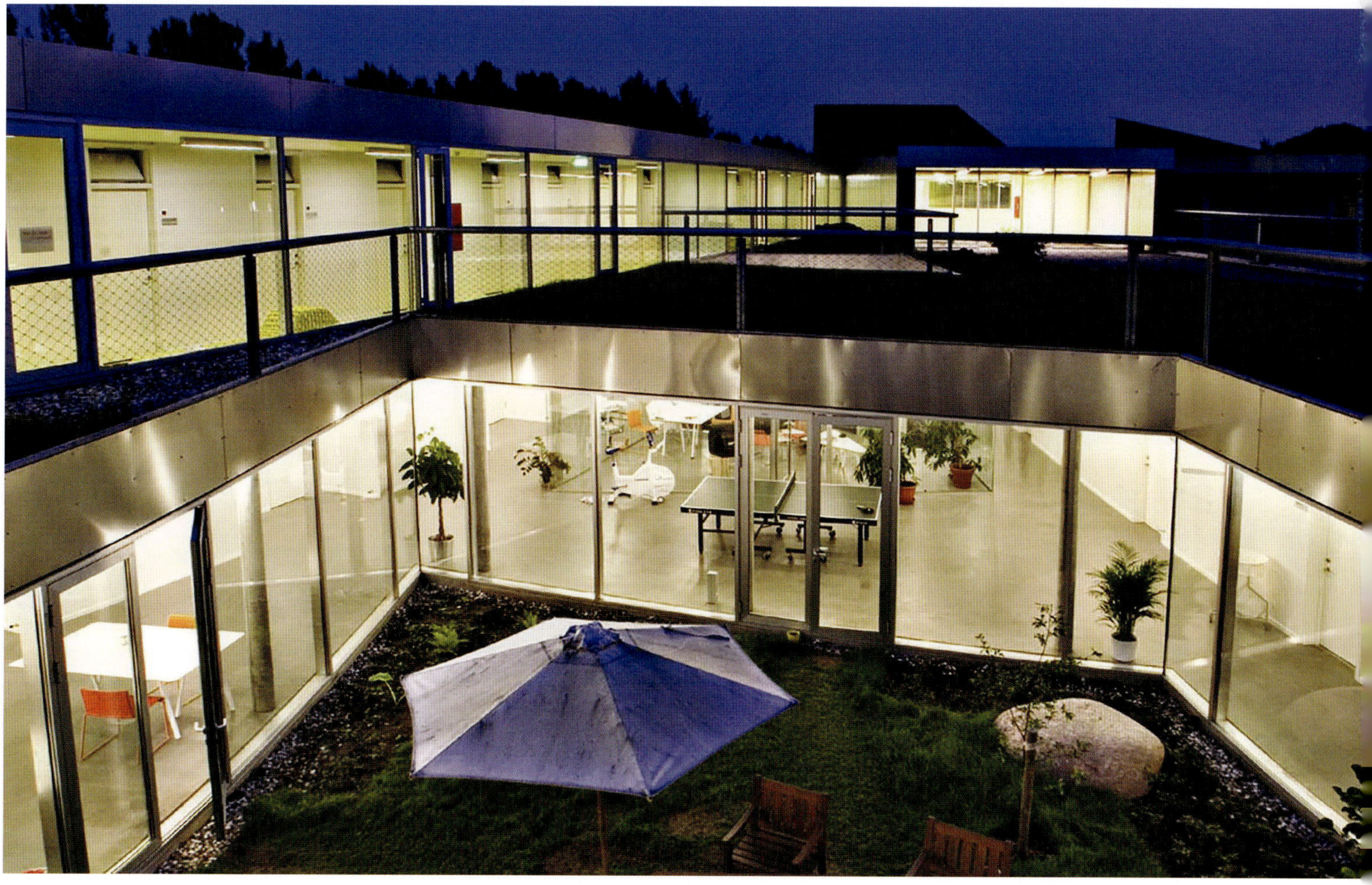

6.8.5 Spaces adjoin courtyards and a roof terrace reinforces visual transparency.

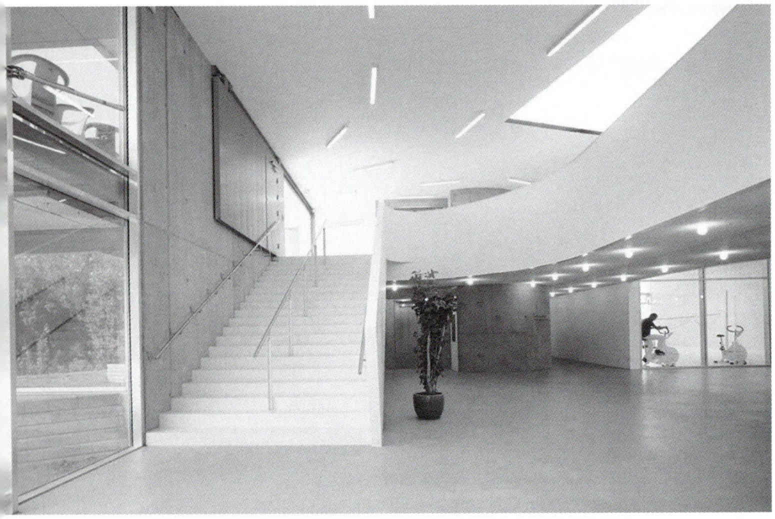

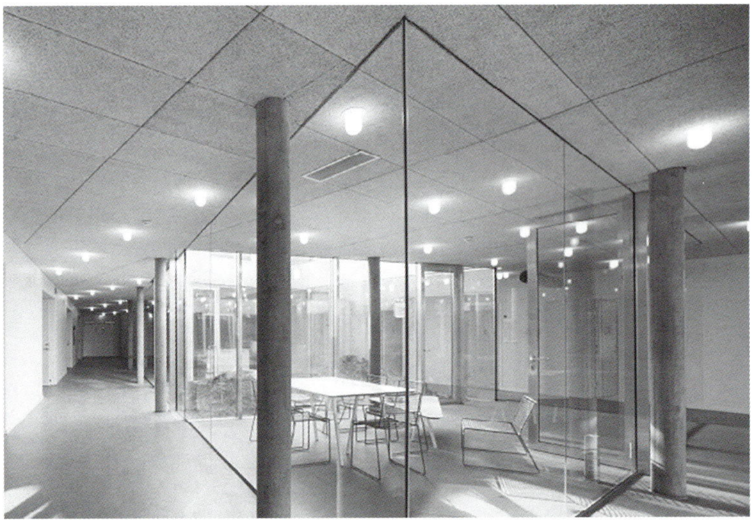

6.8.6 The commons atrium functions as social epi center of the Helsingor campus.

6.8.7 Consultation and conference rooms express openness.

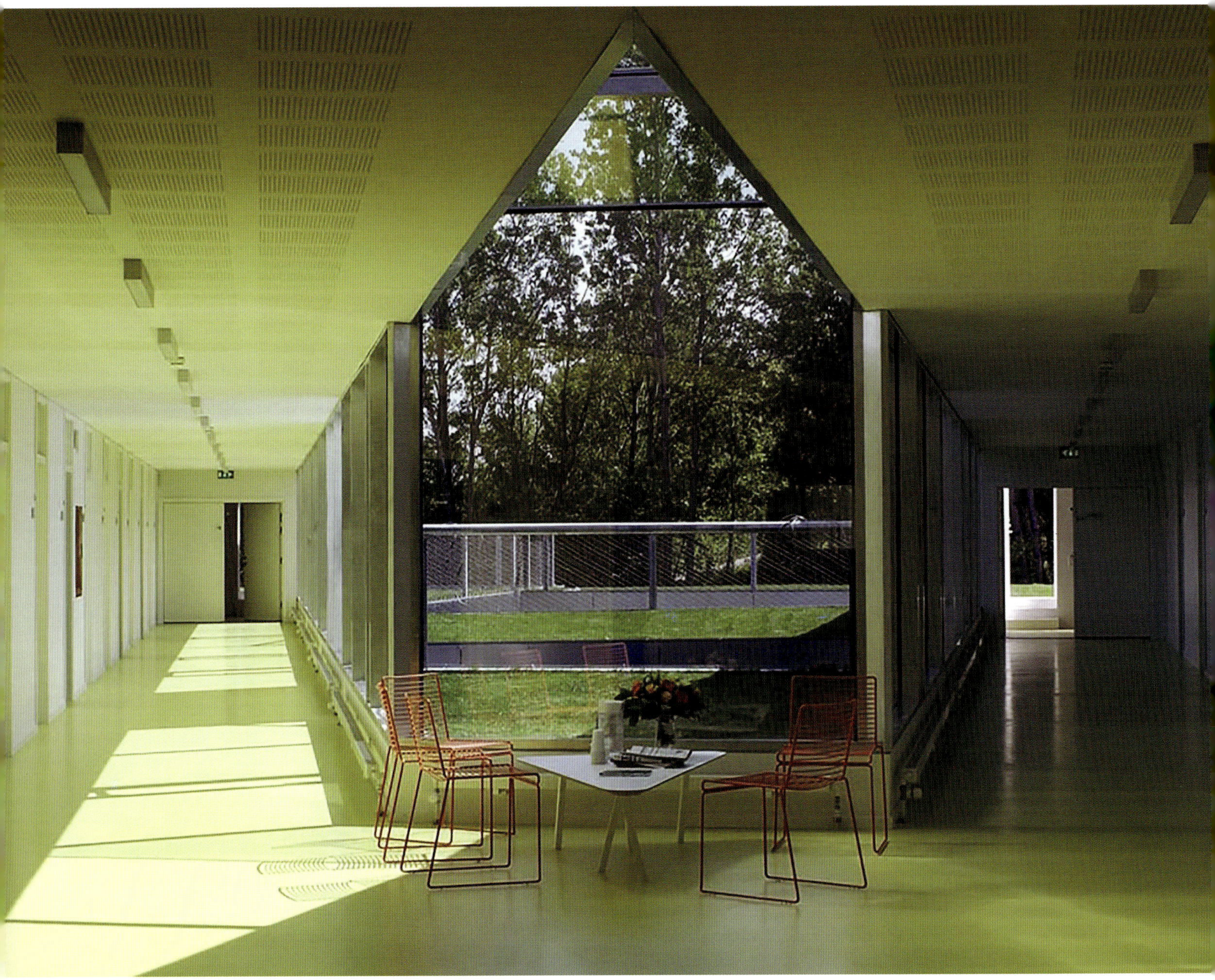

6.8.8 The splayed axis's irregular shape draws natural light into the residential units.

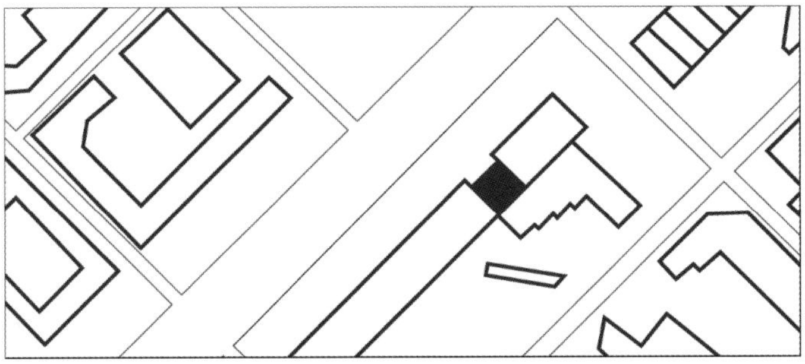

9 Residence and Day Centre for the Mentally Handicapped, Barcelona, Spain

ARCHITECT: Aldayjover Arquitectura Y Paisaje, Barcelona, Spain
LANDSCAPE ARCHITECT: Aroa Alvarez, Ruben Paez, Marilena Lucivero, Barcelona, Spain
CLIENT: GISA, Barcelona
FEATURED MATERIALS: Corrugated steel system; tinted, glazed curtain wall; wood
COMPLETED: 2010
INPATIENT BEDS: 16
SITE/PARKING: 2 acres/10
HOSPITAL/TREATMENT CENTER SIZE: 35,500 square feet
NURSES' WORKSTATION: Open

Context/site

This inpatient and outpatient mental health treatment center was inserted between two existing nine-level apartment buildings, in the historic center of Barcelona, on the Gran Via de les Cortes Catalans. The idea for a facility of this type, as romanticized in the architects' own descriptive brief, would have, ideally, been a rural villa surrounded by picturesque gardens or at the very least to have been located in a far less dense district of the city. Due to the actual site's narrow, rather restrictive site condition, it was decided at the outset to create a series of minivillas by means of a series of stepped roof terraces able to transmit natural light deep into the bowels of a five-level volume. This resulted in 'vertical gardens' providing occupants opportunities for contact with landscape and vegetation in the heart of the city. Its rather nondescript front façade is described by the architects as 'enigmatic', with the decision made for the building to open inward, addressing itself, first and foremost. The public entrance is on the opposing (rear, or back) side and it opens into a small lobby and waiting area (Figure 6.9.1). Given this entry condition overlooking an alleyway only 1.5 meters wide, the programmatic elements were split into two unequal volumes at the lowest level, gradually becoming more equivalent in size, ascending upward. The 'rear' façade opens up dramatically at the uppermost level of the building.

Treatment units on the fourth and fifth levels are deployed around the largest of these outdoor court/terraces (Figures 6.9.2 to 6.9.5a–b). The design team produced a series of descriptive diagrams beginning with the preexisting condition of the zero-lot condition of the block apartment buildings situated to either side. Next, the designer's idea of a park or villa, at ground level, is diagrammed, followed by a diagram depicting various vertical gardens penetrating through the building at every level, allowing for trees and hanging plantings to become dominant elements; next, a plan view diagram depicts the roof terrace as a park-like space in its own right. The following two diagrams (of six in all) depicted the inserted new building, in section, with its centralized courtyard bisecting an otherwise undifferentiated, rectangular volume into two smaller volumes of relatively equal size (Figure 6.9.6).

Building/unit

The day (outpatient) clinic and the residential treatment unit are treated as self-contained entities. Maximum autonomy exists at the upper levels and in their relationship to the largest terraced garden. The day clinic, by contrast, is housed on the ground level. This level also houses building services, the main kitchen, and the administration and supports. It also houses a gym (facing the main street side), the central dining room, therapy workshops, and a light well. The two levels above house counseling offices, group rooms, a living room, and dayrooms and are accessed by means of an exterior staircase, interior vertical lift, and interior staircase. On the two uppermost levels, three semiprivate inpatient bedroom suites are provided, and two private rooms (eight beds per level times two); the inpatient bathroom/shower units on these levels are semiprivate, with the inpatient floors housing additional clinical supports, laundry, housekeeping, linens, and staff workspace. The visual and spatial effect is not unlike a hotel, in terms of the overall aesthetic.

The aim of creating a series of garden courts is further accentuated in the facility's exterior glazing composed of tinted panels of varying shades of green and aqua. These panels reflect off of one another, resulting in further accentuation of these spaces' virtual *greenness*. These provide pockets of seating for social interaction, consults, or quiet contemplation. The plant species were selected

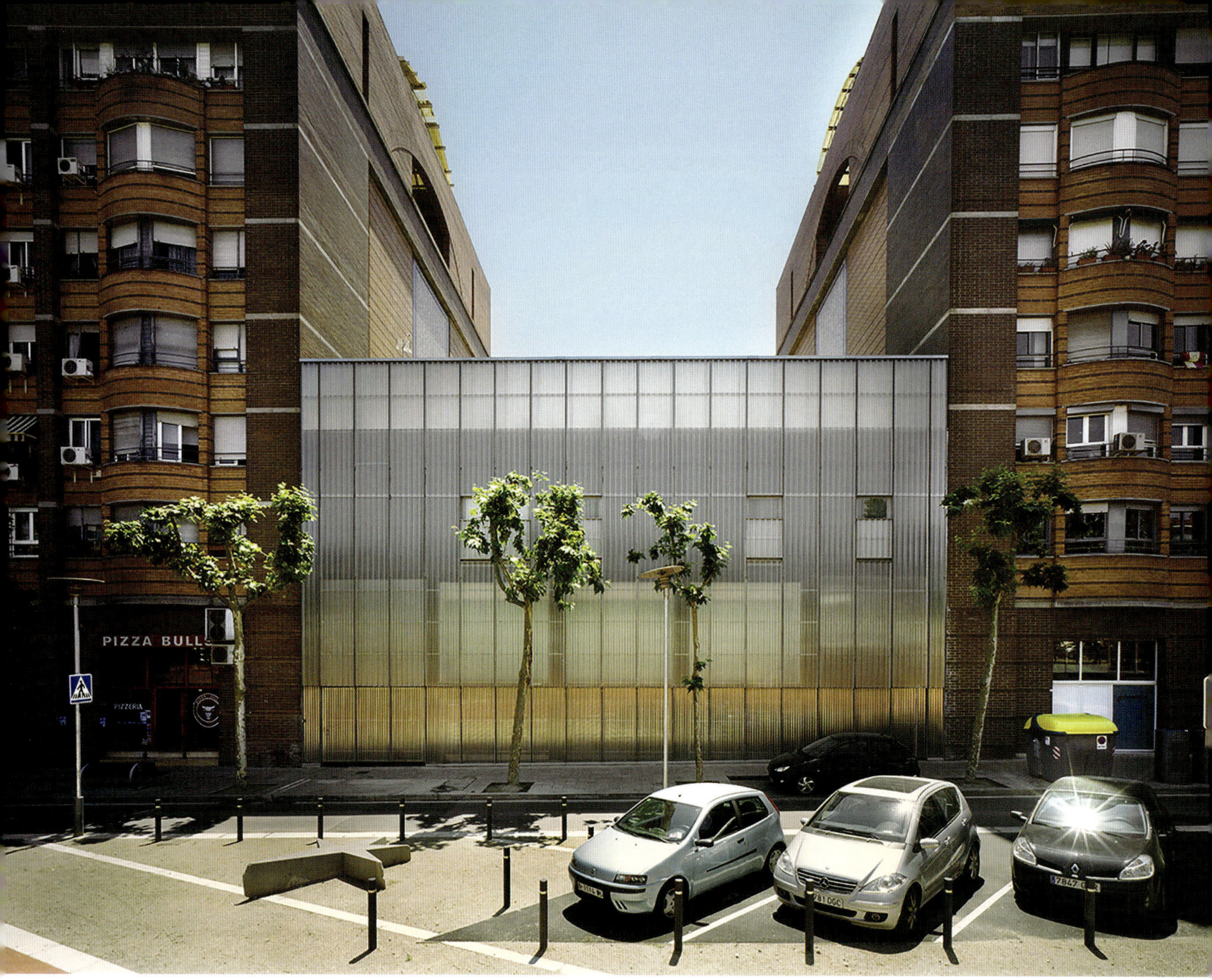

6.9.1 The center occupies an infill site in the urban core of Barcelona.

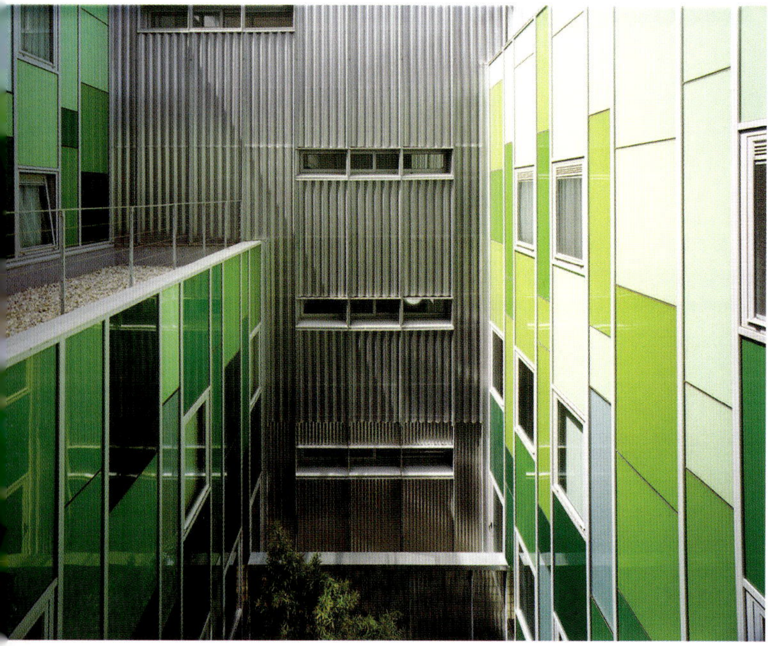

6.9.2 Multiple light courts draw light into otherwise windowless spaces.

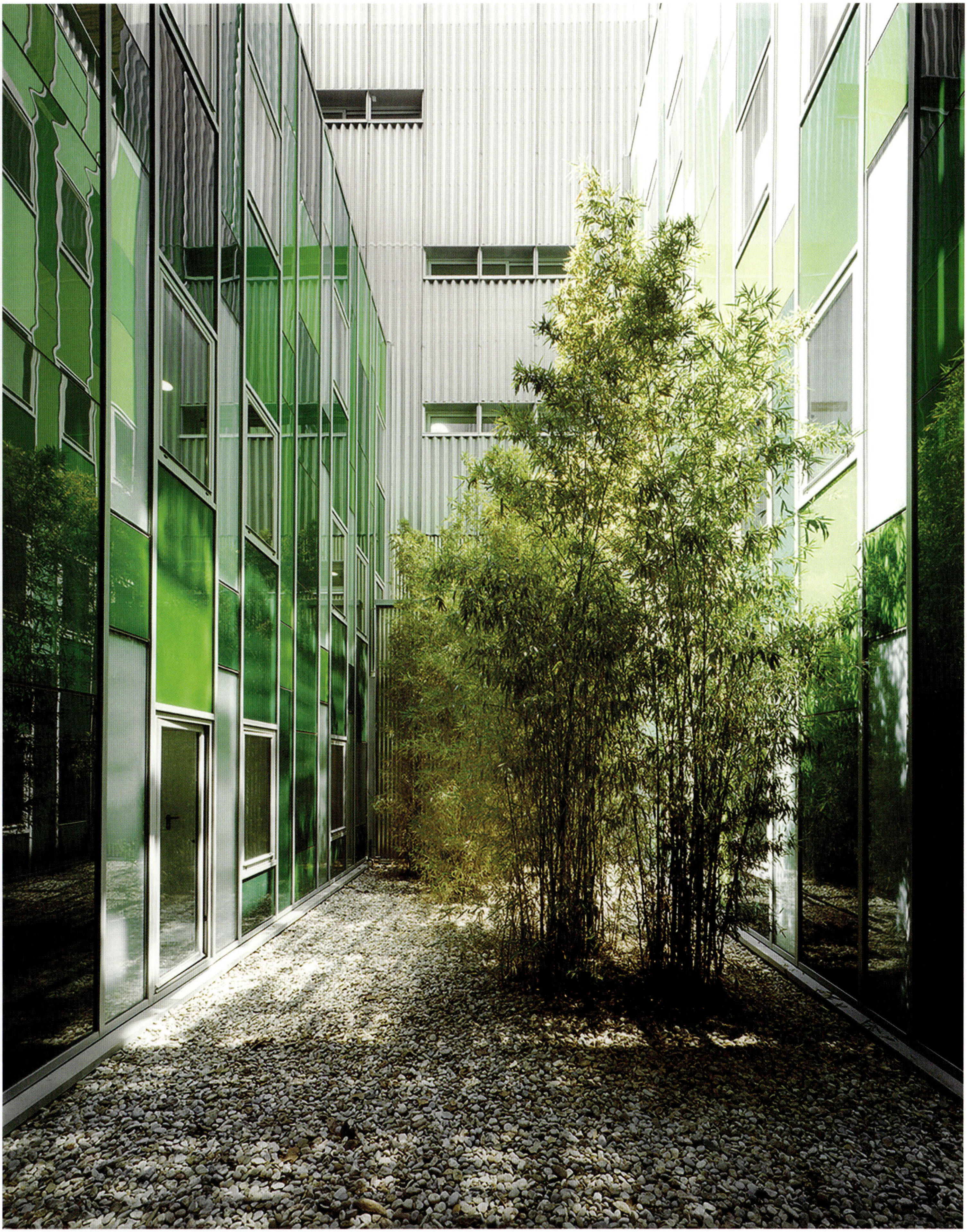

6.9.3 Vegetation was selected in response to microclimate conditions.

for their suitability to local microclimate conditions, as well as the light restrictions imposed by the narrow site footprint (Figure 6.9.7). Even the narrowest of these terraces was reflectively enlivened with plantings, a concept elaborated upon variously as these spaces open up further on the upper floors, culminating with the roof terrace at the top (Figure 6.9.8). This case study demonstrates how an infill building for mental health care can be inventively inserted into a dense urban site – in a section of the city in need of additional mental health services and with scant open space available for their construction. Other self-referential architectural strategies are worth examining on restrictive urban sites in diverse contexts, and especially in situations where an existing building can be restored, repurposed, or expanded.

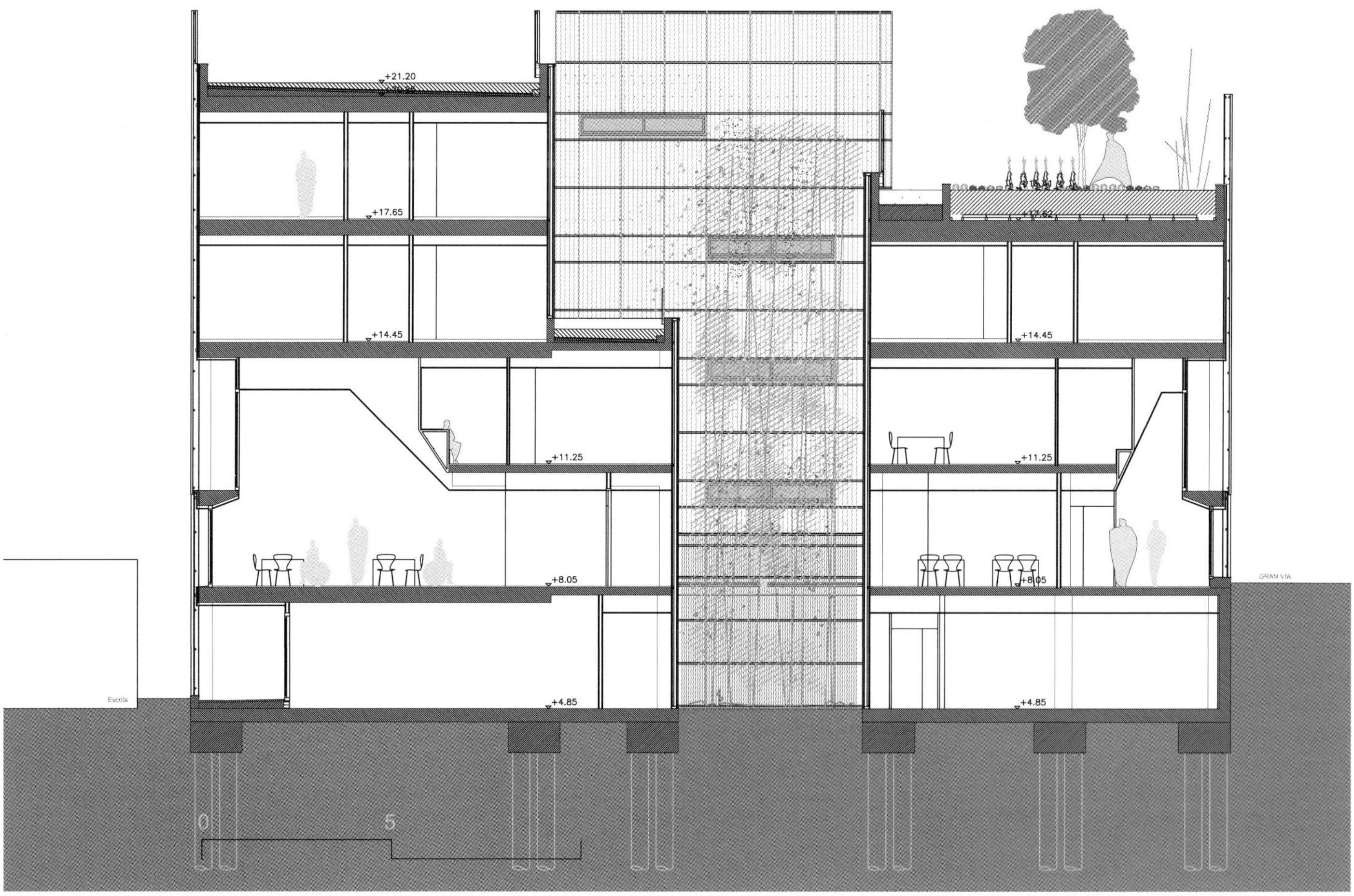

Section

6.9.4 A full-height light court activates the total building envelope.

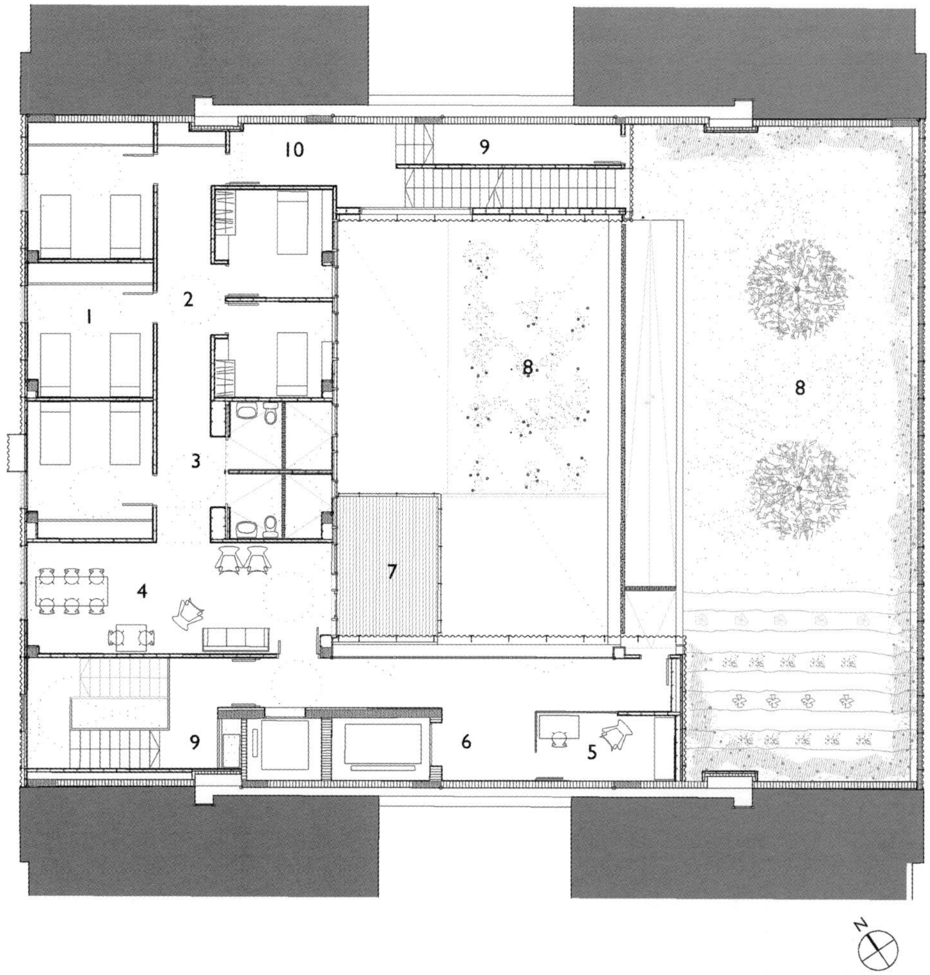

Key:

1 semiprivate patient rooms
2 private patient bedrooms
3 communal bath/shower rooms
4 living room/kitchen
5 nurses' workstation/office
6 lobby
7 terrace/courtyard
8 recreational/vegetable garden
9 vertical circulation
10 emergency stair lobby

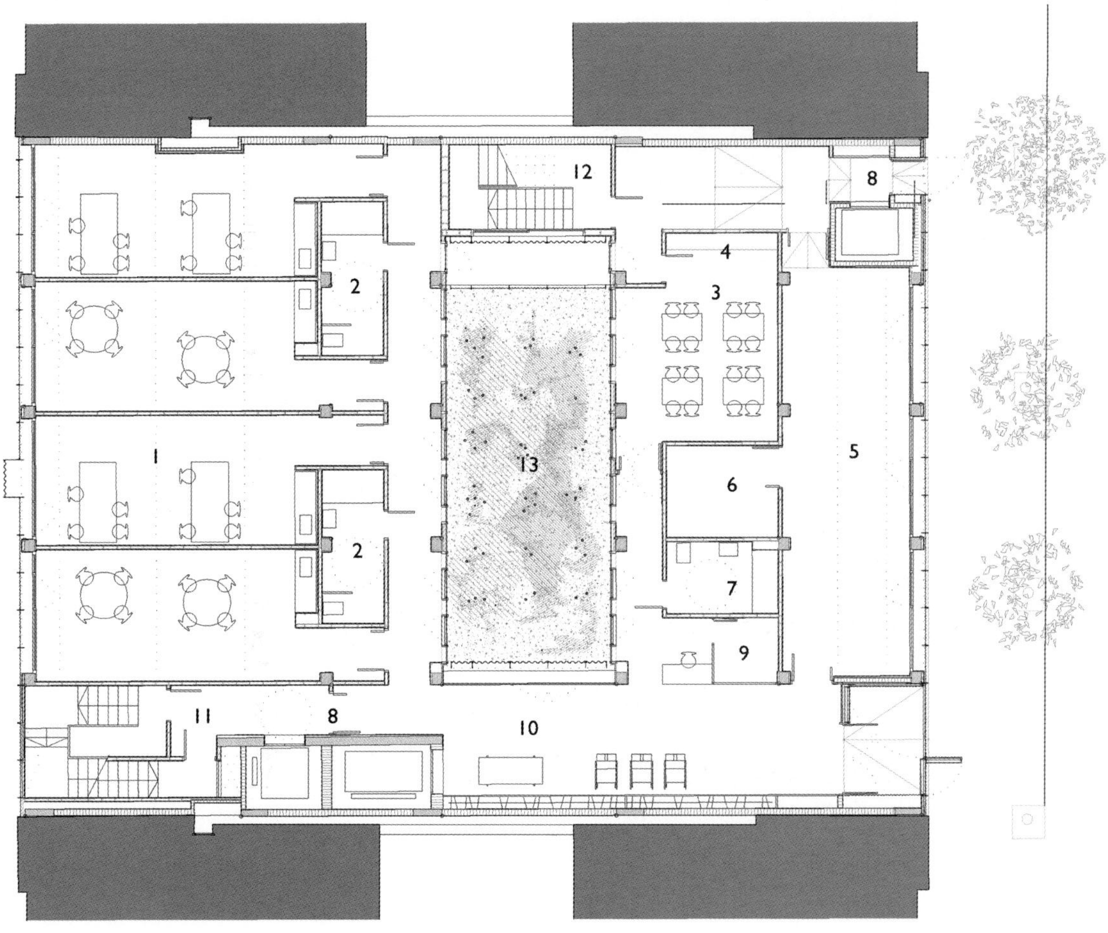

Key:

1 classroom/workshop 1–4
2 adapted bathroom 1–2
3 dining room
4 kitchen
5 rehabilitation gymnasium
6 individual treatment room
7 adapted bathroom
8 elevator
9 concierge
10 main lobby
11 vertical circulation
12 emergency stair
13 courtyard

6.9.5a–b The light court expands as it rises through the building envelope, as do roof terraces.

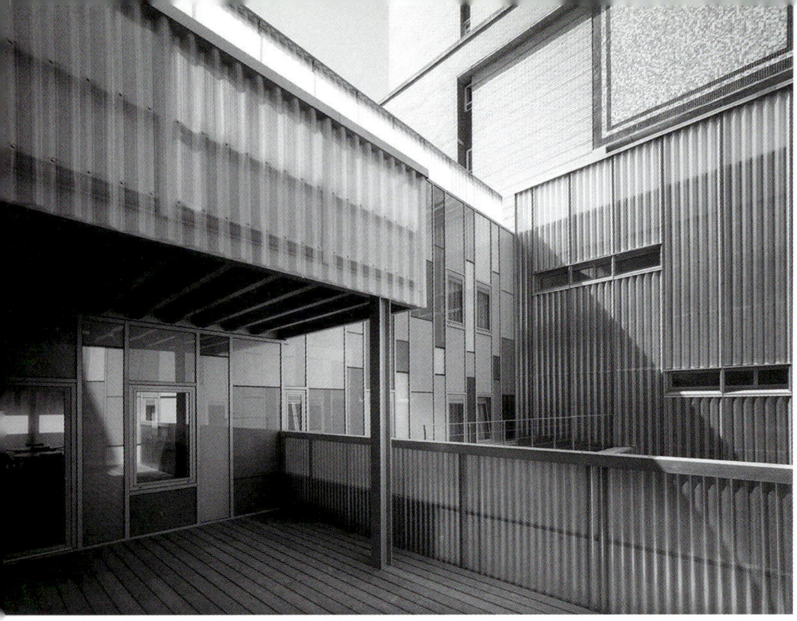

6.9.6 Multiple geometries and sheathing materials intersect in the light court.

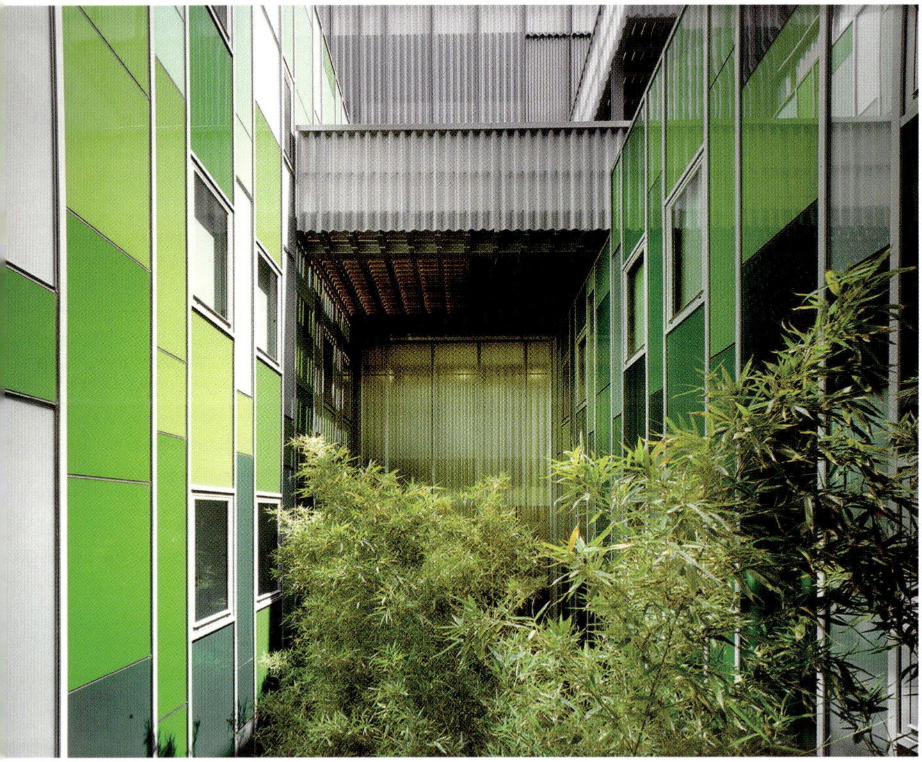

6.9.7 Hues of green-tint translucent window panels reflect off of one another in the light court.

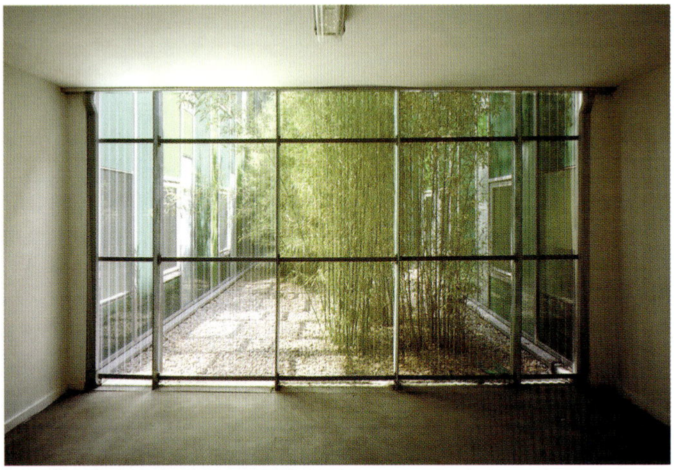

6.9.8 Transparency is expressed throughout interior and exterior spaces.

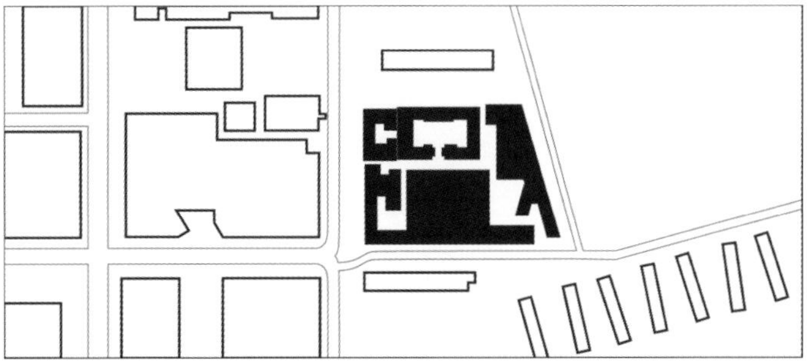

10 De Hogeweyk (Dementia Village), Weesp, the Netherlands

ARCHITECT: mbvda (Molenaar & Bol & Van Dillen), Vught, the Netherlands
LANDSCAPE ARCHITECT: mbvda, Vught, the Netherlands
CLIENT: Hogeway Health
FEATURED MATERIALS: Masonry, glass, precast concrete panel system
COMPLETED: 2011
INPATIENT BEDS: 152
SITE/PARKING: 25 acres/45
HOSPITAL/TREATMENT CENTER SIZE: 65,000 square feet
NURSES' WORKSTATION: Open

Context/site

De Hogeweyk, built and operated by the nursing home provider Hogeway, is a gated urban retirement village for the aged. It is a residential care facility for persons with dementia and mental health comorbidities, and the care philosophy is centered on reminiscence therapy emphasizing cognitive recollection. The treatment model is premised on a professional care staff who themselves do not dress in medical uniforms. Instead, they wear everyday street clothing. This was done to instill a look and feel of everyday life. This facility has been compared by its critics to the 1998 film *The Truman Show*, in its depiction of a faux town (in the film, Seaside, Florida), where virtually every aspect of everyday life is preprogrammed, on a stage set, and observed by a centralized, authoritative big-brother entity.[5] De Hogeweyk, in this regard, is a comparable, tree-lined pedestrian village situated at the edge of Amsterdam. Built adjacent to a warehouse and light manufacturing district, it features shops, restaurants, a movie theater, and a hair salon, and 23 'houses' occupied by a total of 152 residents. However, it is in fact a full-service nursing home. The supermarket cashier and all 'employees' are professional healthcare staff who 'work' incognito. Interestingly, the majority of residents at De Hogeweyk believe it to be a real, genuine village (Figures 6.10.1 to 6.10.3a–b).

Staff encourages all residents to experience this real-unreal world on their own terms, if even in terms of recollections drawn from many decades ago. This allows them to play to their remaining strengths, not their weaknesses, and to socialize freely without the stigma of a traditional nursing home. De Hogeweyk is the first place of its type in Europe, although the Towsley Village Memory Care Center, an earlier faux-village nursing home, has been operating in Chelsea, Michigan, United States, since the early 2000s (Towsley, for its part, is home to 100 dementia patients living in one of four themed 'neighborhoods' complete with a 1950s era soda shop). Similar amenities exist at De Hogeweyk (Figure 6.10.4a–b). It is elaborate in nearly every respect, with its residences set in a roughly orthogonal urban street grid in seven precincts (neighborhoods). These are Stedelijk, for persons used to living in a dense urban area; Goois, with its upscale, rather aristocratic ambiance; Ambachtelijk, for persons drawn from the working trades, including craftsmen/women; Indisch, for individuals from Indonesia or with an affinity with the Dutch East Indies; Huiselijk, for homemakers; Cultureel, for persons with an affinity with theater and cinema; and Christelijk, for persons with a strong religious affinity, Christian or otherwise.[6] This care facility accepts a percentage of patient-residents with a dual diagnosis of dementia together with a mild preexisting psychiatric condition, such as depressive disorder. Somewhat ironically, a nearby, comparatively conventional, high-rise elderly housing block peers directly down into this enclave.

Building/unit

The complex is comprised of one- and two-level structures contemporary in their aesthetic, avoiding most architectural references to the pandering historicism currently so prevalent in North American dementia care facilities (Figures 6.10.5 and 6.10.6). Its exterior spaces are ramped and terraced, with adjoining gardens and seating, lookout points, and ancillary spaces, for use as weather permits. Level changes correspond to the goal of fostering interpersonal social and physical support. Individual living suites feature small private balconies and are relatively spacious, and each unit is able to be personalized to express the occupant's personal artifacts and taste. Dayrooms and social activity spaces feature large windows and flooring of natural oak, with artworks and contemporary

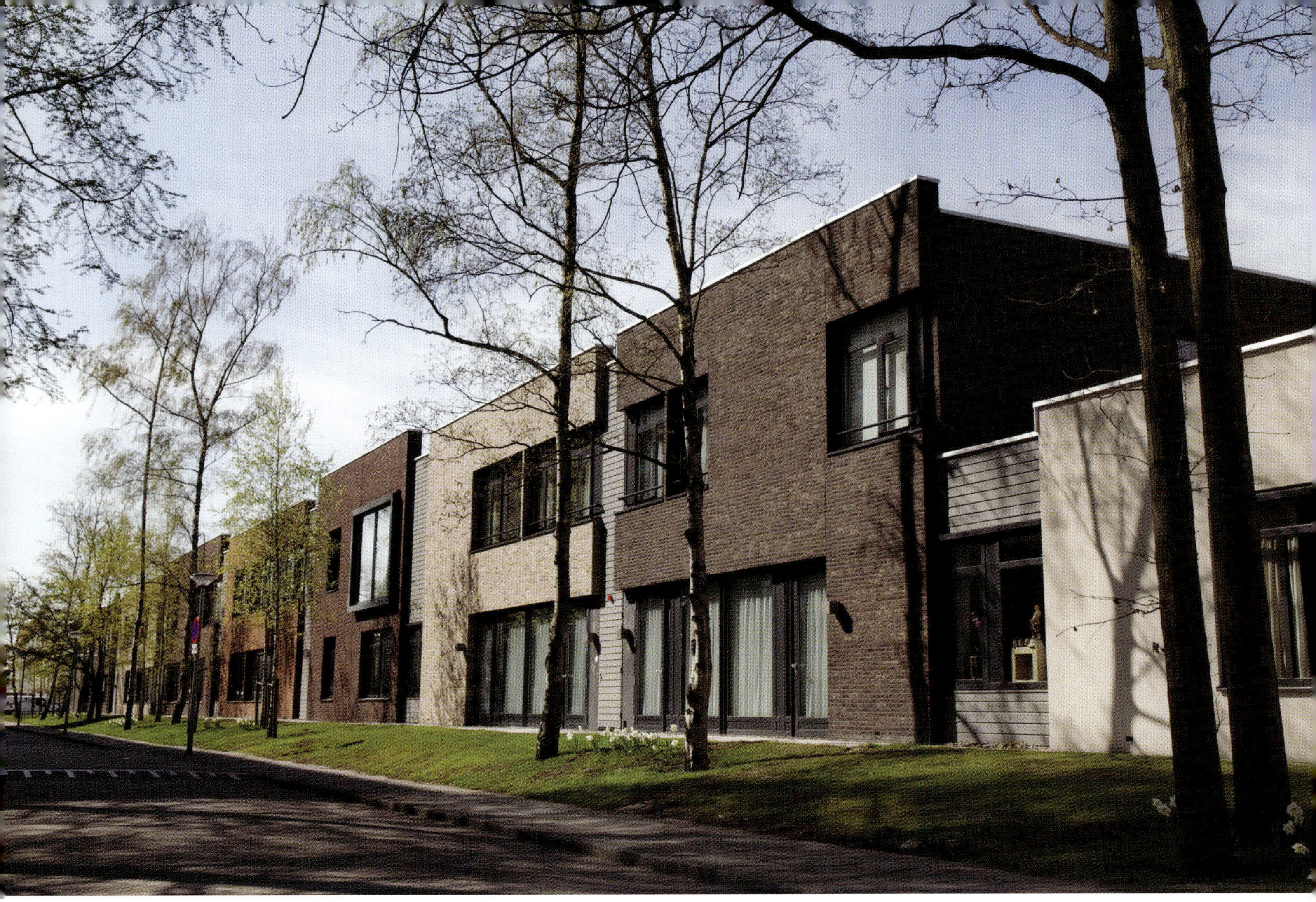

6.10.1 The De Hogeweyk residential community is in metro Amsterdam.

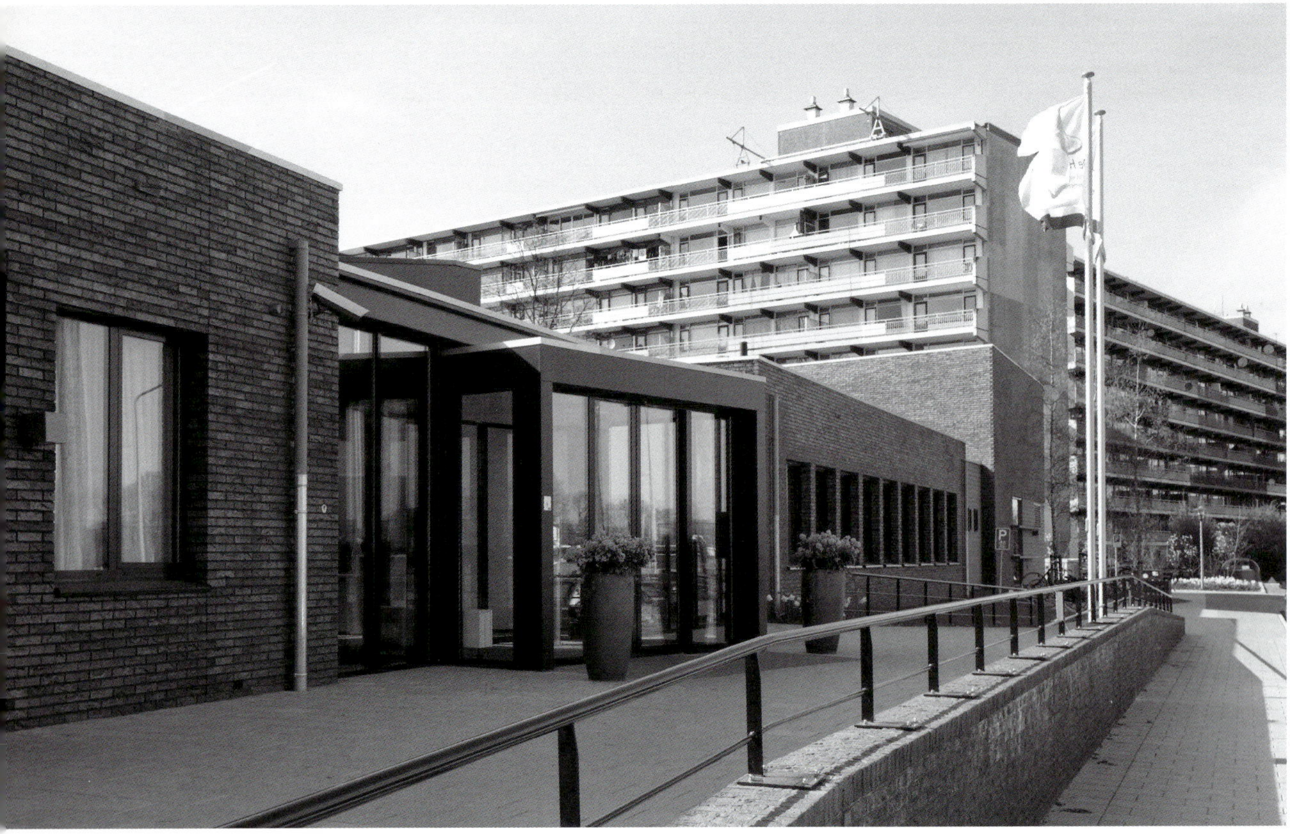

6.10.2 Level changes and varied buildings establish a village streetscape. A large (unrelated) housing block looms in the background.

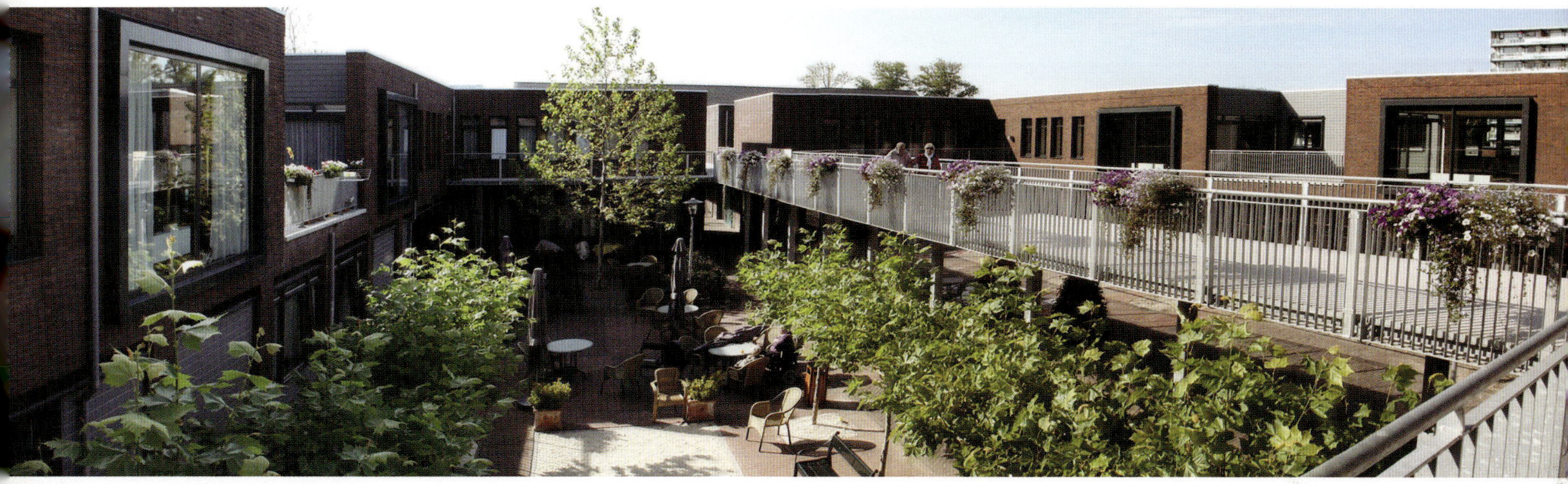

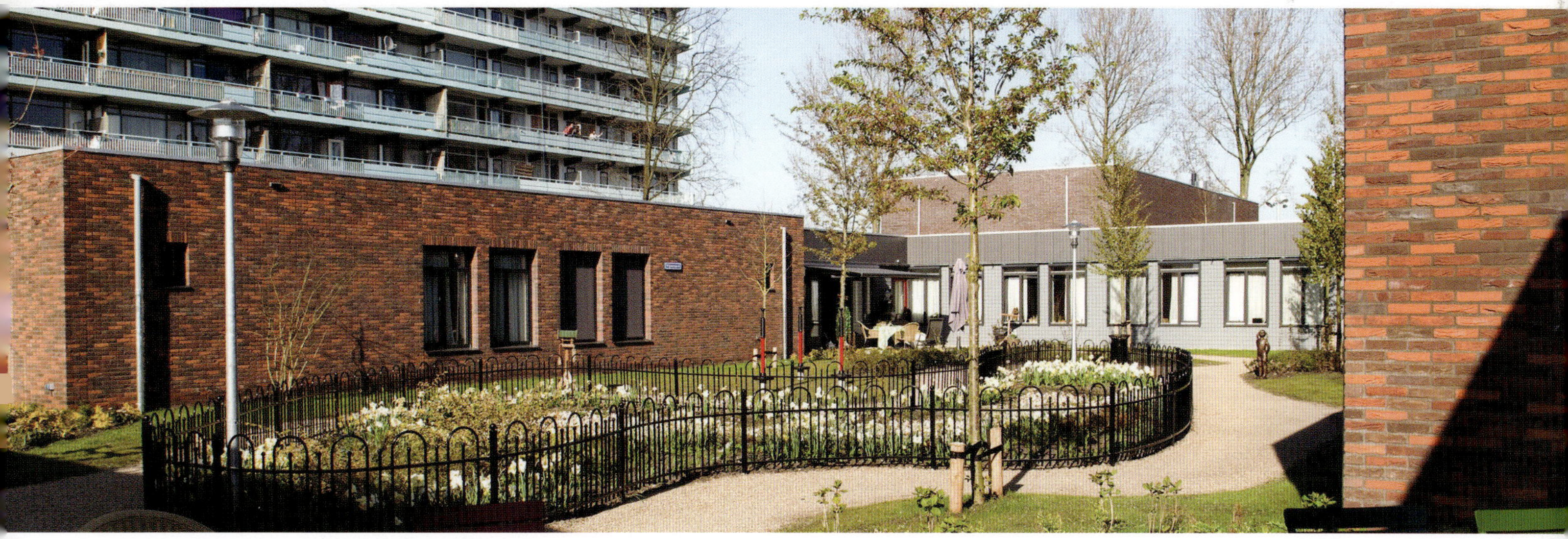

6.10.3a–b De Hogeweyk is one and two levels in height, with residential enclaves connected on the upper level by a pedestrian walkway (top), and ground-level gardens and walking paths (bottom).

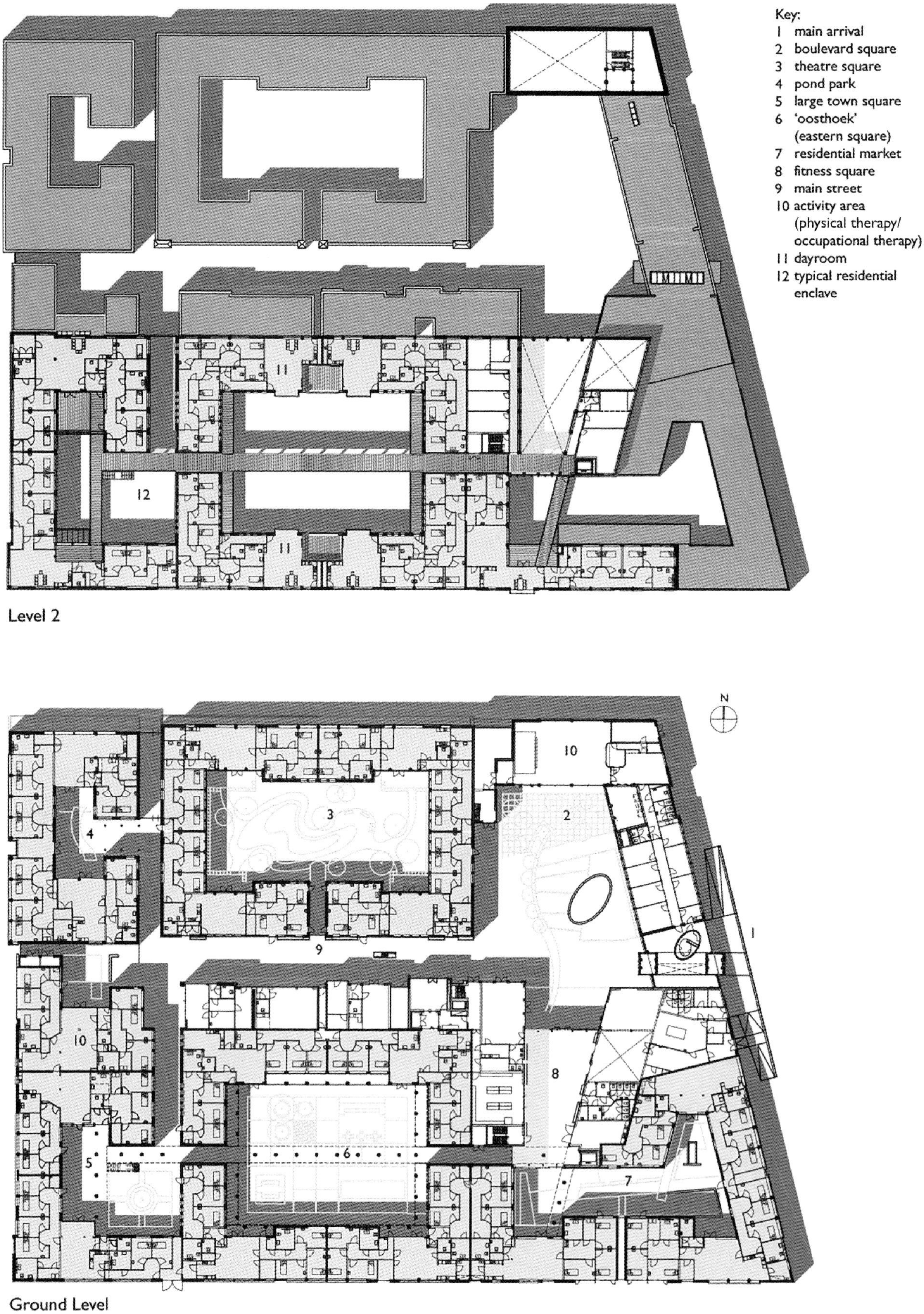

6.10.4a–b Residential units and therapy support areas are arrayed around numerous courtyards, with building footprints kept relatively narrow.

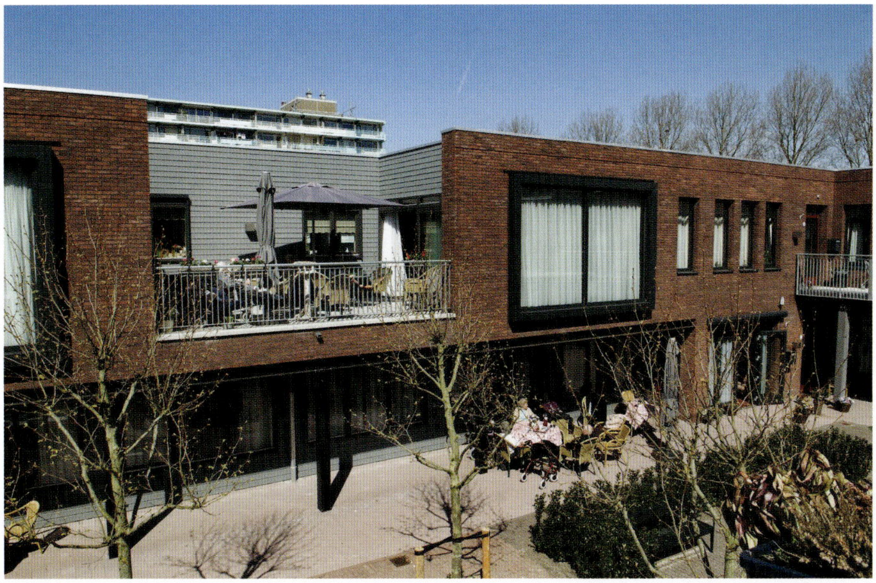

6.10.5 Individual residential units feature 'picture' windows overlooking terraces and balconies.

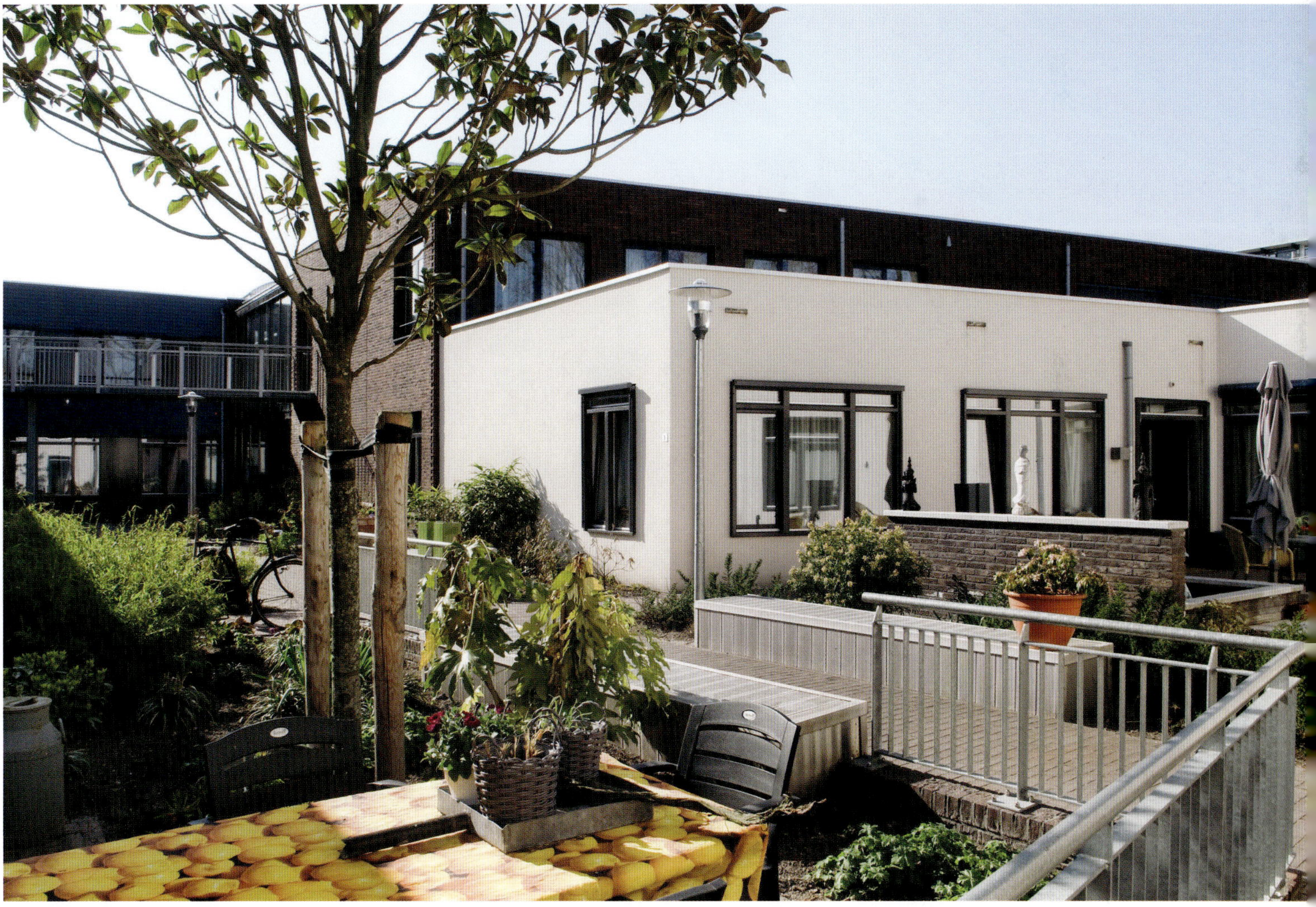

6.10.6 Pocket gardens and patios encourage residents' engagement with the outdoors.

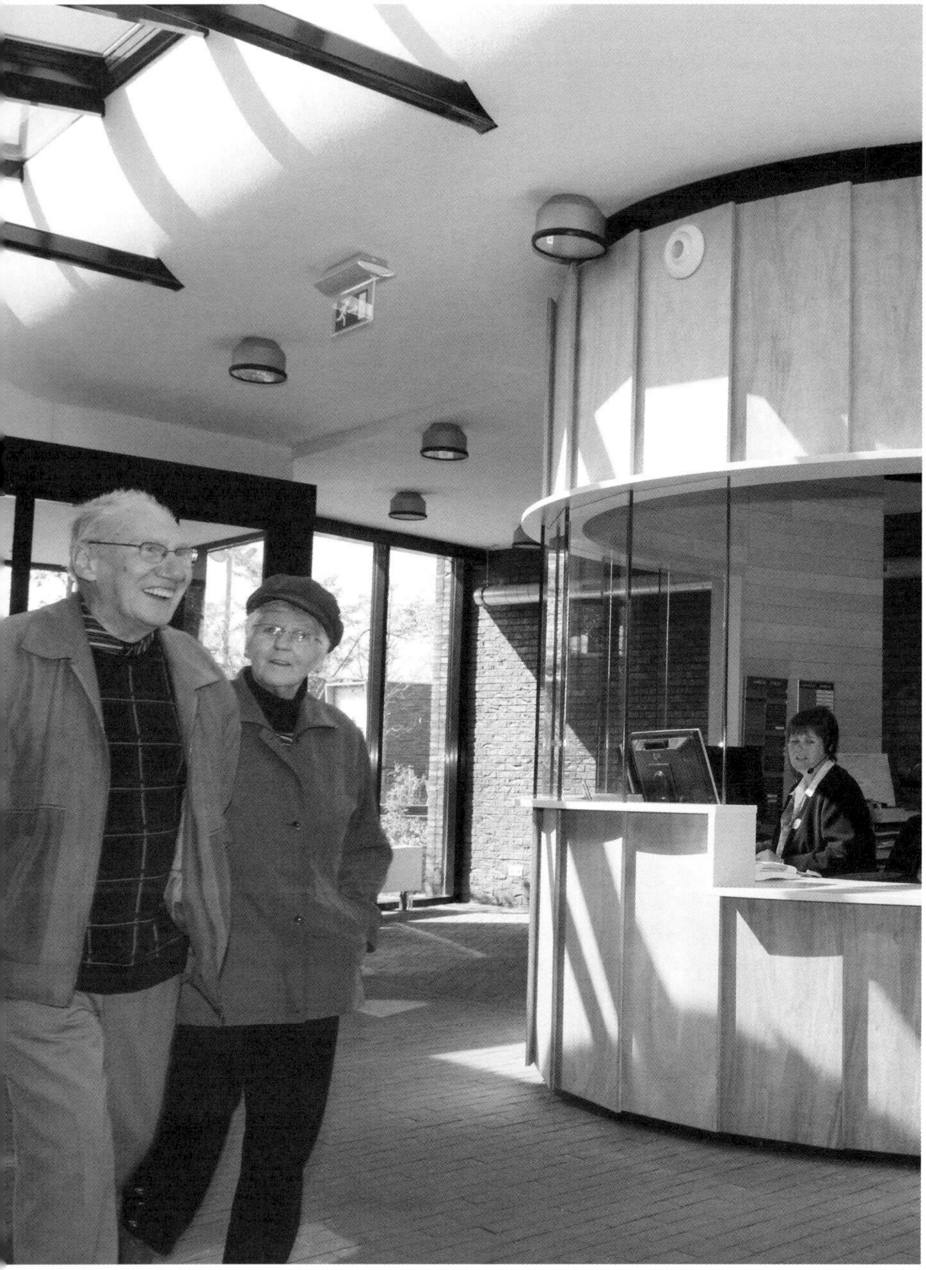

6.10.7 A staff workstation is situated at the ground-level entry portal of each residence enclave.

furnishings, including antiques. Each resident's family assists the staff in staging 'mood boards' adjacent to the front door of each unit. The interiors of the seven residential enclaves differ from one another; this dissimilarity is considered to be a key attribute, although the color palette throughout remains residentialist.[7]

Residents are able to roam semi-independently, and many doors often remain unlocked (although a high-security perimeter wall protects the complex). Each of the seven residences has a staff security station at the front entry (Figure 6.10.7). Activities of daily living include art, music, and recreational therapy. Transparency and direct engagement with nature is of importance – that is, small garden plots, tress, and outdoor spaces for retreat and cognitive decompression; these are features that are too infrequently provided in conventional, hospital-centric nursing homes. Each individual living unit is zoned as three realms: living area, sitting/dining area, and private bedroom with bath/shower unit. Each enclave has a communal dining room and kitchen, while food is typically prepared in the central kitchen, and then transported to the various residences (Figure 6.10.8a–b). Once every 2 years all nursing homes in the Netherlands are required to take part in a national survey completed by residents and their families on the quality of care provided. In a recent iteration of this survey (2015), while the national average satisfaction score was 7.5 points (out of a maximum score of 10), this iconoclastic care facility located at the edge of Amsterdam scored an average of 9.1 points, considered a high rating for a facility of its type.

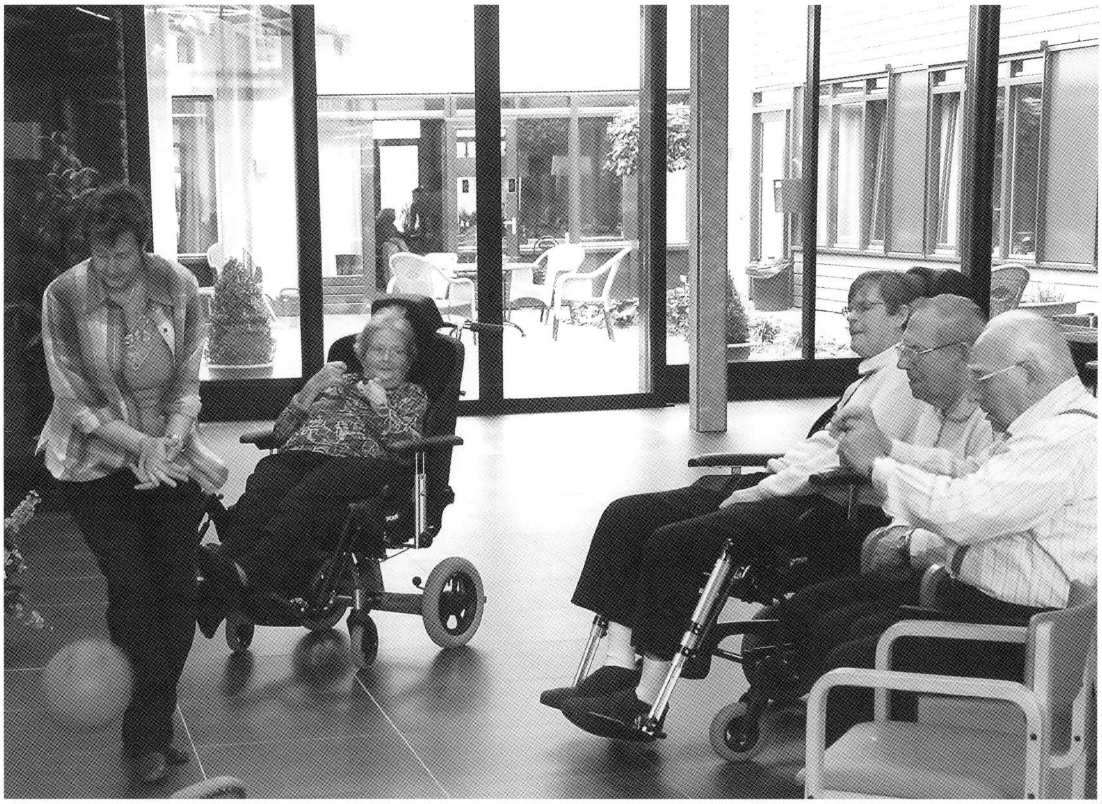

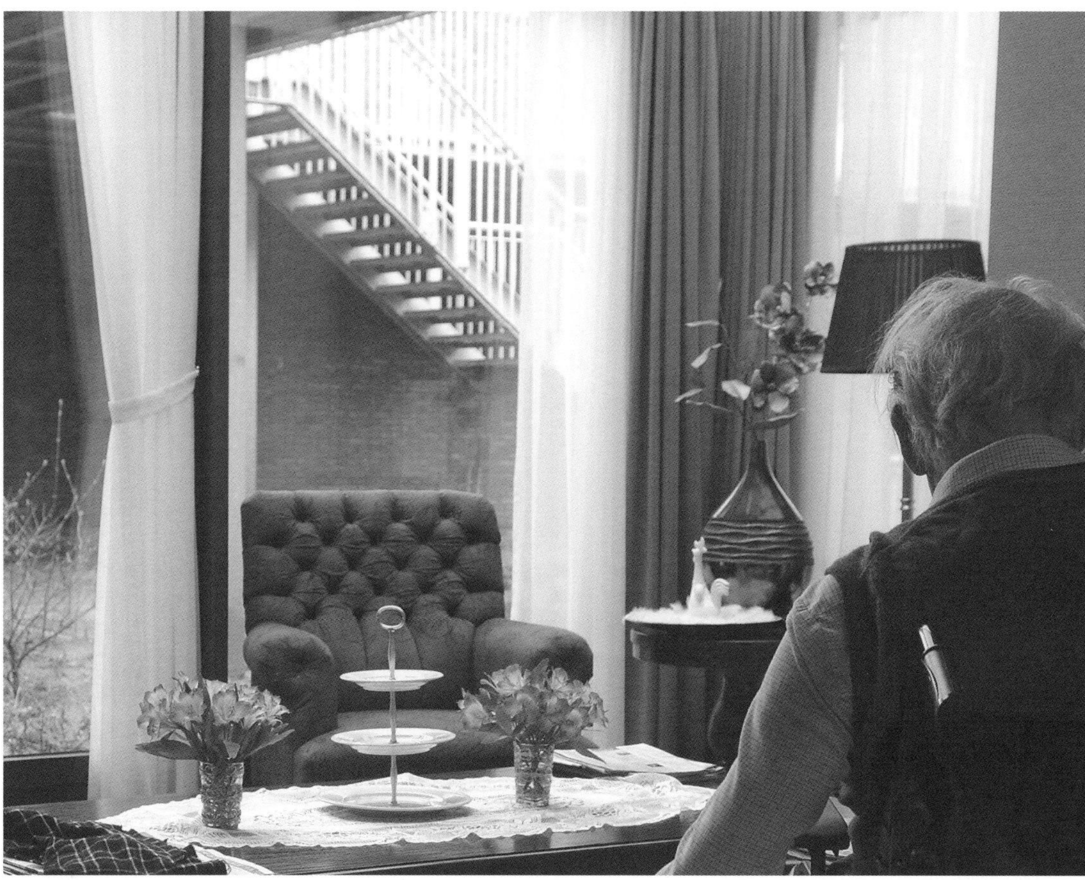

6.10.8a-b Social activity spaces (top) and places for respite are in and near the enclaves (bottom).

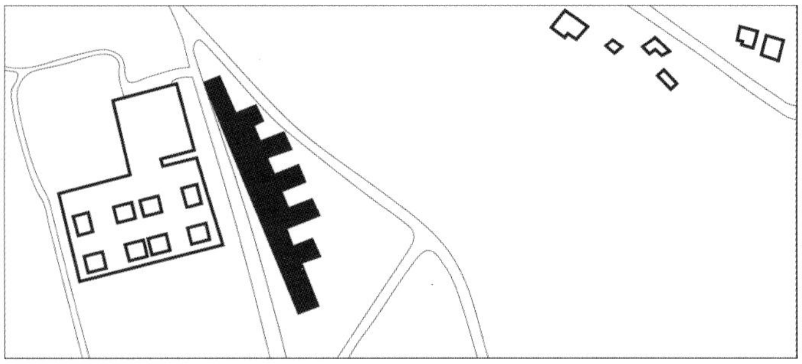

11 Centre for the Mentally Handicapped in Alcolea, Cordoba, Spain

ARCHITECT: Taller de Arquitectura/Rico+Roa, Cordoba, Spain
LANDSCAPE ARCHITECT: Rico+Roa, Cordoba, Spain
CLIENT: Honourable Council of Cordoba
FEATURED MATERIALS: Precast concrete panels, masonry, aluminum panels
COMPLETED: 2012
INPATIENT BEDS: 30
SITE/PARKING: 12 acres/75
HOSPITAL/TREATMENT CENTER SIZE: 54,000 square feet
NURSES' WORKSTATION: Hybrid

Context/site

This residential treatment center is set in a rolling landscape along the Guadalbardo River, near the town of Cordoba, Spain. A residential district is located to the east, directly across the river. Its sloping topography was a prime design determinant. It was decided to expand to the south of an existing psychiatric facility in order to establish a stronger visual relationship with the Alcolea Valley and its dramatic landscape. To the east, the site slopes dramatically and this condition maintains various dramatic views. Five independent wings reach outward, balanced upon a cluster of black, slender, toothpick-like columns, slanted variously as if to accentuate the site's topographic irregularities and the wings' relationship to the earth – reminiscent of the iconic residential work of Le Corbusier and specifically, the Villa Savoye (1928–1931), a modernist residential villa built in Poissy on the outskirts of Paris, designed by Corbu and his cousin, Pierre Jeanneret. This private residence was similarly elevated, appearing to float above the ground plane.

The use of *pilotis* in this manner is uncharacteristic for a psychiatric facility, and symbolizes a break from the neoclassical European asylums that preceded the work of pioneering 20th-century modernists such as Corbu. The open space beneath, created by uplifting these five elements, is not utilized for patient care, however. The architects opted to leave this soil relatively undisturbed. Five residential units reach outward, in unison, and yet are anchored to a shared circulation spine that runs perpendicular and functions as a collector in numerous ways. This facility was the winning entry in an architectural competition held in 2004 and the winning team was allowed input in selecting the site. In addition, this treatment center was among 50 exemplary designs selected from throughout Europe for a 2012 exhibition, 'Vers de Nou Veaux Logements Sociaux 2', organized by the French Ministry of Culture and exhibited at the Cité de l'architecture et du patrimoine, in Paris (Figures 6.11.1 to 6.11.3).

Building/unit

The main level (Level 2) houses the various 24/7 residential units; this level is accessible by an ambulance drive that also allows for the direct transfer of patients. An emerging care clinic and its various supports are housed on this level, with its own entrance. A parking area is also located on this level. The lower level (Level 1) houses central administration and related supports and is set into the slope of the irregular site. The aforementioned main circulation artery runs longitudinally on Level 2 and serves as a main lobby, and this element also functions as a visual buffer (Figure 6.11.4a–b). Each residential unit has a dayroom/activity area connected to a solarium, and the wings bracket full-height windows situated along the main circulation spine. Balconies are provided at the farthest end of each residential unit (Figure 6.11.5). Corridors on the units are double loaded and house a mix of private and semiprivate (two-bed) rooms, with a communal bathroom/shower unit located at one end of each residential unit.

Nurses' stations on residential units are located on the inboard side of the wing, next to the main circulation spine, and they are thereby connected to all of the units plus ancillary staff support and clinical functions. The physical therapy gymnasium straddles an adjoining corridor, and this space opens onto an exterior terrace. A ventilated exterior panelized-cladding system was employed in response to the hot, semiarid local climate conditions, where temperatures can vary significantly by season. This system reduces monthly energy consumption levels while allowing for maximum human comfort. The exterior cladding system was chosen for its low maintenance, durability, on-site assembly affordances, and thermal advantages. This case study recalls certain fundamental

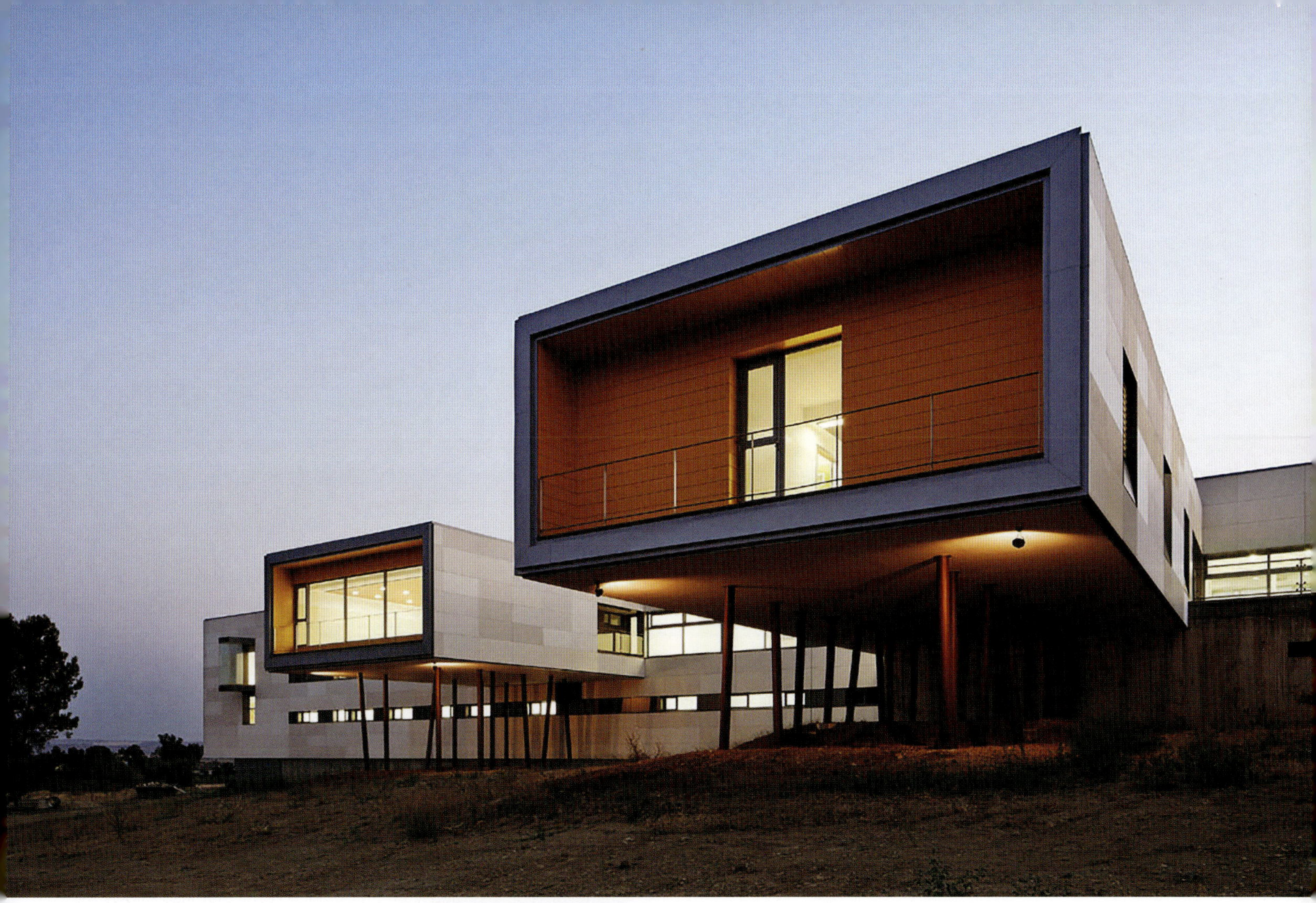

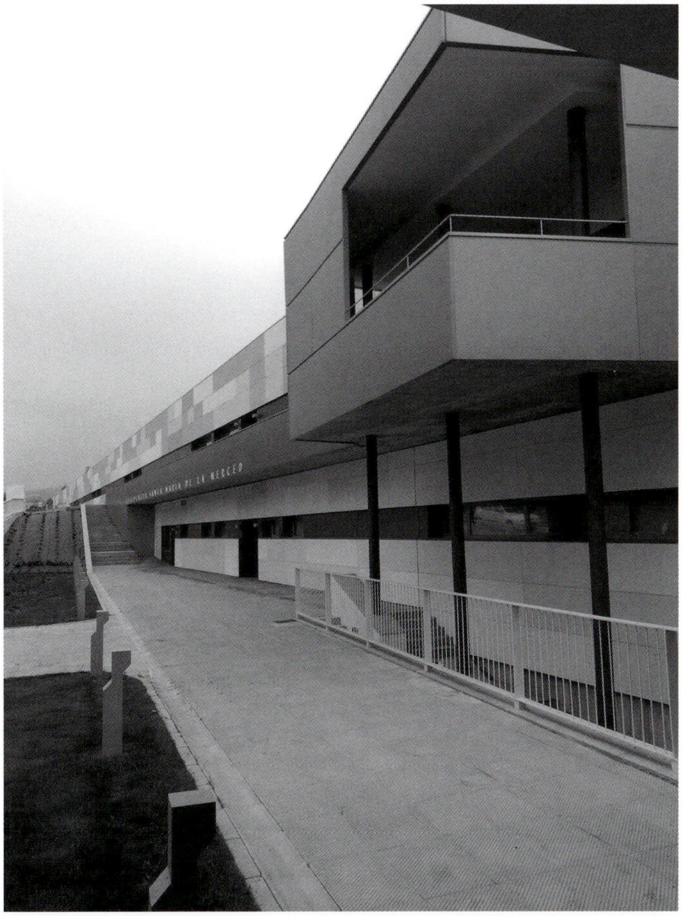

6.11.1 Residential units at the psychiatric treatment center in Alcolea, Cordoba, Spain.

6.11.2 The treatment center features multiple color-coded cantilevered, elements.

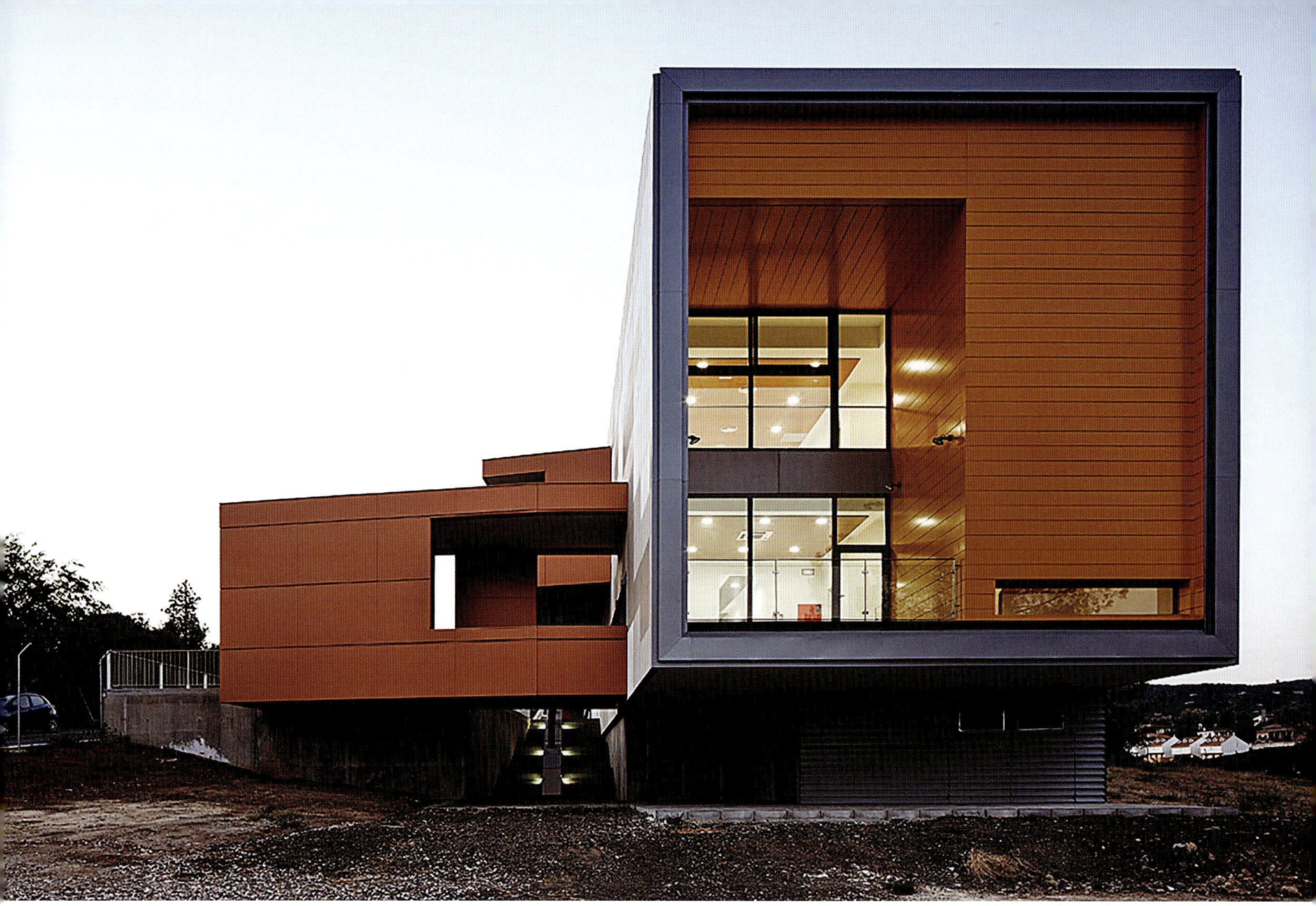

6.11.3 An exterior metal panel system and prefabricated building components are part of a modularized composition.

tenets associated with the International Style, specifically, its minimalism, interior color palate, fenestration, uplift of the residential units so that they appear to float above the grand plane, materiality, and the significant incorporation of off-site premanufactured building technologies (Figures 6.11.6 to 6.11.8).

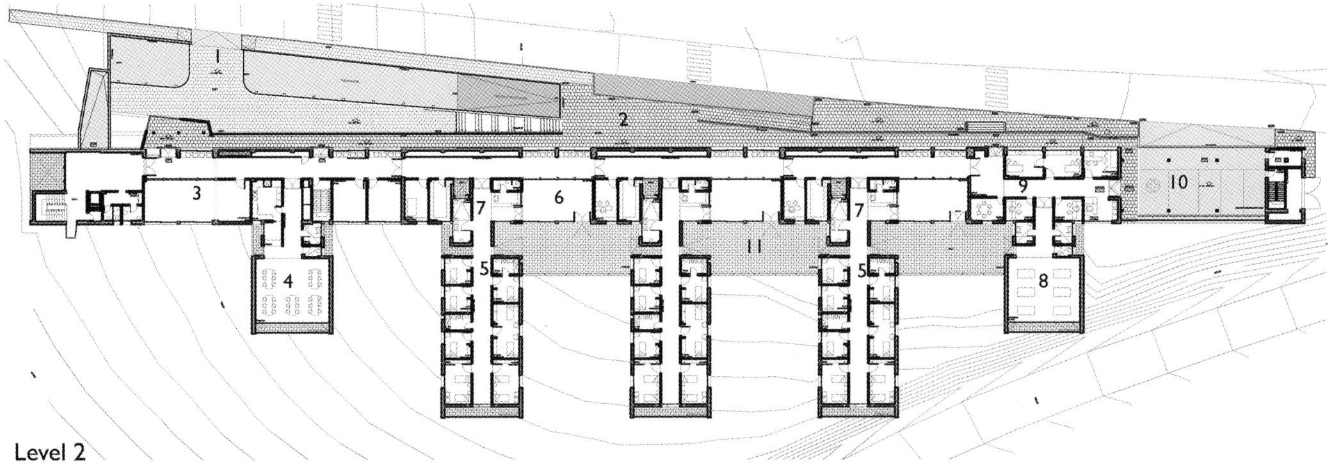

Level 2

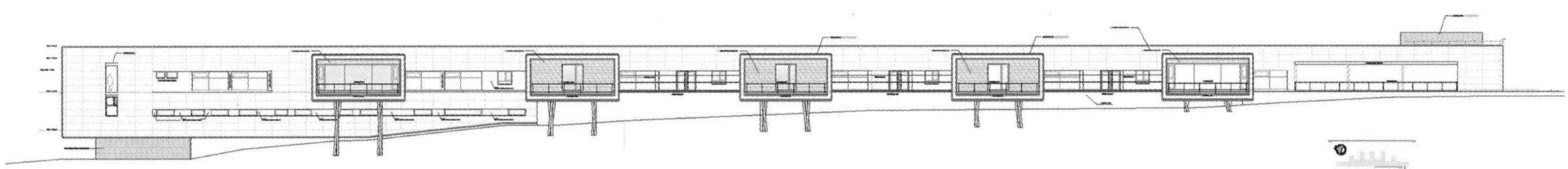

Elevation

Key:

1 main arrival
2 exterior terrace/activity
3 occupational therapy/workshop
4 dining/kitchen
5 inpatient residential unit/ communal hygiene room
6 dayroom
7 nurses' station
8 physical therapy
9 observation rooms
10 covered parking (exterior)
11 exterior terrace
12 common room
13 staff lockers
14 staff restrooms
15 vertical circulation
16 counseling (outpatient)
17 reception/waiting/kitchenette
18 counseling/staff support
19 central administration
20 reception/entrance
21 exterior terrace

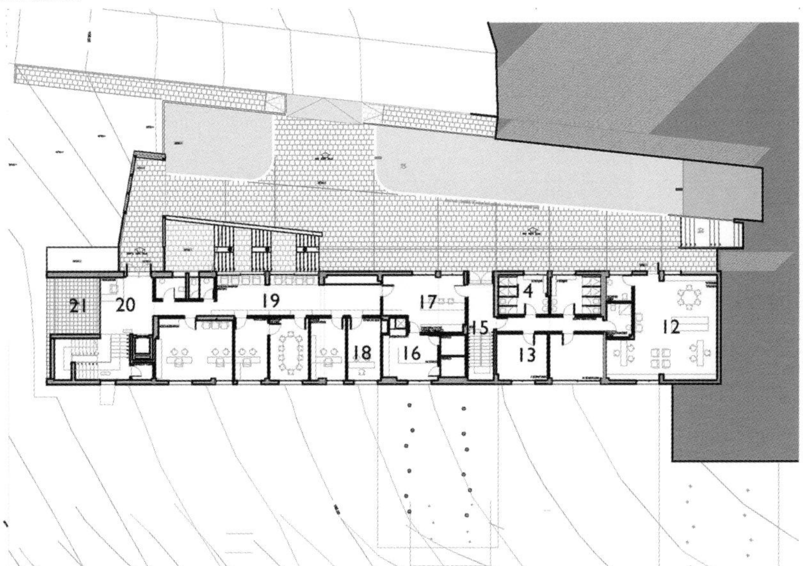

Level 1

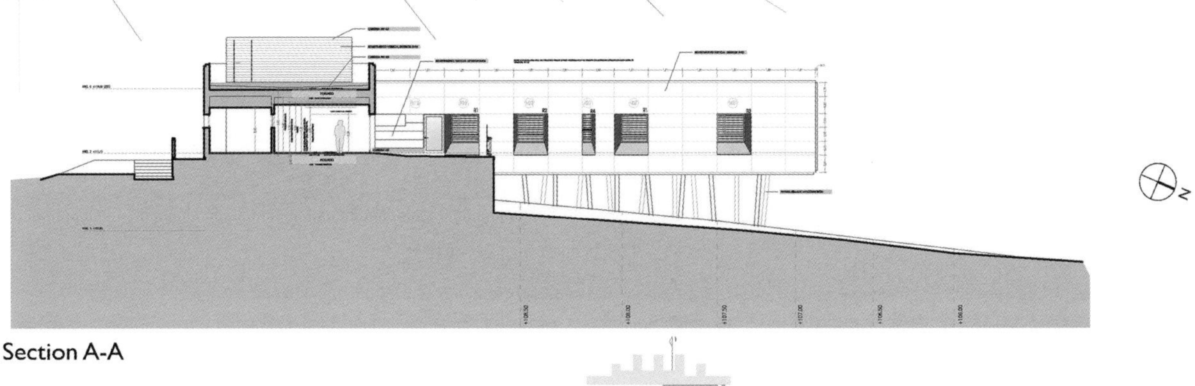

Section A-A

6.11.4a–d A circulation spine connects main programmatic elements, and five cantilevered wings project orthogonally from this element.

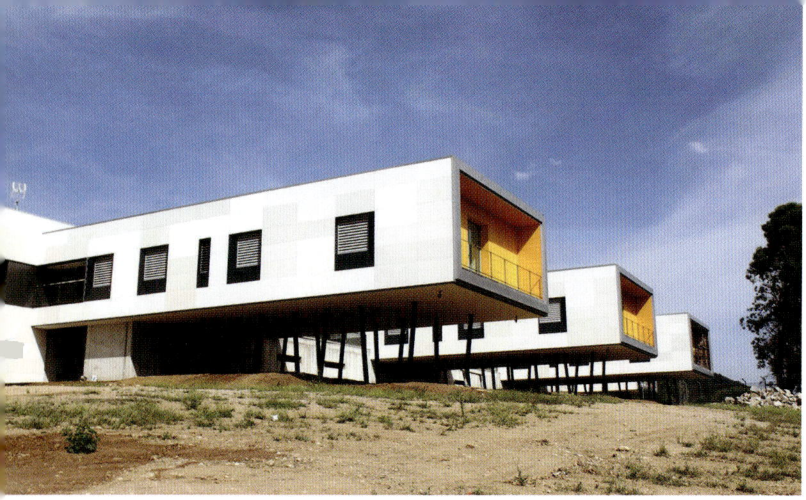

6.11.5 The prefab, panelized inpatient wings rest on slender diagonal black columns.

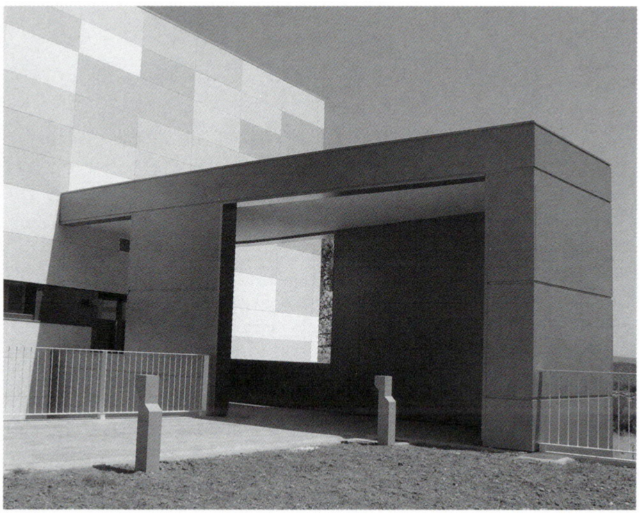

6.11.6 An entrance is color-coded (in sienna panels), heightening its legibility.

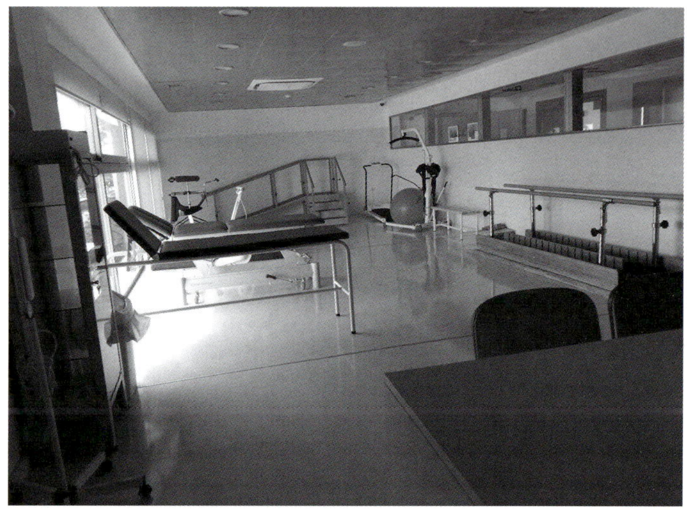

6.11.7 Many therapy/treatment rooms have windows on both inboard and outboard sides.

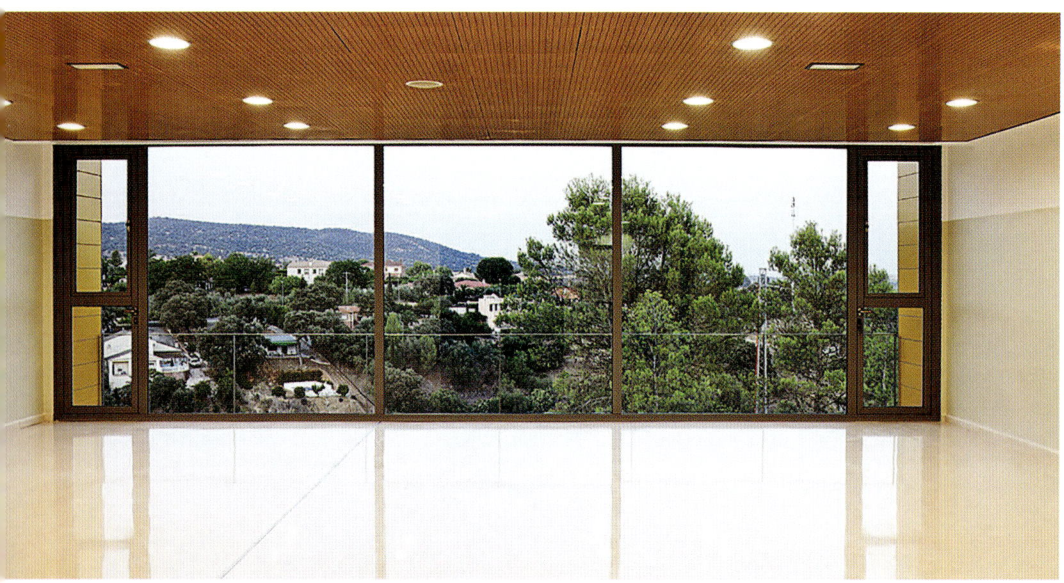

6.11.8 Five cantilevered wings are oriented and proportioned to maximize views of the surrounding landscape.

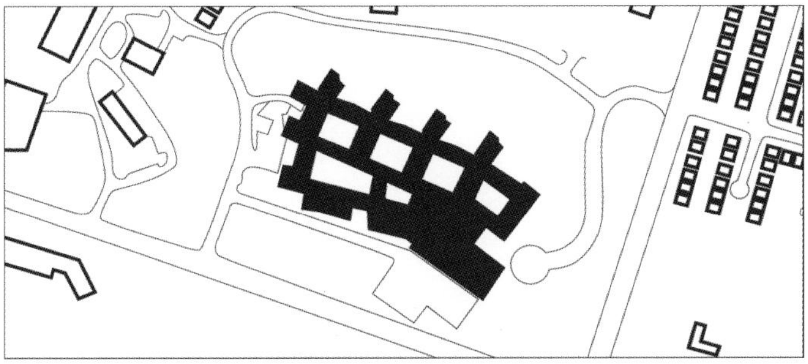

12 Margaret and Charles Juravinski Centre for Integrated Healthcare, Hamilton, Ontario, Canada

ARCHITECT: Cannon Design, Buffalo, New York, USA/architecture+, Troy, New York, USA
LANDSCAPE ARCHITECT: Cannon Design, Buffalo, New York, USA
CLIENT: Province of Ontario Ministry of Health and Long-Term Care/ St. Joseph's Healthcare, Hamilton
FEATURED MATERIALS: Precast concrete panels, glass, masonry
COMPLETED: 2013
INPATIENT BEDS: 305
SITE/PARKING: 42 acres/155
HOSPITAL/TREATMENT CENTER SIZE: 830,000 square feet
NURSES' WORKSTATION: Shielded

Context/site

This Canadian public-private partnership (PPP) regional psychiatric hospital is on the Niagara Escarpment, overlooking Hamilton, next to an upscale residential neighborhood. Remnants of the old, abandoned Hamilton Insane Asylum remain on the site, an institution founded in 1876. Three former buildings of the asylum remain, including the neoclassical, Victorian-era main structure, but all have fallen into disrepair at this writing. The replacement facility centralizes regional psychiatric services as one location, including community education and medical diagnosis and treatment services, and its sizeable forensic unit serves all of southwestern Ontario. Upon opening in 2013, the 450,000-square-foot midcentury hospital on the site, expanded since the 1950s, was demolished. This replacement facility was certified LEED Gold, based on materiality, drought-resistant plant species, incorporation of high-efficiency plumbing fixtures, connections with public transit and bike paths, passive solar building orientation, massing, and reclamation of a brownfield site. The designers' aim was to destigmatize the mental health hospitalization experience by means of a normative architectural vocabulary. The care philosophy emphasizes the role of the family and the community throughout treatment and rehabilitation.[8]

Compositionally, the public face of this large complex appears, as a collection of smaller parts, achieved by means of multiple setbacks, variations in exterior cladding, and varied fenestration, creating the effect from the exterior of a series of visually independent compositional elements, yet interconnected (Figure 6.12.1 to 6.12.3a–d). This public side houses the administration, all outpatient clinics, research functions, café, outdoor terrace, large auditorium, and related clinical and staff supports. This concept was carried into interior spaces, principally in a large atrium that rises four levels. The floor plates here were set back, in effect, to maximize natural light, whereas on the building's more private 'back side', this concept is eschewed in favor of repetitively stacking the inpatient units on top of one another. The back side of the complex is sheathed mainly in red brick masonry, with three security-screened outdoor courts provided at ground level. This zone houses central facility management functions, a loading dock area, and central materials-management unit. The surrounding grounds feature at-grade parking, a circular labyrinth, and multiple seating areas available for use by the general public (Figure 6.12.4).

Building/unit

The main level on the public face of this complex contains the public entrance; this portal connects to a public atrium/food services area and a large auditorium. The public elevator core is located immediately to the left. This atrium provides seating and a reception area and receives natural light from skylights. Directly ahead are links to various outpatient clinics housed in the stepped front side of the complex. Diagnostic services are housed on the main level, including radiology, an MRI unit, women's services, central pharmacy, neurodiagnostics, and cardiodiagnostics. Also housed on this level are the schizophrenia and medical outpatient clinics and community psychiatry. The second level houses outpatient clinics for mood and anxiety disorders, geriatric psychiatry, and neuropsychology; chapel; dental clinic; physiotherapy unit; and inpatient units (on the nonpublic side) for individuals hospitalized for acute mental health, mood disorders, and geriatric psychiatry treatment. The third level houses additional outpatient clinics and residential

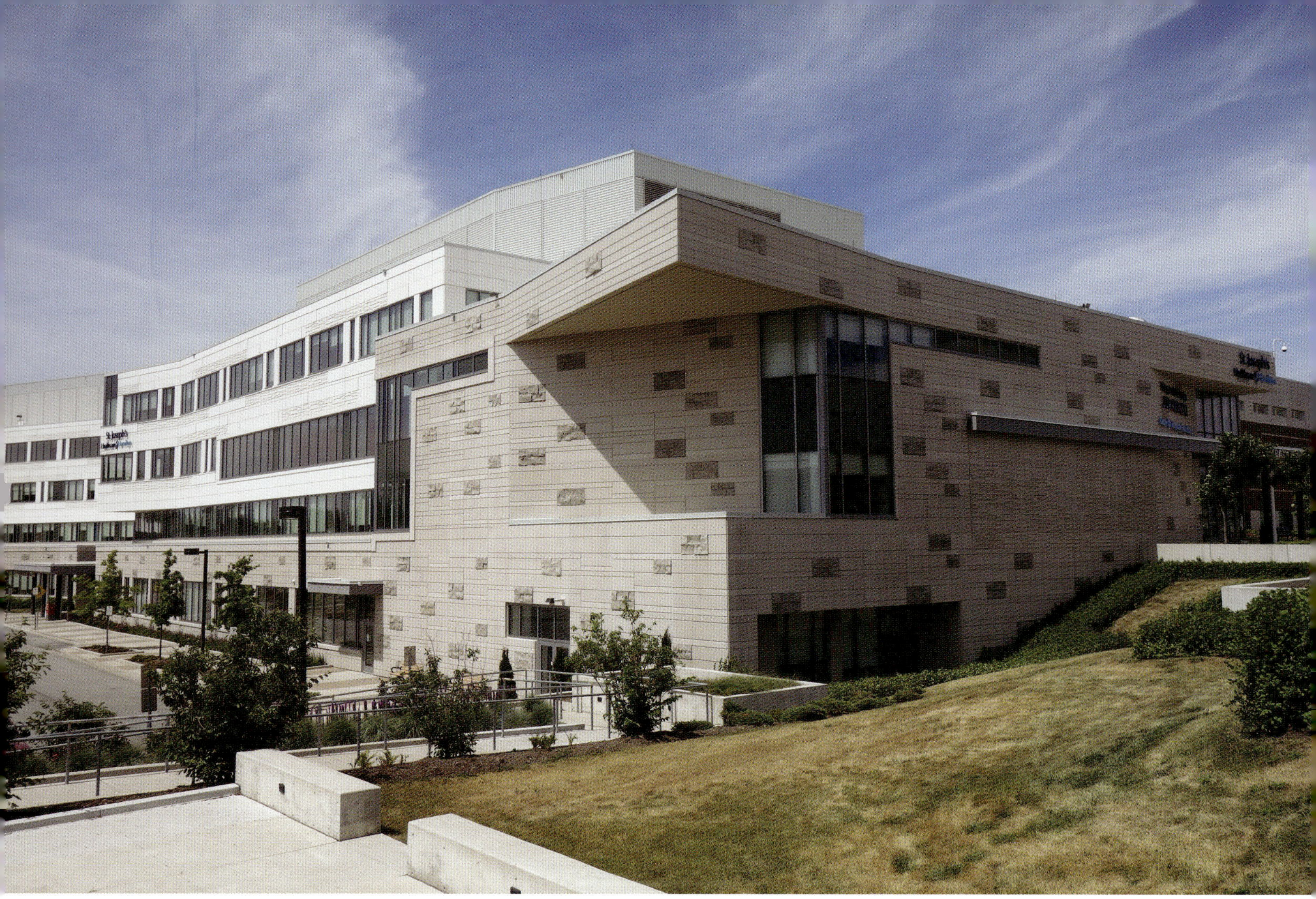

6.12.1 Juravinski Centre in Hamilton, Ontario, is set into a sloping site.

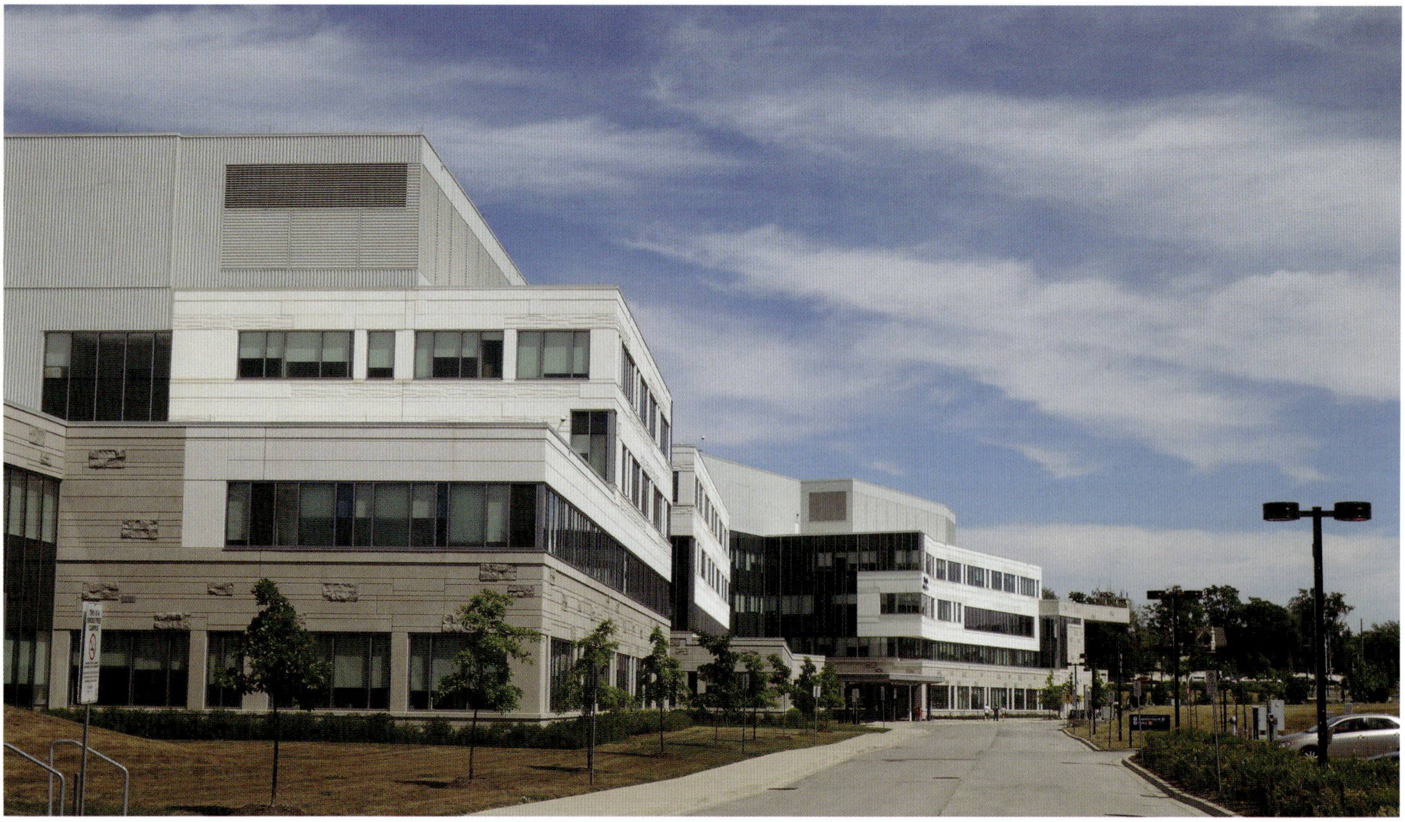

6.12.2 A vehicular drive leading to the public entrance passes by the compositionally diverse constituent parts of a single superstructure.

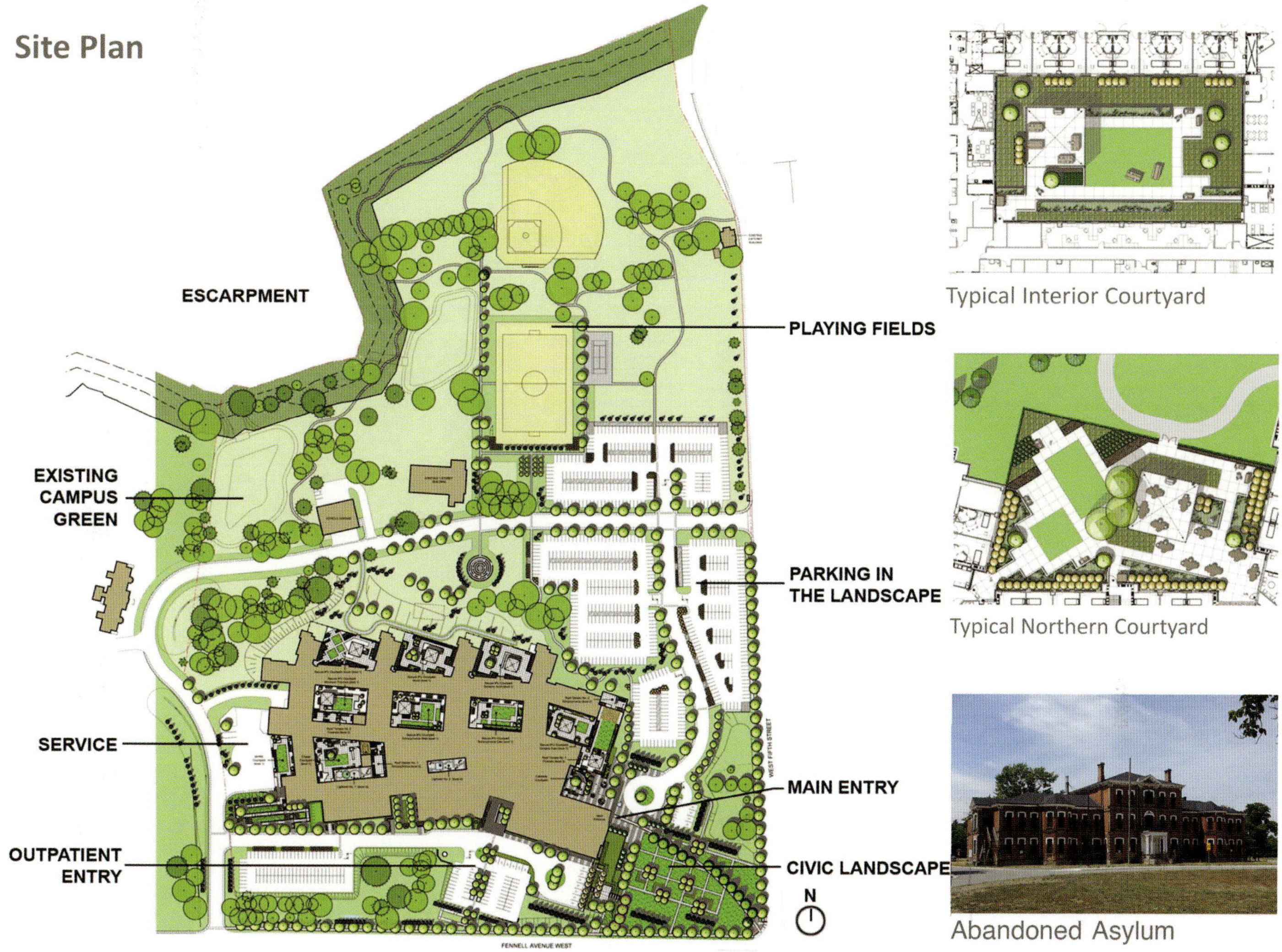

6.12.3a–d The Juravinski Centre was built on the site of a postwar psychiatric institution, since demolished, and the architectural remnants of an abandoned, heritage-protected 19th-century provincial asylum.

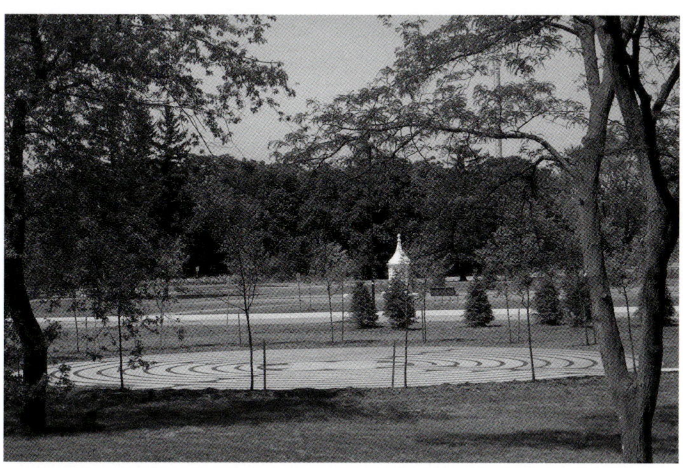

6.12.4 A labyrinth provided on the open-access portion of the grounds is next to an open field and wooded area beyond.

forensic and schizophrenia units. This level houses a library and resources center, athletic and recreational therapy unit and gym, and 'stores', including a hair salon and clothing store. The fourth level houses, on the front (public) side, additional outpatient clinics, with the back side housing additional 24/7 adult acute care psychiatric units. This superstructure's exterior materiality varies significantly between the public and the private sides, in an effort to diminish its formidable overall scale and volume (Figures 6.12.5 and 6.12.6a–b).

Each patient room is provided with a private bath/shower unit. Unit nurses' stations are centrally positioned at the intersection of connecting corridors, in plan. Patient rooms are deployed along these double-loaded corridors on three of four paths created by a biaxial overall unit configuration. Patient rooms overlook the surrounding suburban landscape, and a fourth occupied zone on each unit houses staff supports and therapy functions (e.g., dayrooms, group rooms, dining areas/food preparation staging, and

Key:

1 arrival forecourt
2 arrival vestibule
3 lobby/reception
4 elevators
5 restaurant/dining (public)
6 exterior courtyard/dining
7 diagnostic services (radiology/MRI/women's services/ultrasound/ECT/TMS/neurodiagnostics/cardiodiagnostics)
8 medical outpatient clinic
9 pharmacy
10 community psychiatry services
11 specimen collection
12 clinical lab
13 mailroom/central support
14 shipping/receiving
15 materials management
16 long-term storage
17 morgue
18 facility management unit
19 central storage
20 central kitchen
21 central server room
22 environmental services
23 Cleghorn Schizophrenia Clinic
24 registration/health records
25 retail pharmacy
26 cafeteria/support

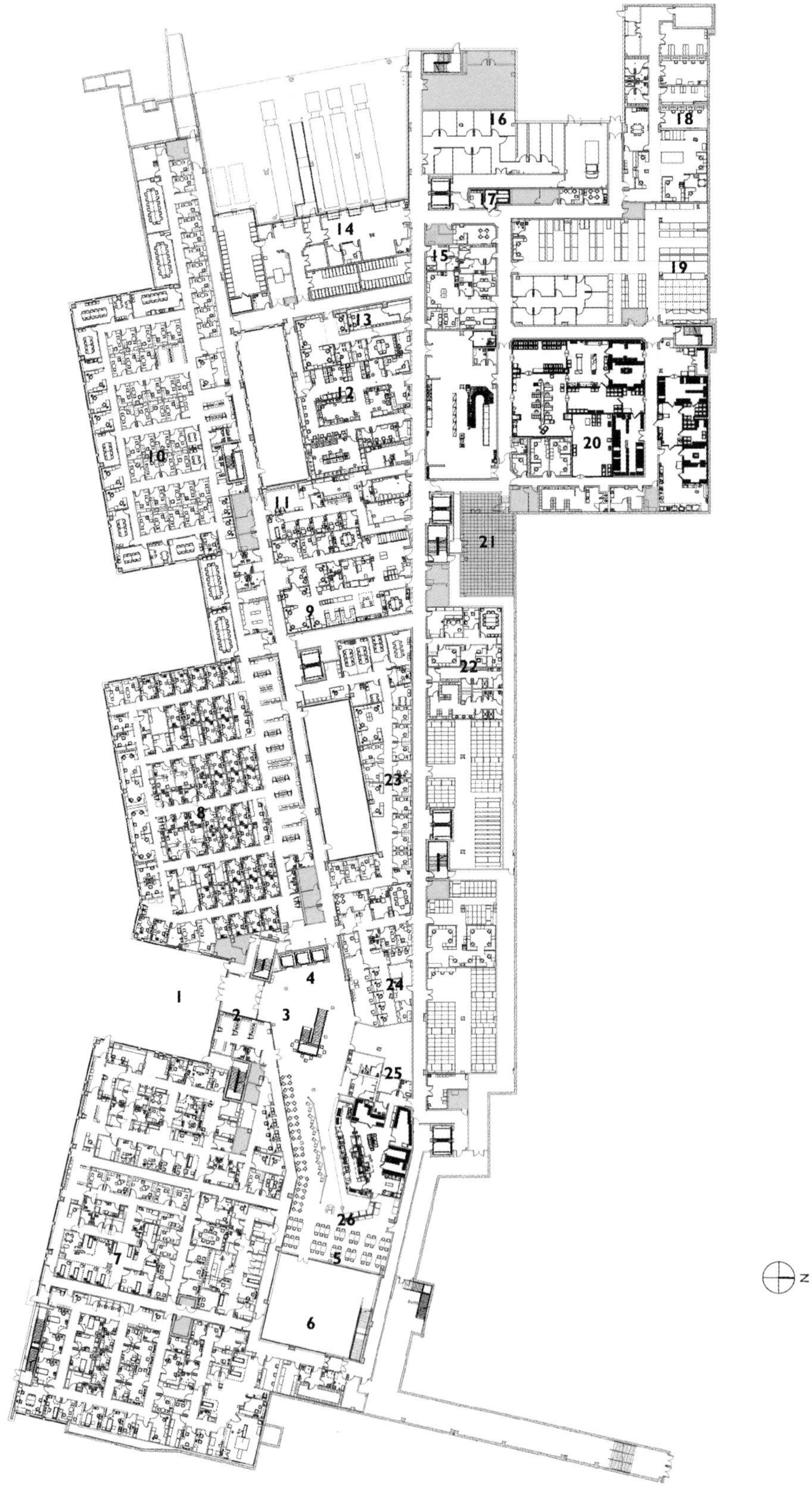

Main Level

6.12.5 The footprint is dominated by a pair of diagonal axes, one of which is partially splayed to the left, in plan.

Key:
1 forensic inpatient unit
2 music therapy suite
3 schizophrenia inpatient unit
4 schizophrenia research unit
5 finance/administration
6 peer support and patient advocate center
7 mental health/ wellness resource center
8 schizophrenia IPU
9 schizophrenia IPU
10 clothing store
11 salon
12 patient library
13 coffee shop
14 schizophrenia outpatient clinic
15 OH&S/infection control
16 human resources
17 department of psychology
18 psychotherapy center
19 spiritual care
20 athletic and recreation center
21 museum
22 information and learning center
23 conferene center
24 auditorium
25 exterior courtyard

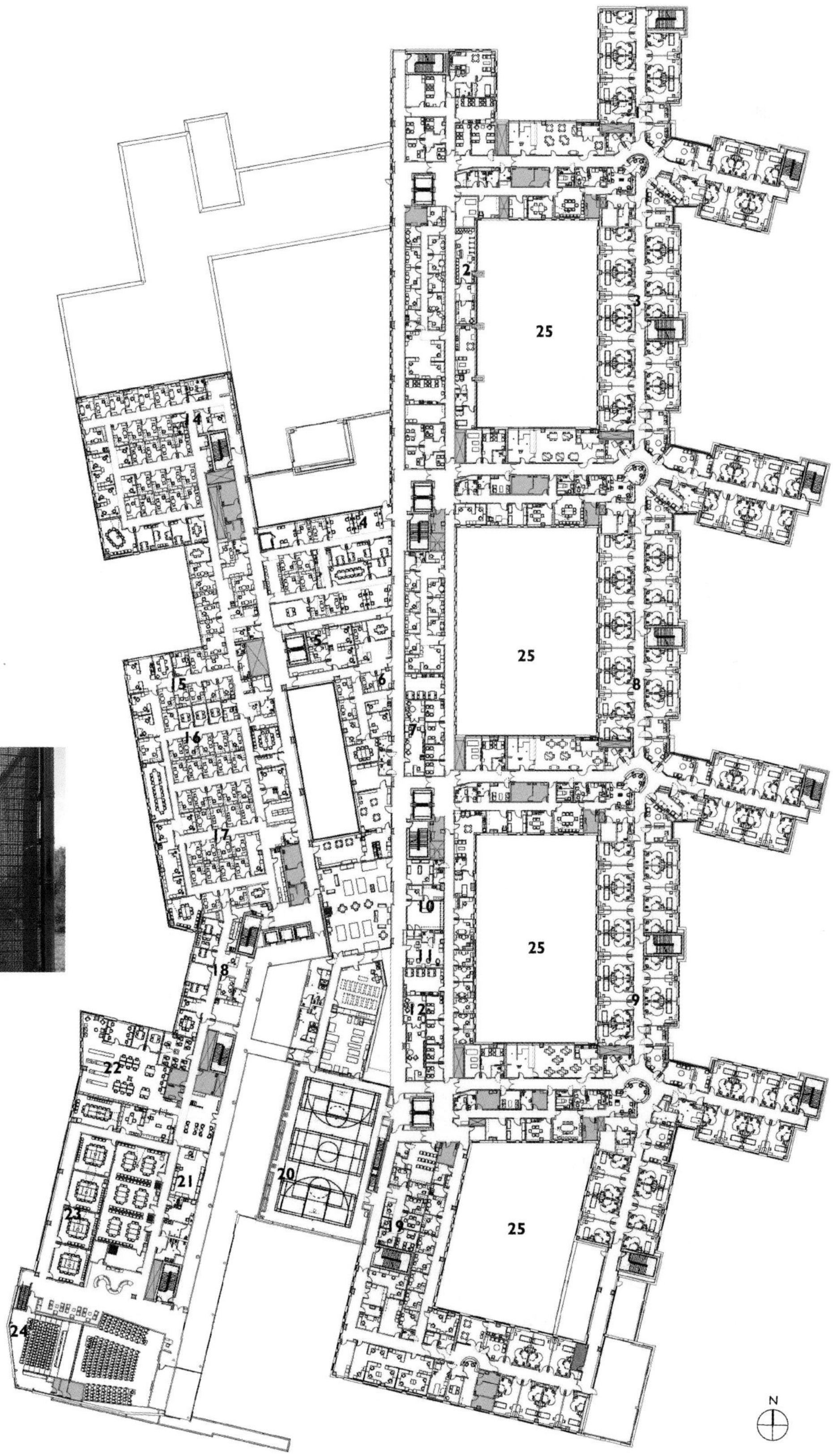

Level 3

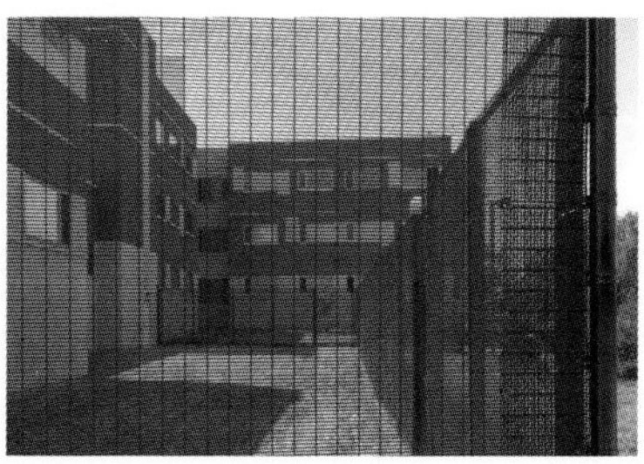

6.12.6a–b On various upper levels, inpatient units are located to the right side, configured around courtyards, with outpatient units, outreach education, and research units to the left.

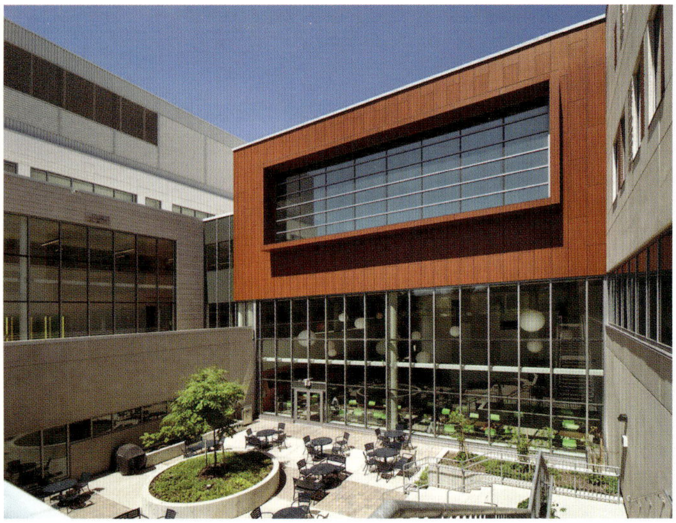

6.12.7 The main public dining area in the atrium adjoins a large terrace, enclosed on three sides by the superstructure.

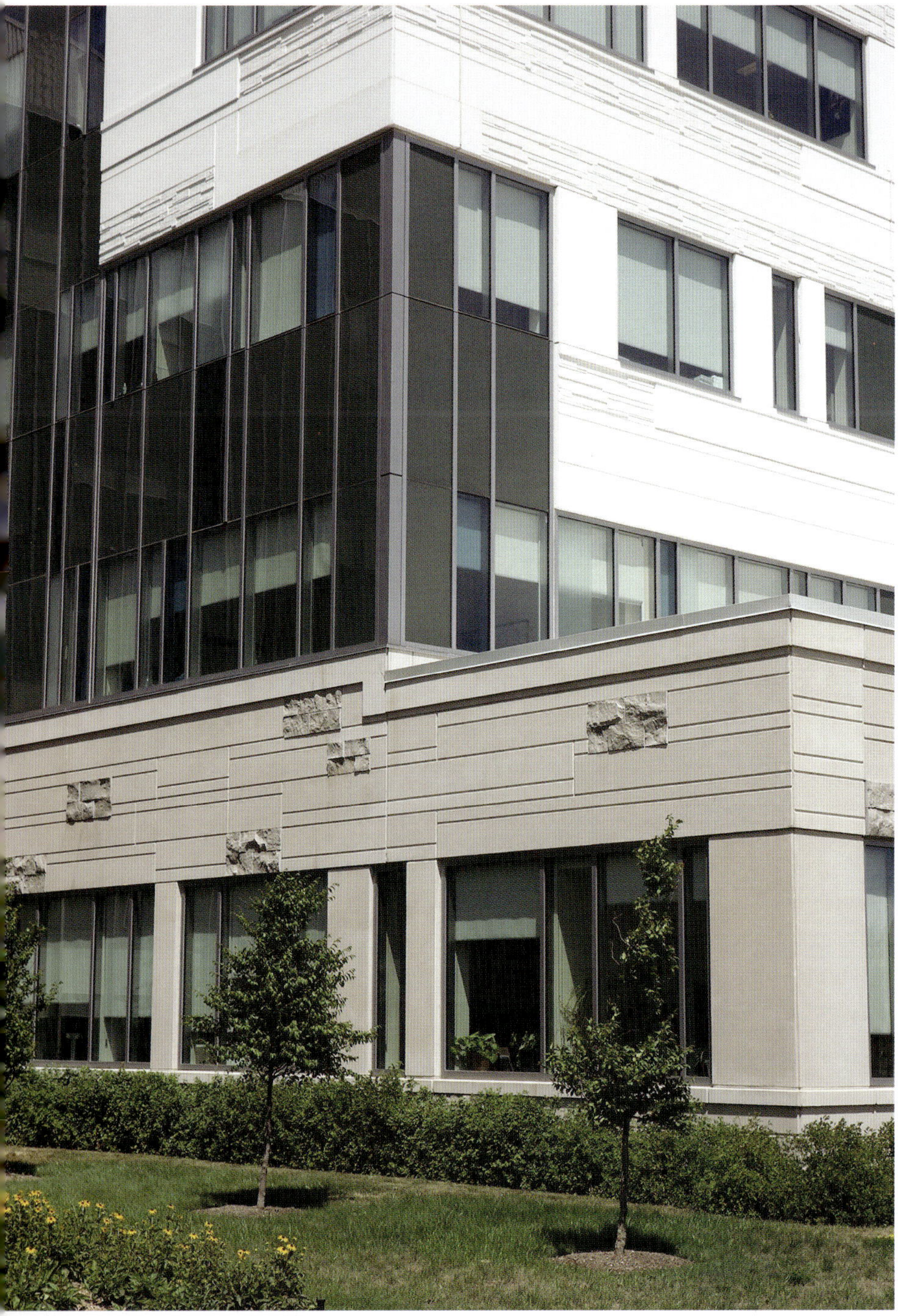

6.12.8 Varied materials, massings, and fenestration break up the formidable scale of the superstructure.

unit offices). The master plan acknowledged therapeutic value of natural light and ventilation, and in response, courtyards are carved out of the center of the footprint. However, the patients are often restricted in their freedom of movement to directly experience the outdoors and this is mostly a function of the large overall scale of the complex and the number of floor levels, with the main exception being three security-enclosed ground-level courtyards for patients' use. Opportunities for future expansion exist in designated portions of the upper floor plates on the front side of the superstructure (Figures 6.12.7 to 6.12.9). This replacement facility stands in contrast to the decentralized footprints of many recent psychiatric hospitals built in Europe and Australia.

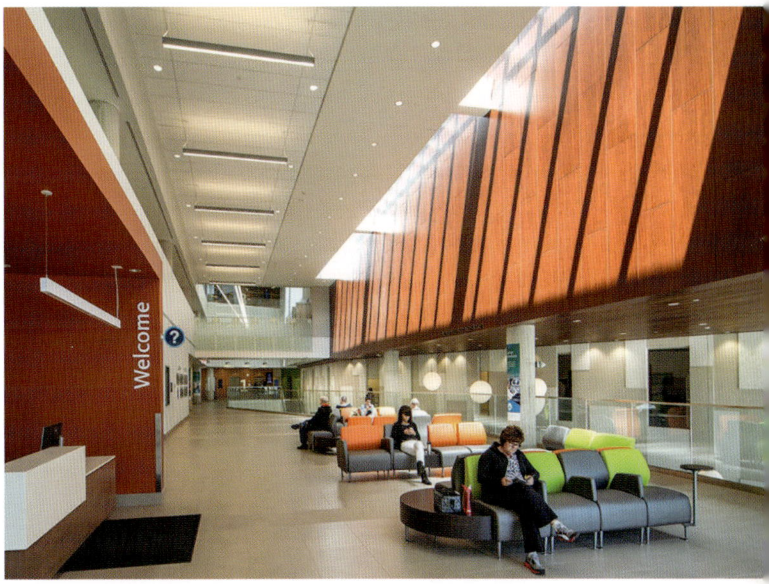

6.12.9 The main public waiting/reception area in the arrival atrium features light (skylights and bright color bands.

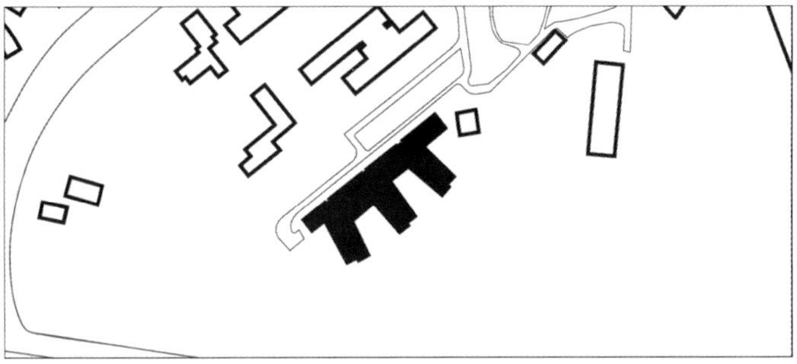

13 High Care Clinic, Oegstgeest, the Netherlands

ARCHITECT: de Jong Gortemaker Algra (dJGA), Rotterdam, the Netherlands
LANDSCAPE ARCHITECT: dJGA, Rotterdam, the Netherlands
CLIENT: Stichting Rivierduinen
FEATURED MATERIALS: Masonry, glass panels
COMPLETED: 2012
INPATIENT BEDS: 36
SITE/PARKING: 12 acres/35
HOSPITAL/TREATMENT CENTER SIZE: 28,765 square feet
NURSES' WORKSTATION: Hybrid

Context/site

The High Care Clinic is an inpatient psychiatric hospital for persons with severe mental health needs. This replacement facility is located on an old country estate surrounded by allied psychiatric facilities. It was built next to Castle Actor, dating from 1307. From 1895 until the 1970s, it was used as an asylum. Presently, it is the administrative center for the board of directors of the Mental Health Rivierduinen Organization. To the south of the site is the University of Leiden campus district. To the east is Rijnlands' Revalidatie Centrum Hospital, which is next to a special education school for children and adolescents with learning and behavioural difficulties. The High Care Clinic campus is approximately 38 kilometers from Amsterdam. The complex is configured as more private on the back side, while presenting its public face, when approached in a vehicle or on foot, on the front side (Figure 6.13.1). The building itself symbolically functions as a protective perimeter wall to a large extent – not unlike the formidable barriers that once surrounded neoclassical asylums in the Netherlands and elsewhere in Europe. By contrast, here, the type of protective wall created is integral to the building composition and not set apart from it. Its façade is moderately imposing, especially for a building of its modest overall scale. It is fabricated of red masonry, with an irregular, somewhat jagged roof line. In silhouette, it appears broken at only three intervals. These minimalist, planar elements, in white stucco, slice through, breaking the wall's cadence as if to signify the presence of the three inpatient residential units situated immediately behind the wall/façade (Figure 6.13.2).

This one-level building is centralized, configured in plan as a central spine with three projecting wings – housing three inpatient residential units and associated clinical supports. Parking is provided in a central zone at the site perimeter. Rhythmically repetitive, modestly scaled windows in the outer wall-*cum*-façade are arranged in a seemingly random pattern. In a way, these devices function as foils, countering the dominance of the wall, obliquely referencing the instability of the patients inside, or perhaps the incoherence of the society this place ostensibly separates its patients from during treatment. The façade protects from an uncertain world beyond yet simultaneously functions as a datum, a definitive boundary facilitating informal internal connections with nature, relative openness, and a sense of being cloistered. Considerable theraserialization occurs within this inner realm, as abundant natural light enters while providing views outward into four semi-enclosed courtyards, and beyond. The first of these contains a basketball court; two exterior courtyards at the midsection in plan are, in comparison, passive spaces yet able to be activated for recreational use; the fourth functions as a wooded retreat area and therapy garden. Courtyards are buffered by a row of mature trees and new supplemental plantings, in turn buttressed by a translucent 10-foot-high perimeter security fence (Figure 6.13.3 and 6.13.4).

Building/unit

The design strategy rejects comparisons to the drab double-loaded corridors of the old asylum by staggering the primary circulation element, in plan. This was done by slightly rotating walls and tilting them, then rendering them in white and off-white hues. Natural light activates these rotated, variously skewed planes by means of skylights, particularly on the inboard side of the spine. The effect is one of informality as opposed to rigid institutionalism. Walls and floor patterns flow from exterior to interior, to improve spatial orientation and to prevent the perception of a

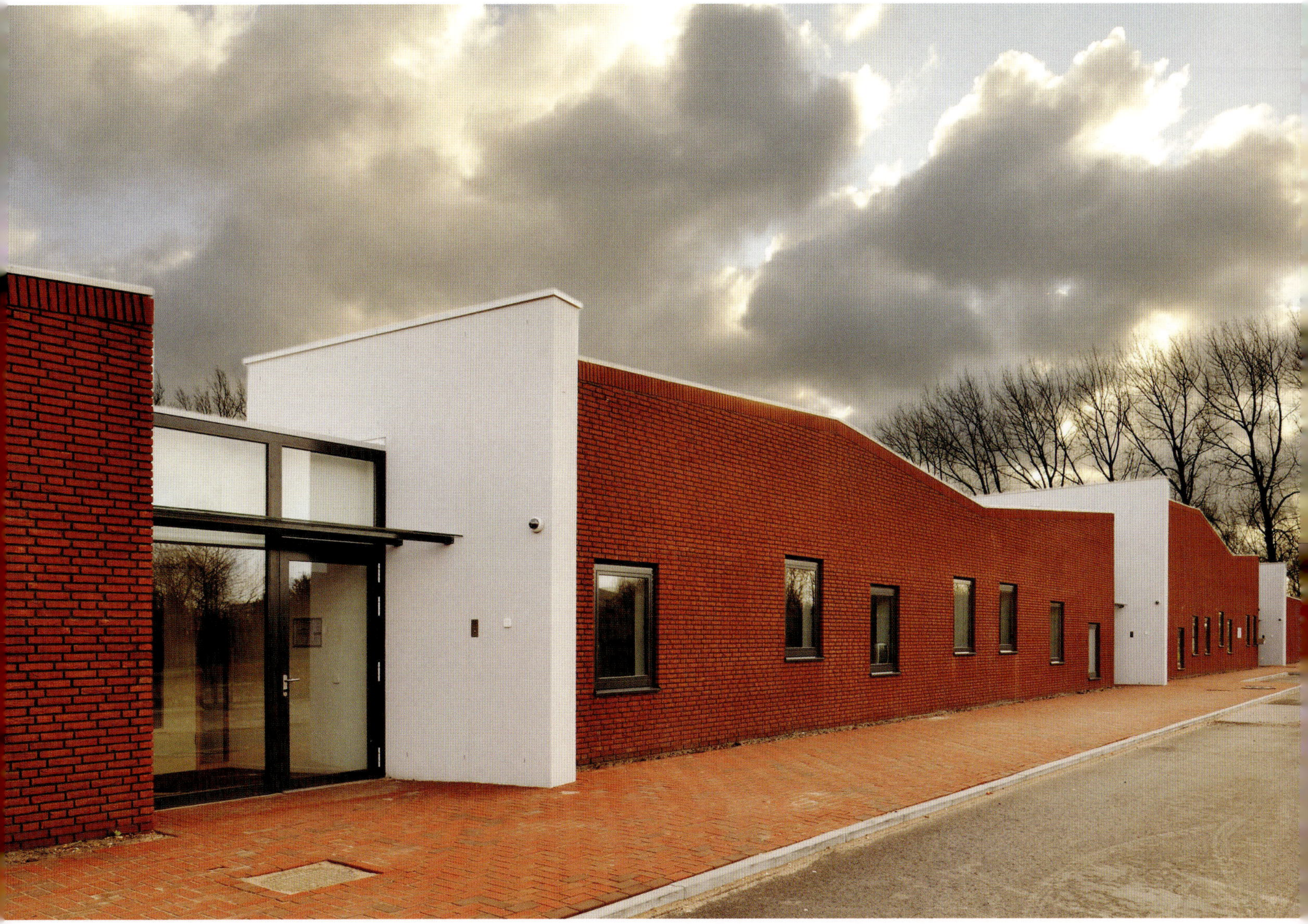

6.13.1 The public façade of the High Care Clinic is formidable yet modestly scaled, obliquely referencing the outer perimeter walls of old European asylums.

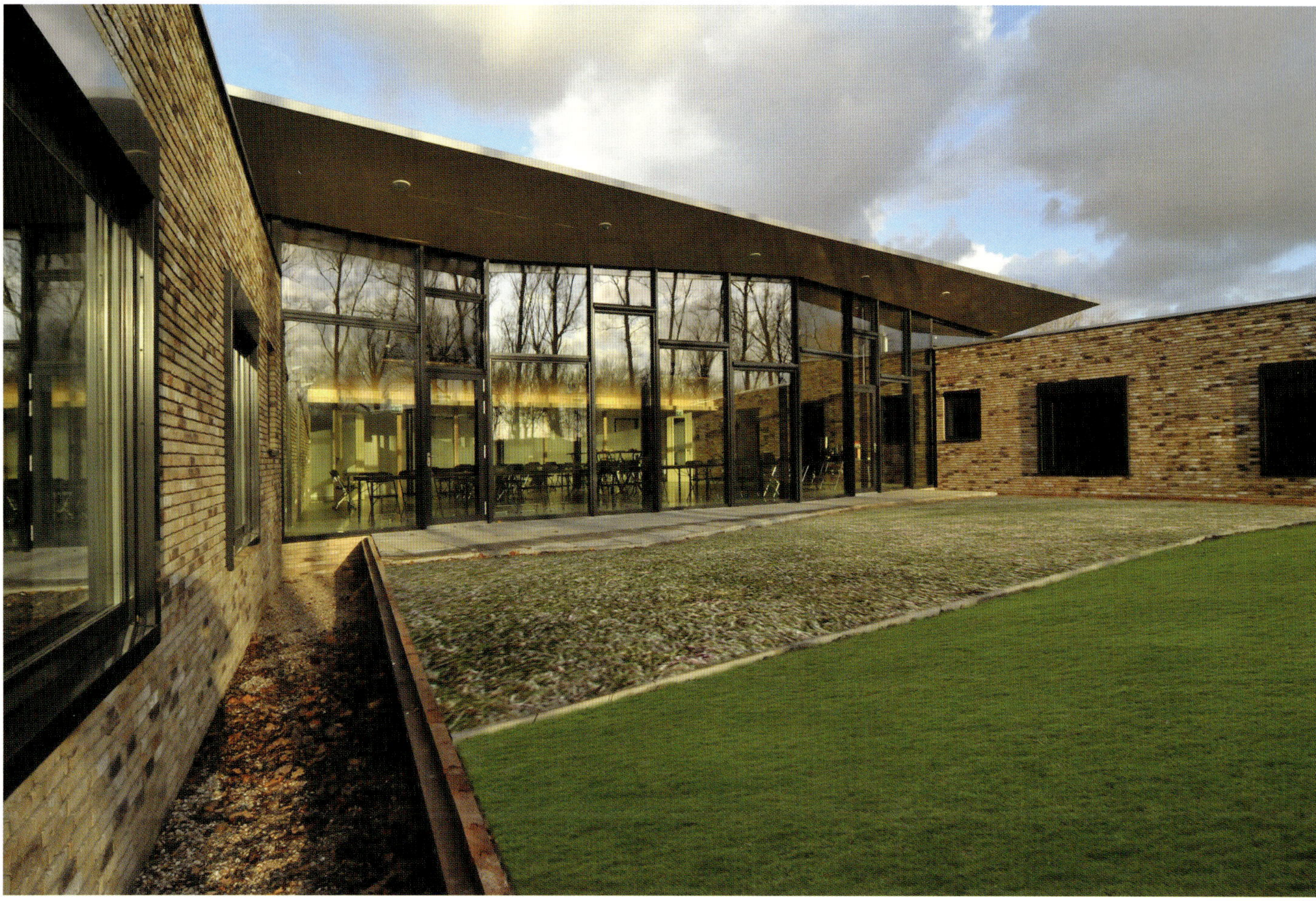

6.13.2 Interior courtyards, with lawns and informal therapy/activity areas, are dissimilar from the front façade's more resolute imagery.

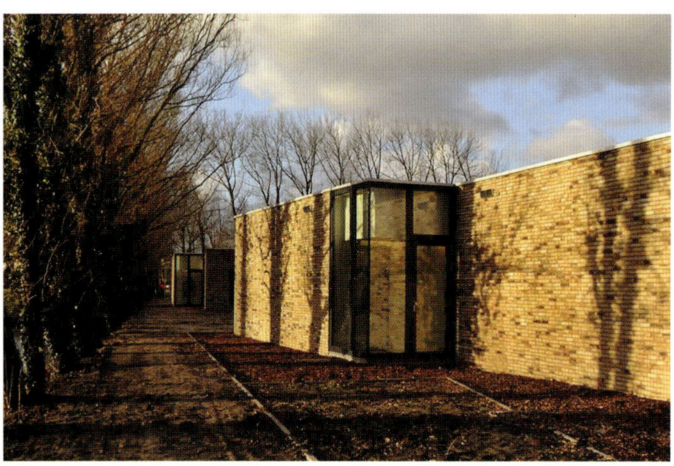

6.13.3 The back side of the campus is quasi-residential, and residential units overlook a wooded area.

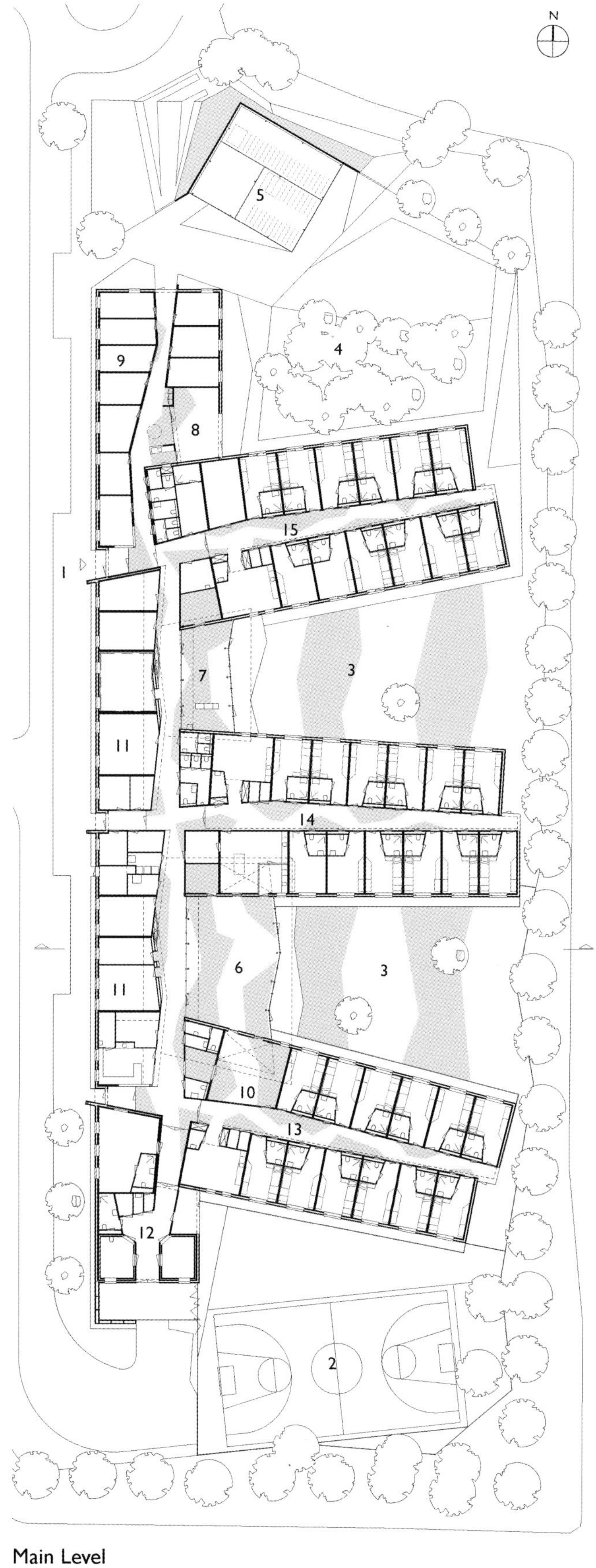

Key:
1 main arrival
2 ball court
3 courtyard
4 wooded retreat
5 garden
6 dining
7 dayroom/activity
8 art therapy
9 administration
10 kitchen
11 counseling/staff support
12 central support
13 residential treatment unit 1
14 residential treatment unit 2
15 residential treatment unit 3

Main Level

6.13.4 The plan is dominated by a circulation 'street' with three fingers – outstretched hands – wings flanking open green spaces.

stark, clinical corridor. Circulation spaces are configured so that no opposing walls stand strictly parallel to one another. The communal spine, connecting various sections of the building, is thereby transformed into a meandering sequence of interconnected mini-zones.

These informal zones afford opportunities for social interaction and consultation among the staff, as well as staff, patients, and visitors. Forms, materials, views, natural light, and plantings reinforce strong connections to the semirural site. The courtyard-facing side of this irregular, highly trafficked main artery is transparent except for being interrupted by three entry portals to the inpatient units. A main dining room, multipurpose space, and group therapy room feature full-height windows facing outdoors, articulated by lifted and tilted roof planes. With their accentuated overhangs, these elements appear to float above the building's anchoring base, themselves functioning as compositional foils. Throughout, black anodized-aluminum frames accentuate the window gridwalls (Figures 6.13.5 and 6.13.6).

The circulation spine houses the administrative and medical staff offices and numerous group and individual therapy/treatment spaces. Residential units are double loaded in plan, with doors to patient rooms staggered to foster greater visual and auditory privacy; each bedroom has a private bathroom/shower unit, located on the inboard side along the main corridor. At the furthermost end of each unit the two facing bedrooms are staggered, in plan, with an emergency exit at the end, in between; this establishes a view sight line extending outward into the landscape. The outer edge of the campus on this side parallels a small creek. Patients' rooms have large operable windows with deep sills, overlooking a courtyard. Each room is provided with a large storage unit and a work area with a table, positioned along the same wall as the patient bed, near the bath/shower unit. A color palette of blue, black, and white is used interchangeably to accent ceilings, walls, and floor surfaces. The bed-desk headwall is banded with a black wainscot and a black-and-white midlevel height band. Some patient rooms feature full-height glass doors in lieu of a large picture window. A quiet/seclusion room is located on the innermost (inboard) end of each residential unit, directly across from the nurses' station and miscellaneous staff supports (Figures 6.13.7 and 6.13.8).

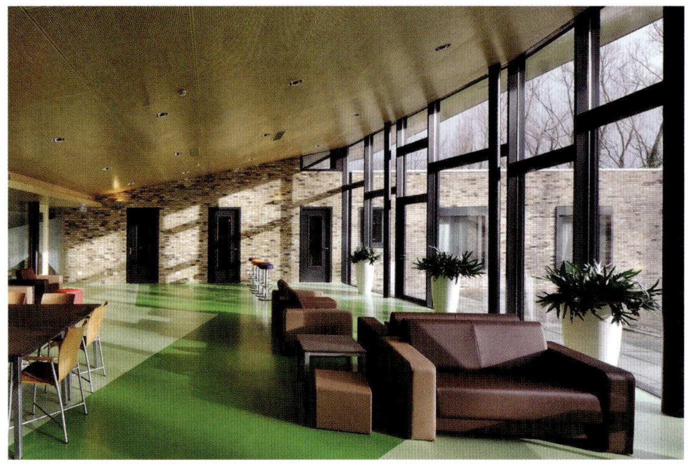

6.13.5 The sloped ceiling of a dayroom/activity space accentuates its relationship to an adjacent courtyard.

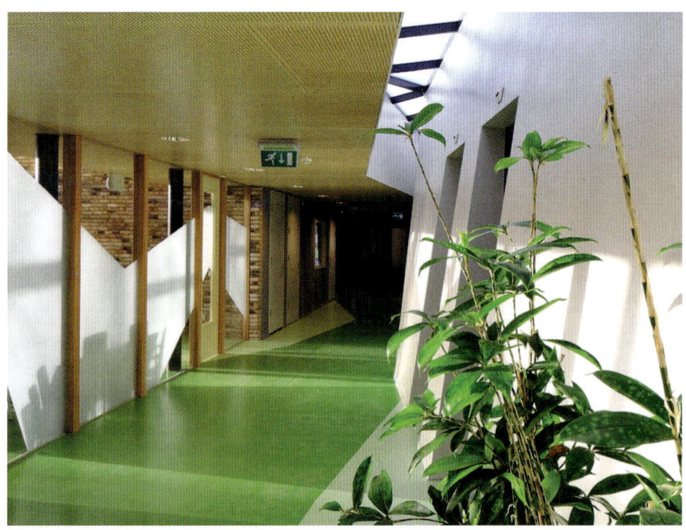

6.13.6 Walls in the circulation spine/street tilt and rotate, with flooring coded to reinforce indoor plantings, accentuating the therapeutic role of nature.

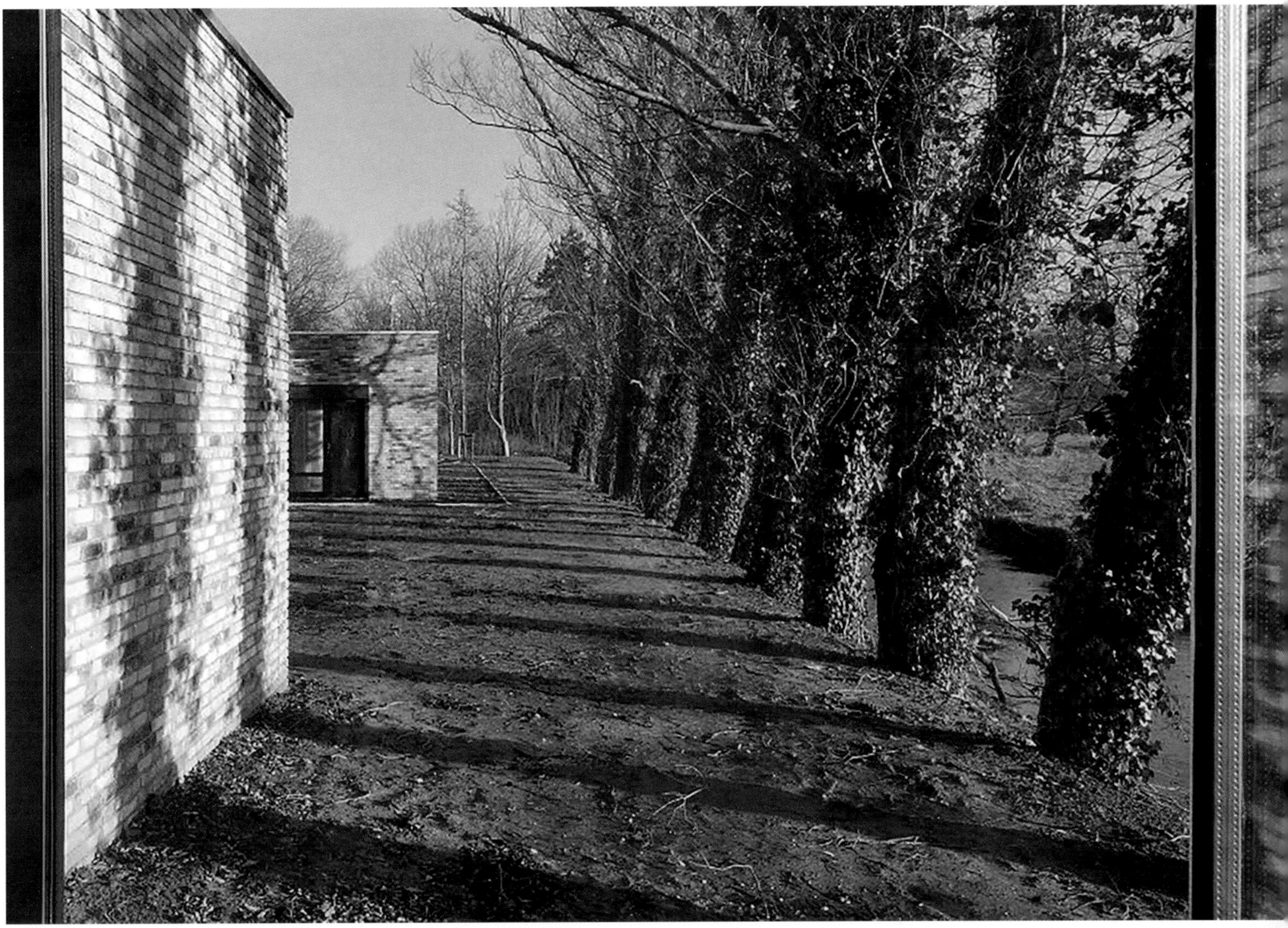

6.13.7 The rear perimeter of the High Care Clinic campus looks out to trees, a stream, and woods beyond.

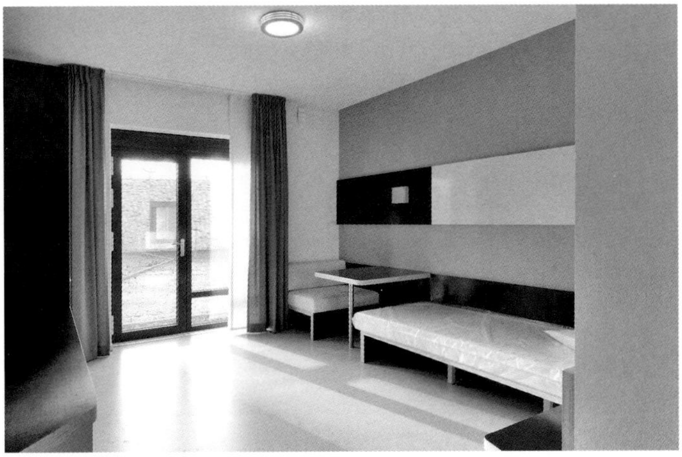

6.13.8 Patient rooms feature private doors connecting to an exterior terrace, banded walls, and built-in furnishings.

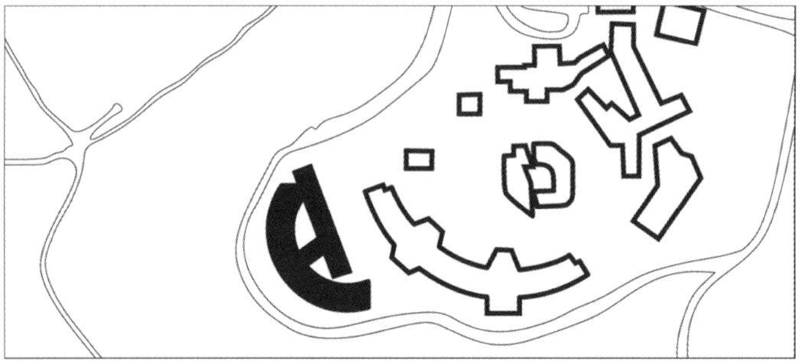

14 The Lowry Unit, Prestwich, Manchester, UK

ARCHITECT: Gilling Dod Architects, Lancashire, UK
LANDSCAPE ARCHITECT: Gilling Dod Architects, Lancashire, UK
CLIENT: Greater Manchester West Mental Health NHS Foundation Trust
FEATURED MATERIALS: Standing-seam steel roof, precast concrete panels, glass
COMPLETED: 2016
INPATIENT BEDS: 30
SITE/PARKING: 10 acres/14
HOSPITAL/TREATMENT CENTER SIZE: 46,000 square feet
NURSES' WORKSTATION: Shielded

Context/site

The Lowry Unit is a forensic psychiatric hospital located on the Prestwich Hospital site northeast of Manchester, United Kingdom. It was commissioned under Procure 21+ and was the latest part of the NHS's long-term redevelopment of its Edenfield Secure Hub Site. Inpatient alcohol and chemical dependency recovery services are provided in Prestwich and in neighboring communities. The adjacent Edenfield psychiatric hospital is a medium-security forensic facility, and the new moderate-security level facility is autonomous, having established a unique architectural identity. Nearby are the Rockley House Hospital and the recently built Junction 17 mental health care facility, both also part of the Prestwich Hospital campus district. The obsolete Prestwich Asylum was built in the mid-19th century, neoclassical in design, on a site remote from the rapidly industrializing city of Manchester, intentionally once removed from what were perceived as the daily trials and tribulations of the Victorian Age. Its grounds were expansive and the complex was completely walled and fortress-like. The new facility is named for the well-known British artist Laurence Stephen Lowry, who died at age 88 in 1976. He lived and worked in the region and is honored in a mural installation at the main entrance, with human figures symbolizing everyday-life qualities so characteristic in his paintings.

The site occupied by the Lowry Unit is shared with the Dovedale and Rydal Wards of the Edenfield facility, and its principal arrival axis is shared with their parking areas, which lead to the drop-off zone at the public entrance to this new facility. A wall extends outward into this arrival zone, functioning as a form of identification signage, perhaps symbolizing an extended 'helping hand' to the incoming patient. Building information modeling (BIM) software was utilized in the design, manufacture, and on-site construction processes. This pertained to all of the building's anatomical systems and prefabricated subsystems, and it allowed for a faster building-delivery time line than would have otherwise been the case. This allowed fabrication of numerous building componentry off-site. The site is a rolling landscape, and the exterior perimeter green space that wraps around this facility is protected by a semi-transparent security fence, relatively unobtrusive in appearance (Figures 6.14.1 to 6.14.4a–b).

Building/unit

This facility is one level, and the aim is to establish a residentially scaled, noninstitutional image to counter the stigma associated with the local psychiatric institutions of the past. A 'front building' houses administrative, art therapy, counseling, and gym/fitness rooms; various staff supports; and central facility management support. An arcing building to the rear, connected via an umbilical link, houses two 15-bed inpatient residential units. These mirror one another, in plan. Their configuration is reminiscent of panoptical asylums, but further reference to this precursor remains faint, mainly because this facility is minuscule by comparison and provides a relatively high degree of nature and landscape connectivity. The bisecting, diagonal element that connects the front building with the semicircular inpatient unit element yields a pair of courtyards of roughly equivalent size. These allow for close visual supervision and respite, and are available for counseling. The building partí here, too, functions as a protective wall. Two inpatient units house nearly identical spaces and supports, including living room/dayrooms, nurses' stations and staff work zone, dining and dietary functions, and the unit medication dispensary. Natural light is transmitted into semipublic and public interiors, with varied ceiling configurations further accentuating the presence of Daylight. As for

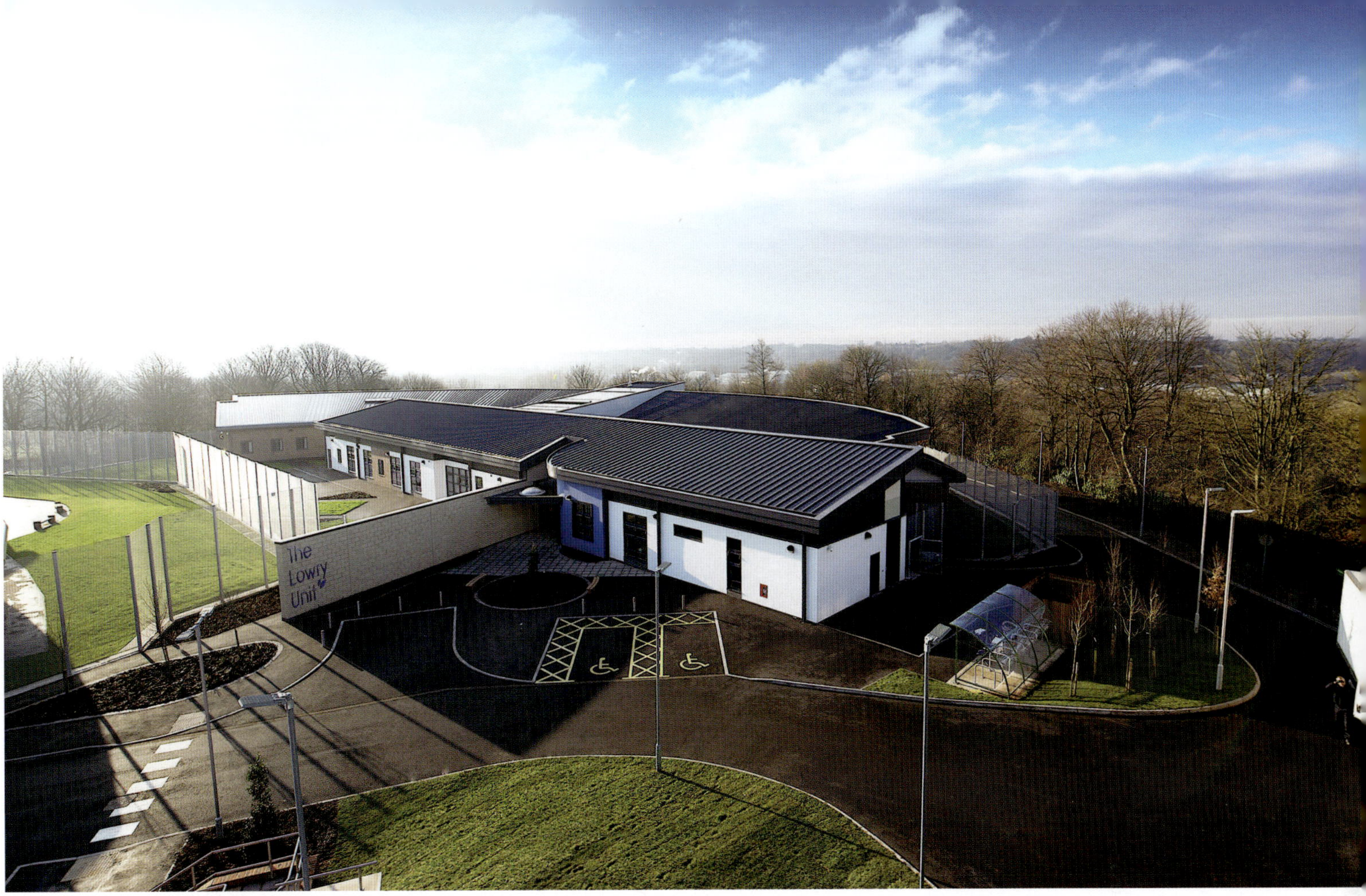

6.14.1 Visitors encounter a symbolic 'outreached hand' when approaching the Lowry Unit.

ceilings in the living/dayroom, various material changes occur; full-height windows are in the patient rooms and throughout the living and counseling spaces. The gym/fitness room features a full wall mural reminiscent of characteristic themes and motifs in Stephen Lowry's artwork, and numerous, similarly themed murals are viewable along corridors throughout (Figure 6.14.5).

The building's pervasive radiality extends horizontally, as its main corridors wind through and around spaces, their fluidity reinforced by inventive color-coding. Patient rooms are private, each with its own bath/shower unit located on the inboard side, along the corridor. The primary circulation artery is double loaded, with the doors of patients' rooms generally aligned directly across from one another; skylights are positioned at key intervals along this artery, culminating in an ascending ceiling in a recreational therapy space. Each patient room is provided with dormitory furnishings, consisting of bed and headboard and a small side table. A desk, chair, bookshelves, and a storage closet are provided along another wall. Windows are operable, with curtains, walls are color-coded, and wood-grain-finished floors are present throughout the unit. Extensive client consultations were held with the administration and the staff to eventually occupy this facility on a daily basis. This information was translated into numerous core design concepts, including an emphasis on the inventive display of works of art, including sculptures in the exterior courtyards. These artifacts are displayed in a secure two and interior environment, and in high-activity interior spaces, where an accentuated sound-absorbing ceiling and wall surfaces mask unwanted noise (Figures 6.14.6 to 6.14.9).

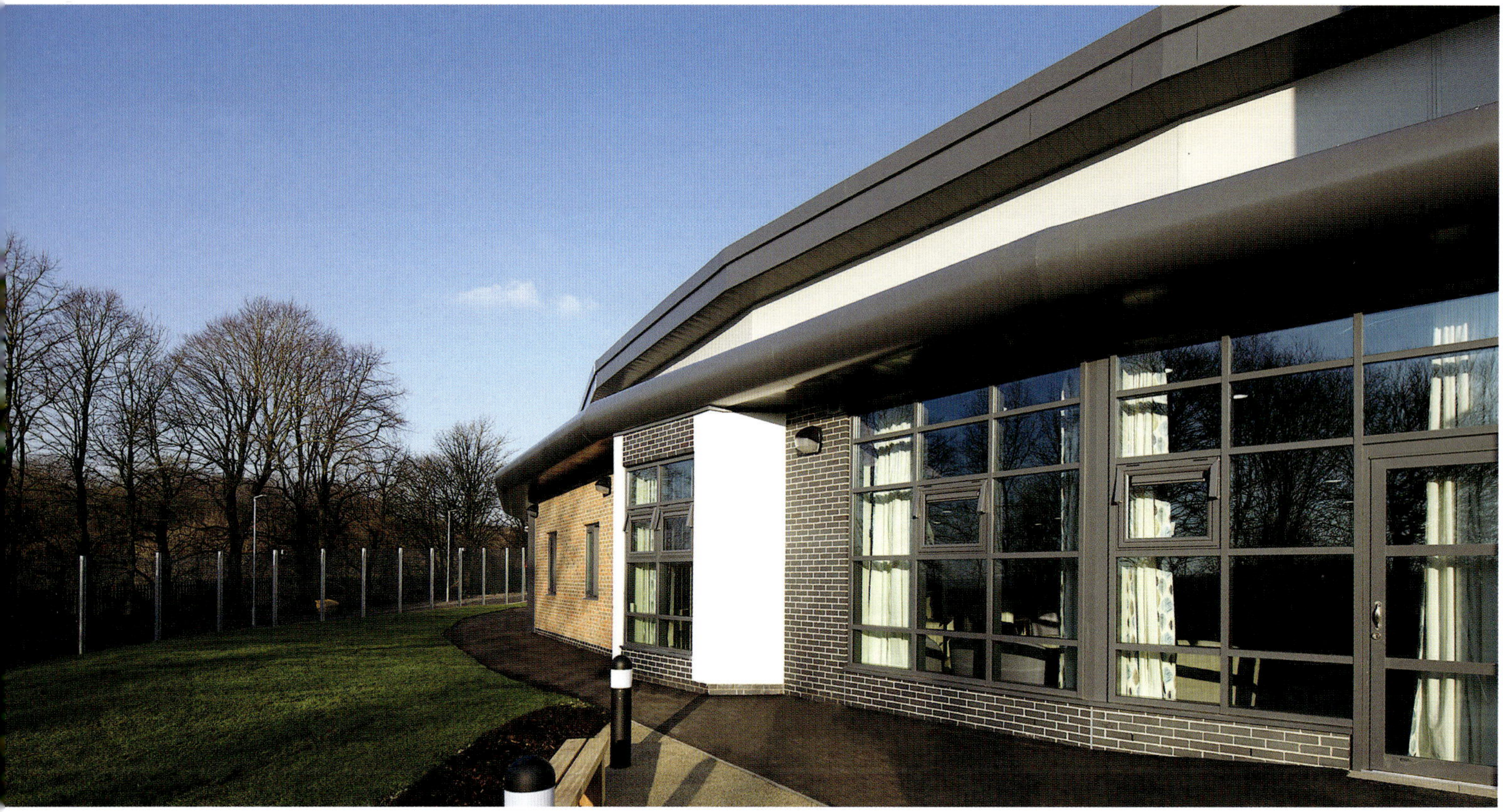

6.14.2 The curvilinear structure features sweeping forms, horizontality, operable windows, and a quasi-residential aesthetic.

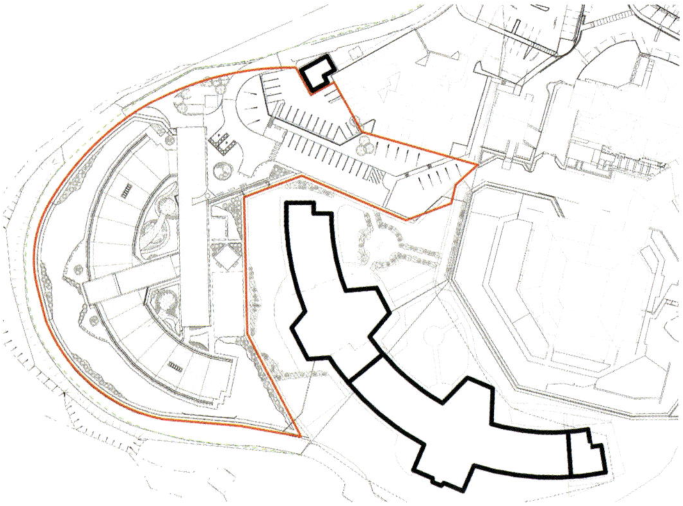

6.14.3 The Lowry Unit's immediate campus context.

BIM Rendering

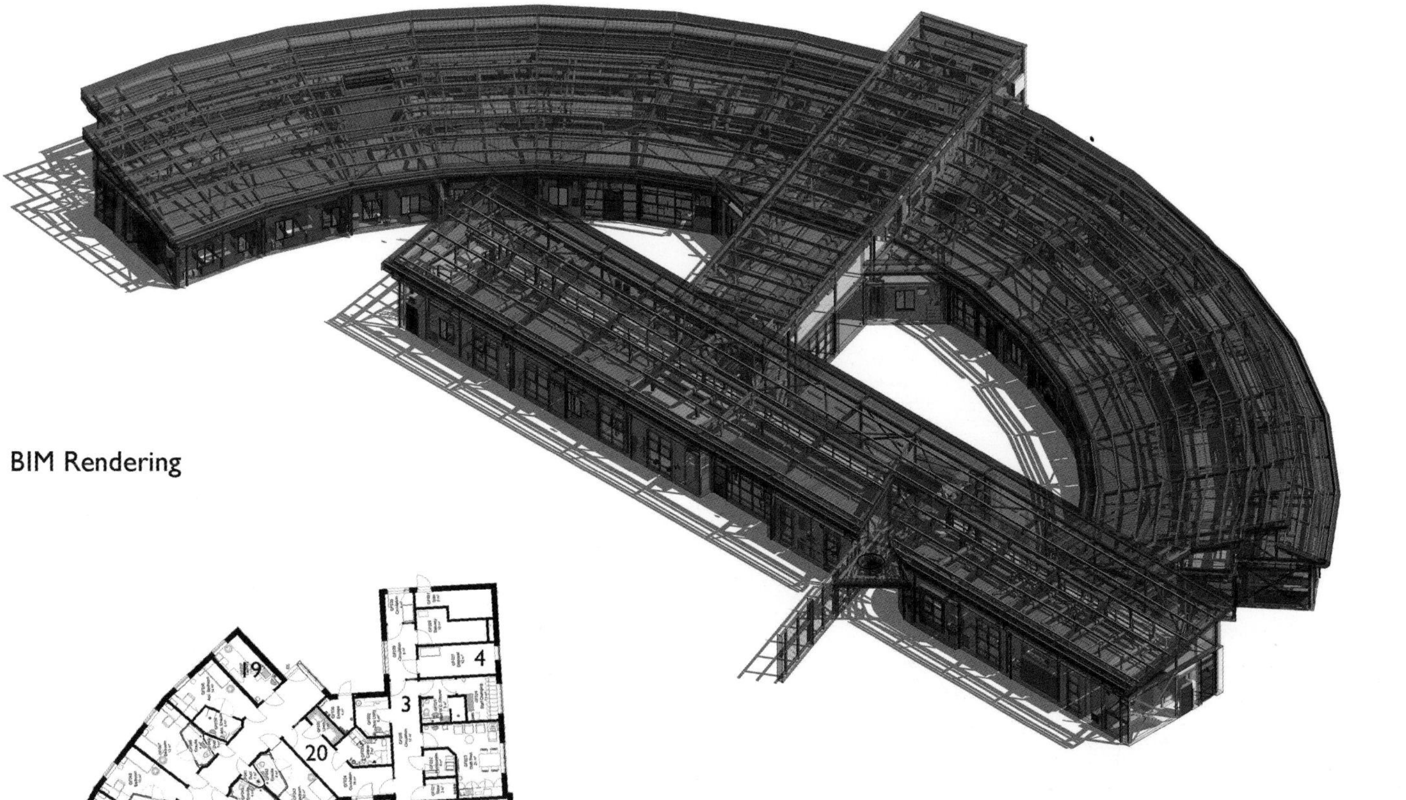

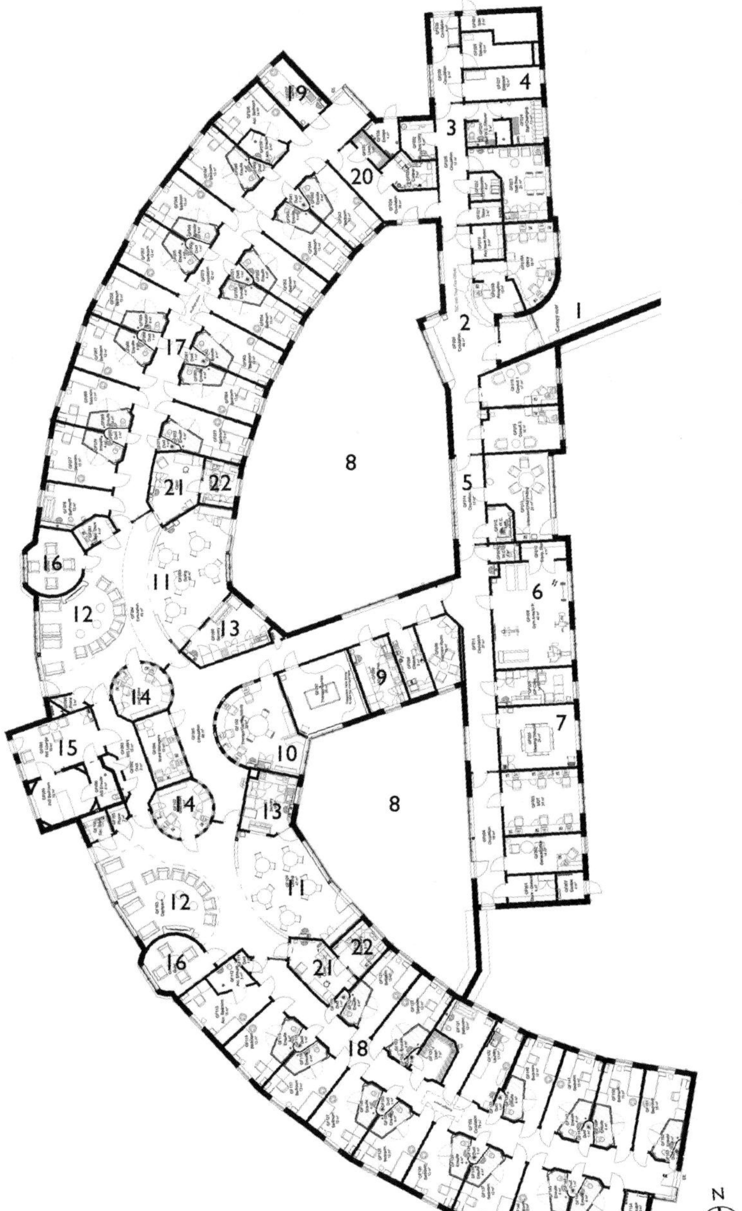

Main Level

Key:
1 main arrival
2 reception
3 administration
4 facility management
5 treatment/consultation
6 physical therapy/gymnasium
7 treatment/staff support
8 courtyard
9 ADL kitchen
10 treatment/activity
11 dining
12 dayroom
13 kitchen/servery
14 nursing/clinical support
15 seclusion unit
16 quiet room
17 acute care unit 1
18 acute care unit 2
19 laundry/linens
20 housekeeping
21 clinical support
22 pharmacy/dispensary

6.14.4a–b The curvature of the Lowry Unit's two residential wings is juxtaposed against a thin linear element (administration and therapy/treatment), and a diagonal connector (therapy/unit supports).

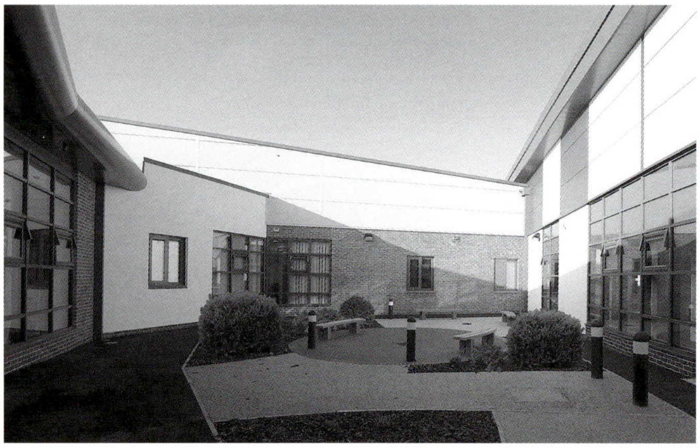

6.14.5 In a view of the (south) courtyard, looking toward the diagonal connector, seating, ground plantings, and paths are visible.

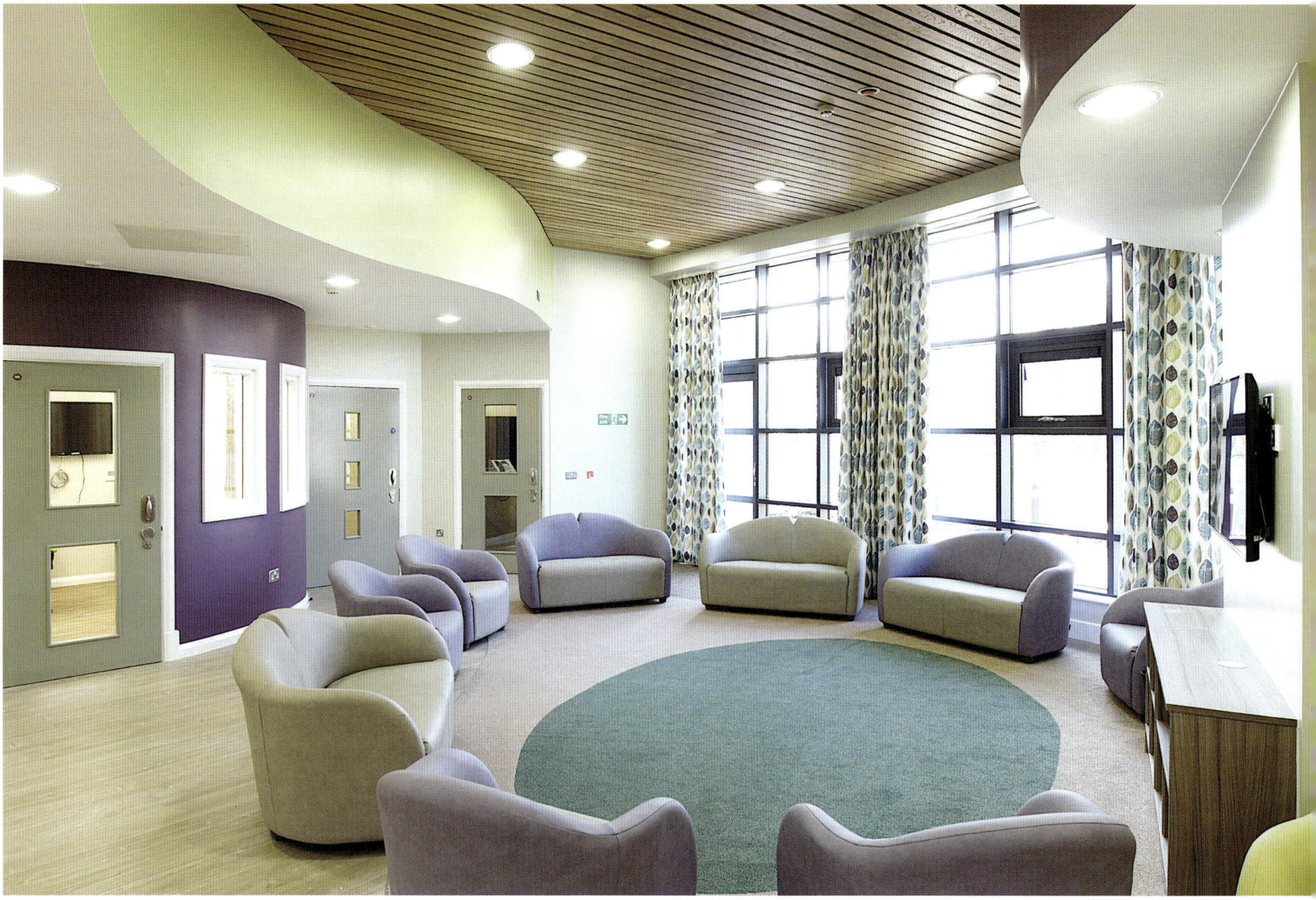

6.14.6 Group therapy rooms are spacious, with muted colors and curvilinear walls, ceiling, and floor surfaces.

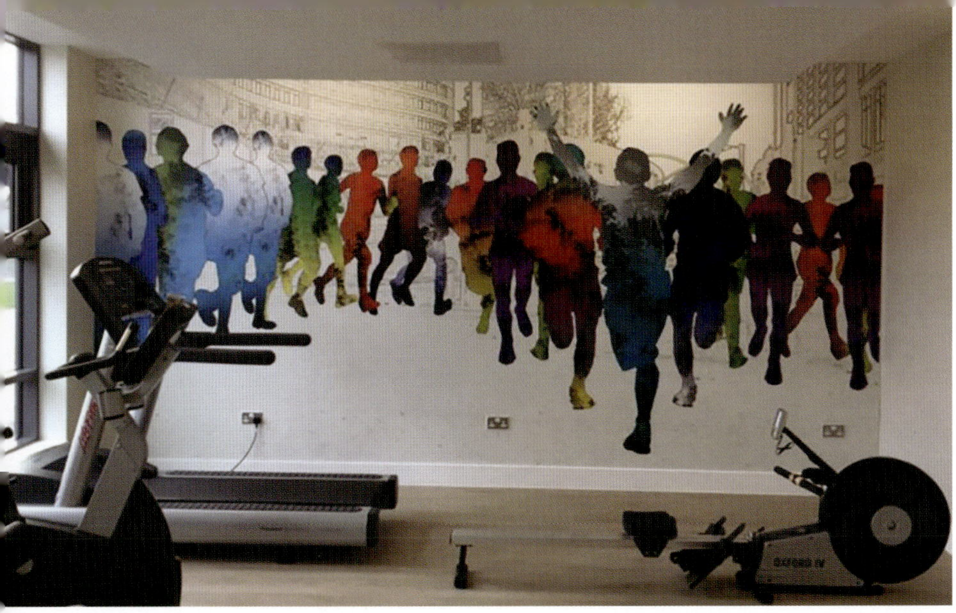

6.14.7 A recreational therapy room features a wall mural inspired by the Lowry Unit's artist namesake.

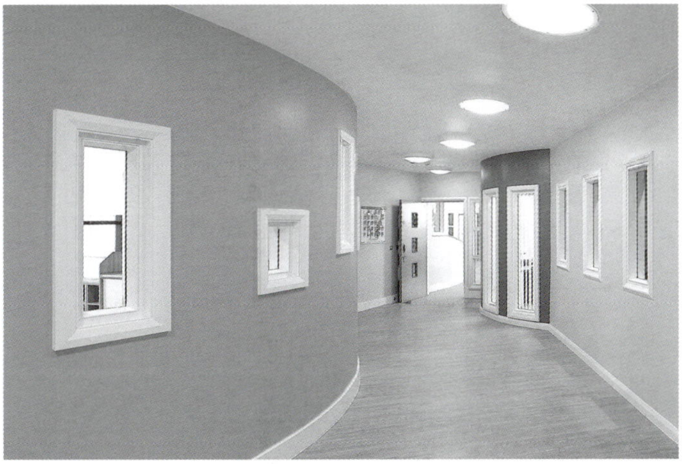

6.14.8 Corridors in various therapy/treatment areas feature curvilinear walls with residence-scaled windows and muted colors.

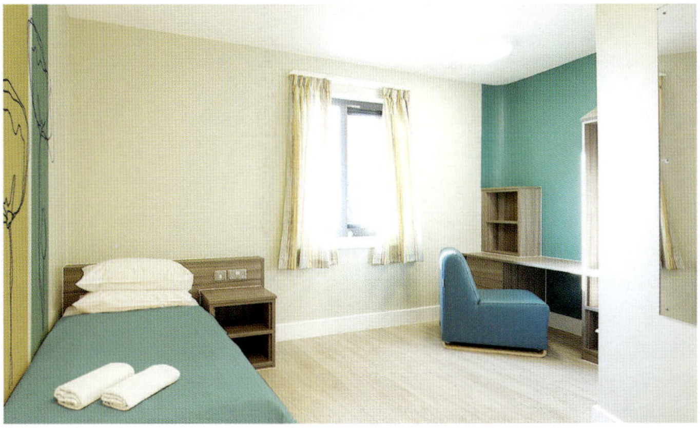

6.14.9 Patient rooms feature built-in furnishings, operable windows, and a private, diagonally shaped bath/shower unit.

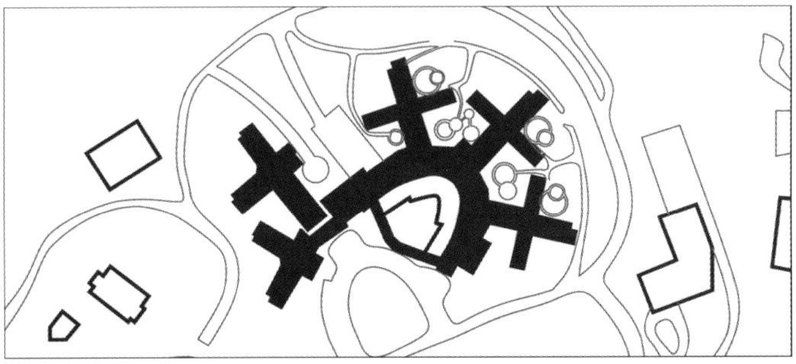

15 Worcester Recovery Center and Hospital, Worcester, Massachusetts, USA

ARCHITECT: Ellenzweig, Boston, Massachusetts, USA/architecture+, Troy, New York, USA
LANDSCAPE ARCHITECT: Horiuchi Solien, Inc., Falmouth, Massachusetts, USA
CLIENT: Massachusetts Department of Mental Health
FEATURED MATERIALS: Precast concrete panels, masonry, steel, glass
COMPLETED: 2012
INPATIENT BEDS: 320
SITE/PARKING: 44 acres/175
HOSPITAL/TREATMENT CENTER SIZE: 320,000 square feet
NURSES' WORKSTATION: Shielded

Context/site

The Worcester Recovery Center and Hospital (WRCH) was launched in 2005 when the State of Massachusetts, on an emergency basis, commissioned a replacement campus for individuals with serious mental illnesses, with emphasis on reintegration into the community with inpatient and partial hospitalization. The campus was built to replace the obsolete Worcester State Psychiatric Hospital, located immediately next door and near the University of Massachusetts Medical Center. The new campus was to reject the intuitionalism of the 19th-century asylum. A portion of the old asylum was retained, however, and the new campus obliquely acknowledges its physical presence (yet not its harsh legacy). It serves 260 adults and 60 adolescents and includes psychiatry, psychology, social work, and occupational therapy with nursing care, and medication education, as well as individual therapy, group therapy, and family counseling. The sweeping curvature of central 'main street' serves as the focus of the public realm and provides connections to five treatment units radiating outward obliquely from this spine. Residential units (wings) are three levels in height, with interior layouts nearly identical from floor to floor (Figure 6.15.1 and 6.15.2a–b).

The inpatient population consists of long-term residential patients and includes adolescent and adult forensic bed units. Components of daily life and treatment revolve around three principal realms: five individual *houses*, each connected to a discrete *neighborhood*, and in turn collectively linked to a *downtown* center. The campus plan was developed to draw patients outward from their specific residential unit and into the public realm, into exterior spaces that populate the zones between the five radiating units and various recreational therapy spaces. The planning process for this campus included the involvement of over 300 stakeholders, including community representatives, patients' rights advocates, the administration, psychiatrists, and a phalanx of specialized consultants, planners, and designers. The main 'street' five residential units function semi-independently, in terms of their general openness (within limits) and aesthetic (normative); the intent was to eschew any semblance of punitive or institutional architecture – and reject the now-demolished, forbidding walls of the old asylum. The grounds were landscaped with trees, paths, gardens, and informal seating areas (Figures 6.15.3 to 6.15.5).

Building/unit

The patient circulates from his or her residential unit into the nearest 'neighborhood', a zone of shared clinical services with emphasis on activities of daily living. Interdisciplinary care teams formulate an individualized program for each patient consisting of therapy, rehabilitation, and psychopharmacology. This concept of moving from private to public realms corresponds to being at times alone while at other times out immersed in social interactions (Figure 6.15.6a–b). The architects (architecture+) conceived of a campus whereby patient access to the *downtown* is available on a privileged (earned) basis, with 'downtown' functioning as an active zone with aggregated resources shared by the entire campus. Throughout the campus, spatial zones are configured to psychologically reinforce in patients that they live within a broader community that encourages them to look outward and to eventually emerge from this clinical inpatient setting into everyday normative life beyond.

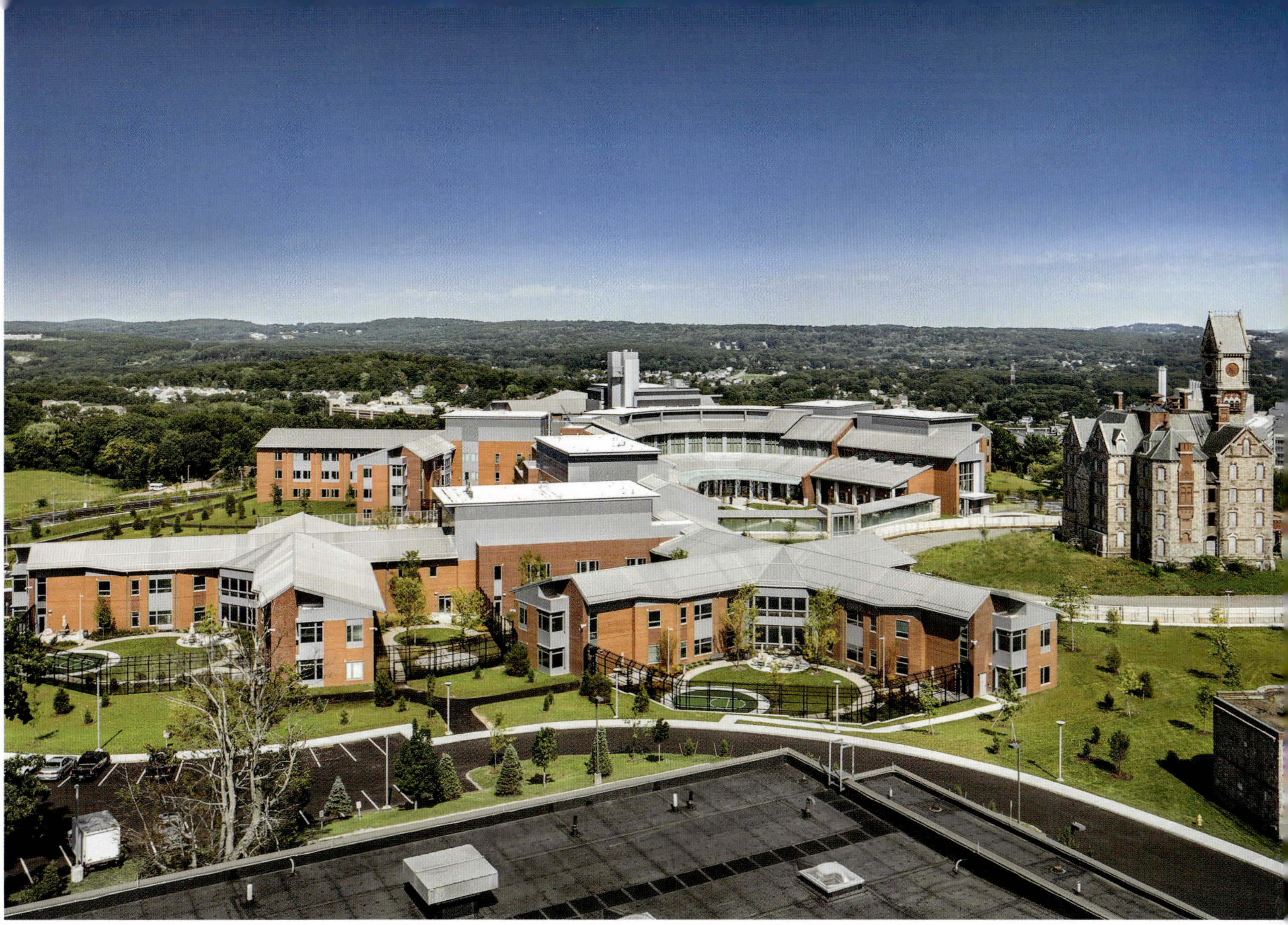

6.15.1 The Worcester Recovery Center and Hospital shown in relation to the heritage-protected remnants of the state-run asylum it replaced.

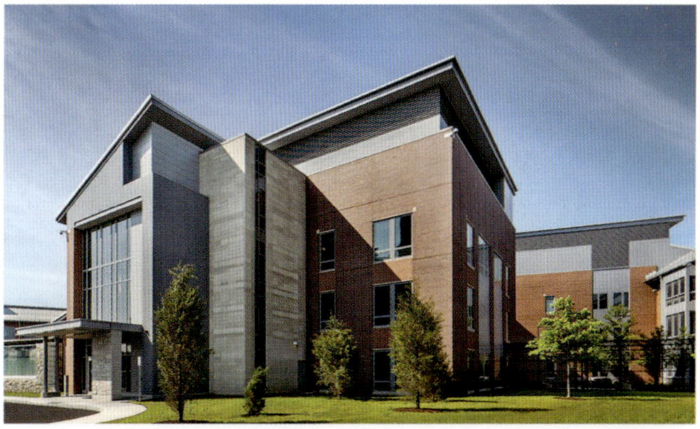

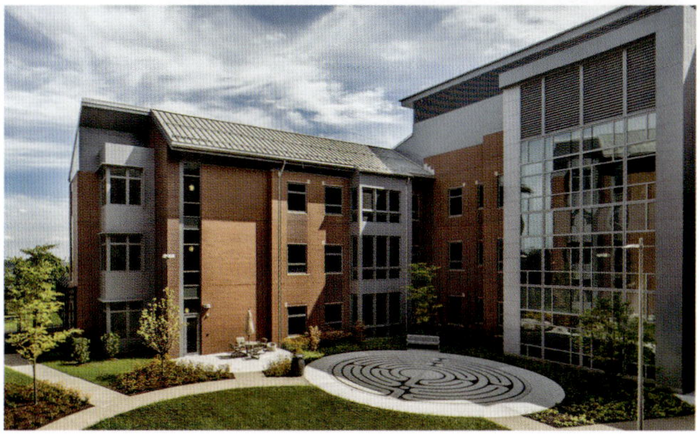

6.15.2a–b Residential units and exterior spaces provide opportunities for activities contemplative in nature compared to the publicness of the commons/courtyard at the campus center.

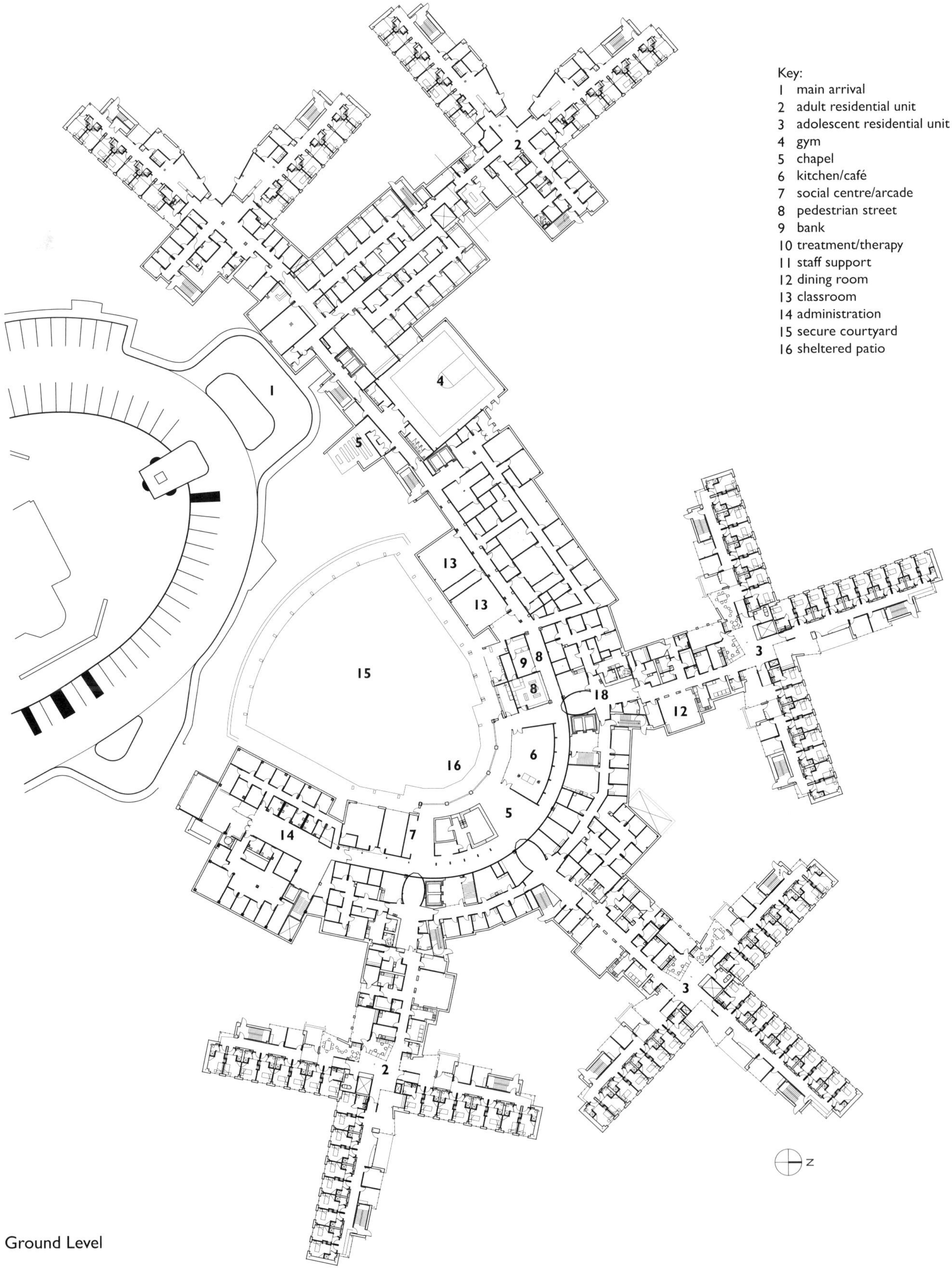

6.15.3 This replacement facility wraps around the old asylum, with a curvilinear spine connecting all constituent parts (neighborhoods) into a unified whole, with the commons (town square) at center.

Key:
1 entry to unit from adjacent unit
2 dining
3 housekeeping/support/charting
4 kitchen
5 team/conference
6 nurses' workstation
7 staff/administration
8 activity/recreation
9 screened porch
10 consultation
11 quiet room
12 residential unit

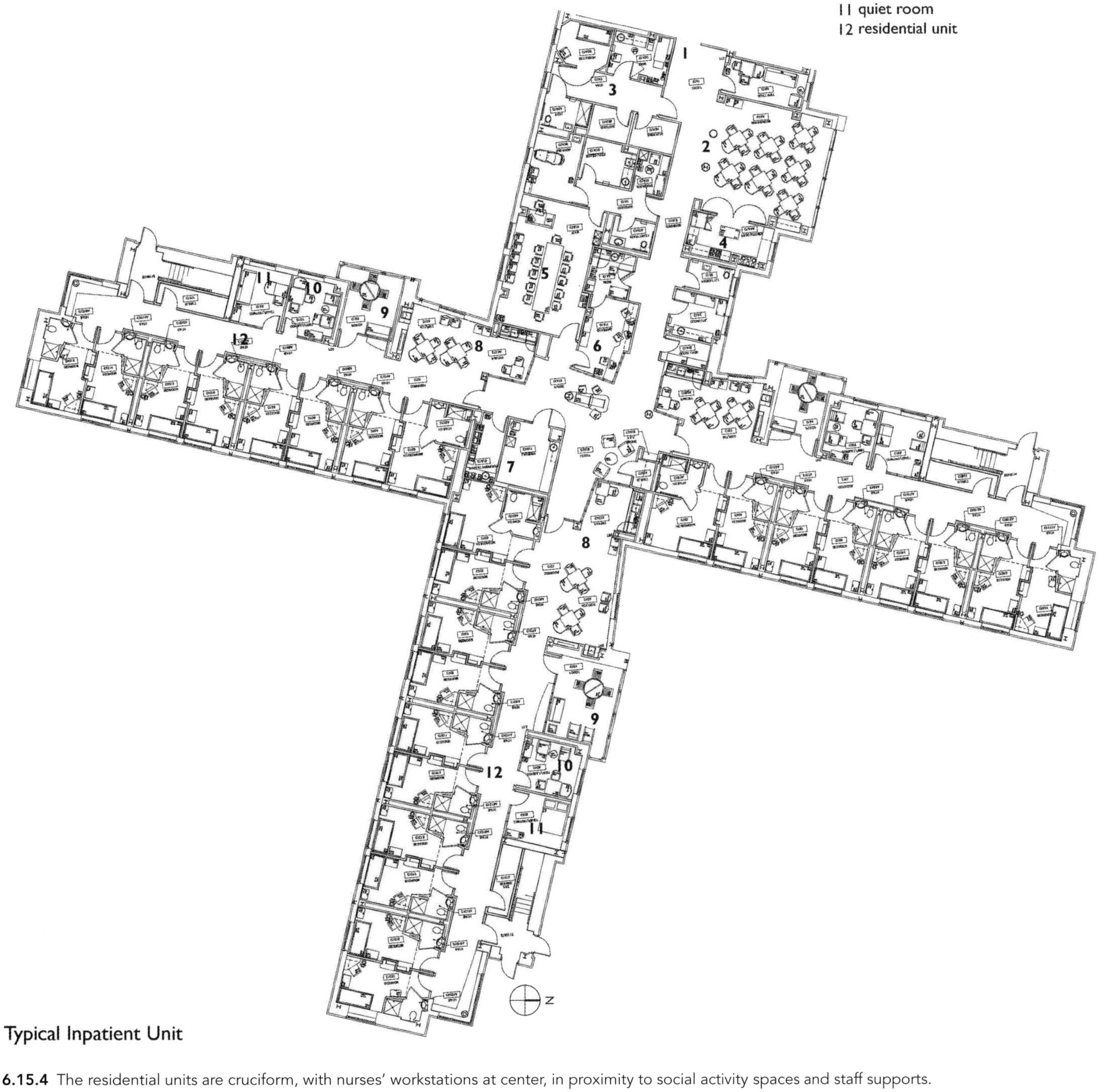

Typical Inpatient Unit

6.15.4 The residential units are cruciform, with nurses' workstations at center, in proximity to social activity spaces and staff supports.

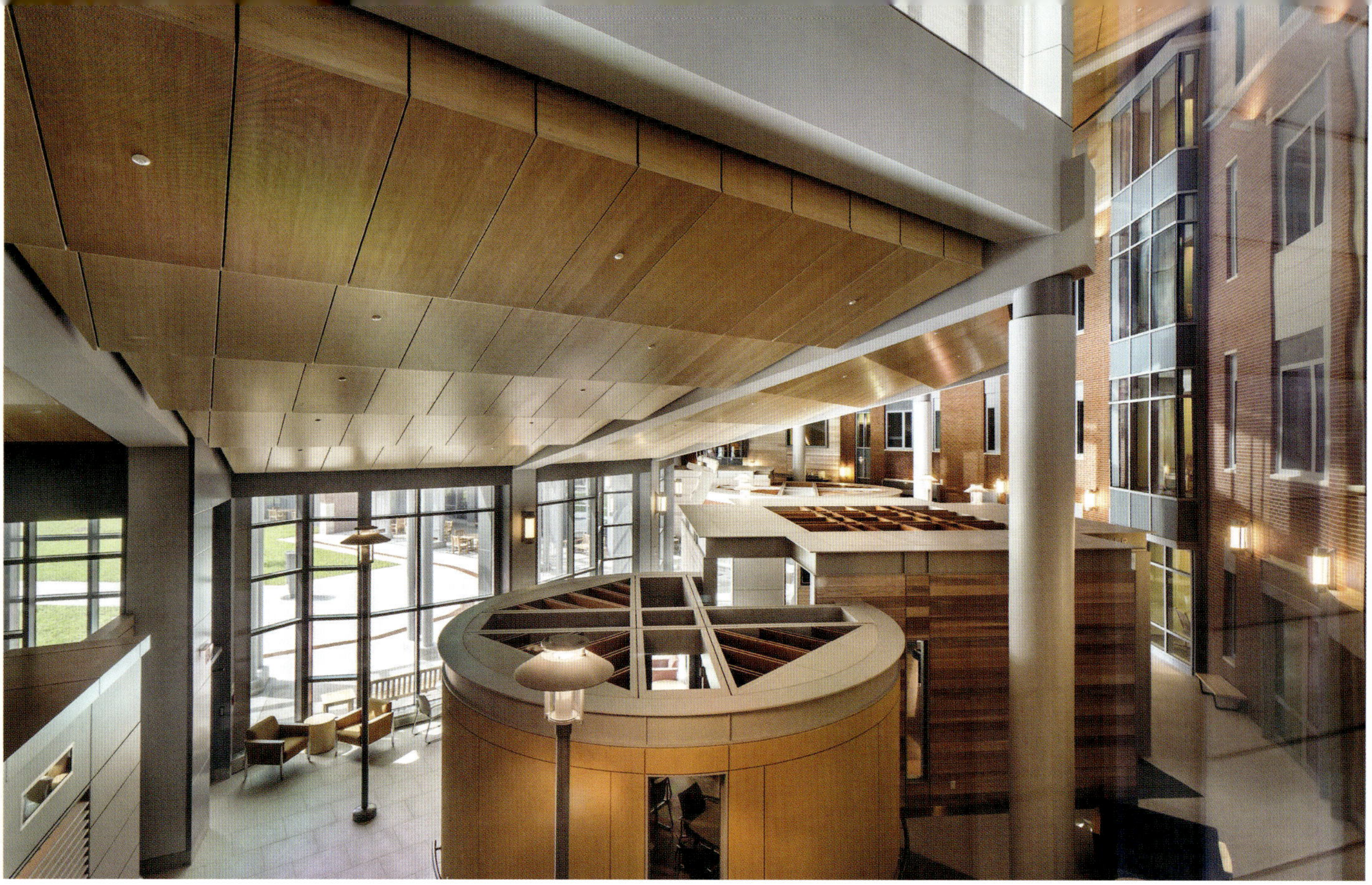

6.15.5 Freestanding pavilions are placed within a superordinate volume at the heart of the public realm.

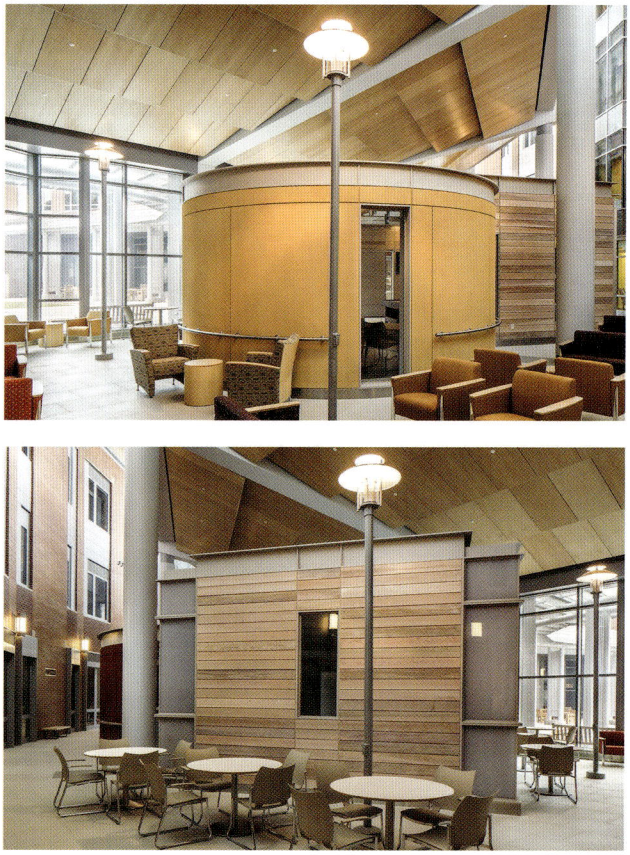

6.15.6a–b The autonomous pavilions house a bank, clothing store, and other 'everyday' activities, along a 'main street'.

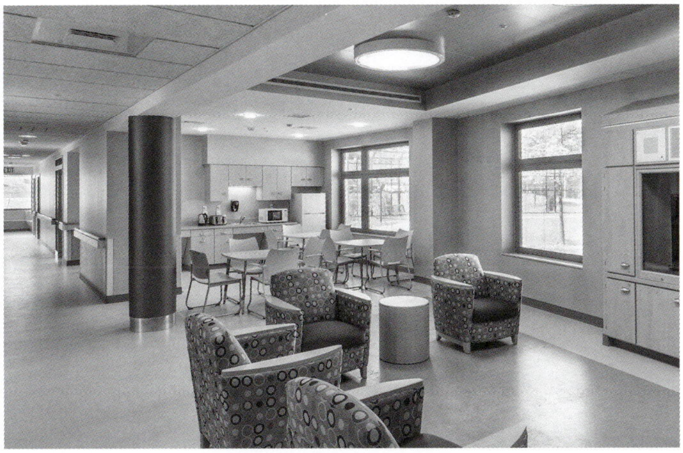

6.15.7 The dining areas on residential units are informal, with varied furnishings, and a satellite (remote) kitchen.

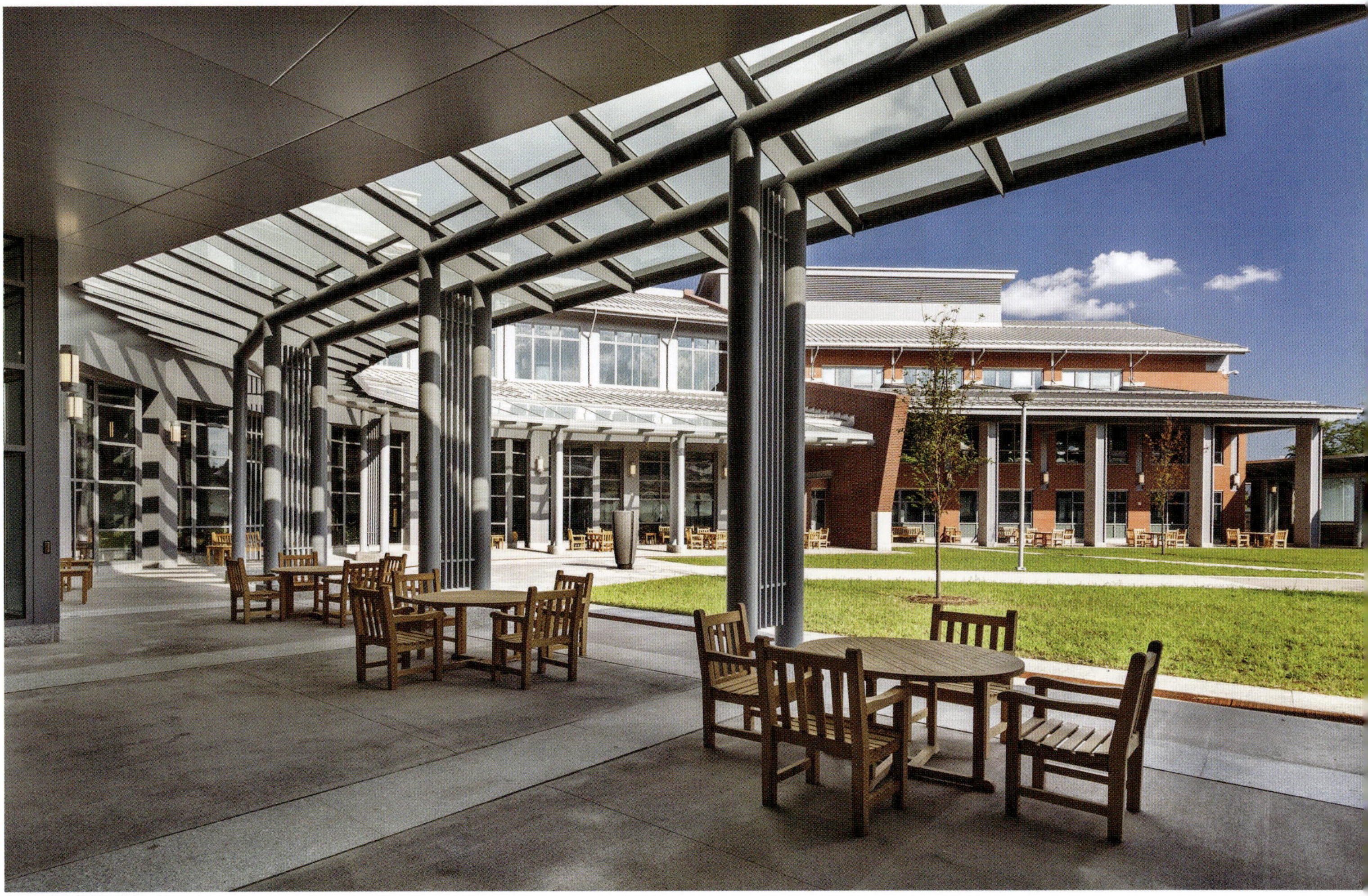

6.15.8 The main commons (square) is flanked by a sheltered terrace and skylight canopy.

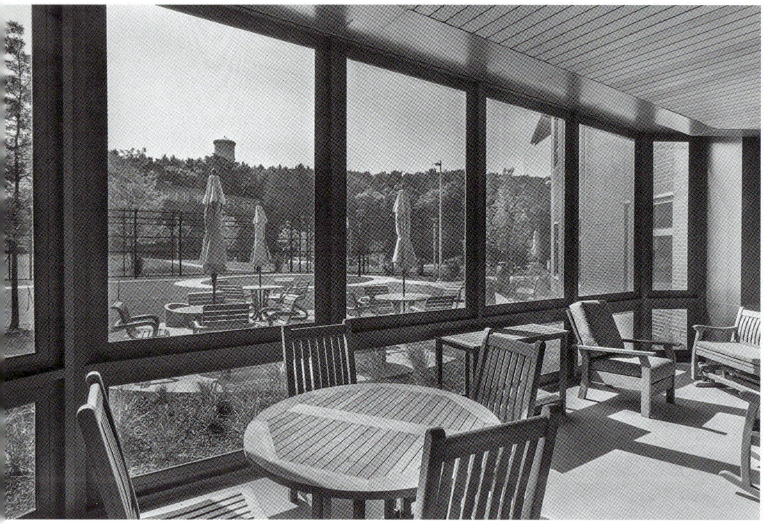

6.15.9 Activity rooms overlook exterior spaces, functioning as extensions of the interior realm.

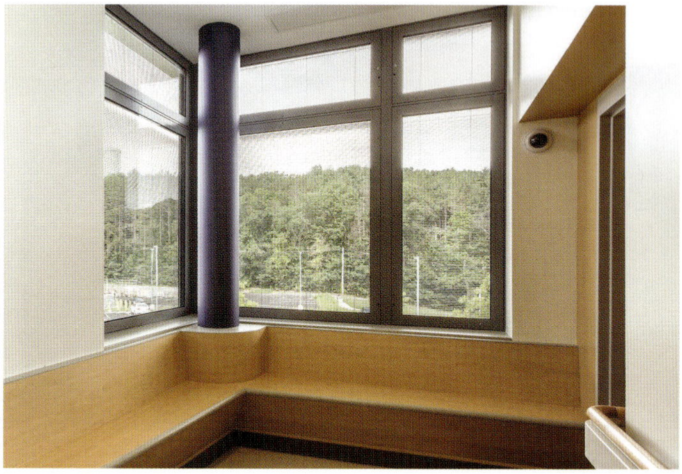

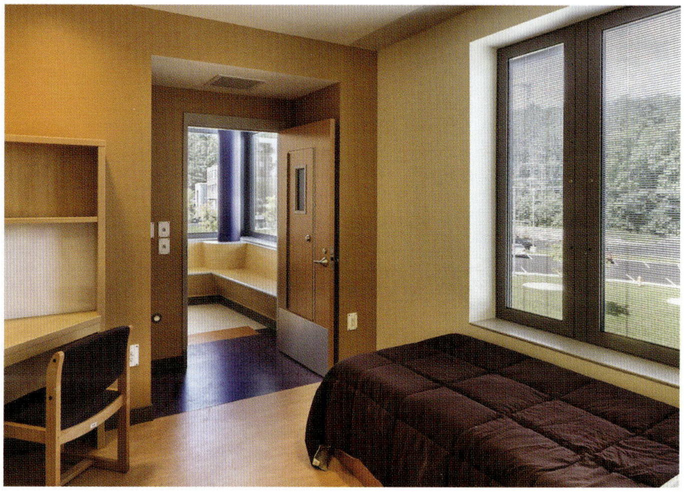

6.15.10a–b A window seat (outer alcove space) is located next to a patient room, with bed positioned beneath a large operable window. Note the inset (security) door.

The daily treatment regimen encourages the patient to take an active role in this process. The central 'village green' is more 'municipal' and public by nature, and recalls the imagery of a main square in a New England village. Located in this zone, the stained-glass windows of the nondenominational chapel were designed at the University of Massachusetts Adolescent Continuing Care Unit, in collaboration with a commissioned artist who resides in North Carolina.

In the residential units, patient rooms are private and clustered in proximity to an active (social) zone, and a passive (quiet) zone, with a living room/dayroom at the center. Each grouping of bedrooms consists of 8–10 patients residing within a larger, 26-bed unit. Patient rooms have dormitory furnishings, including a desk, storage shelving, and a bed positioned along the outer perimeter wall, with large, operable windows and sill heights low enough to allow full view sight lines. Doors to the patient room are multifaceted – that is, designed with an *insert door* to counter the occurrence of an adverse event taking place within the room. The nurses' station is semisequestered (physically bracketed/protected) due to a high-security requirement throughout the five neighborhoods (i.e., five groupings of three units each). As mentioned, the 'downtown' realm is the most socially active and public with its 'street' and 'square' at the center (Figures 6.15.7 and 6.15.8). This realm consists of a café, arcade, store, bank, meeting rooms, theater, music room, and health club, surrounded by more passive activities – the aforementioned chapel, greenhouse, as well as a library, and art therapy room. These are configured as small freestanding structures within a larger pavilion – not entirely unlike small elements placed within a commercial big-box store's overall envelope. The WRCH received LEED Gold certification for innovative water conservation measures, health-promoting interior living and treatment spaces, low-maintenance and long-life materials of construction, reduced environmental emissions and waste recycling programs, smart building-management IT-systems integration and commissioning process, and rainwater harvesting campus irrigation system (Figures 6.15.9 and 6.15.10a–b).

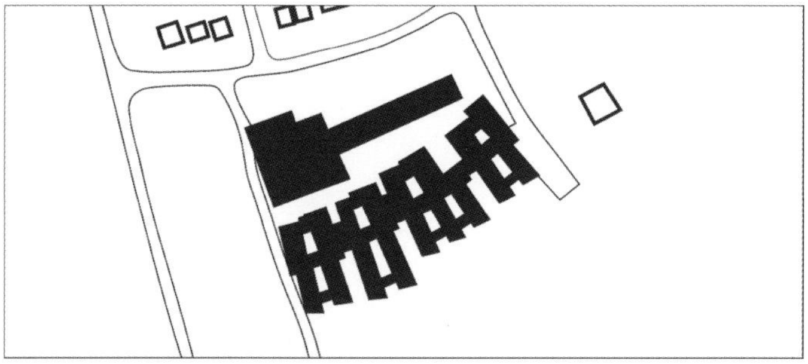

16 Ferndene Children and Young People's Centre, Northumberland, Prudhoe, Newcastle-upon-Tyne, UK

ARCHITECT: MAAP (Medical Architecture and Arts Projects, Ltd.), London, UK
LANDSCAPE ARCHITECT: MAAP, London, UK
CLIENT: Northumberland, Tyne and Wear NHS Foundation
FEATURED MATERIALS: Masonry, slate, glass, wood
COMPLETED: 2011
INPATIENT BEDS: 44
SITE/PARKING: 300 acres/55
HOSPITAL/TREATMENT CENTER SIZE: 74,000 square feet
NURSES' WORKSTATION: Hybrid

Context/site

Set in a rural landscape near Newcastle, England, this treatment center provides pediatric (ages 4–18) mental health and rehabilitation services, with length of stays varying from a few weeks to 3 years. The planning and consultation process took 2 years and included the appraisal of numerous buildable sites across the region. Ferndene was built on a portion of open space on the venerable Prudhoe Hospital campus. Prudhoe is a former psychiatric hospital dating from 1913. Over many decades, it had fallen into a state of dilapidation and is currently nearly fully abandoned, although the old buildings remains just to the east, and the grounds' open space and natural setting was deemed to be equally viable in the 21st century; additionally, the NHS still owned the land. In response, a one-level residential hospital was constructed with the aim of a boarding school–inspired campus, informal in appearance and aesthetic, in a natural setting. Locating the Ferndene campus on this particular site allowed for program consolidation and also the option of retaining and repurposing the existing heritage buildings to new, allied uses.

Ferndene was seen by the NHS as the benchmark for a new generation of pediatric mental health care facilities in the United Kingdom. Works of art, natural color palettes, sustainability, ecological awareness, and connections to place and local history were of priority. These priorities are visible beginning at the main entrance and continue throughout the campus. The design response balances security standards (low security) while fostering a normative atmosphere of 'domesticity'. This was of high importance in the eyes of the facility's (future) daily users, throughout the consultation process (Figures 6.16.1 and 6.16.2). Fixtures, equipment, and material palettes, safe and durable without appearing overtly institutional, were integrated into the composition. Four inpatient units provide 24/7 services (Figures 6.16.3 and 6.16.4): Riding, a 6-bed unit for assessment and treatment; Redburn, a 14-bed unit for treatment of early onset psychosis and complex mental illness (plus four intensive care beds for emergency use); Fraser, a 12-bed unit for individuals with severe developmental and learning disabilities; and Stephenson, an 8-bed low-security unit for treatment of mild to moderate learning disabilities. Since young persons with learning disabilities often exhibit a propensity to also suffer from depression and psychosis, for this reason these services were colocated on the campus, and an integrated service model was implemented. This model is equal parts therapy based and rehabilitation based, with the goal of increasing the probability of discharged patients' success in everyday life following hospitalization.

Building/unit

The architectural team visited the Hazelwood School in Glasgow and Richard Murphy's Harmeny School in Edinburgh, Scotland, both youth-centric facilities set in naturalistic surroundings. The design team also visited Chalkhill, in West Sussex, and the North Wales Adolescent Unit. The initial (generative) design concept was a *hand with fingers* represented by inpatient residential units fanning out from a central activity building, referred to as the *palm*. A public-to-private gradient was established at the main entrance, beginning with a positive first impression for patients and visitors (Figure 6.16.5 to 6.16.8). Circulation within various 'fingers' parallels courtyards with gardens and transitions from the public realm to group therapy and social and recreational zones to the relative privacy of the residential units. The living/dayrooms are located at the 'fingertips' nearest the woods. Throughout, flexible spaces were of priority. From the architects' brief,

> The range of patient ages and needs, from long-term severe learning disabilities to detainees under the UK Mental Health

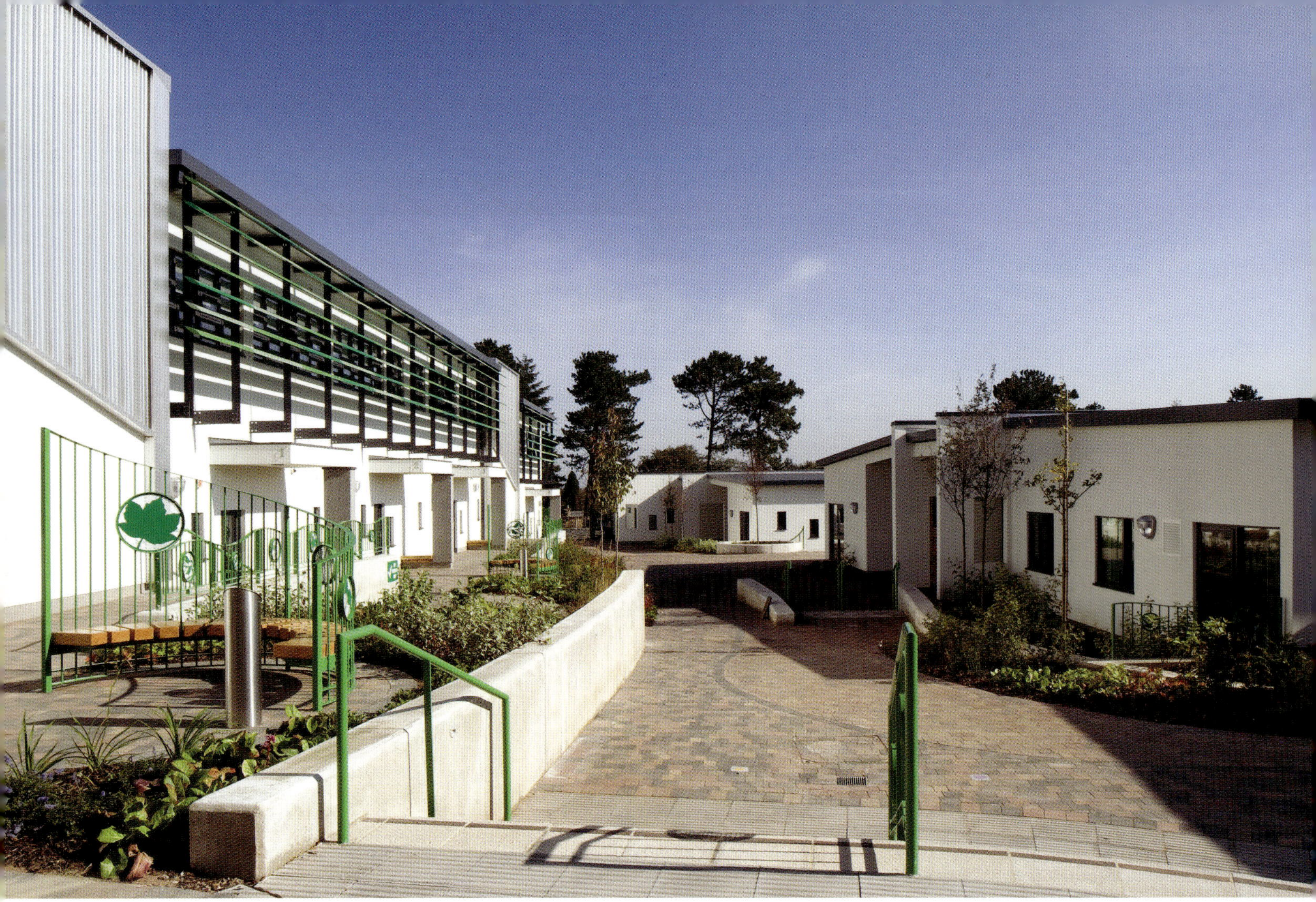

6.16.1 A terraced arrival courtyard at the Ferndene Centre connects the therapy/treatment and residential unit realms.

> Act, led to a number of physical challenges. It was agreed that shared amenities to foster an atmosphere of site-wide integration should be paramount, although separation of patient groups to offer safe and secure boundaries would also be of necessity . . . the challenge was to not create a sense of incarceration, with high walls and fences.

The main artery is referred to as the 'street' and is actually a semipublic forecourt partially shielded from the outer world on one side by the activity center, a building that houses social, therapy, and recreational supports. The separation of the residential from the nonresidential realms distinguishes 'home' from 'school' living/activity zones. As for the residential realm, located across from the activity center, it is accessed via the forecourt. Every patient room is private, with a private bath/shower unit located on the inboard side along the corridor. Bedrooms are clustered along single-loaded corridors overlooking 'pocket' courtyards. There, artworks and places to sit informally are provided, informed by the site's topography and enhanced with plantings. Residential wings double as a security perimeter, precluding the need for a surrounding, freestanding, impenetrable perimeter barrier. The nurses' station on each unit is a hybrid type, insofar as it combines a shielded area with a nearby decentralized staff work zone. Patient rooms are finished with a built-in bed, window seat, desk, and storage closet. The windows are operable, and color-accented walls provide visual relief (Figure 6.16.9a–b). As for eco-sustainability features, most spaces are naturally ventilated and transmit ample light, thereby minimizing overreliance on conventional HVAC systems. Ferndene received a BREEAM 'excellence rating' for its building-management system, a system operated off-site from NHS headquarters in Gosforth, for its role in reducing carbon emission levels. All floor finishes are 100% recyclable and paint finishes are 100% VOC free. Reclaimed slate was used to clad some building exteriors, numerous other recycled building materials were used in construction, and a bank of solar panels is situated atop the main activity building. Also, the provision of birdcages and constructed habitats will, it is anticipated, provide support to local endangered animal species on the campus.

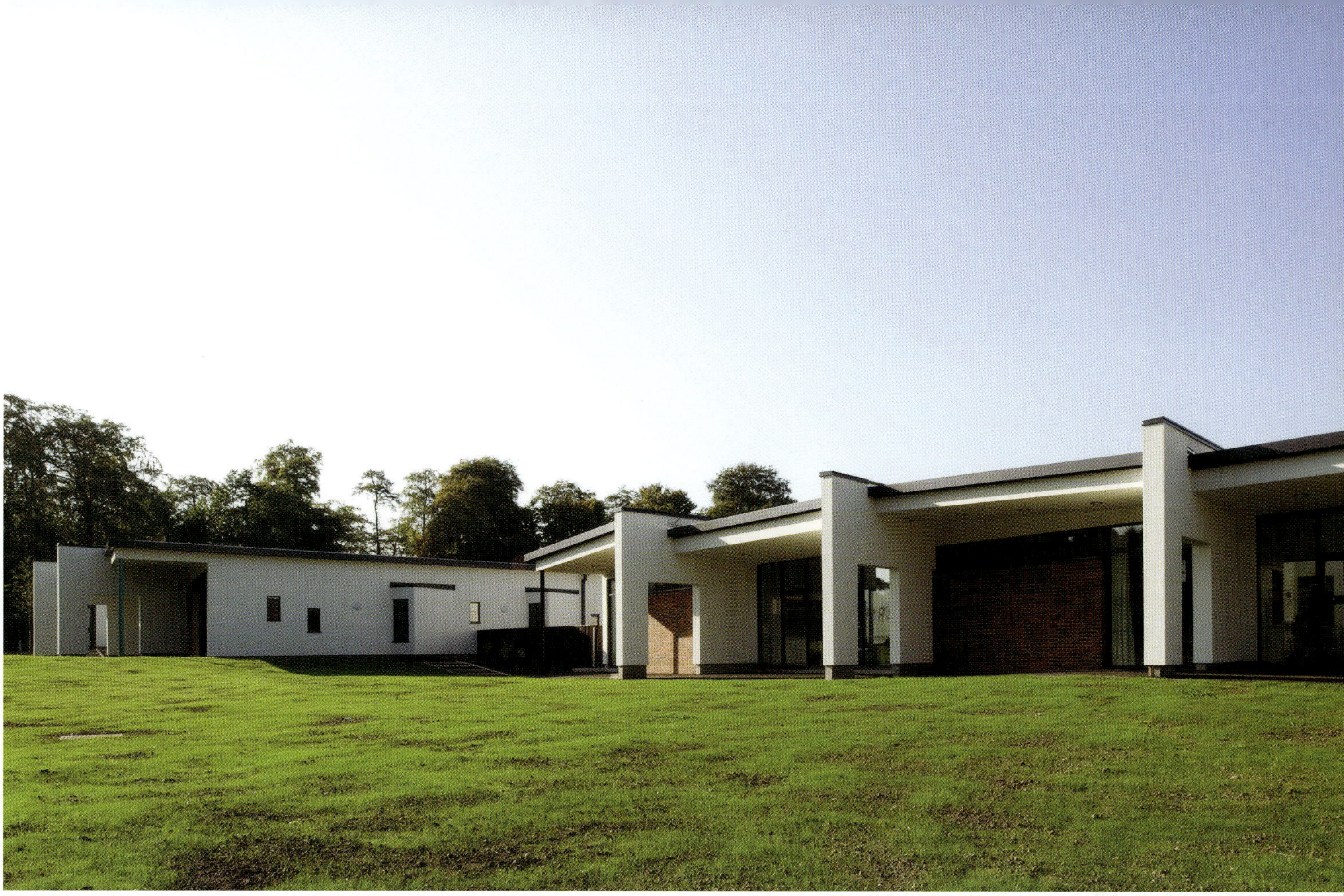

6.16.2 Ferndene Centre is low scaled with extended roof eaves affording sheltered space for patients' use outdoors.

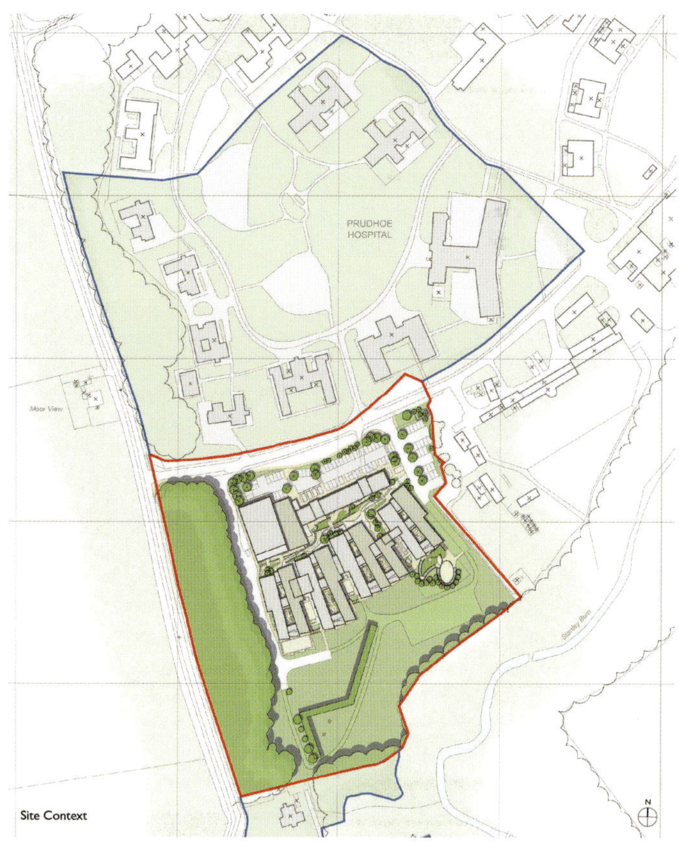

6.16.3 Ferndene Centre was built next to the old (since repurposed) Prudhoe Hospital, on a portion of the grounds owned by the NHS.

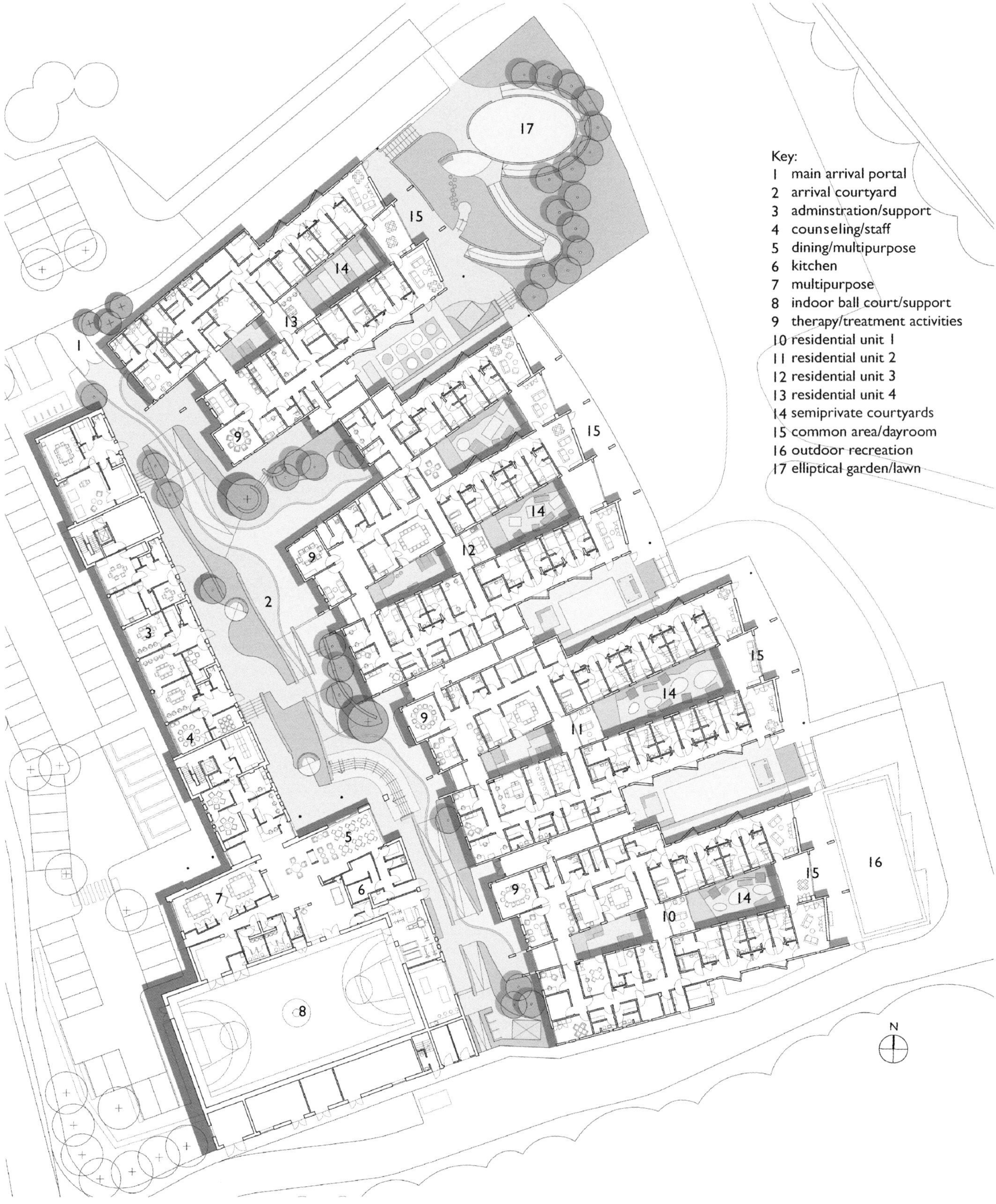

Site Plan/Main Level

6.16.4 The therapy/treatment building is located at left (in plan), residential units to the right, with arrival/connecting courtyard at the center.

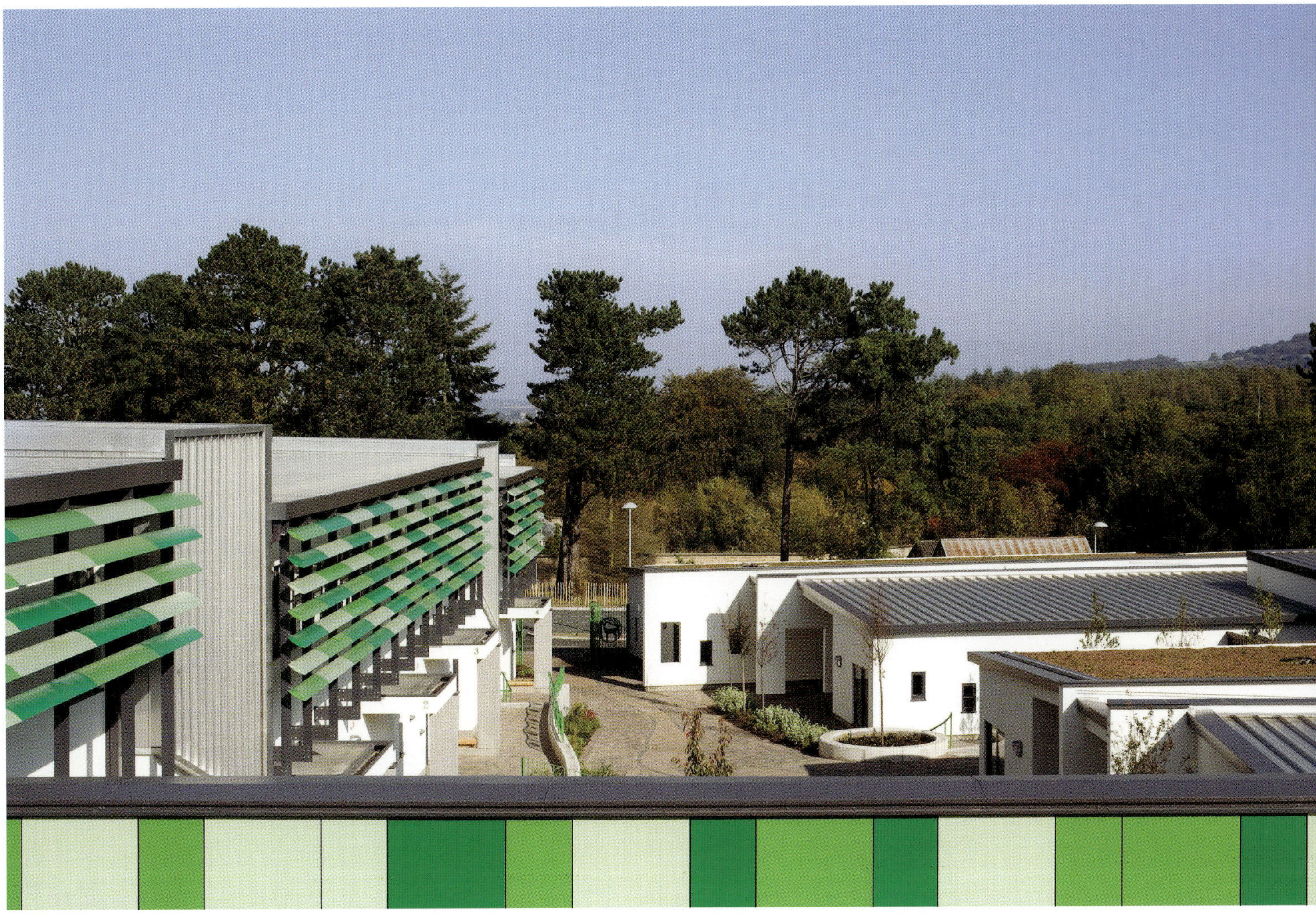

6.16.5 Residential units are one level, with stepped massings, directly across from the therapy/treatment/administration building with its green-tinted sunscreens.

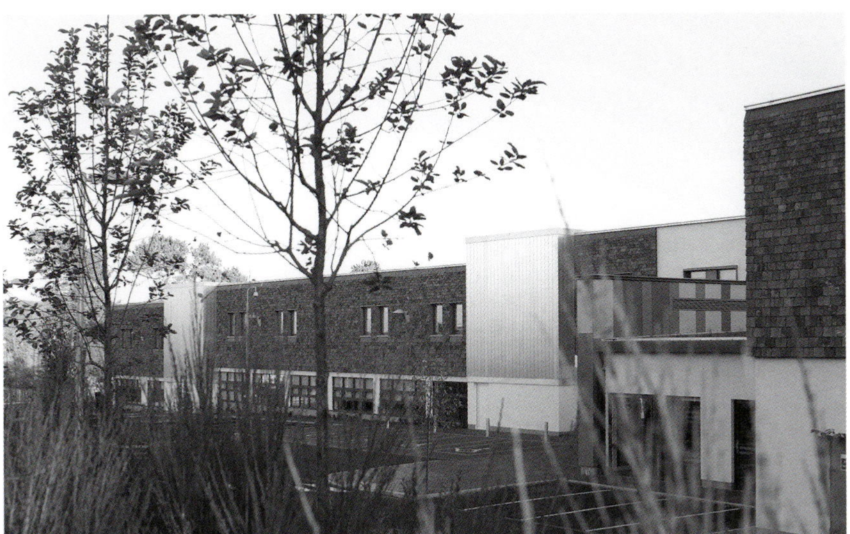

6.16.6 The therapy/treatment areas adjoin exterior spaces for patients' use.

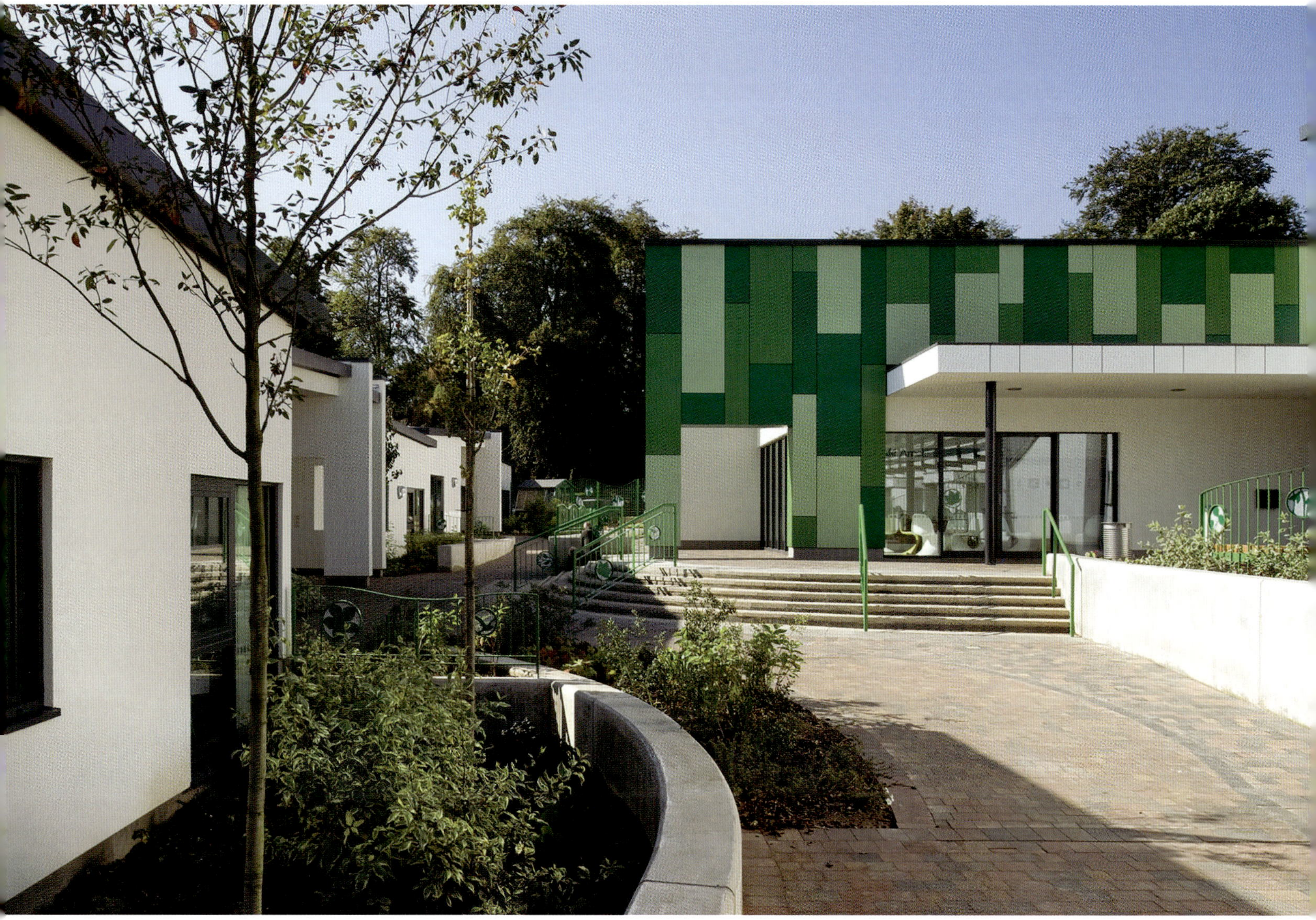

6.16.7 The arrival forecourt features ground plantings, level changes, and inviting imagery.

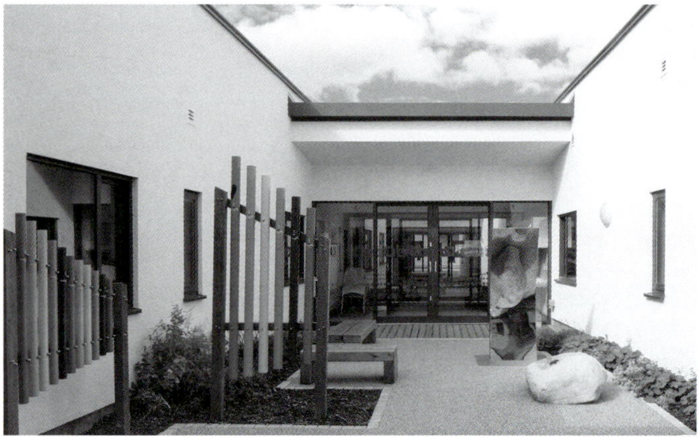

6.16.8 Exterior pocket courtyards are situated between the wings of the residential units.

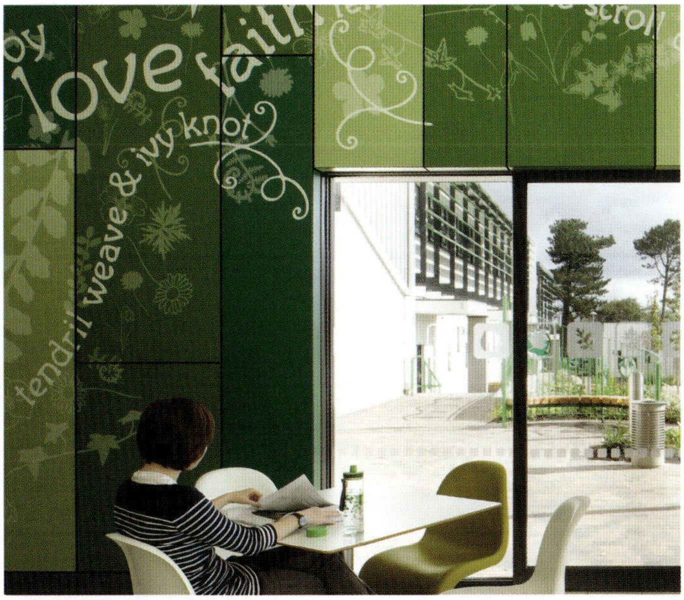

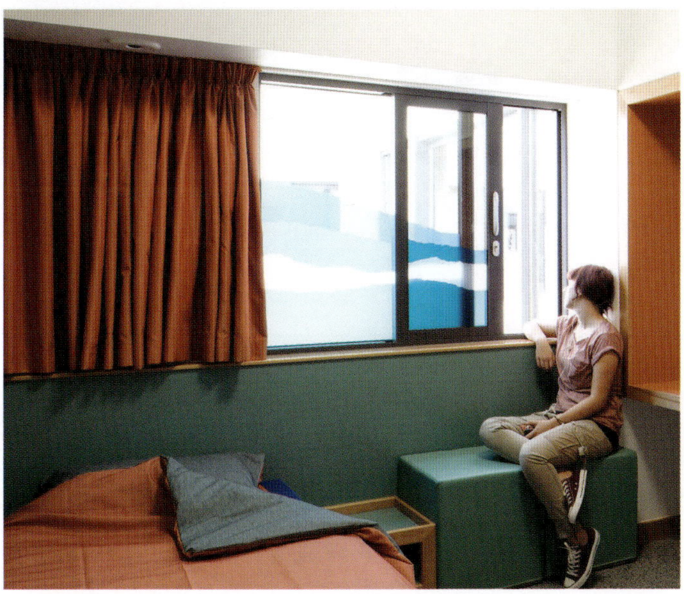

6.16.9a–b Activity areas on the residential units feature wall graphics and doors connecting to the exterior (top), and patient room furnishings are built-in, with operable windows (bottom).

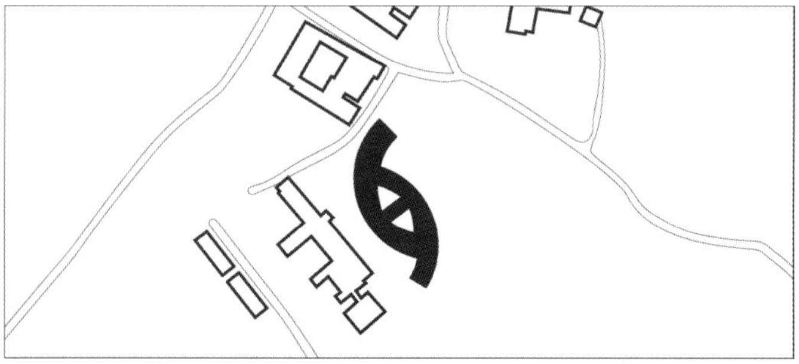

17 Junction 17, Prestwich, Greater Manchester, England, UK

ARCHITECT: Gilling Dod Architects, Lancashire, UK
LANDSCAPE ARCHITECT: Gilling Dod Architects, Lancashire, UK
CLIENT: Greater Manchester West Mental Health NHS Foundation Trust
FEATURED MATERIALS: Composite timber cladding
COMPLETED: 2013
INPATIENT BEDS: 24
SITE/PARKING: 12 acres/32
HOSPITAL/TREATMENT CENTER SIZE: 52,000 square feet
NURSES' WORKSTATION: Shielded

Context/site

Junction 17 is located near the Lowry Unit and the Edenfield Centre near Manchester, United Kingdom. After considering multiple sites, it was decided to build on the same site as the facility it replaced – the McGuinness Unit. This 1962 facility had fallen into obsolescence because it lacked adequate patient privacy, was grim in atmosphere, fostered chronic absconding attempts, had inadequate therapy and activity zones, and a history of violent patient incidents. It has experienced stigmatized as a psychiatric care environment, plagued in later years with high readmittance rates, and its physical setting had increasingly fostered poor staff retention rates and low morale. It also lacked sufficient bed capacity for out-of-area patient referrals, suffered from an obsolete HVAC system and poor acoustics, and was fraught throughout with fire code hazards. Junction 17 was built quite literally in its shadow. When completed, the old building was demolished and that site transformed into a new circular drive, parking area, arrival court, and green space. With the McGuinness Unit now gone, the site was far less constricted, save for the continued presence of the Gardener Unit and John Denmark Unit, both immediately located to the west of the Junction 17 facility.

This replacement facility provides mental health assessment and treatment for persons aged 13–17 at high risk to themselves and others, and persons who suffer from learning disabilities that manifest in various behavioural disorders, including eating disorders, depression, psychosis, bipolar disorder, substance abuse, and dual diagnoses. The treatment program consists of activities of daily living, cognitive-behavioural therapy, family therapy, and art and music therapy. The new facility was inserted into an indisputably tight site. This was accomplished by developing a crescent-shaped footprint in order to weave it around existing buildings in close proximity, also making for a challenging construction sequence, where every measure had to be taken to ensure ongoing construction activity would not interfere with ongoing operations in nearby buildings (Figures 6.17.1 and 6.17.2). The new building's sweeping curvilinearity was therefore no accident, serving a dual purpose. Its sweeping footprint was determined by the site's narrowness as much as by a rejection of the institutionalism of what it replaced. Junction 17 could be everything its predecessor was not. It could be informal, achieving connectivity with nature in a normative, quasi-residential atmosphere, and above all be human scaled, all unachievable in the old hospital.

Building/unit

Upon arrival, one encounters a series of diagonal wall planes that appear to project outward. One such planar element signals the main entrance, although from this specific vantage point it is difficult to envision the overall curvature of the building. Inside, curvature reduces the perceived length of otherwise long corridors, as it is impossible to look from one end directly to the opposite end. This device allowed interior space to wrap around itself, to an extent, insofar as two courtyards were carved out at the center, bisected by a symmetrically positioned connector element that houses dining, kitchen, therapy/counseling, and related staff supports. The nurses' stations are positioned at opposing end points where the corridors intersect, with a third workstation positioned at the center. Overall, the circulation diagram is a racetrack, in plan, with multiple routes available to navigate from a highly trafficked Point A to a Point B destination. The main level houses administration and central supports (Figure 6.17.3a–c). Most rooms are situated along the double-loaded circulation segments, with the exception of the main arrival zone, as this parallels a courtyard. Spaces feature color accents and residential-like operable windows

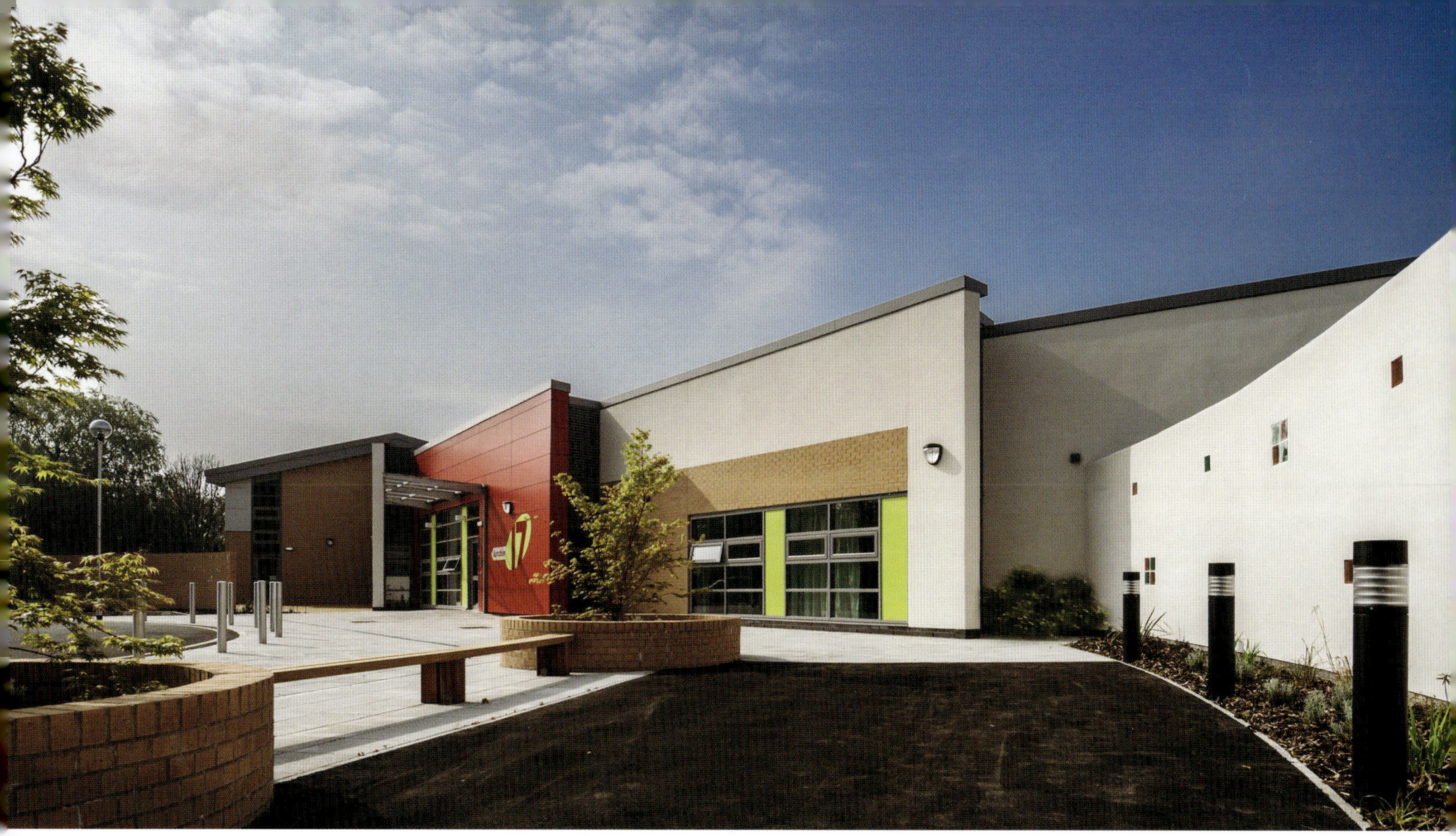

6.17.1 The front façade at Junction 17 pediatric psychiatry center consists of segmented, angular wall planes.

6.17.2 The partí consists of two intersecting, interlocking arcs, yielding extended wings, with a double-loaded connector at midsection.

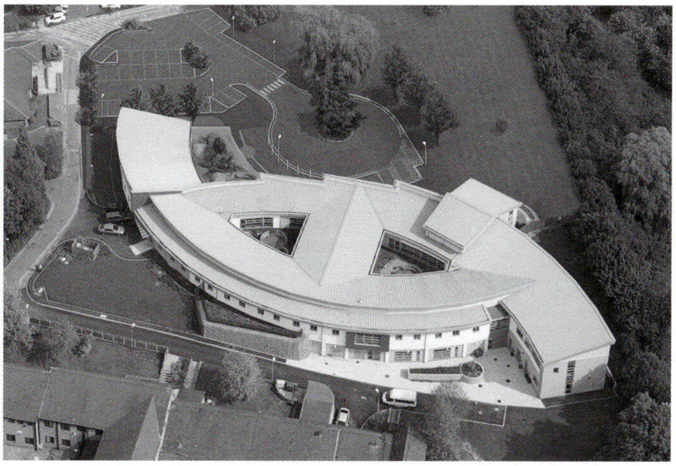

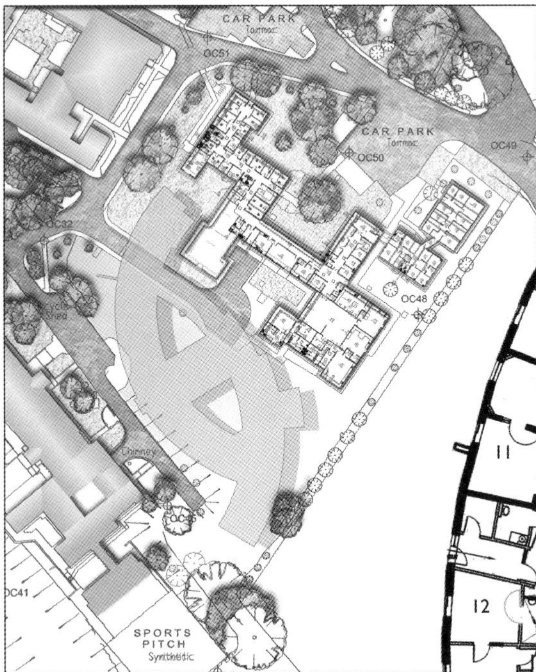

Site Plan

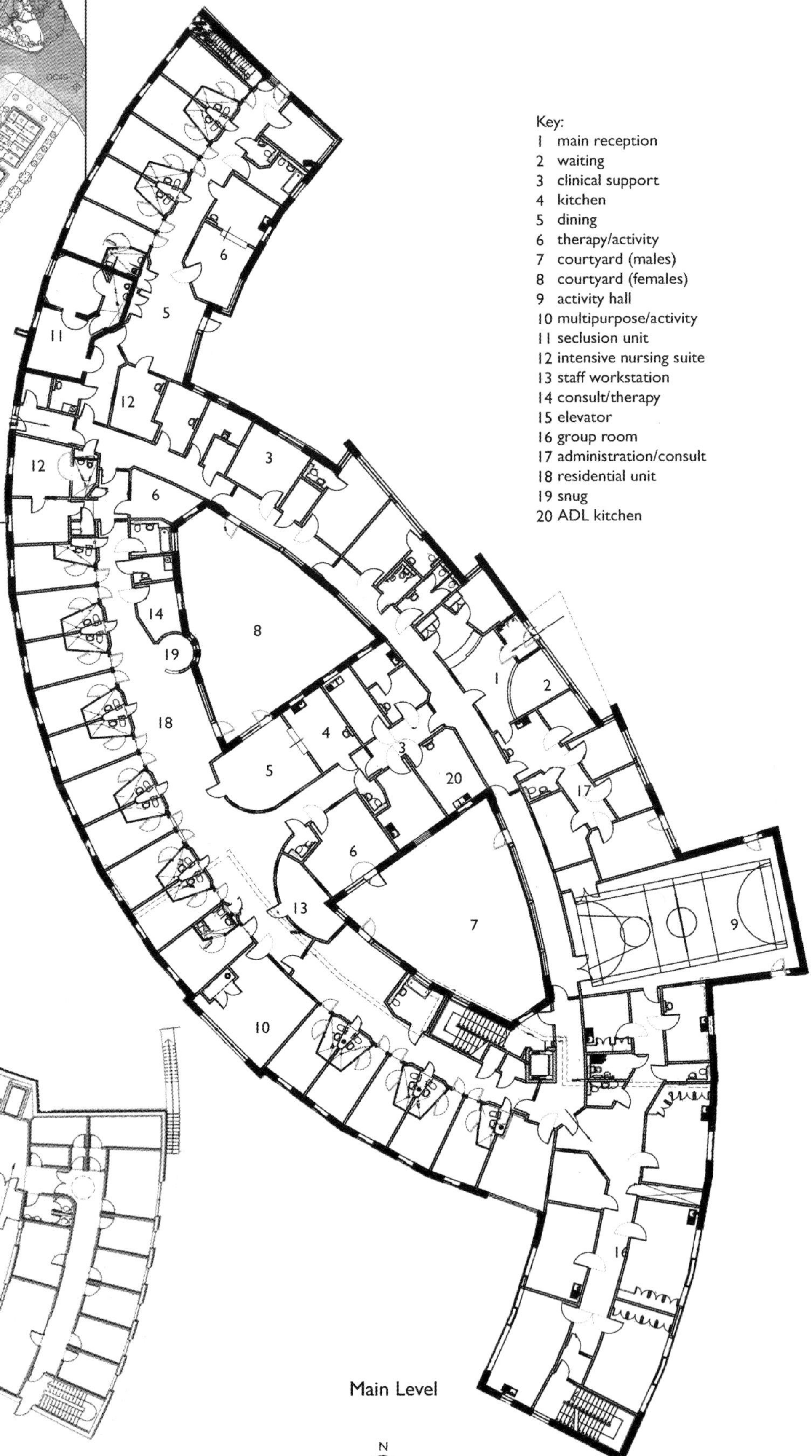

Key:
1 main reception
2 waiting
3 clinical support
4 kitchen
5 dining
6 therapy/activity
7 courtyard (males)
8 courtyard (females)
9 activity hall
10 multipurpose/activity
11 seclusion unit
12 intensive nursing suite
13 staff workstation
14 consult/therapy
15 elevator
16 group room
17 administration/consult
18 residential unit
19 snug
20 ADL kitchen

Main Level

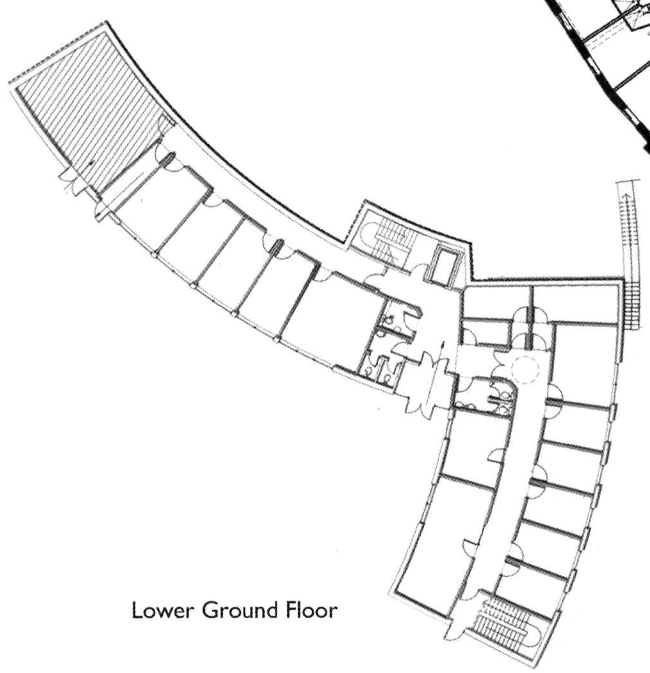

Lower Ground Floor

6.17.3a–c Patient rooms, each with private bath/shower unit, are housed on the inboard side of an inner arc. Therapy and related support spaces are housed in a midsection connector.

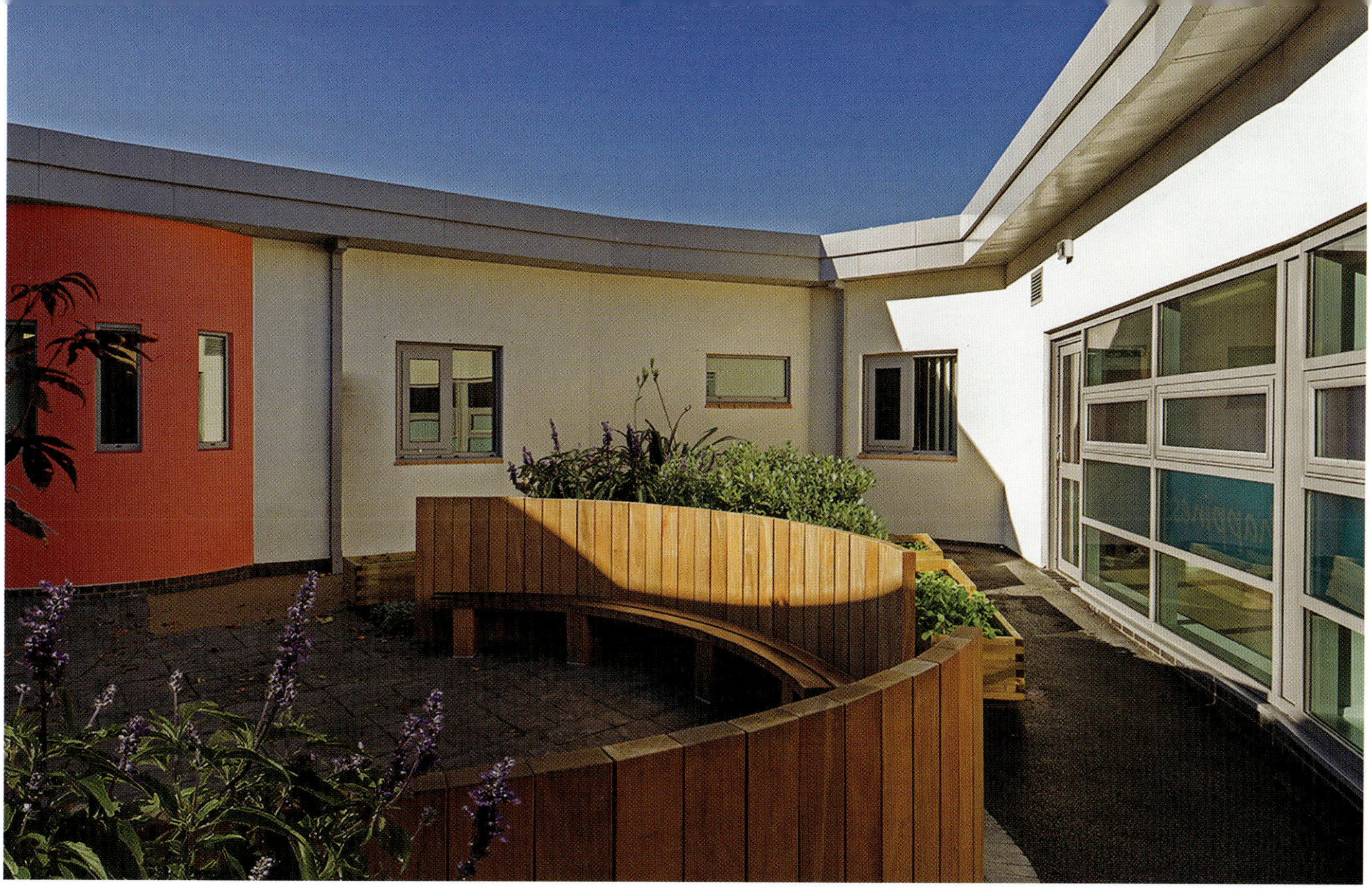

6.17.4 Junction 17's two protected, exterior courtyards are landscaped, with various built-in seating configurations.

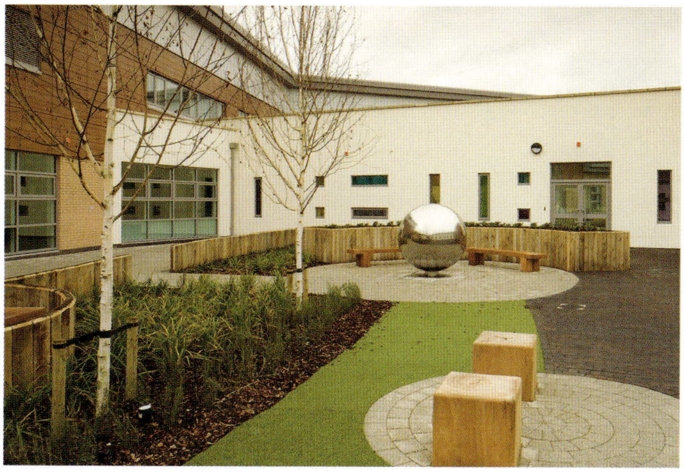

6.17.5 Works of art, ground plantings, and walking paths are integral elements in the courtyards.

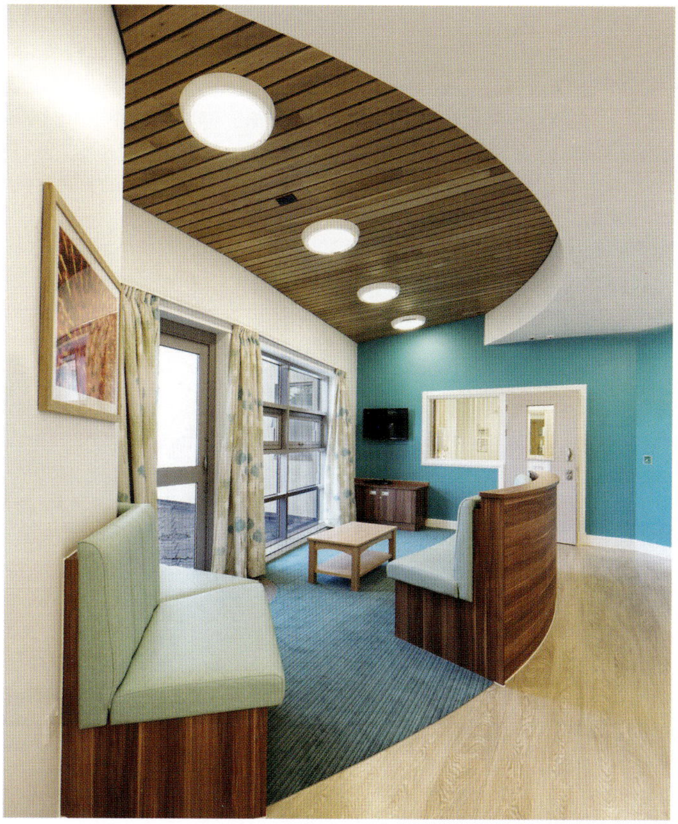

6.17.6 Informal consult/respite spaces are provided on residential units, with furnishings designed to withstand intensive use.

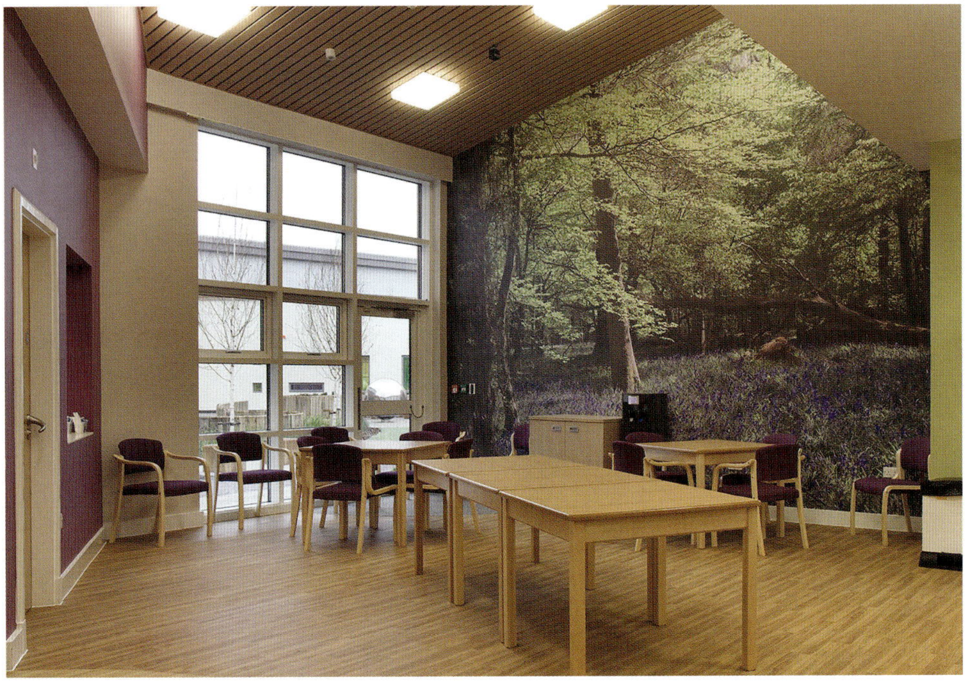

6.17.7 A wall mural adds visual interest to a multipurpose room.

(Figure 6.17.4). The recreational therapy area breaks the curvature at one end, where a gymnasium prominently juts outward and upward into a larger volume.

Patient rooms and seclusion rooms are on the outer perimeter on the far side from the courtyards (Figure 6.17.5). Hard and soft surfaces are choreographed; outdoor built-in furnishings provide places for socialization and informal consults. Dayrooms and multipurpose rooms feature radial seating, floor and ceiling patterns, and a mixture of built-in and moveable furnishings (Figure 6.17.6). Nature-themed wall murals are in the recreational therapy and social activity spaces (Figure 6.17.7). The patient room features a built-in bed and headboard, desk, and next to the desk a storage unit bin for personal belongings (Figure 6.17.8). In 2014, a postoccupancy assessment was conducted, and it was found this replacement facility contributed to, in the first 12 months of operations, a noticeable reduction in the rate of aggressive outbursts and patient self-abuse incidents. Additionally, a reduction in the average length of patient stay was identified, together with a reduced number of other types of acute adverse incidents, and incidents of absconding, as well as an improved level of staff morale and staff retention. These outcomes were attributed by the architects and the facility's administration, in part, to the openness and residential ambiance at Junction 17, as well as, indirectly, to the immediacy of its courtyards, lack of punitive fences or other intrusive security barriers, and the amenity of patient rooms, including the provision of a private bath/shower unit in each room.

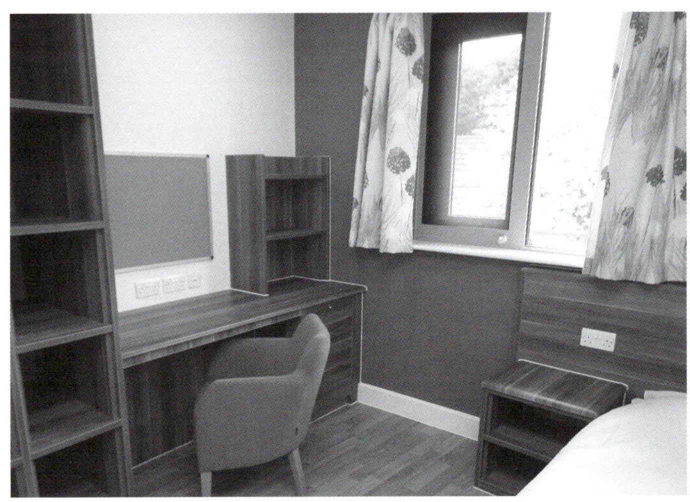

6.17.8 Patient rooms feature built-in amenities, operable windows, and color-coded perimeter walls.

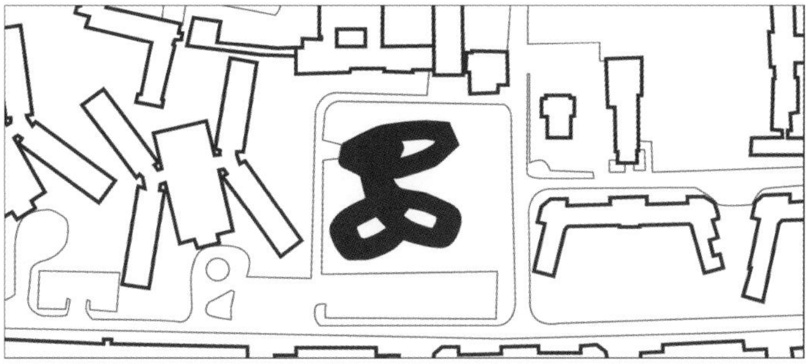

18 Linn Dara Child and Adolescent Centre at Cherry Hill Hospital, Dublin, Ireland

ARCHITECT: Reddy Architecture + Urbanism, London, UK
LANDSCAPE ARCHITECT: Reddy Architecture + Urbanism, London, UK
CLIENT: Health Service Executive Dublin Mid-Leinster
FEATURED MATERIALS: Spandrel glass exterior panels, masonry, steel
COMPLETED: 2012
INPATIENT BEDS: 24
SITE/PARKING: 6 acres/50
HOSPITAL/TREATMENT CENTER SIZE: 32,500 square feet
NURSES' WORKSTATION: Shielded

Context/site

This specialized psychiatric hospital, for patients aged 2–18, consolidates services previously scattered at locations regionally on a single site, part of Ireland's 'Vision for Change' program to treat young persons with mental illness. Treatment is provided for severe psychiatric disorders including schizophrenia, depression, and mania. Other conditions treated include eating disorders, such as bulimia and anorexia. It is located in a suburban area on the outskirts of Dublin, near the panoptical, infamous Cloverhill Prison, with its five immense wings that radiate from a single, centralized control station. The design strategy at Linn Dara, in contrast to the starkness of that high-security prison, was to provide an inviting, informally configured, community-based building for children and adolescents. Initial client consultations and sketch proposals centered on the importance of natural light, ventilation, and maximizing views to the surrounding landscape. Also important was the integration of original works of art, green roofs, a winter garden, and courtyards as safe havens for patients, visitors, and staff. The facility footprint was inspired by local plant species and organic forms found in nature. What evolved from these influences was a rather playful, sweeping building with bright colors symbolizing qualities quite contemporary compared to the rigid institutionalism of bygone European asylums.

Linn Dara is among the first of a new wave of mental health facilities constructed in Ireland in the past decade, based upon a new service provider manifesto, one compatible with a new architectural attitude on how mental health care settings should look and 'feel'. A deinstitutionalized aesthetic was now widely acceptable by the parent governing agency and was also supported by the local community. The goal of breaking from the stigma of the past resulted in barely a straight line anywhere, a strategy premised on not providing any *sharp edges*. To the architects, rounded, softer corner conditions were an obvious way to reject the stigma of mental illness. The neoclassicist right corners and taught formalism of the 19th-century asylum was rejected as much as the stark, orthogonal minimalism of the modernist 1950s through 1970s period. Psychiatric institutions in both periods dehumanized their occupants, in some shared but sometimes radically different ways. On its own merits, Linn Dara is a three-level building with sweeping curvature – leading the eye around the next corner and from one color-themed segment of façade to the next – a building that achieves relative transparency throughout (Figure 6.18.1 and 6.18.2). The forms vary somewhat in height, visually minimizing the overall mass. Child and family caregiver teams, an adolescent care team, adolescent day hospital, staff training unit, and the administration unit are housed in this rather biomorphic building, with internal realms connected by means of a looping circulation system.[1]

Building/unit

The partí weaves in and out of itself, further articulated by a façade of grid panels that strategically wrap shapes at first appearing playful but upon closer inspection are quite strategic. The colorful grid articulates each floor level while providing human scale. Opaque panels of differing colors code the different segments – with some façade segments banded in entirely the same color inset panel (yellow) while others are sheathed in red and orange panels, with sweeping horizontal bands of beige panels (Figure 6.18.3 and 6.18.4a–b). This fenestration strategy, if it had been rendered only in gray scale tones, for instance, would have likely appeared too institutional. By contrast, the brightly colored panel segments together with the horizontal color banding serve as effective antidotes. The entry portal at the center is recessed yet recessed yet identifiable, on approach, and relatively transparent – that is, breaking from

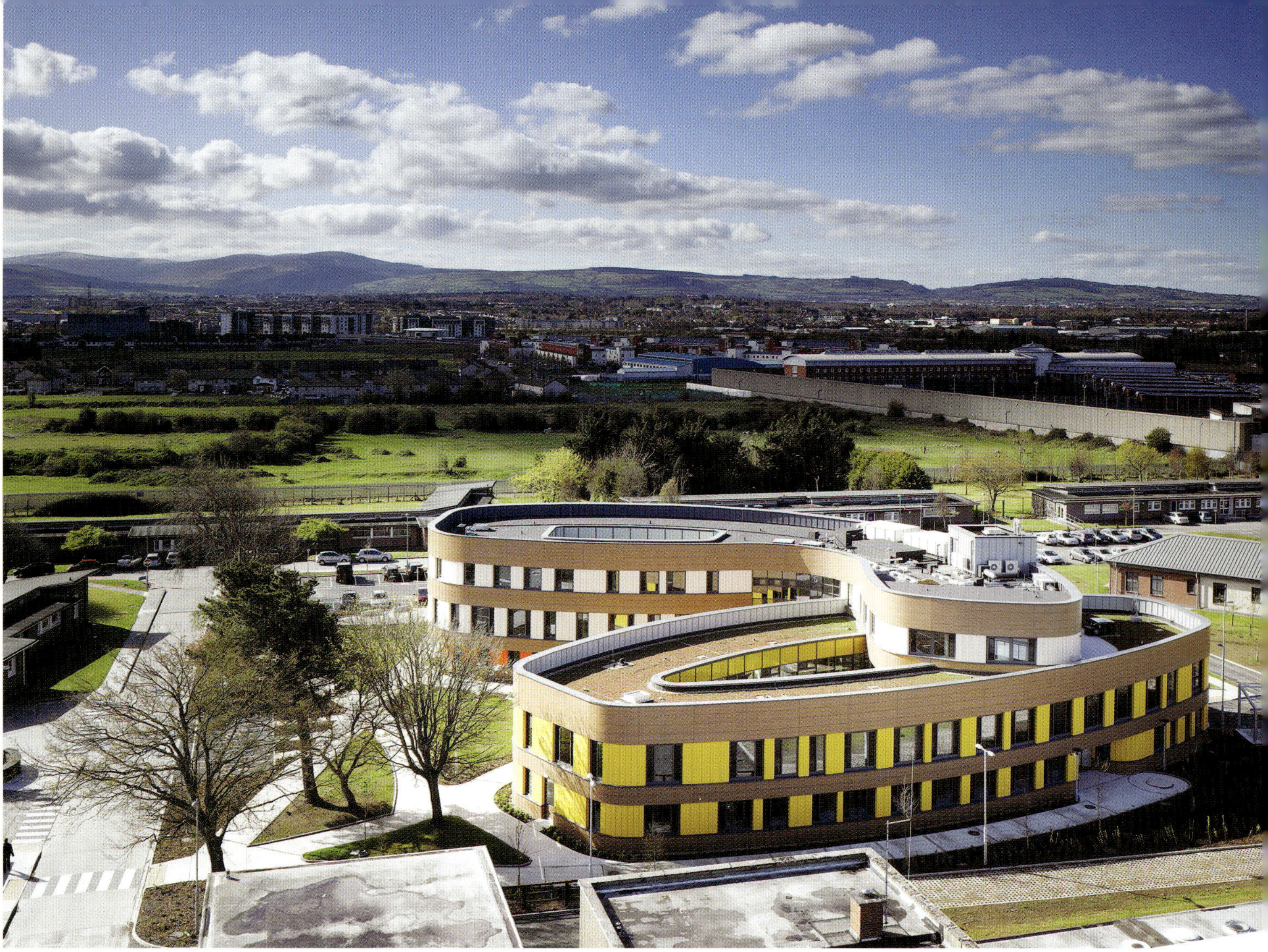

6.18.1 The curvilinearity of the Linn Dara Centre in Dublin, Ireland, distinguishes it from its exurban context.

surrounding motifs and sweeping forms, and for these reasons it is important to the overall composition. Open courts are similarly driven by the curvature, influencing paths and the placement of small pockets of seating. The enclosed front courts leading from the main entry area establish themes carried throughout the interior (Figure 6.18.5 and 6.18.6). Various departments and program sections, coded in differing colors, support the four themed 24/7 residential units: Buttercup Suite, Lily Suite, Clover Suite, and the Bluebell Suite.

This 24-bed facility houses two 11-bed residential units, one for older adolescents up to age 18, and a second unit for younger patients, plus a two-bed acute care unit. Attached to these units is a six-room classroom building, housing an art therapy/crafts room, home economics classroom, occupational therapy room, a sports hall/gymnasium, and an outdoor hard court for sports. A family apartment is provided on-site for overnight stays on the first night of a child's admittance. Interior corridors are single loaded in many places, with large windows facing the open courtyards. Full-height murals of nature scenes are on walls of the four inpatient units, and the nurses' station on each unit is shielded, with a sliding glass window (Figure 6.18.7 and 6.18.8). A central elevator core and staircase is located at the intersection of the two principal wings. The patient rooms are all private, with communal-type hygiene amenities located at the end of the corridor on each unit (Figure 6.18.9a–b). Eco-sustainable features at Linn Dara include a geothermal system, and an underfloor heating system, allowing for flexibility as future space needs evolve. Use-activated lighting was incorporated and building information modeling (BIM) was utilized extensively to design this geometrically complex structure. The use of BIM enabled the contractor to work rather expeditiously, with greater precision on-site. Judges at the 2013 WorldArchitectureNews.com (WAN) awards program recognized this psychiatric facility for young persons for its design inventiveness, and it also garnered recognition in the form of an Irish Health Care Centre Building of the Year Award (2013).

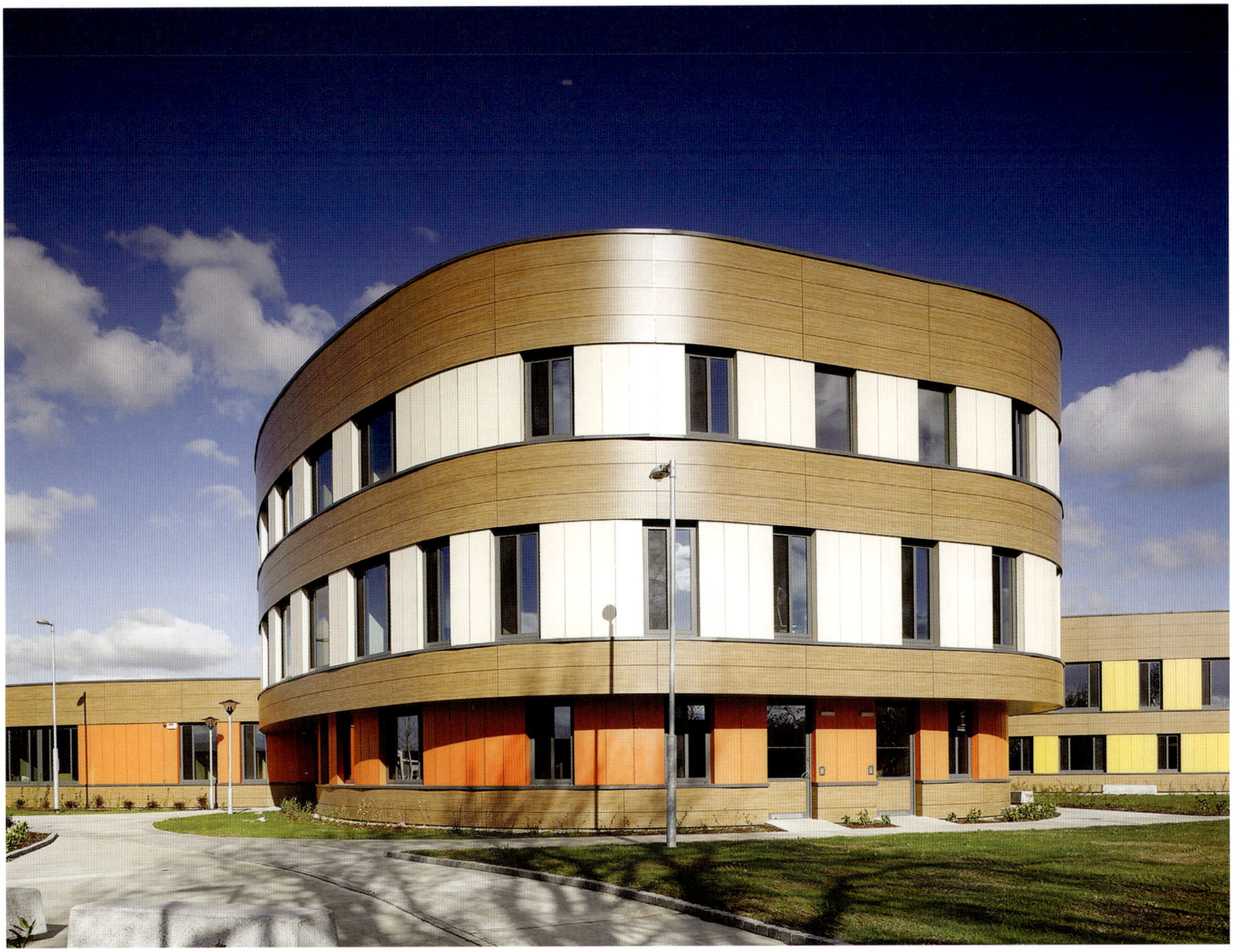

6.18.2 Multiple bands of color-accented panels inject scale and horizontality.

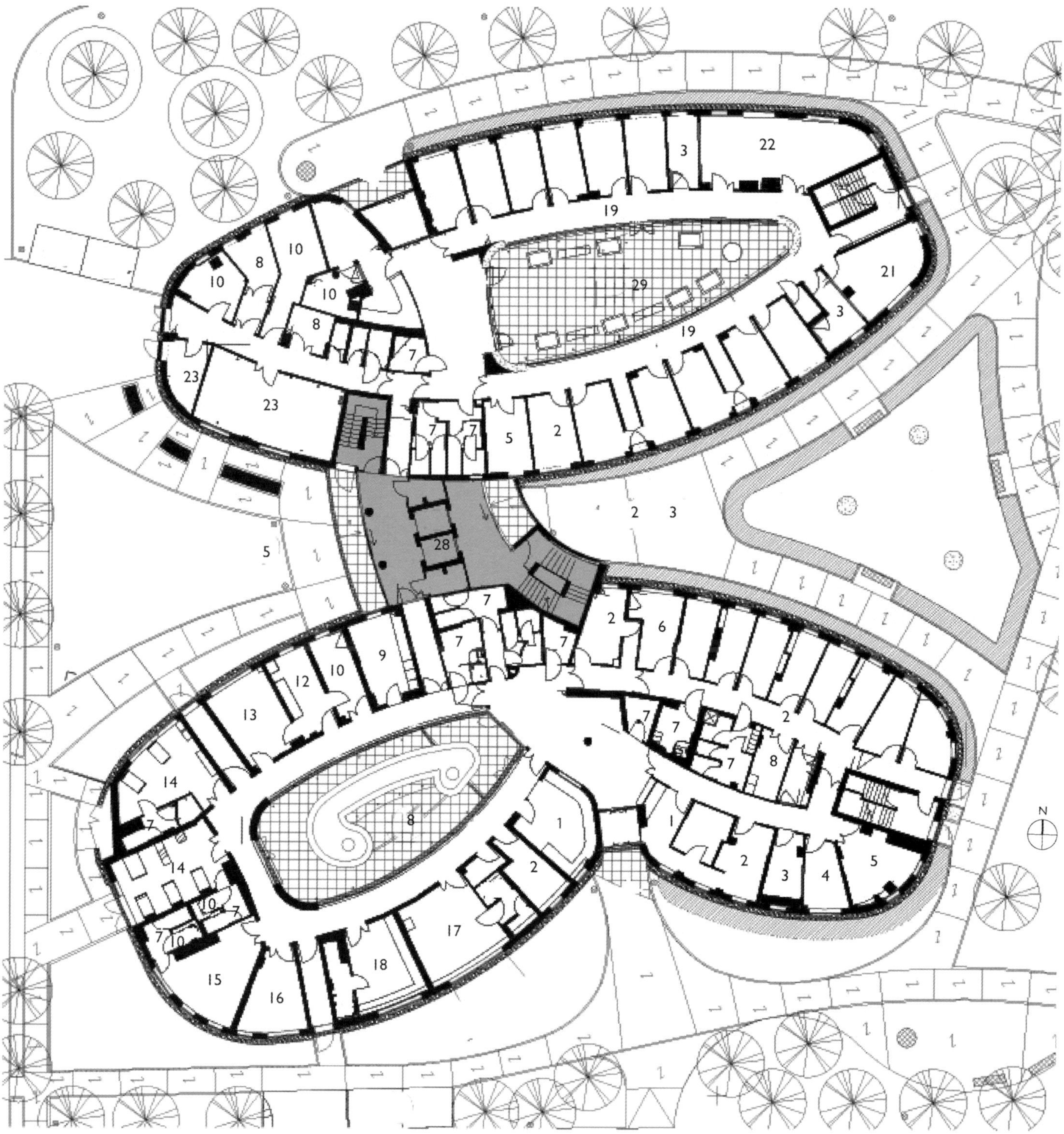

Ground Floor

6.18.3 Treatment units wrap around courtyards and central support cores, with principal zones linked by a common circulation system.

Key:
1 nurses' station
2 office
3 observation room
4 interview room
5 treatment room
6 staff room
7 patient toilets
8 staff toilets
9 housekeeping/laundry
10 training kitchen
11 store
12 kitchen
13 dining
14 woodworking/art therapy room
15 group room
16 occupational therapy
17 classroom
18 computer room
19 multipurpose
20 consulting office
21 family room
22 group room
23 plant room
24 team meeting room
25 meeting room
26 library
27 training room
28 elevator
29 courtyard
30 green roof
31 roof terrace (staff only)

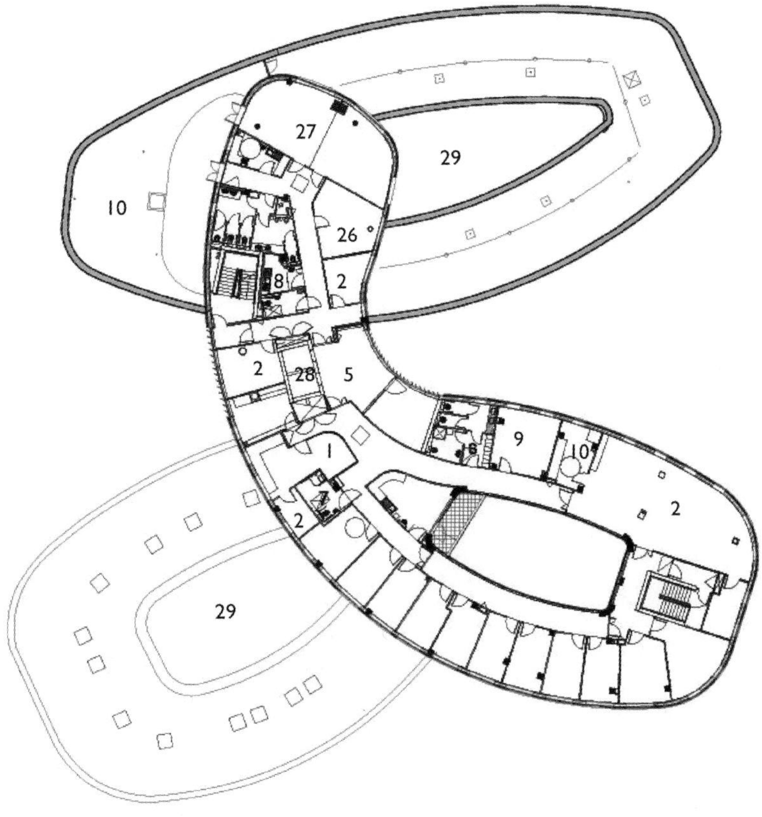

Level 2

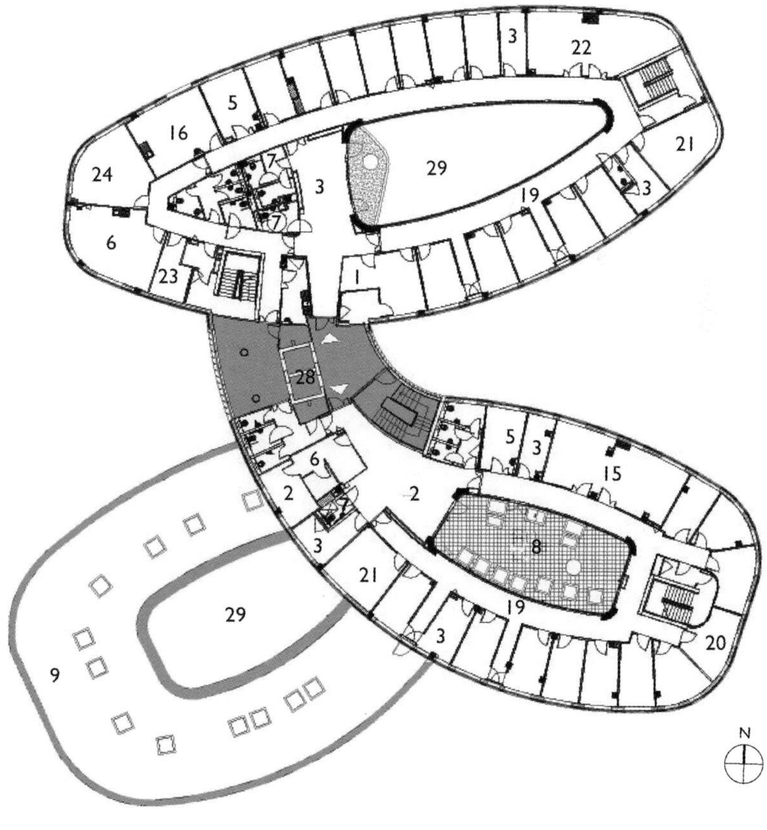

Level 1

6.18.4a–b In plan, three compositional modulations are revealed, undulating in width, weaving in and out as a function of floor level.

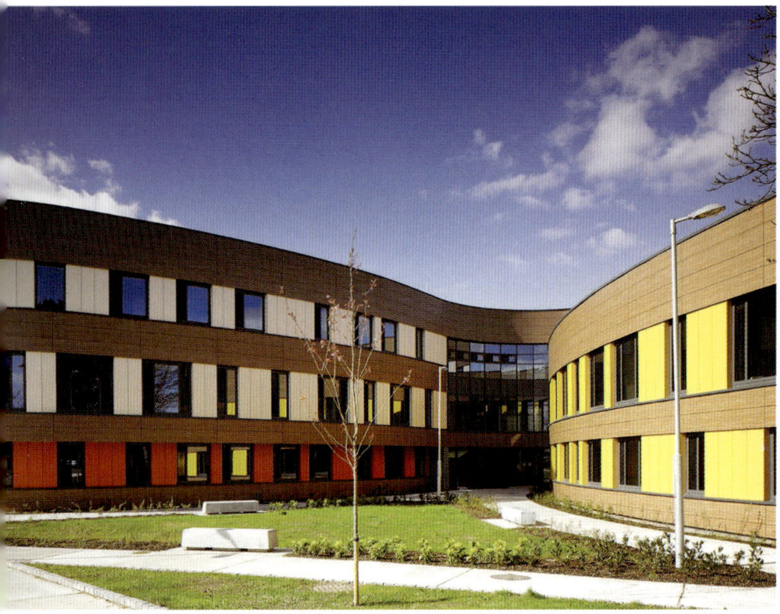

6.18.5 Sweeping forms, banding, and color lead the eye to a 'neutral' element at the intersection of two principal zones.

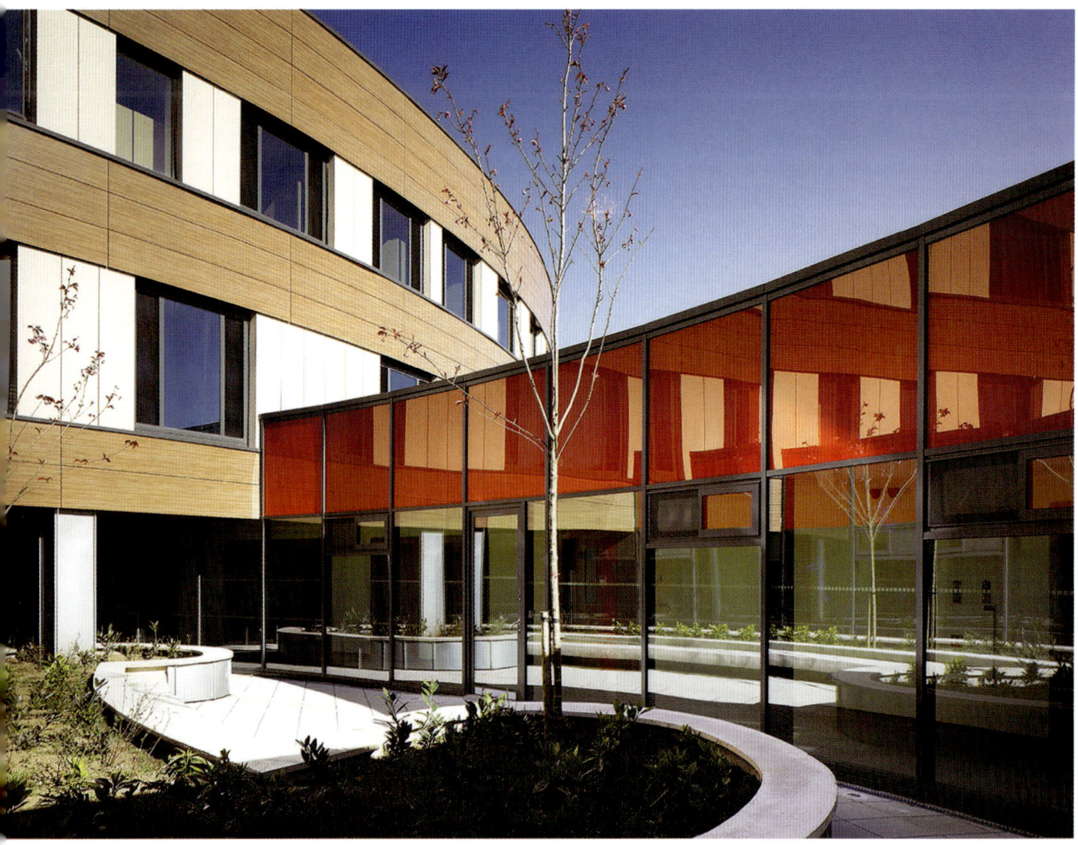

6.18.6 Intersecting geometries yield layered juxtapositions of compositional elements.

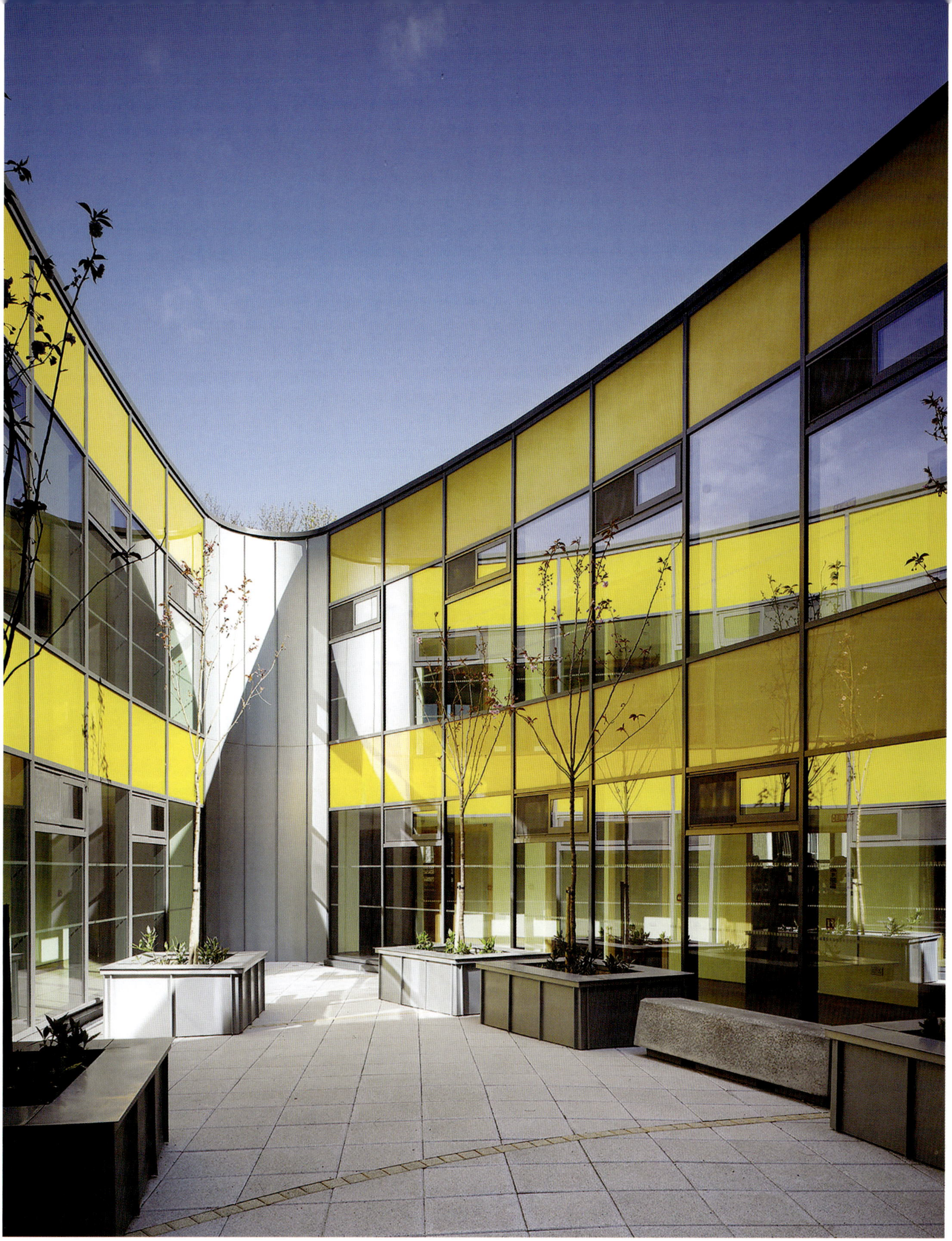

6.18.7 Translucent panels and sweeping forms establish a distinct image in a courtyard at the Linn Dara Centre.

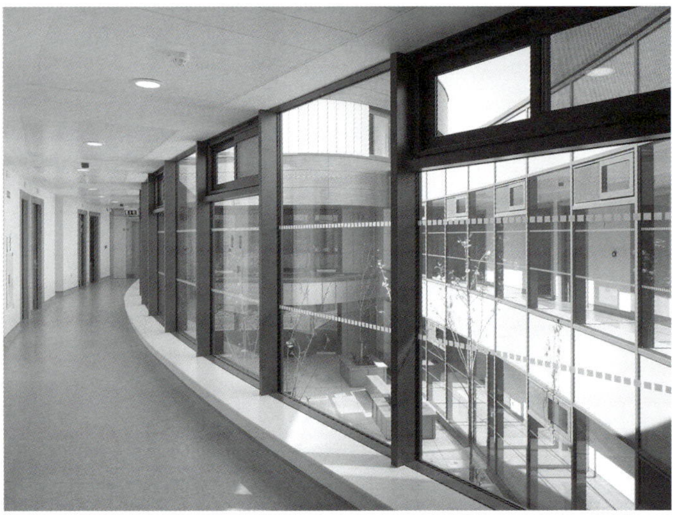

6.18.8 Circulation arteries feature expansive windows (with operable insets) overlooking courtyards, creating a mutually reinforcing effect.

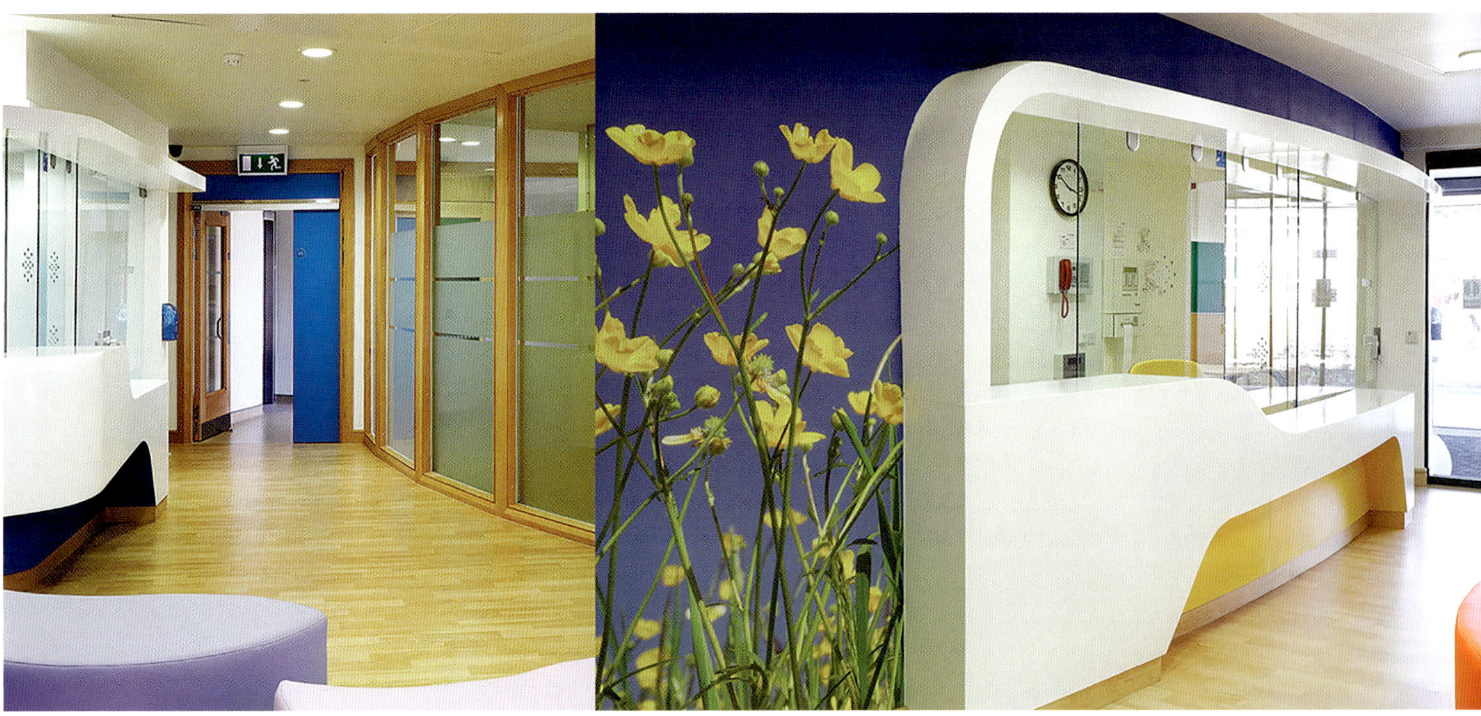

6.18.9a–b Interiors of residential units (left) and staff workstations (right) are secure without compromising aesthetic.

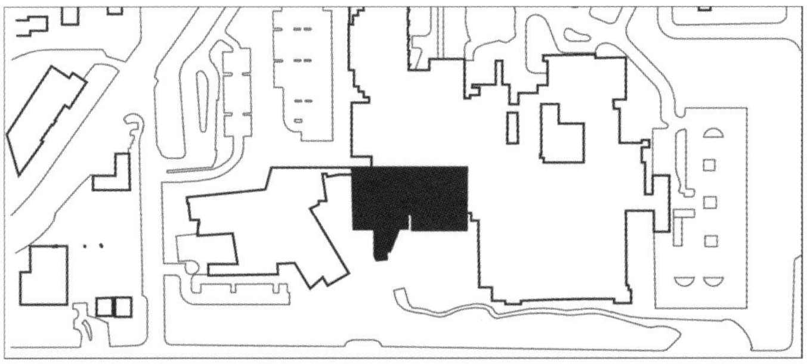

19 Seattle Children's Hospital Psychiatry and Behavioral Medicine Unit, Seattle, Washington, USA

ARCHITECT: ZGF Architects, Seattle, Washington, USA/Medical Planning: architecture+, Troy, New York, USA
LANDSCAPE ARCHITECT: ZGF Architects, Seattle, Washington, USA
CLIENT: Seattle Children's' Hospital Research Foundation, Seattle, Washington USA
FEATURED MATERIALS: Glass, steel, precast concrete, masonry
COMPLETED: 2015
INPATIENT BEDS: 41
SITE/PARKING: 15 acres/450
HOSPITAL/TREATMENT CENTER SIZE: 22,200 square feet
NURSES' WORKSTATION: Shielded

Context/site

The Psychiatry and Behavioral Medicine Unit (PBMU) at Seattle Children's Hospital is housed on Levels 4 and 5 of an acute care facility located near the University of Washington main campus. Services provided consist of assessment and treatment for attention deficit hyperactivity disorder (ADHD), autism spectrum disorders, depression and anxiety disorders, eating disorders, and complex mental health problems occurring in tandem with medical-surgical conditions. Outpatient services include telepsychiatry, neuropsychology, group therapy, and consultation regarding previously undiagnosed symptoms. Inpatient and outpatient services are provided for patients aged 3–18 in psychiatric crisis based on a referral process, with most inpatient stays of 8 days or less in duration. Prior to the renovation of the space currently occupied by the PBMU, it had operated at 98% capacity in 2013 and 102% capacity in 2014. However, the facility had become obsolete, overcrowded, and lacked supports relative to the current level and scope of psychiatric care that the unit wished to provide. Before, patients were, at times day and night, forced to use the public hallways when seeking seclusion and respite, as there was extremely limited private space anywhere on the unit. Social activity and therapy/treatment spaces at the old facility were equally inadequate, and little direct contact with nature was available on-site.

The new PBMU provides a much more supportive treatment environment through the use of uplifting, playful design elements versus the minimalist, detention-like modern psychiatric hospitals of the past. The main design challenge at Seattle Children's was to provide a high level of care in a safe, protected environment with the aim of promoting each patient's self-dignity and respect through prescriptive treatment and rehabilitation (Figures 6.19.1a–b and 6.19.2). In Phase 1, completed in 2014, 23 beds were opened, with a dining area, comfort rooms, group rooms, a classroom, recreational facilities, and designated area for an autism spectrum disorders program. These spaces project an inviting image, with bold, bright colors and curvilinear furnishings set against blue and beige wall surfaces. In 2015, Phase II opened, bringing the total bed capacity to 41 beds on two levels of the hospital. An internal staircase now enabled the staff and patients to circulate between both levels interdependently without having to leave the unit. The new PBMU was designed using LEAN planning principles, a facility-planning method proven in numerous instances to increase the probability of improved behavioural health outcomes by drawing upon the prior experiences of the direct caregiver staff. This helped identify and minimize extraneous spaces and inefficient spatial adjacencies, and to establish a functional connection with the acute care hospital of which it is a component part, while retaining its autonomy.[2]

Building/unit

The inpatient unit on Level 4 houses 16 beds, with bedrooms clustered into two pods, one to each side of a central nurses' station, with a seclusion room in proximity. The perimeter zone houses a classroom and group room (Figure 6.19.3a–b). Functions located in the inboard side of the floor consist of staff support, a family lounge, counseling offices, and a communal kitchen/dining room near the center. On Level 5, 25 beds are deployed in two configurations: a linear grouping consisting of eight beds, and in two clusters of four beds positioned to either side of the dayroom/living room and dining space. The beds on this level are arranged

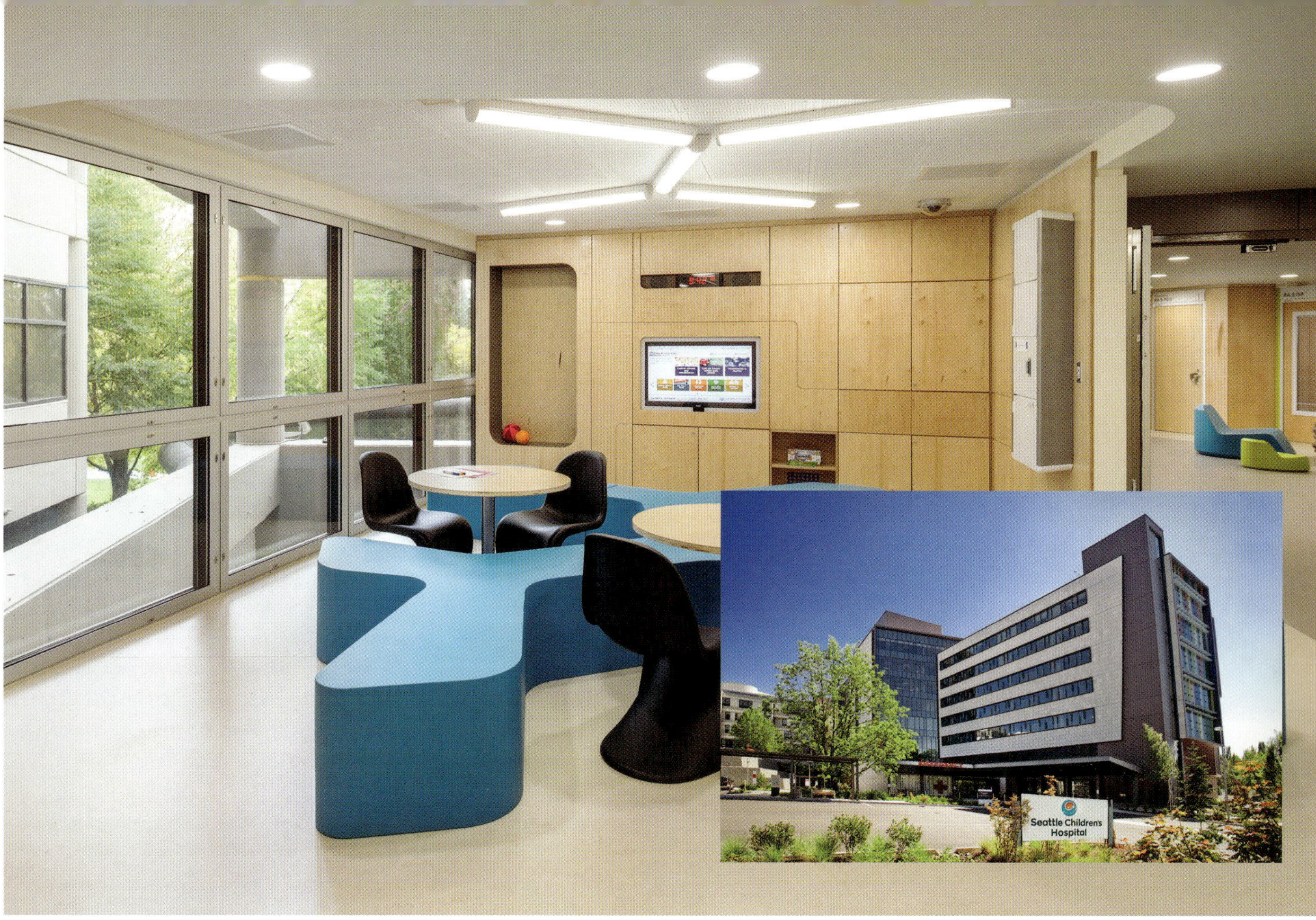

6.19.1a–b Seattle Children's Hospital Psychiatry and Behavioral Medicine Unit occupies two levels of an acute care medical center facility.

nearly the same as those on the level immediately below. As mentioned, both levels have seclusion and 'chill' spaces. The nurses' stations are partly shielded in a manner that facilitates direct communication with patients and their families, while not compromising staff safety. Wayfinding is enhanced using landmarks in the form of color-accented walls, signage, furnishings, and varied lighting effects. Natural wood paneling; colorful, curvilinear furnishings with rounded edges; and natural light contribute to a significantly deinstitutionalized aesthetic throughout compared to before (Figures 6.19.4 to 6.19.6).

All patient rooms are private, and depending on room orientation, have large windows overlooking either a stand of trees, the medical campus, or a nearby residential neighborhood. Each bedroom has a private bath/shower unit, located inboard along the corridor, with access only from the corridor directly outside the patient room. One bed is placed parallel to the window wall, with a second bed positioned orthogonally along the bath/shower unit wall. Built-in storage bins are provided below. This second bed is

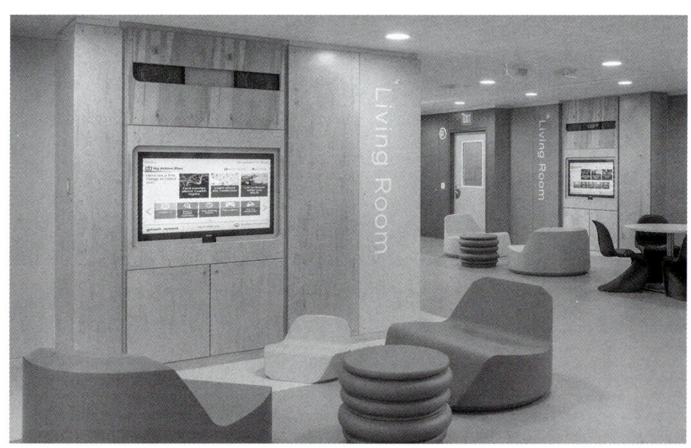

6.19.2 Playfully shaped, durable furnishings animate interior spaces throughout.

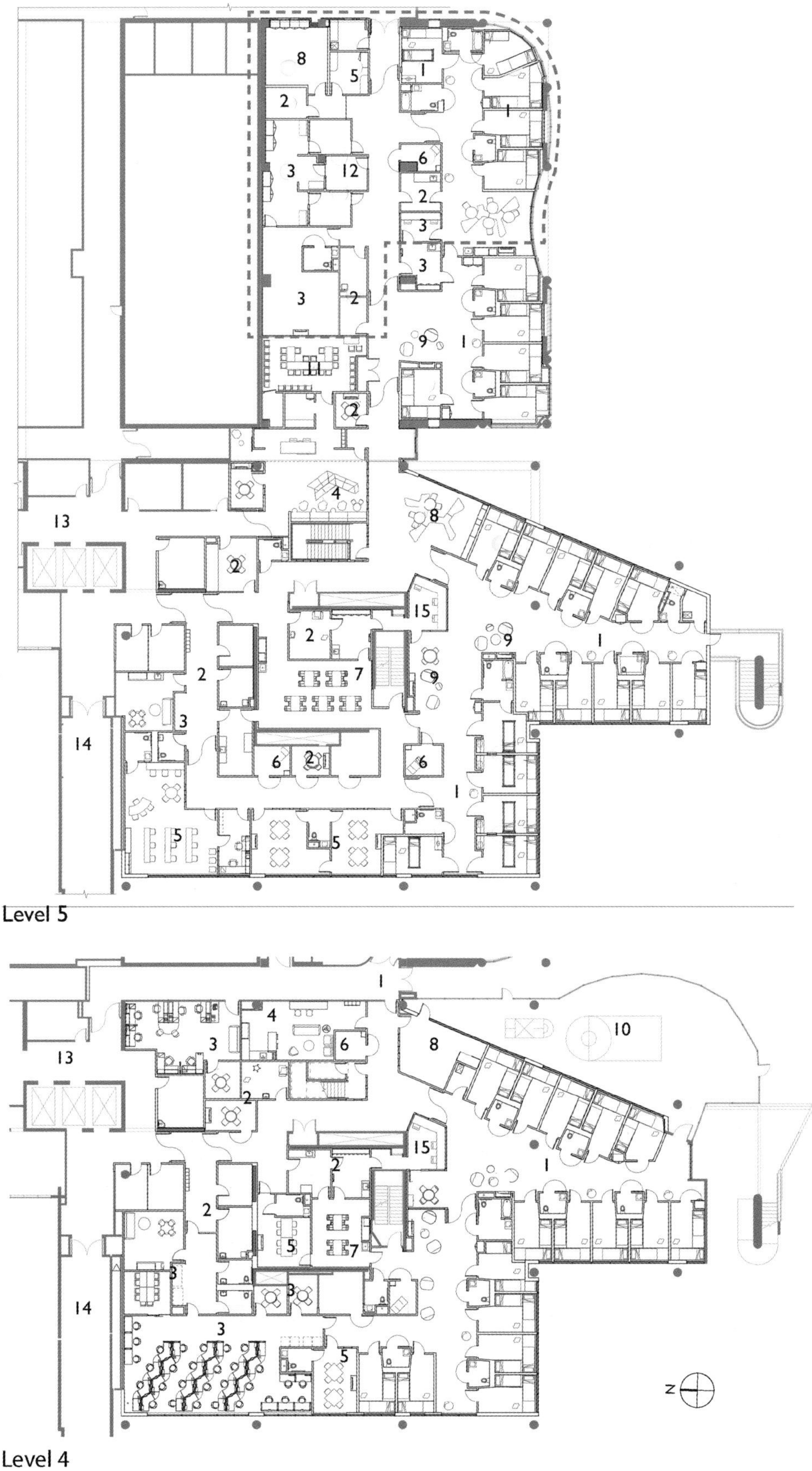

Key:
1 patient room
2 patient support
3 staff support
4 family lounge/waiting
5 group room/classroom
6 comfort space
7 dining/multipurpose
8 recreational activity
9 patient dayroom
10 reception/exterior secure play area
11 conference
12 RSD therapy
13 elevators
14 access to hospital
15 nurses' station

6.19.3a–b The unit's two levels are linked internally, functioning as a semiautonomous entity within a 'mothership' hospital.

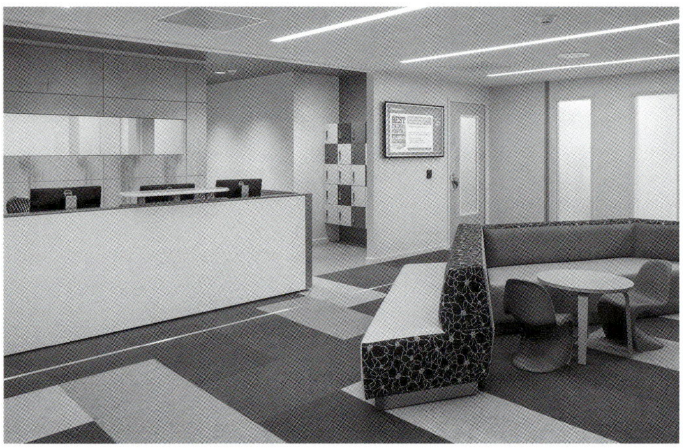

6.19.4 Furnishings throughout the unit are designed to withstand intensive use by patients.

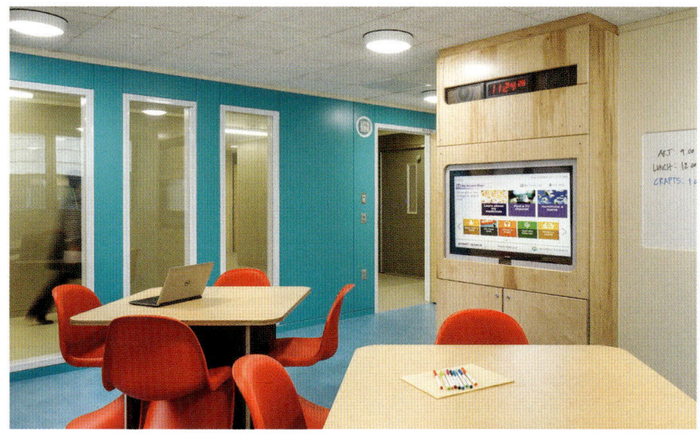

6.19.5 Colors, video monitors, and wood panels are coordinated in social activity spaces.

provided for use by parents and significant others' during overnight stays, as it is common for a parent to stay with the child at key points during his or her hospitalization (Figures 6.19.7 and 6.19.8). The door and entry threshold to the patient room is recessed 4 feet from the corridor and this is noteworthy insofar as this affords an additional measure of personal privacy because the patient bath/shower unit is only accessible from the corridor side – with no door directly connecting from the bedroom. All patient rooms on Levels 4 and Level 5 are located on the south side of the unit. This case study demonstrates both the challenges of working within an existing hospital envelope as much as the possibilities associated with taking an existing generic shell and remaking it into a progressive psychiatric assessment and treatment environment for young persons and their families.

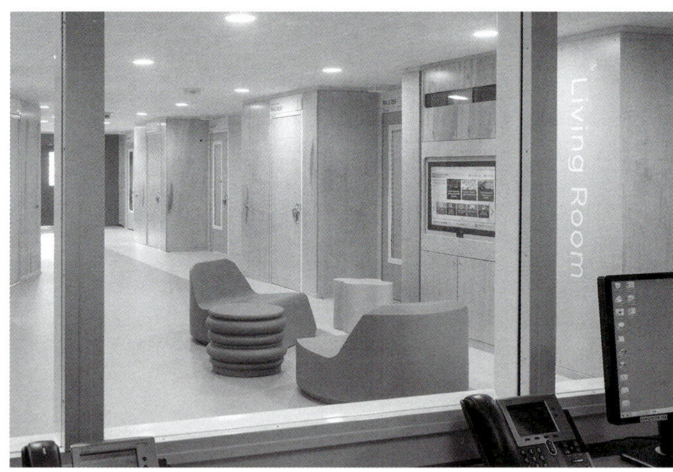

6.19.6 Patient room doors are recessed, and staff workstations are protected (secure) without compromising visual connectivity.

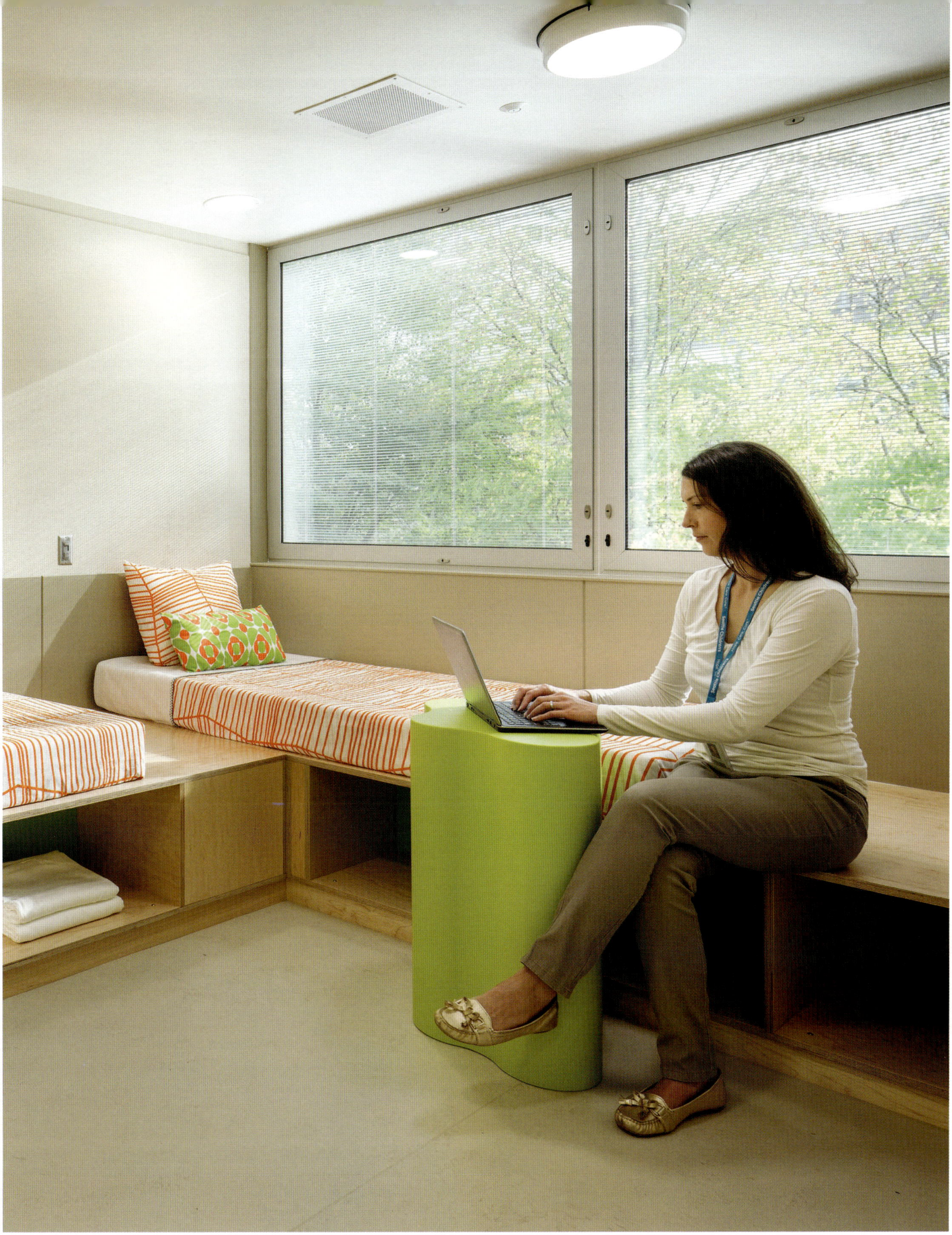

6.19.7 A second bed for overnight use by a visitor is stationed along the window wall of the patient rooms.

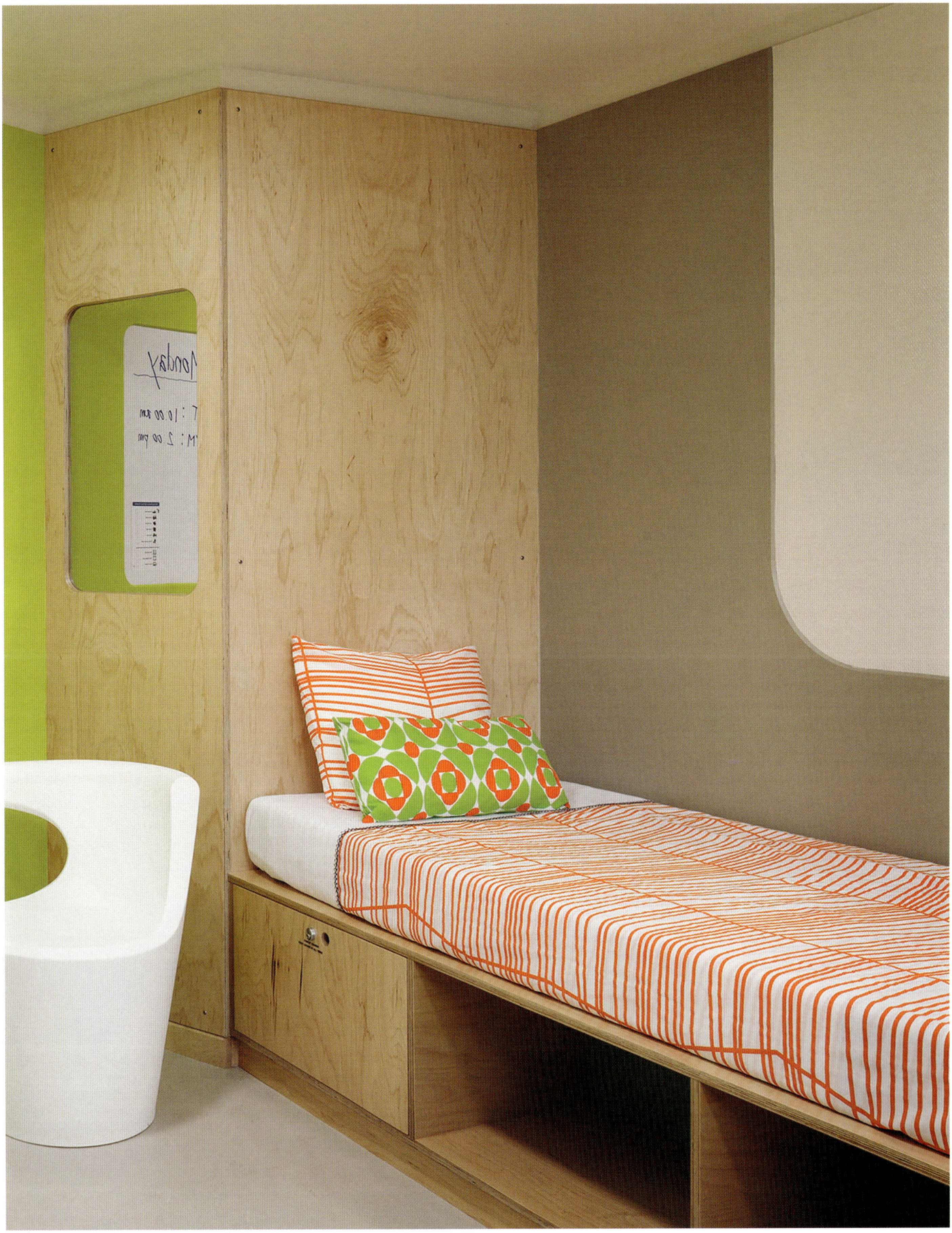

6.19.8 Patient room beds are built-in, with storage bins provided below.

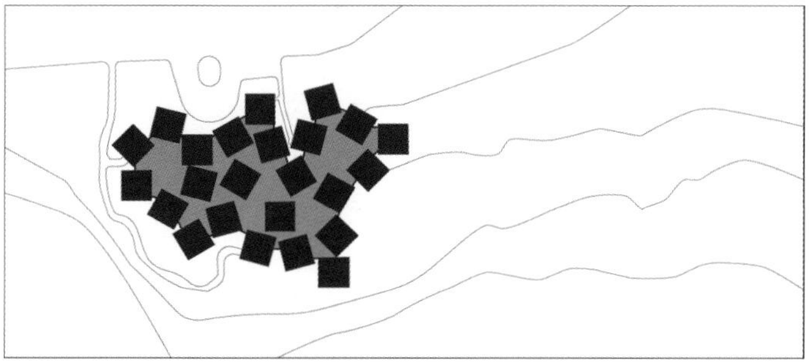

20 Children's Centre for Psychiatric Rehabilitation, Hokkaido, Japan

ARCHITECT: Sou Fujimoto, Architect, Tokyo, Japan
LANDSCAPE ARCHITECT: Sou Fujimoto, Architect, Tokyo, Japan
CLIENT: Hokkaido Health District
FEATURED MATERIALS: Masonry, concrete, glass, wood sheathing
COMPLETED: 2006
INPATIENT BEDS: 50
SITE/PARKING: 10 acres/40
HOSPITAL/TREATMENT CENTER SIZE: 42,500 square feet
NURSES' WORKSTATION: Hybrid

Context/site

Architects in Japan, not unlike elsewhere, typically receive their earliest commissions through friends and family members. But it is that rarest occurrence when one's father commissions his 20-something-year-old son to design a total inpatient psychiatric hospital. Fujimoto's father was a psychiatrist, although the client was actually a close colleague of his father who ran a large post-World War II modern psychiatric hospital in the same region, and who commissioned Fujimoto for this project. This 24/7 mental health facility was built on an open, rolling site in northern Japan, a site exposed to formidable Siberian winds from the north. Completed in 2006, it signified the finality of a series of healthcare projects Fujimoto designed in the early phase of his career. The site is located near the interchange of the Hokkaido Expressway, next to Fujimoto's '7/2 House' (2008) and near to the Minernba Hospital and Fujimoto's own Dormitory for the Mentally Disabled (2003). The setting is rural, with farms and sweeping vistas of nearby mountains. He conceived this project as an urban-residential (home-like) amalgamation, a duality expressed in its rather oblique randomness. What at first appears a formal strategy of discombobulation is in fact guided by a deliberate strategy to rearrange a set of identical cubes (residential units) to approximate the scale and ambiance of a remote rural village in in an expression of rural 'microurbanity'. Fujimoto outright rejected the rigid, grid-based geometry of the archetypal modern psychiatric hospital – with its long, austere, double-loaded corridors. He equally rejected the a patient leaving one's bedroom and immediately being thrust into a public corridor zone without transitional space in between, likening this to being thrust out into the middle of a busy highway and left to fend for oneself.

Fujimoto proceeded to design a quasi-normative environment that simulates the condition of a small village, complete with its narrow, winding streets; varied spatial relationships; and unexpected vistas. He considered this strategy a positive means to promote social cohesiveness and mutual support among the patients, caregiving staff, and patients' families. The result was an informal arrangement of numerous cubes arrived at through successive approximation (Figures 6.20.1 and 6.20.2). As repetitive cube elements were repositioned, iteratively, this would yield various new juxtapositions, allowing the staff, patients, and family members to consider how various modular elements might be ordered relative to one another without requiring long corridors. This process resulted in multiple informal, smaller-scaled living and treatment zones. During the planning and consultation process, staff psychiatrists and other key stakeholders expressed a collective desire for an anti-institutional environment and for a residential treatment environment supportive of residents' self-choice and individuality. However, many prominent staff members, including a number of senior-level psychiatrists, did not expect *this* degree of 'informality' and subsequently voiced their difficulty in being unable to 'let go' of certain old-school preconceptions. That said, many on the staff initially expected a more conventional architectural outcome but became amenable, in time, to the alternative concept arrived at by their architect (Figures 6.20.3 and 6.20.4).

Building/unit

The emphasis on a *softer*, or more organic, informal expression, versus a strongly axial one, is clearly evident. From the exterior, the complex appears as a group of people huddled together in close conversation, or members of some type of sports team working out a play on the field (Figure 6.20.5a–b). At the same time, it appears almost monastic, with its nearly entirely white exterior and strategically placed, minimally sized windows. Various public and semipublic spaces are situated in between the 25 house cube elements – especially those facing outward – have full-height windows and

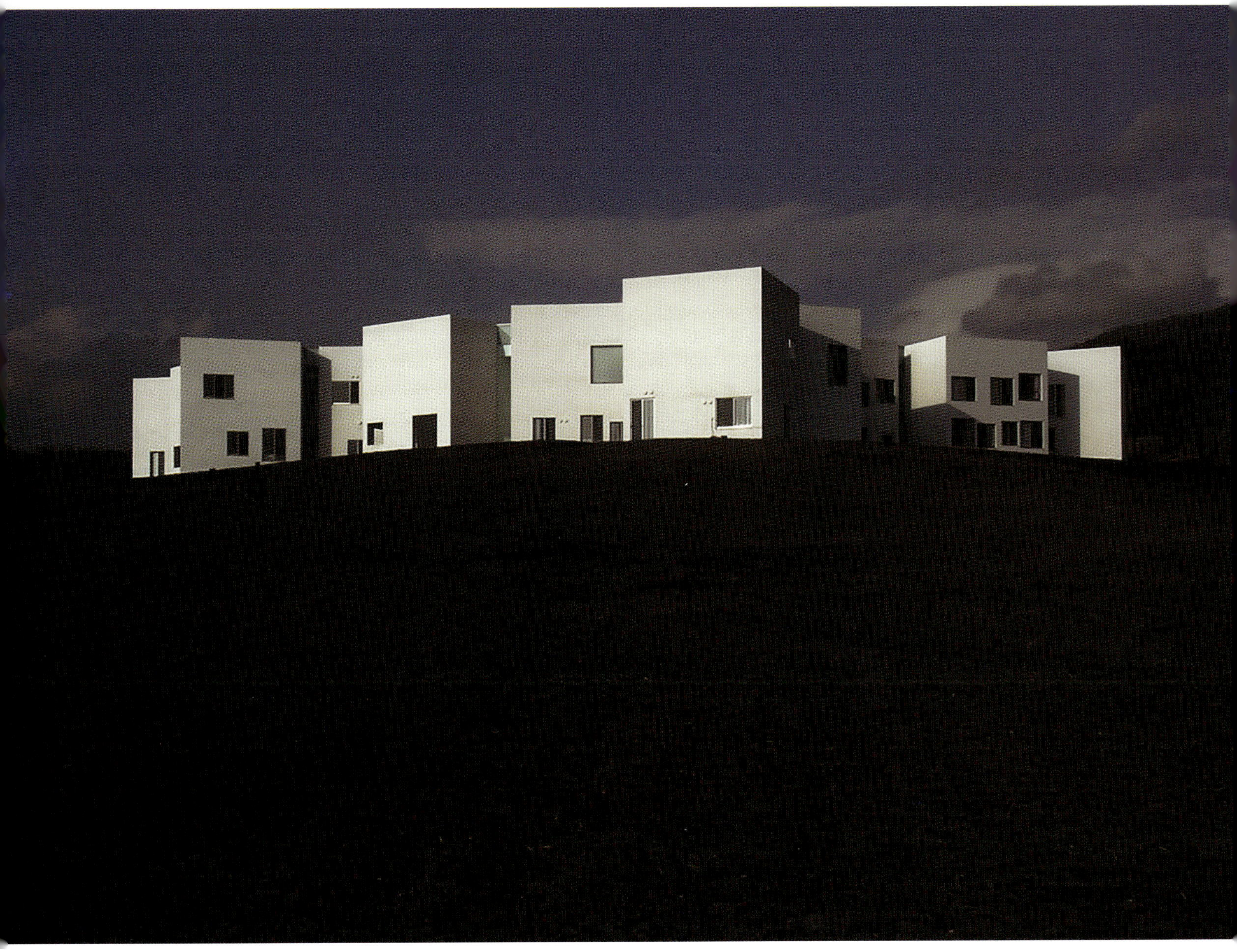

6.20.1 Exterior view of the constituent parts of the Children's Centre for Psychiatric Rehabilitation in Japan.

adjacent spaces for social activities. These elements are enclosed by a somewhat suppressed, independent roof, allowing the cubes to 'variously pop up' above the roof line. This resulted in a completely enclosed contiguous building. A single main entrance is provided for the public, and one for staff; there are no outdoor courtyards. Instead, as these boxes were rotated, sometimes in a dramatic push-pull manner, some appearing to nearly collide with one another. Again, this playful kineticism represented a clean break from the stasis of the modern psychiatric hospital, because those places were definitely not about such 'random' geometric experimentation. The planning process usually began and ended with everything conforming to a superordinate artesian grid – the mainstay of modernists, and the Miesian-influenced modernists, in particular, who designed psychiatric and other hospital types in the post-World War II period (see Chapter 2).

At the Children's Centre, the majority of support functions are housed on the 'main level', with inpatient housing occurring on both the main and second levels (Figure 6.20.6). Some spaces are two levels in height, with small, tucked-away alcoves off to one side, with a corresponding lower ceiling height, ostensibly to invite idiosyncratic uses by the patients. Daylight enters the corner edges of these elements, providing views out to the open rural landscape. In these units, patients are housed either in a private bedroom or in a semiprivate (four-bed) suite, with bath/shower units in proximity. A postoccupancy assessment was conducted with the staff, not long after this facility in Hokkaido opened. It was found that the staff

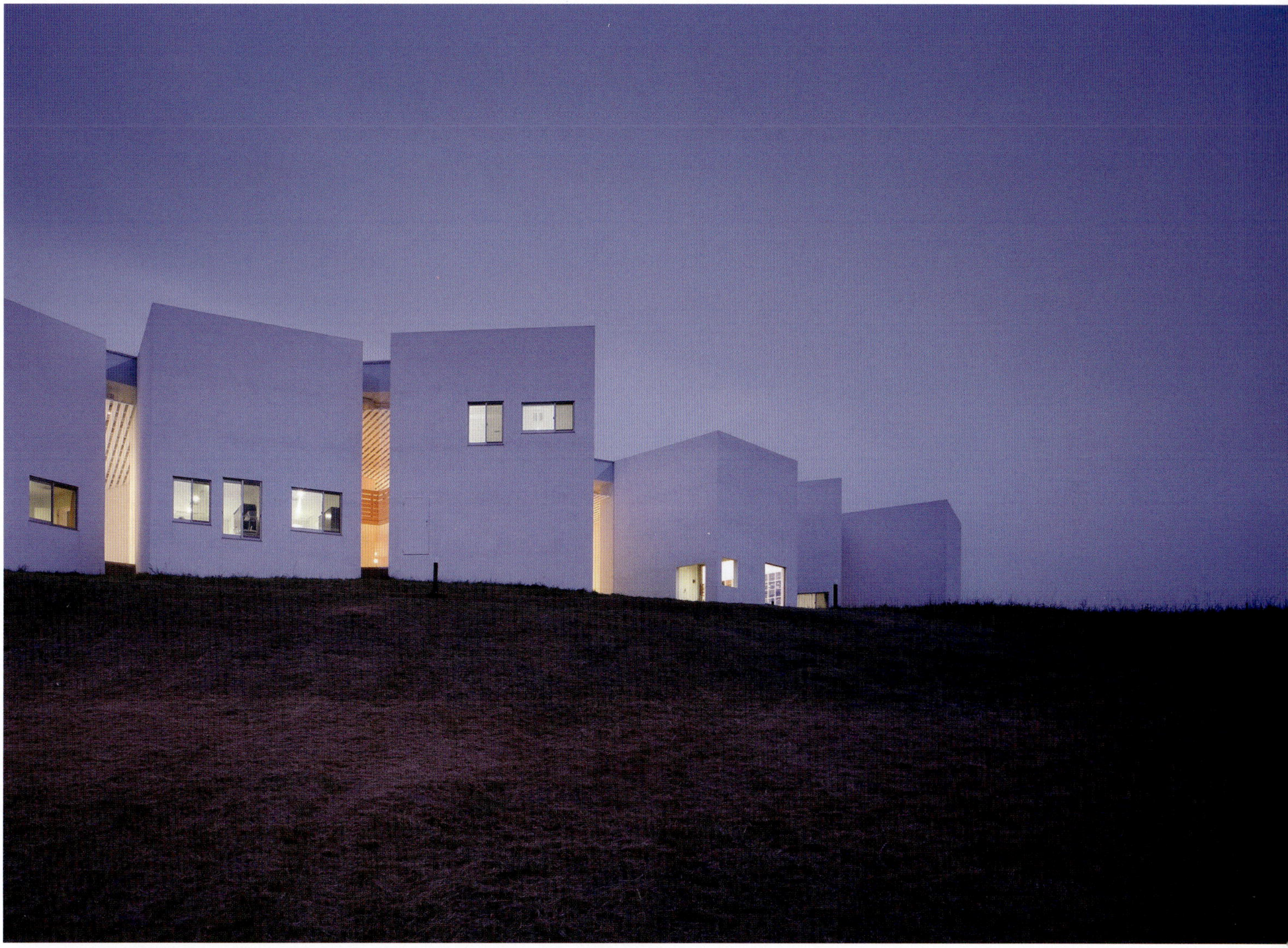

6.20.2 Fenestration and connections with landscape are minima on the outward side of the treatment center.

at first had difficulty adjusting to the architectural informality of the new building but soon adapted their caregiving approach accordingly and in time were able to develop a new, more individualized treatment program. This outcome led to numerous other positive outcomes, most of which had been unforeseen. In the intervening years, the architect has expressed some reservation, however, that his building did not relate as well to the immediate landscape as it might have. Since then, he has placed greater emphasis on blurring the boundaries between interior and exterior realms in his work, as Fujimoto's career has evolved into one of considerable prominence in Japan and beyond (Figures 6.20.7 and 6.20.8).

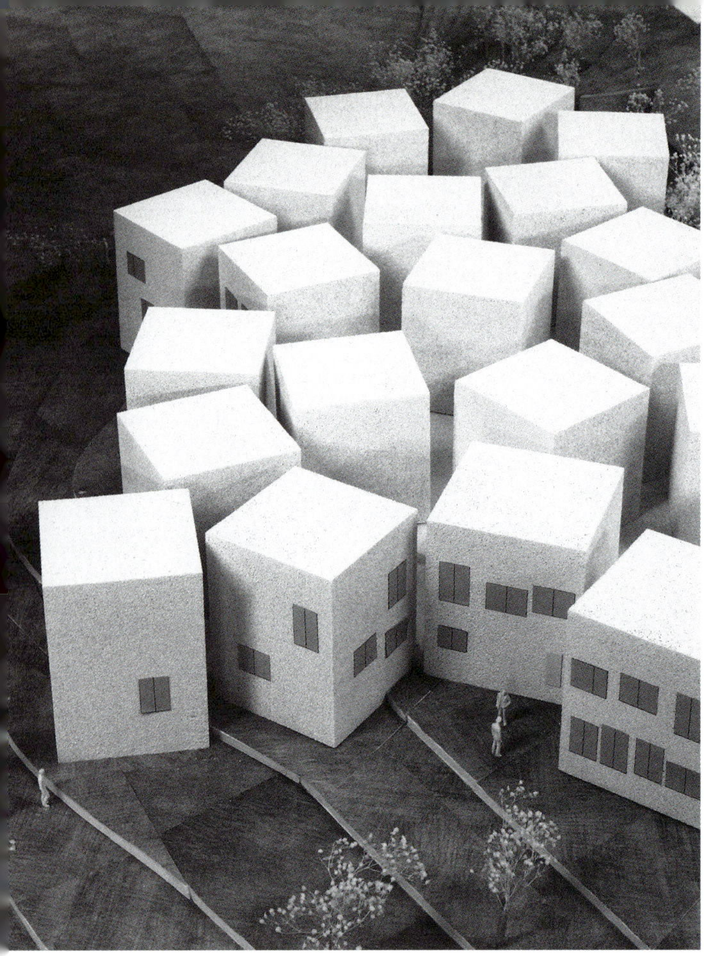

6.20.3 A series of cubes were rotated iteratively until an optimal formal composition was reached.

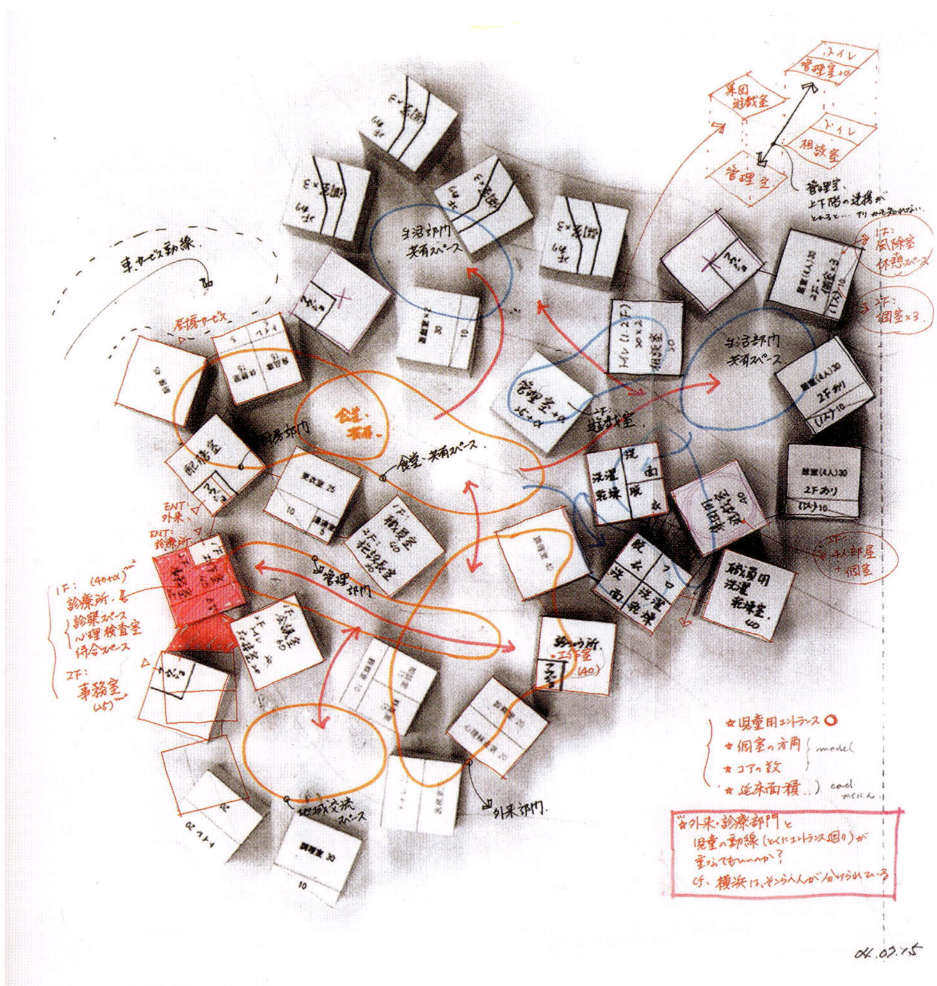

6.20.4 Illustration of the iterative push-pull process that characterized the design process.

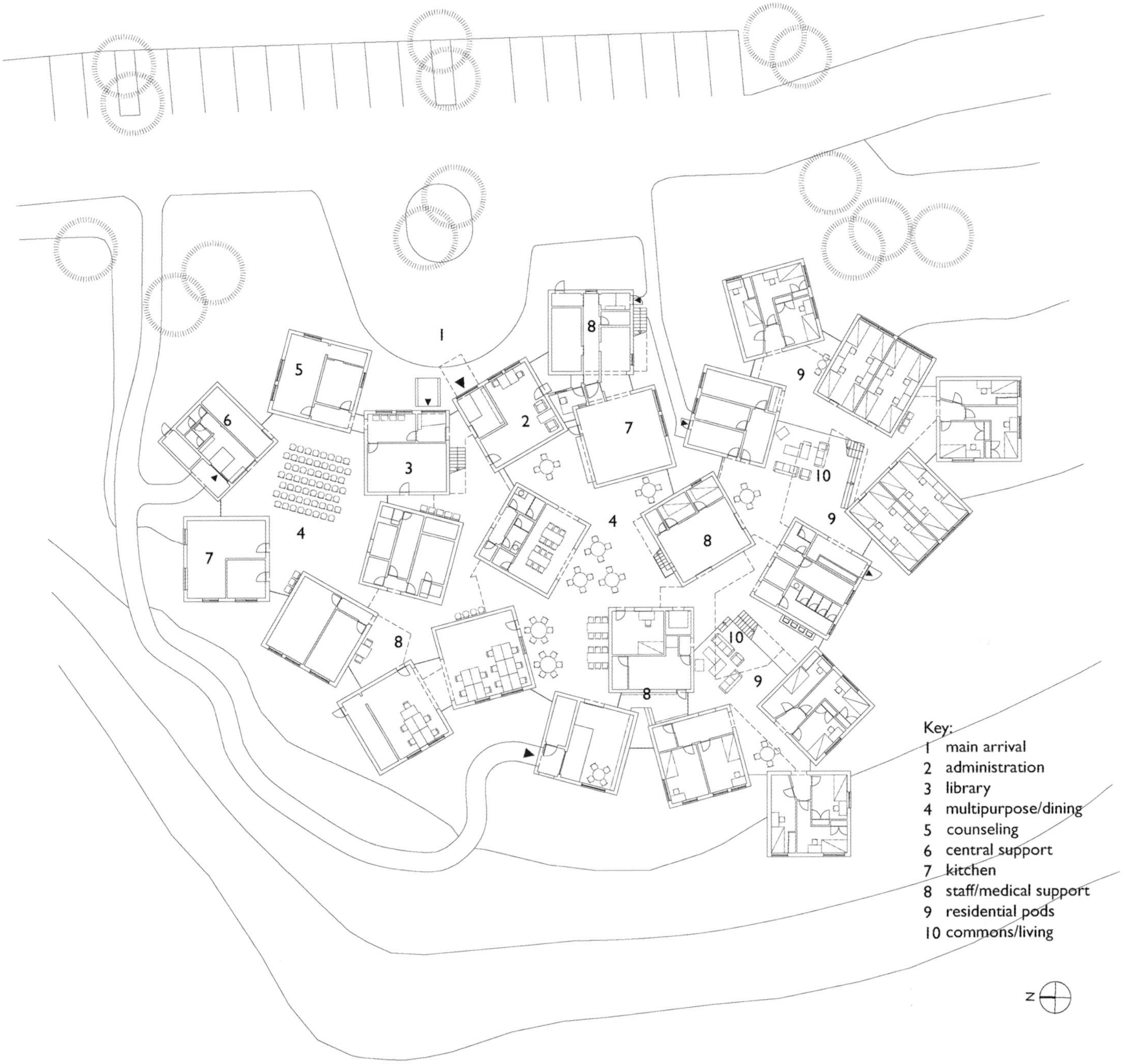

Key:
1 main arrival
2 administration
3 library
4 multipurpose/dining
5 counseling
6 central support
7 kitchen
8 staff/medical support
9 residential pods
10 commons/living

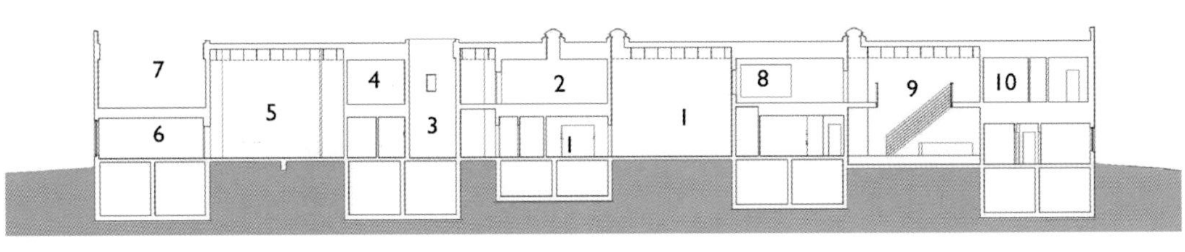

Key:
1 dining
2 conference
3 courtyard
4 dayroom
5 multipurpose
6 kitchen
7 mechanical
8 study room
9 social activity area
10 residential

6.20.5a–b The cube residences are depicted here, as well as the resulting 'exterior' spaces around them, enclosed beneath a unifying roof that allows the cubes to rise above.

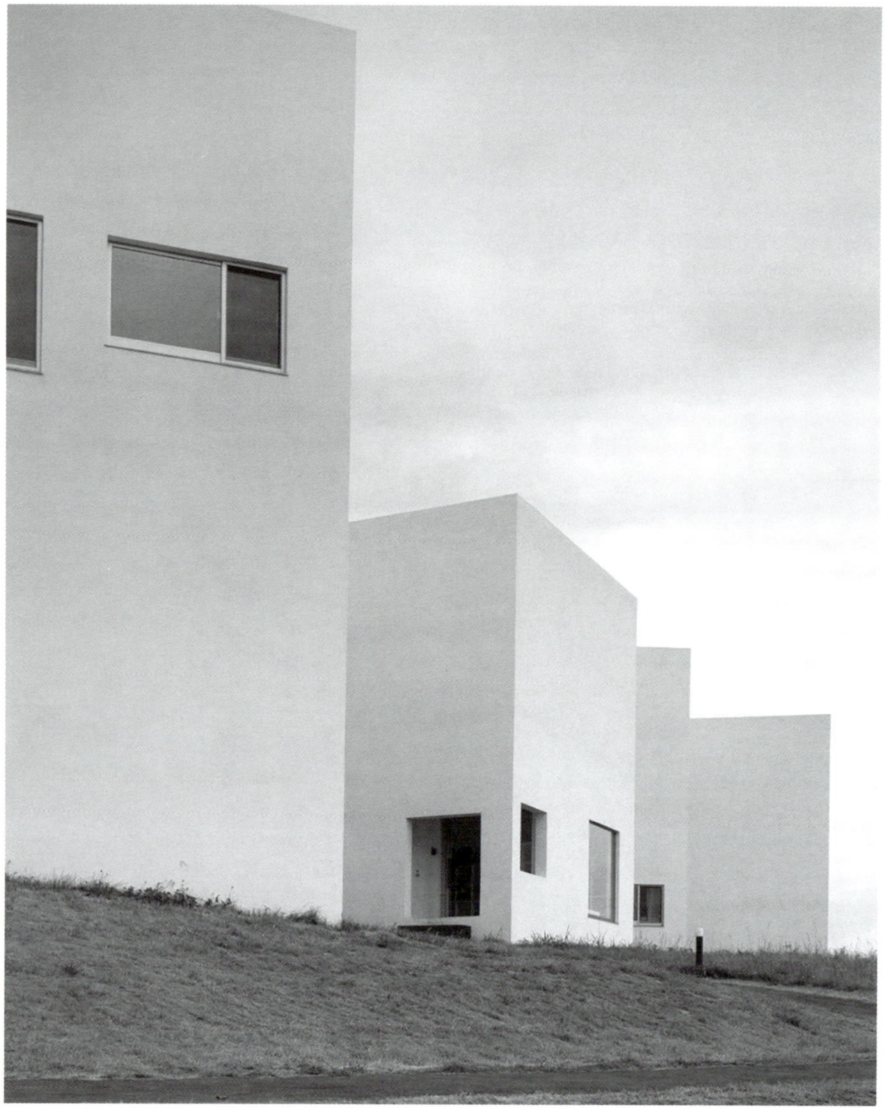

6.20.6 The formal composition is minimalist.

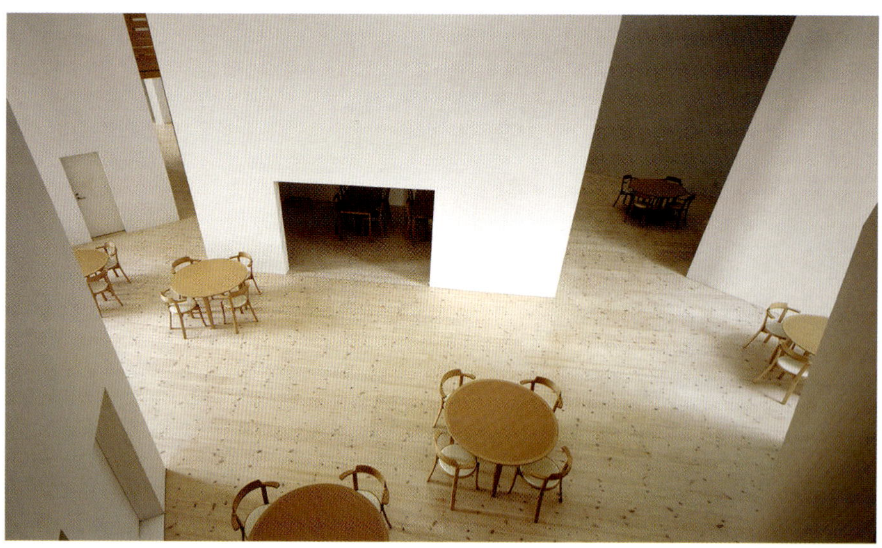

6.20.7 Interior social spaces vary in height and proportion as a function of the cube residence push-pull design strategy.

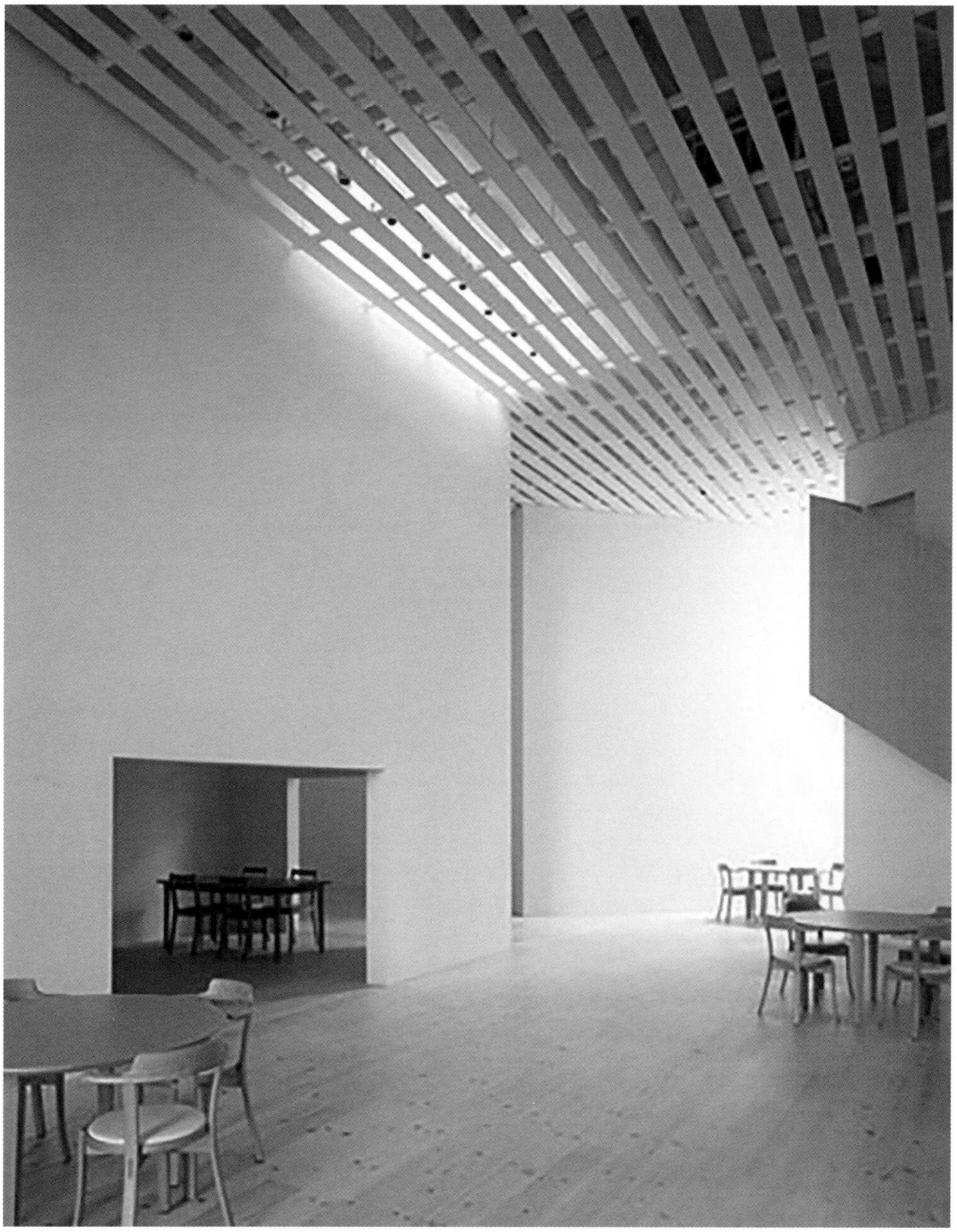

6.20.8 A multipurpose space and pocket alcove in Sou Fujimoto's Children's Centre for Psychiatric Rehabilitation in Japan.

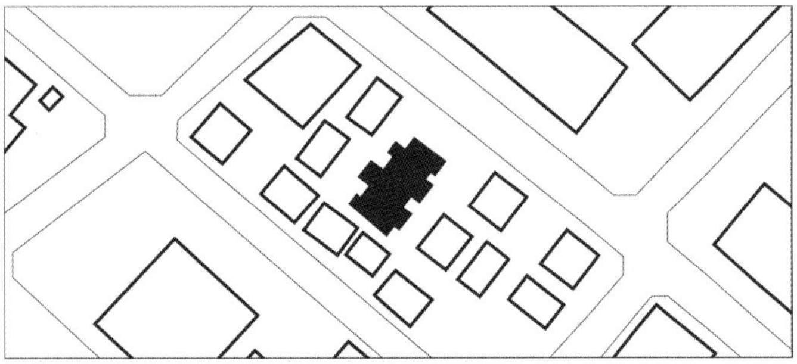

21 Sowa Unit, Saitama, Japan

ARCHITECT: Kensuke Watanabe Architecture Studio, Tokyo, Japan
LANDSCAPE ARCHITECT: Kensuke Watanabe, Tokyo, Japan
CLIENT: Not provided
FEATURED MATERIALS: Cast-in-place concrete, bamboo flooring, glass panels
COMPLETED: 2010
INPATIENT BEDS: Outpatient treatment
SITE/PARKING: 1.5 acres/8
HOSPITAL/TREATMENT CENTER SIZE: 8,400 square feet
NURSES' WORKSTATION: Open

Context/site

The Sowa Unit is an outpatient mental health clinic for adult patients aged 18 and older, located in the densely developed suburb of Saitama within metropolitan Tokyo, in a residential district an hour's train ride from Tokyo's urban center. The architectural strategy was to design a normative clinic environment in a fragmented neighborhood context context of mixed-use commercial, residential, and industrial buildings. The client sought a clinic: inviting, human scaled and somewhat referential. The tight site, with its direct abutments, necessitated expressing the building's 'parts' as six bandwidths, these are then shifted relative to one another in accord with their individual internal functions. Recent precursors include Peter Eisenman's Greater Columbus Convention Center, in Columbus, Ohio (1993); Herzog & de Meuron's M.H. de Young Museum, in San Francisco (2005); the Four Sport Scenarios Stadium, in Medelin, Columbia (2010), by Giancarlo Mazzanti + Felipe Mesa; an indoor swimming pool in Litomysl, Czech Republic (2010), by Architekti DRNH; the Marcel Sembat High School, Sotteville, lès Rouen, France (2011), designed by archi5 with B. Huidobro; and the Zamet Center, in Rijeka, Croatia, designed by 3LHD (2014).

These buildings (albeit all larger in scale) share with the Sowa Unit a strategic shifting of contiguous bandwidth elements of varied functions, materiality, and level of transparency (Figures 6.21.1 and 6.21.2). The principal material of construction is cast-in-place concrete, with formwork exposed on both exterior and interior. A second prominent material was the use of bamboo flooring throughout, further accentuated by full-height glazing at the ends of various bands. The Sowa Unit's bandwidths, when viewed from the front elevation, reveal relatively little about the building's internal functions. This is because the sight lines from within the building do not address the streetscape elevation, while the ends of bands sometimes are windowless, and as such are not oriented to any specific neighboring building. Instead, this clinic's internal spaces and zones tend to be self-referential, maintaining physical separation, autonomy, from the facility's broader site context. The bands accommodate circulation, a waiting area, administration offices, conference rooms, and various support and treatment rooms. The result is a simple, understated, elegant building – an oasis – amid a rather chaotic urban context, a building whose neutrality in relation to its fragmented context succeeds and in this regard, need not call out attention to itself.

Building/unit

Extensive consultations were held with the client, a mental health specialist who sought a building not disconnected from the surrounding city, yet one relatively easy to access via public transit, auto, or on foot. The arrival and entry foyer are residential in scale; this space leads to the main staircase and elevator and connects to the upper level. A café and dining/multipurpose space are located in proximity, as is a kitchen and small dining area. A second lounge and multipurpose space is located adjacent to a set of restrooms and a quiet room. An exterior patio and garden is located to the rear on the first level. The second level houses various group and individual counseling rooms and therapists' offices, the administrative suite, staff workspace, and staff conference room. The ends of some bandwidths remained unarticulated, used as storage and as restrooms. Ceiling heights vary from first to second levels, adding varied interest. A sense of spaciousness characterizes the entire clinic (Figure 6.21.3a–b). Its compositional elements, materials, and finishes are consciously muted and minimalist without becoming repetitive. This strategy also made it possible to avoid long corridors and keep the building relatively easy to navigate, a condition extremely unlike the typical large modern psychiatric hospitals in Japan today.

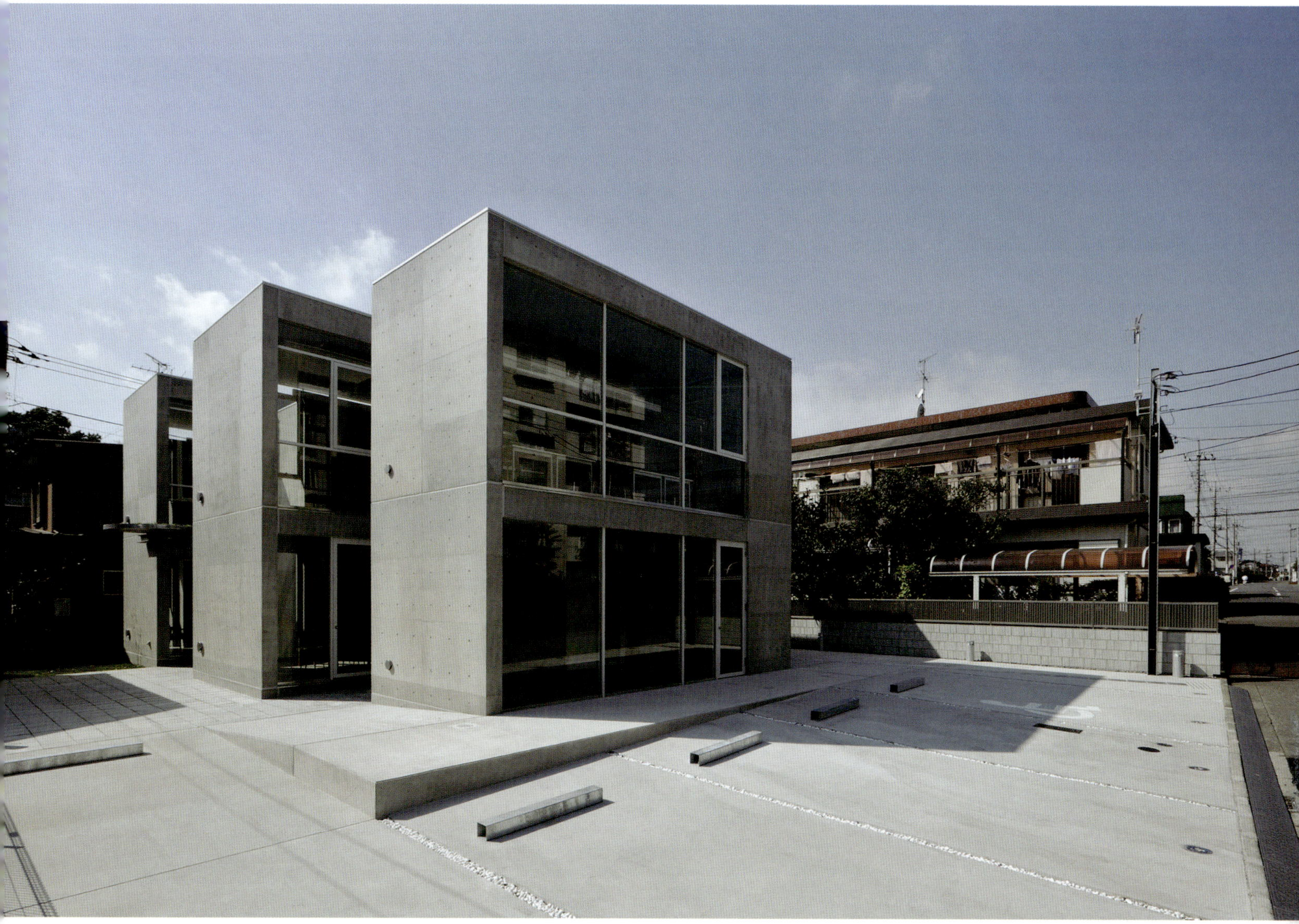

6.21.1 The Sowa Unit is located in a fragmented urban district in metro Tokyo.

From the outside, the composition al forms appear to have been placed on a tray, extending into the parking area (Figure 6.21.4). The spaces created by the bands function as implied 'rooms', viewable places without compromising one's privacy. This shifting occurs in an A/B pattern (mass/void relationship) and viewed at night, these interior spaces glow, although this condition was considered by some staff and patients as sacrificing patients' confidentiality to a degree. Doorways feature projecting circular canopies, a motif repeated on the second level, where this same motif cleverly doubles as a raised platform garden. Furnishings and equipment are minimalist and the clinic's overall visual openness further highlights its bamboo floors. In summary, this clinic's rather fragmented, restrictive site provided limited outward views of therapeutic value and necessitated the importance of creating an internalized world, as expressed in its inwardness achieved by means of a design strategy of establishing microcourts to draw in natural light. And as mentioned, subdividing the functional program in this manner into a series of smaller elements avoids the unfortunate pitfall of the vast majority of clinics of this type. The Sowa Unit's self-referentialism and relative neutrality within a messy urban context resulted in a tranquil, serene place within a fast-paced, chaotic mega-city (Figures 6.21.5 to 6.21.8).

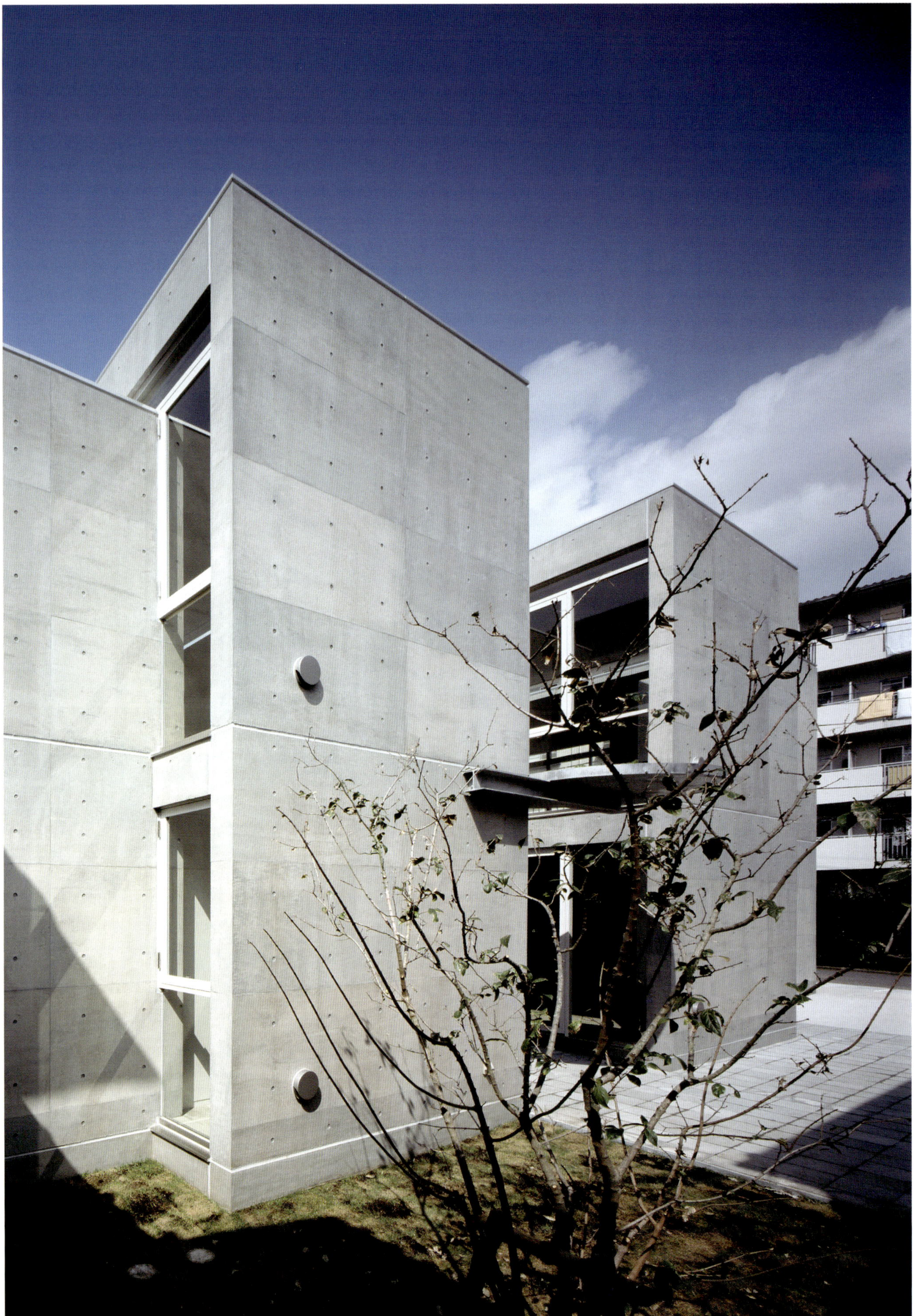

6.21.2 Multiple linear bands in turn yield exterior pocket spaces.

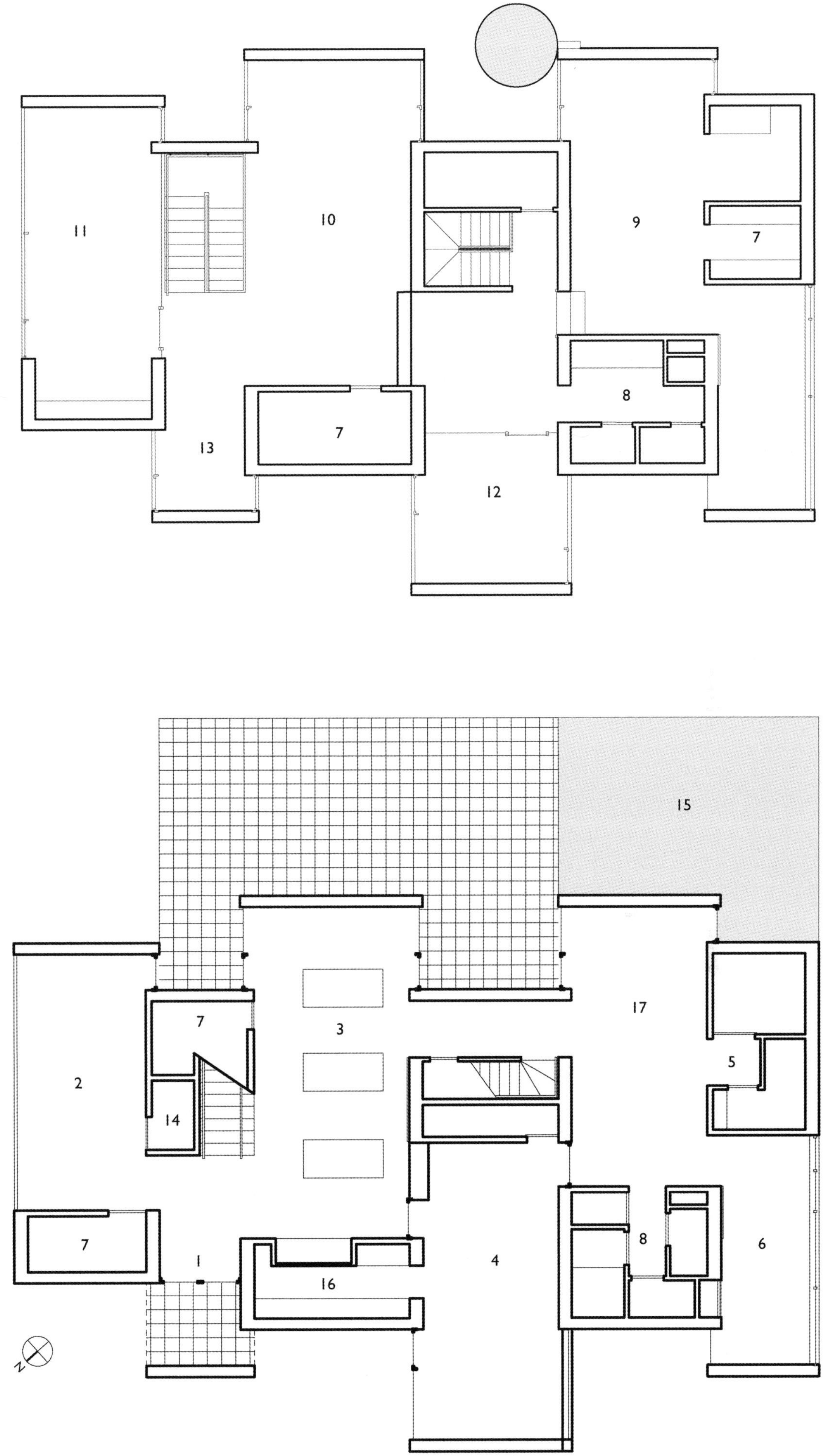

Key:
1 main arrival
2 café
3 dining/multipurpose
4 kitchen
5 lockers/lounge
6 quiet room
7 storage
8 restroom
9 administration/support
10 multipurpose
11 staff/counseling/training
12 conference
13 social alcove
14 elevator
15 garden
16 reception
17 lounge/multipurpose

6.21.3a–b Linear bands are pushed/pulled, resulting in a compact footprint with no long corridors.

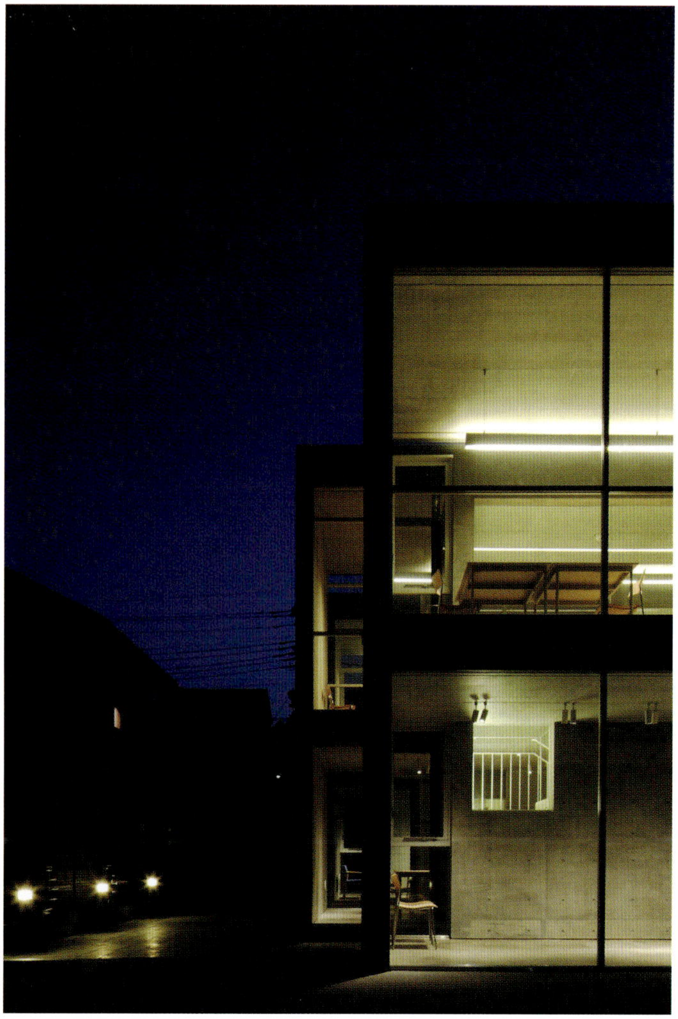

6.21.4 The end points of linear bandwidths are transparent.

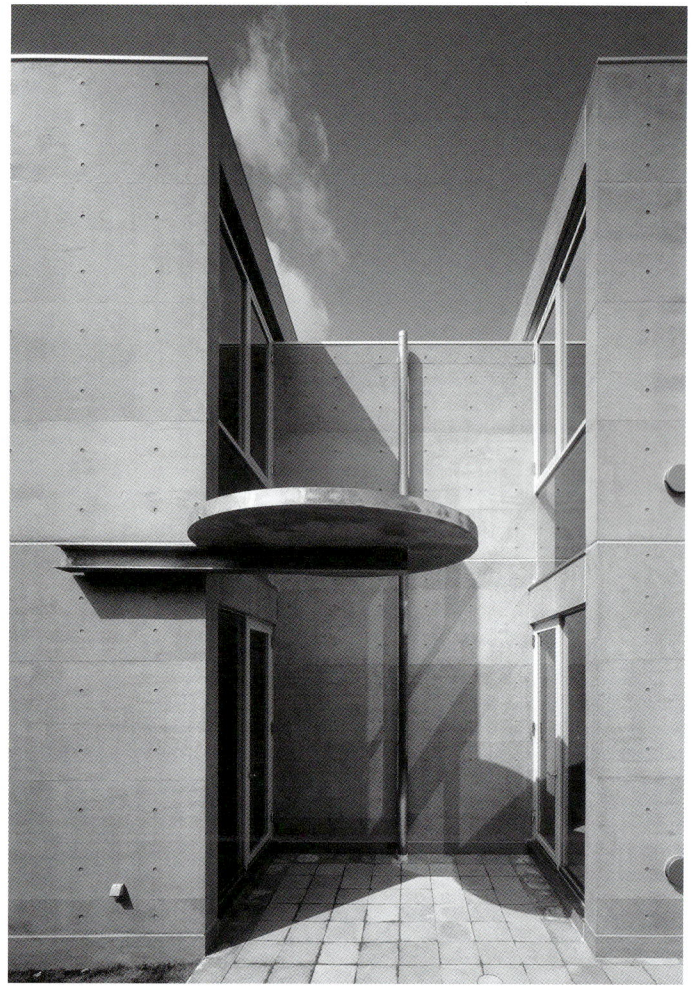

6.21.5 A circular canopy occurs above an exterior entrance.

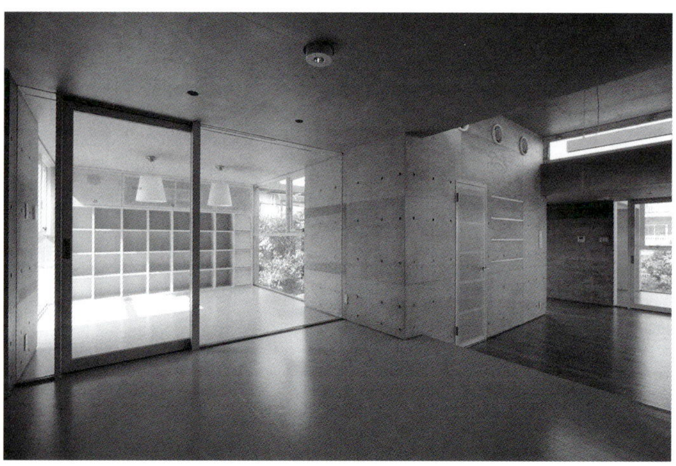

6.21.6 Interior spaces are minimalist throughout this outpatient clinic.

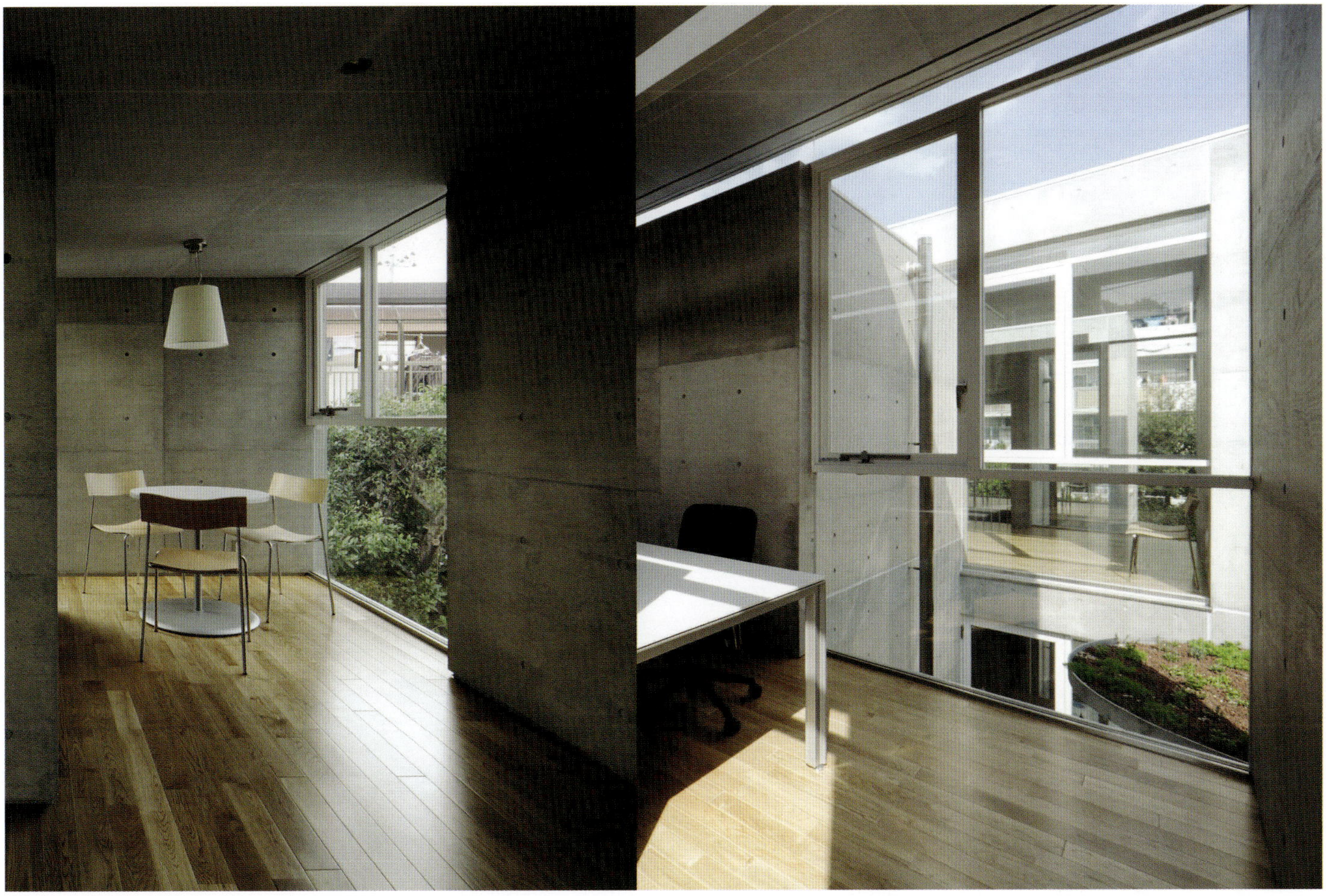

6.21.7a–b Bamboo flooring in the staff break room (left) and in a counseling office (right).

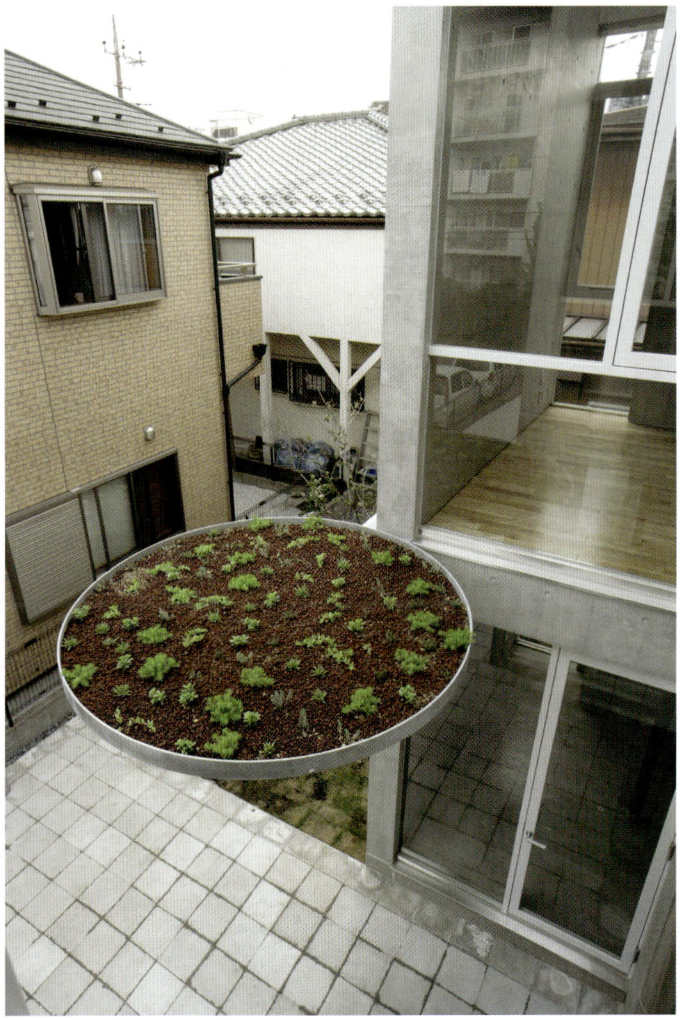

6.21.8 The circular (entry) canopy doubles as a planter, viewed from the upper level.

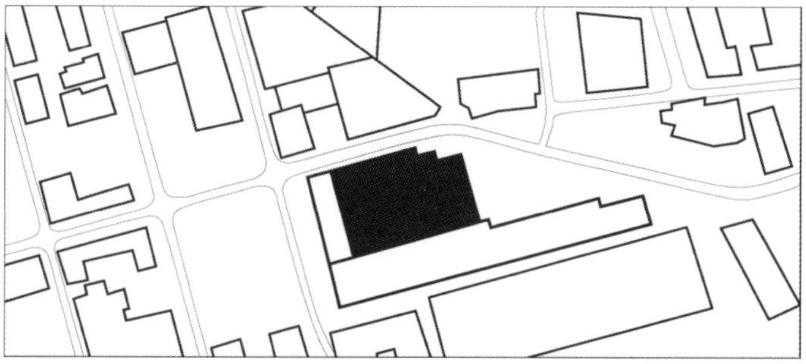

22 Village Family Health Team Clinic, Centre for Addiction and Mental Health, Toronto, Ontario, Canada

ARCHITECT: ARK Architects, Toronto, Ontario, Canada
LANDSCAPE ARCHITECT: None
CLIENT: Centre for Addiction and Mental Health, Toronto
FEATURED MATERIALS: Glass panels, inset photomurals
COMPLETED: 2012
INPATIENT BEDS: Outpatient treatment
SITE/PARKING: 4 acres/20
HOSPITAL/TREATMENT CENTER SIZE: 6,500 square feet
NURSES' WORKSTATION: Open

Context/site

This urban outpatient clinic is located in the rapidly evolving Liberty Village neighborhood, 2 miles from the main campus of the Centre for Addiction and Mental Health (CAMH, see Chapter 4). The Village Family Health Team established in Toronto this community-based clinic devoted to primary care, as well as mental health and substance abuse assessment and counseling (for persons who do not otherwise have a primary care physician). Five additional clinics of this type have since opened in metro Toronto. Primary care and sickness-prevention services offered on-site consist of a clinic for flu, cancer screening, prenatal care, well-baby clinic, chronic disease management for metabolic disorders, hypertension, and nutritional health. Mental health services include eating disorders, substance abuse, gambling addiction, depression, schizophrenia, and bipolar disorder. This storefront clinic is housed at street level in a converted factory in the downtown core, three blocks from the Lake Ontario waterfront. The intent was to integrate it into a rapidly densifying urban context – a neighborhood undergoing rapid gentrification and expansion, including the construction of numerous high-rise condominium point towers (Figure 6.22.1).

As seen from the street, the clinic's large storefront windows announce its presence, without conveying the institutional imagery of a psychiatric hospital or 'clinic' *per se*. This direct visual connection with the streetscape extends to a pharmacy also viewable from the sidewalk, and into the reception area inside. The sign-in counter is located at midsection, in plan, and a row of examination rooms are organized to either side of a central waiting area, thereby subdividing the clinic into two distinct diagnostic and treatment zones. The net effect of this subdivision into two zones was the minimization of corridor lengths. The smaller of these two zones is an L configuration, whereas the larger zone is a racetrack configuration that reconnects to the main reception/waiting area. Minimized travel distances to the farthest points in the clinic contribute to establishing the patient's cognitive frame of reference, and it being perceived by the public as a quasi-commercial storefront operation versus a 'hospital' – with their myriad internal departments and tedious, complex circulation systems. This was of utmost priority from the outset. Additionally, healthcare facilities difficult to locate and navigate can easily become disorienting and stressful, further overwhelming persons coming in off the street suffering from mental illness and addictive disorders (Figure 6.22.2).

Building/unit

Upon entering, one sees directly ahead the reception/sign-in counter; this is the main staff workstation for clinical operations. A waiting area is located directly behind the reception/sign-in counter, and two triage rooms for emergency walk-in patients and a second staff workroom are near in proximity. Functions housed in this clinical zone include the high-risk examination rooms, minor procedure rooms for primary care, restrooms, clean/soiled linen, and Pod A – a battery of nine contiguous rooms devoted to primary care and mental health counseling and treatment. A conference room and open-plan staff work zone are located at the far end of the main arrival axis. This zone houses Pod B – a second grouping of contiguous rooms (in this case seven), also for integrated primary and mental health patient care. A rectangular space in the corner of this zone allows for future expansion (Figures 6.22.3 to 6.22.5). Representations (scenes) of nature are injected throughout the interior by means of a series of thematically linked photomurals. These installations are full height in size and installed as behind Plexiglas panels with each independently affixed to a wall. The designers' intent was for one or more of these photomurals to be viewable from literally anywhere within the public zones. Additional

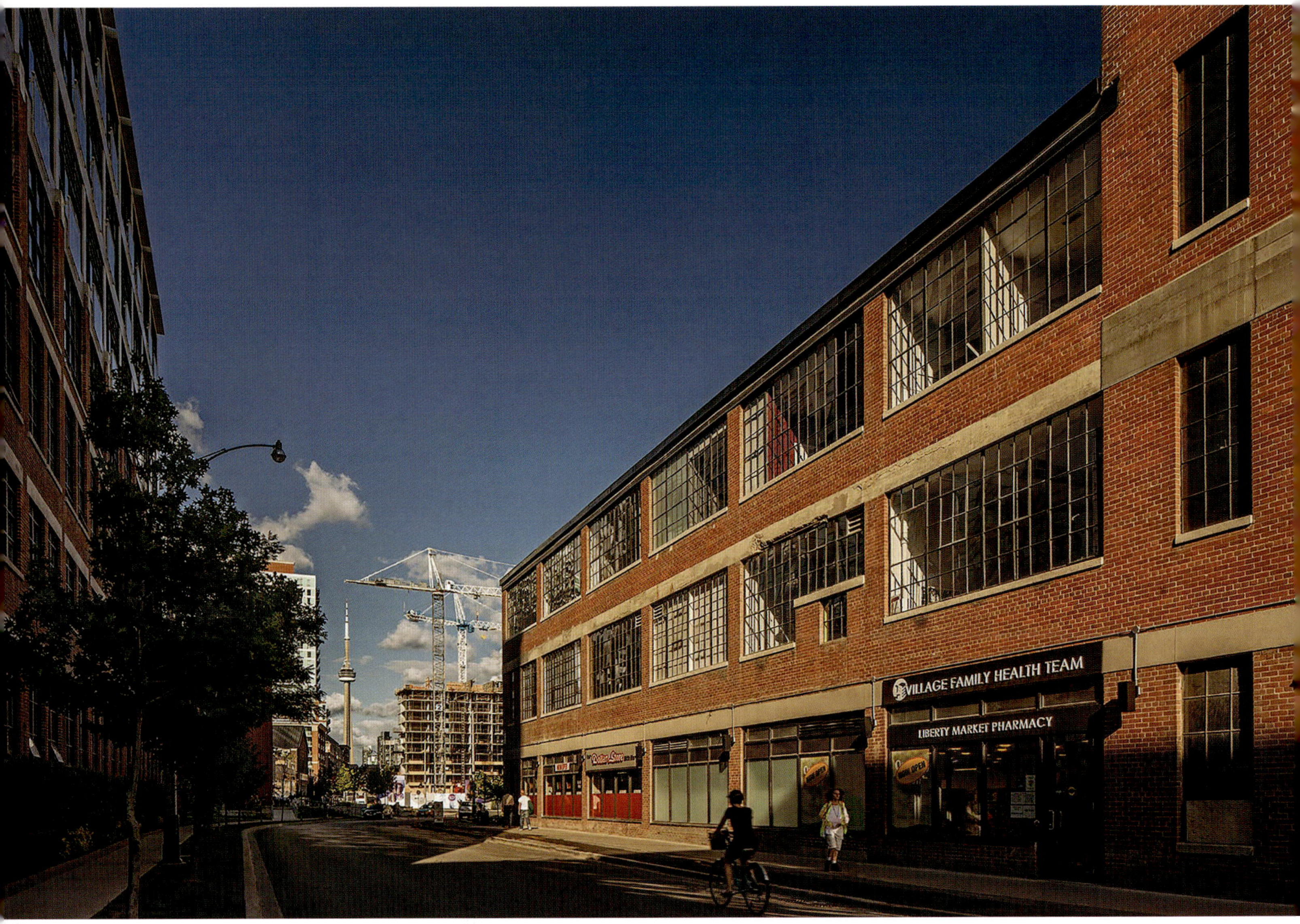

6.22.1 This storefront primary care, psychiatric, and addiction disorders clinic is located in Toronto's downtown core.

photomurals are positioned behind the reception/sign-in counter and in the main waiting area.

Murals are also located in the staff conference room, at corridor intersections, and in architecturally windowless internal corridors. Forest and seashore scenes of the four seasons are depicted, with their content somewhat abstracted, as they straddle the line between figuration and abstraction (surrogate representations; see Chapters 4 and 5). This is the most unique aspect of this clinic, visually and experientially, because the patient encounters a series of themed nature representations in a serialized manner (yet not theraserialized, as this would have required actual physical indoor/outdoor inter connectivity). Here, in a way *softer* and much more ambient than is often the case when nature surrogates are used in 21st-century healthcare environments, psychiatric or otherwise. This is because nature-themed murals in most hospitals and other clinical settings are often portrayed in vivid full-life 'technicolor', as if to be boldly perceived as 'real', or as somehow immediate – *to project you into the scene to the fullest possible extent* – quite literally (without actually doing so). Here, this is not the overarching intent: it is far more about pure surrogation, yet without any attempt to superficially overhype its representational content as some near-approximate substitute for reality. This thematic series of panel installations is to be read and interpreted, essentially, more as a series of abstract paintings and in terms of their collective impact, not unlike viewing an artist's showing of a series of new paintings at a gallery opening (Figures 6.22.6 to 6.22.8).

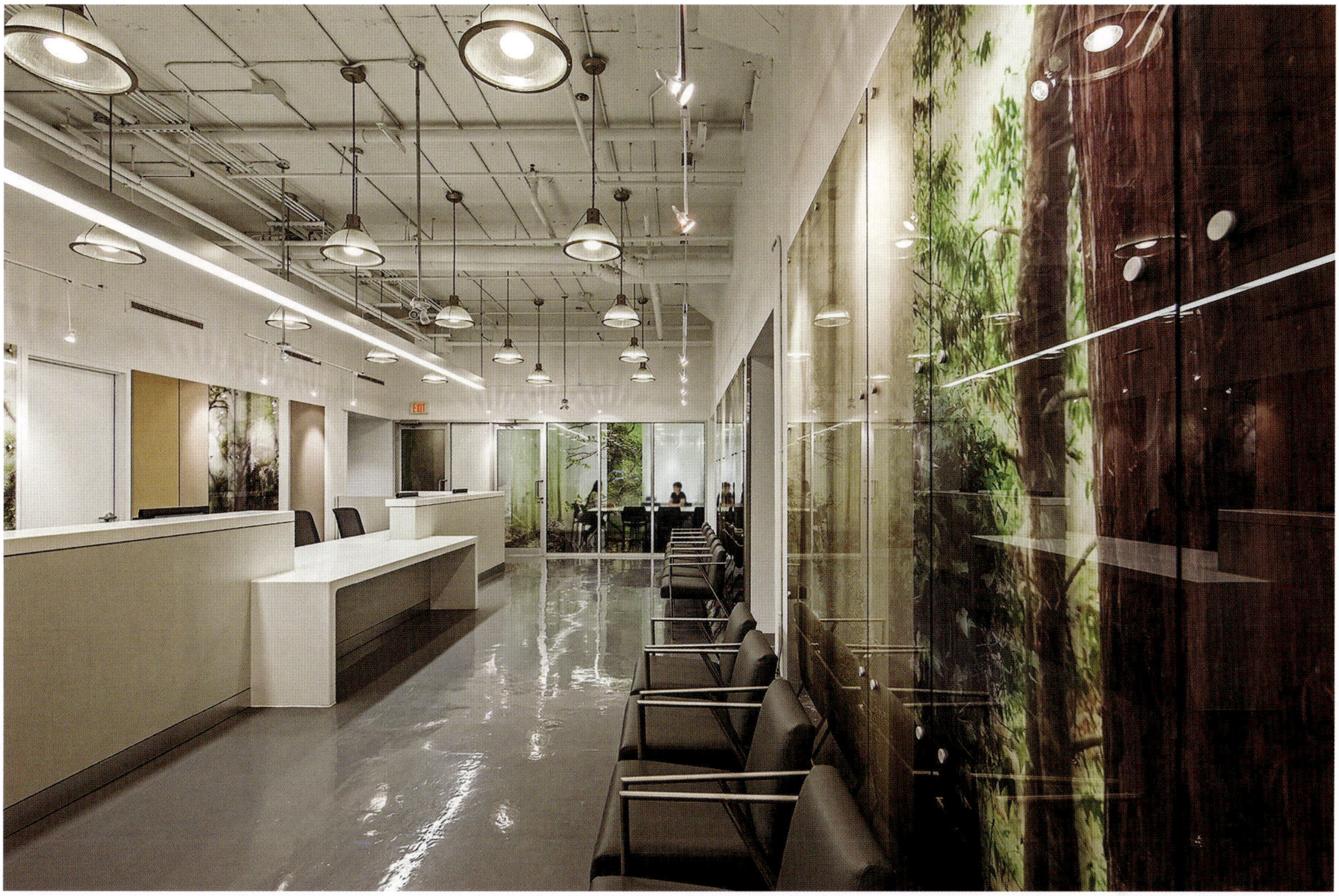

6.22.2 The sign-in/reception/waiting area is directly visible from the main entrance.

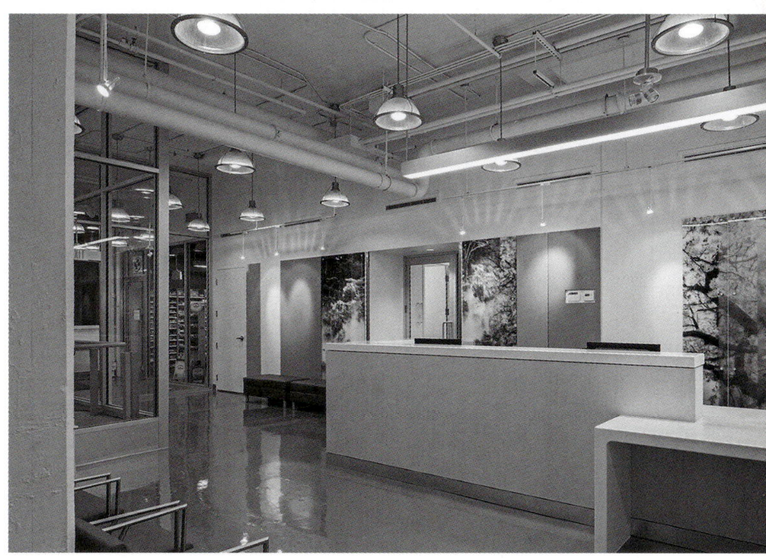

6.22.3 The sign-in counter is located in the center of the clinic.

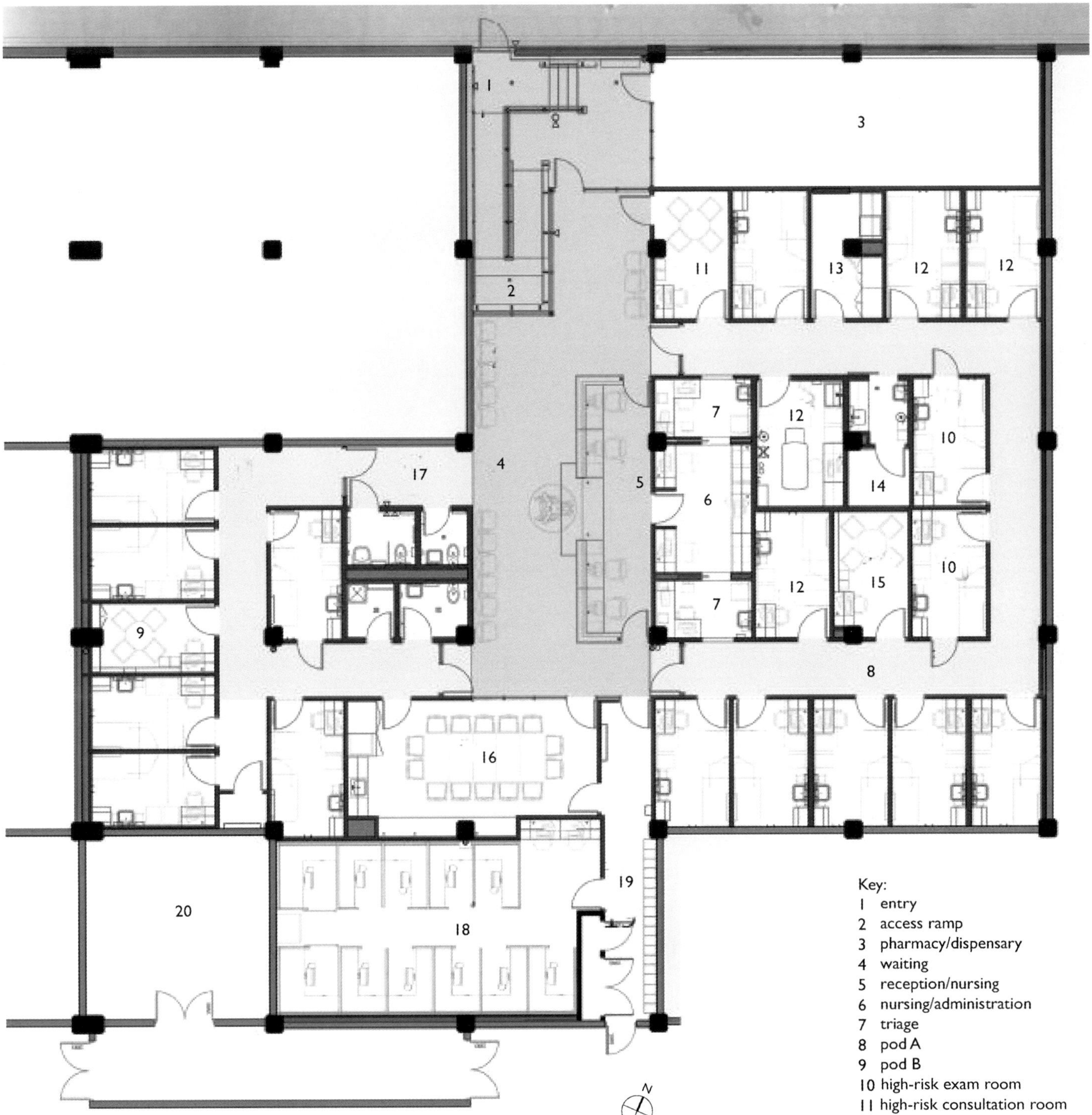

Key:
1 entry
2 access ramp
3 pharmacy/dispensary
4 waiting
5 reception/nursing
6 nursing/administration
7 triage
8 pod A
9 pod B
10 high-risk exam room
11 high-risk consultation room
12 minor procedures
13 clean utility/medication
14 soiled utility
15 social worker
16 boardoom/multipurpose
17 restroom
18 staff work area
19 staff entrance/lockers
20 future expansion

6.22.4 Consult and procedure rooms are configured as two clusters flanking an arrival axis.

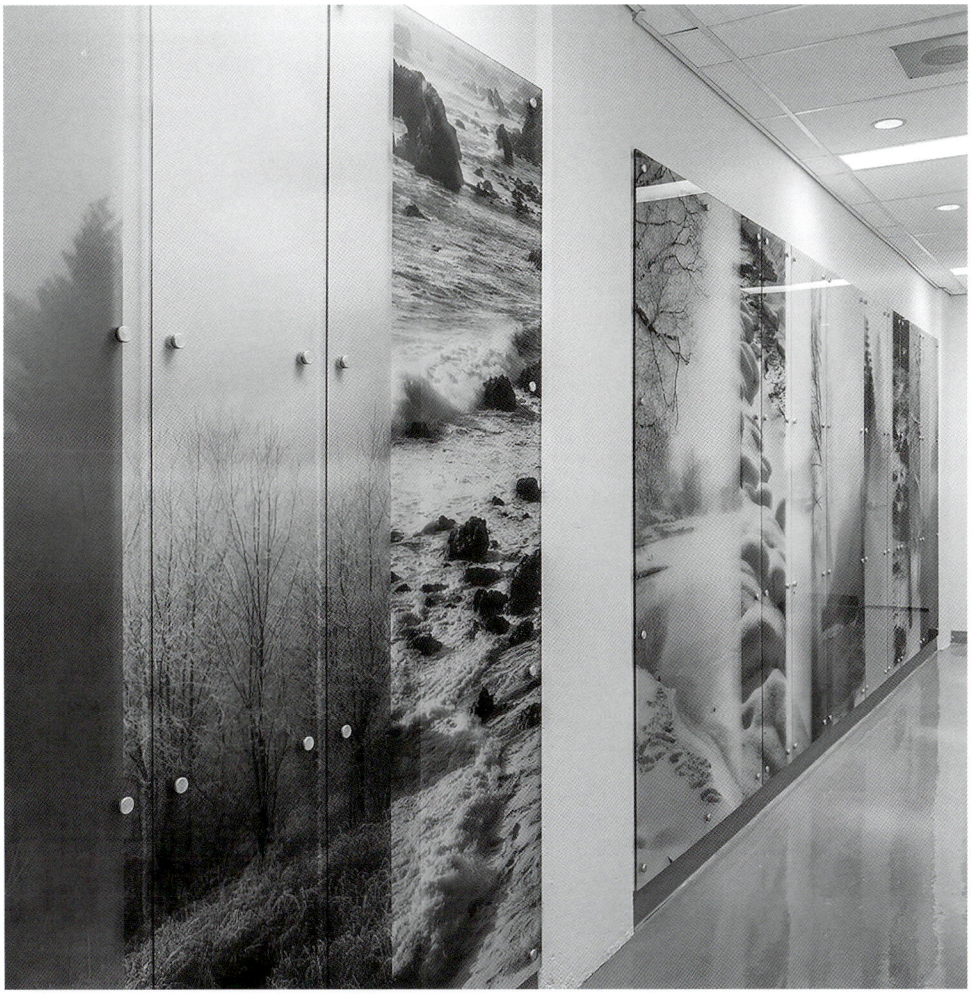

6.22.5 Numerous large photomurals activate interior spaces throughout.

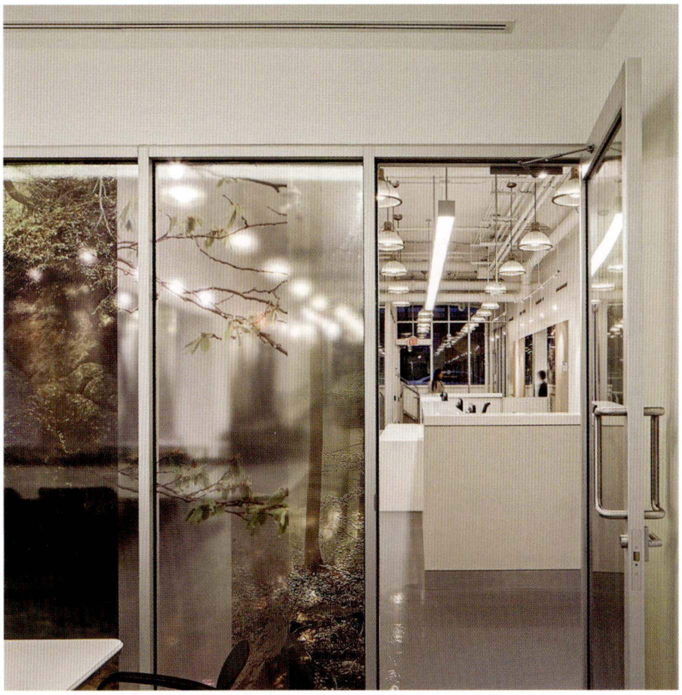

6.22.6 Transparency, combined with nature-themed photomurals, fosters visual continuity.

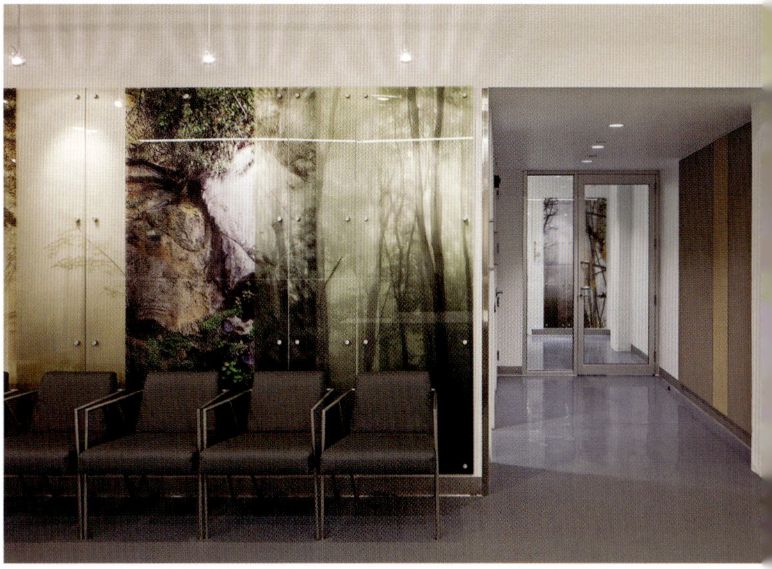

6.22.7 Scenes depicted in the murals are of local natural environments in various seasons.

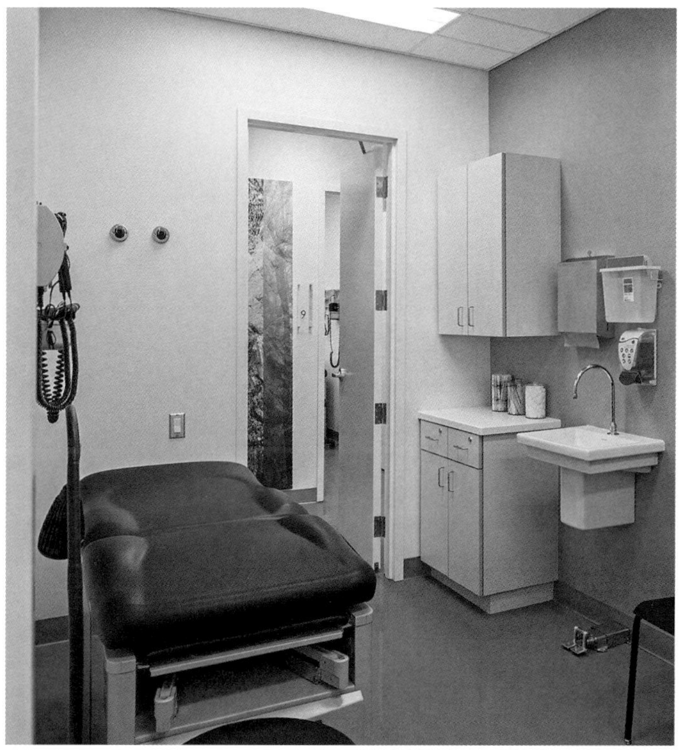

6.22.8 Examination rooms are adaptable in support of the multiple types of services provided.

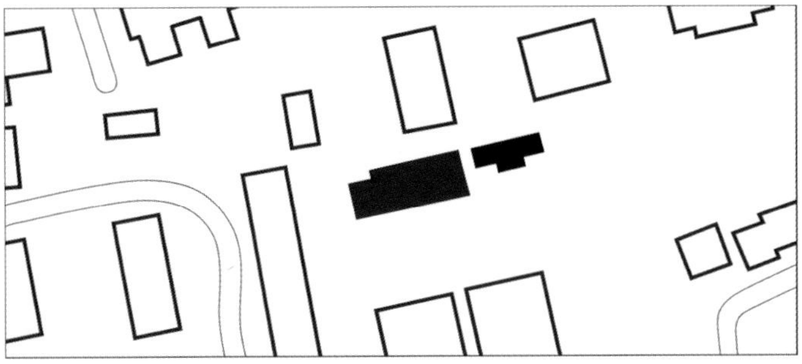

23 Sydenham Garden Resource Centre, London, UK

ARCHITECT: Architype, London, UK
LANDSCAPE ARCHITECT: Architype, London, UK
CLIENT: Sydenham Garden Resource Centre, London, UK
FEATURED MATERIALS: Timber structure, horizontal wood cladding, green roof
COMPLETED: 2011
INPATIENT BEDS: Outpatient treatment
SITE/PARKING: 4 acres/15
HOSPITAL/TREATMENT CENTER SIZE: 4,500 square feet
NURSES' WORKSTATION: Open

Context/site

Sydenham Garden is a mental health rehabilitation center that employs creative and therapeutic activities to aid people with significant diagnoses in London, predominately in the boroughs of Lewisham and Bromley. More than 30 participating healthcare organizations refer patients to Sydenham's Adult Mental Health (AMH) group therapy program. Therapeutic gardening is the focus of the treatment program. Numerous horticultural therapy opportunities are available for individuals experiencing mental health difficulties, with the majority of patients recovering from schizophrenia, depression, anxiety disorder, Korsakoff's syndrome, cardiomyopathy, social phobia, bereavement, acute stress, PTSD, cancer treatment, eating disorders, learning disabilities, and bipolar disorder. In 2010, the architectural firm Architype began client consultations to design a building and compact campus to expand its treatment programs and further establish its presence in the city. A second aim was to demonstrate a major commitment to eco-sustainability in the form of restoring this site's preexisting natural ecosystems to the maximum extent feasible.

At the site's northern edge, adjoining a bowling green and pavilion, the center's public entrance and arrival sequence is accessed from a parking area, pedestrian lanes, and nearby public transit stops. The building's flat roof is landscaped, underscoring its mission as an environmentally sustainable entity, and as a means to connect the center to numerous surrounding outdoor amenities. This green roof also functions as an attractive overlook for the residents of nearby apartment blocks in the immediate vicinity (Figures 6.23.1 and 6.23.2). Extensive client and daily user consultation process resulted in local residents becoming active volunteers at the center after its opening. From the interior of the main building, views are provided of the center's surrounding gardens, and this 'vernacular' building was integrated into its immediate context by means of its small scale, materiality (wood sheathing), and wrap-around porches providing semisheltered outdoor space – as valued transitional space used for group and individual consults (Figure 6.23.3). Synergies between this structure and the immediate landscape are at the core of Sydenham's appeal. Further, its location within a predominately residential area, and the site's preexisting nature preserve condition, called for an unassuming residential-like structure that simultaneously would convey a welcoming image.

Building/unit

The main building's exterior sheathing is *thermowood* and it contributes to the residential, vernacular aesthetic. This was viewed by the client as important in creating a suitable atmosphere for horticultural therapy. This structure is a timber-stud frame building with triple-glazed windows and doors. Space is provided for community organization meetings, the center's administration, and for group and private therapy. A main kitchen and dining room are prominently located, and workspace for coworkers and volunteers is provided nearby. Interior surfaces feature organic, nontoxic paints and stains. Ceiling panels are cement bonded, manufactured free of chemicals, and reduce noise while reinforcing a naturalistic aesthetic. The flooring consists of natural linoleum of linseed oil and jute, with bamboo preoiled tiles with recycled tire matting at the main entrance. Direct access is provided to the multifaceted gardens outdoors (Figure 6.23.4a–b). These therapy gardens are linked to the structure via a footbridge traversing a small pond. Once in the gardens, a variety of horticultural therapy spaces unfold as one moves from zone to zone via a stone walkway leading to a greenhouse. Throughout, 'coworker' patients work in small teams, and individually, tending to a mix of vegetable

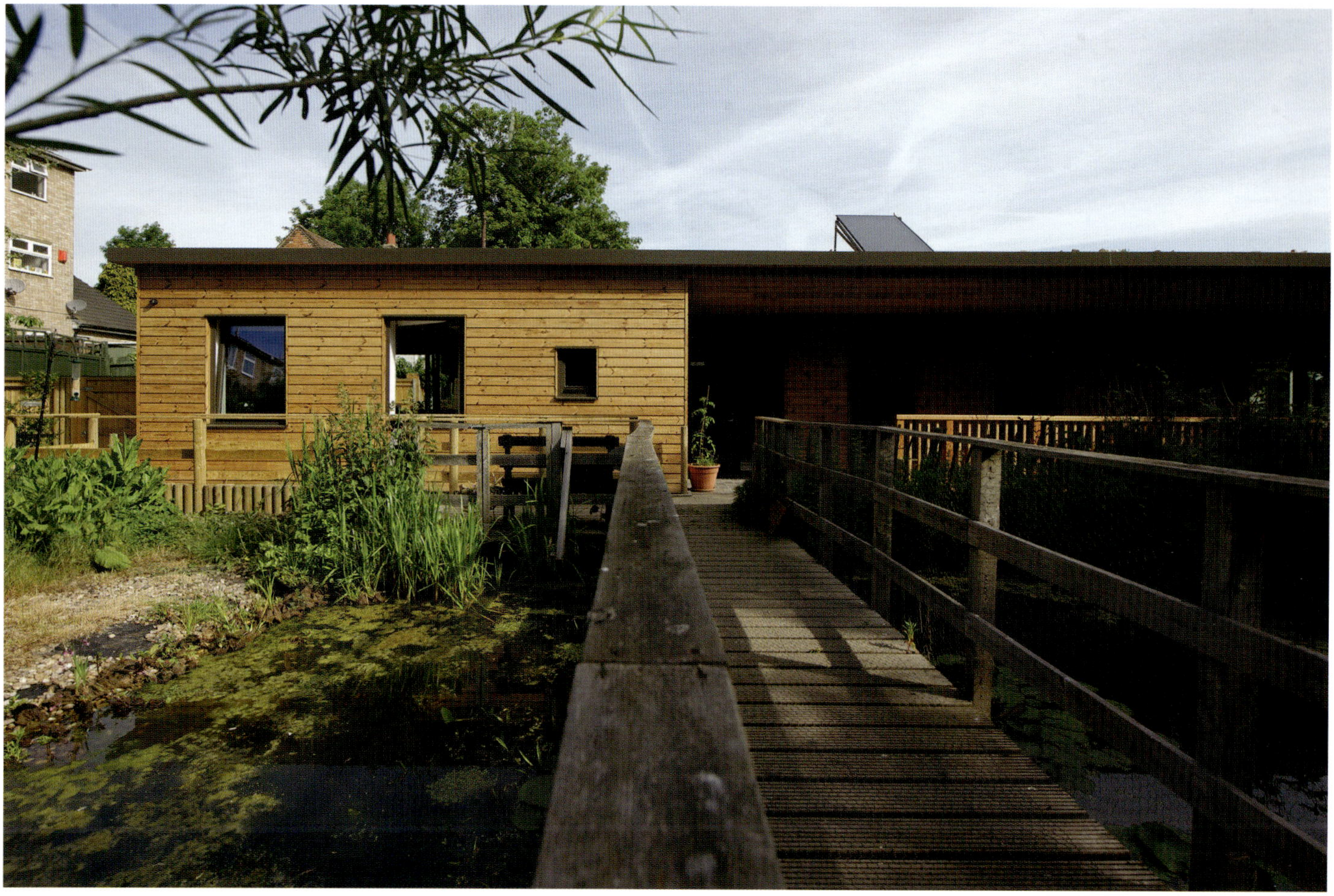

6.23.1 Approach/footbridge leading to the Sydenham Garden Resource Centre in London.

gardens and plant nurseries, at grade, in elevated plots, and in the potted-plant nursery.

As mentioned, open-air, wrap-around decks of the main building provide protection from the elements (Figure 6.23.5). The building and its immediate environs policies are in part determined by coworker 'patients' who are actively involved in organizational policy decision making, while being encouraged to set personal goals toward their own rehabilitation recovery timetable. All coworker patients attend sessions in therapeutic horticulture and arts and crafts weekly, for up to 18 months. The center links its coworkers with complimentary programs in the wider community, including employment, volunteering, and sustainable hobby interests. In the 2015–2016 budgetary year, 403 patients were referred, with 67% attending during this time period. Based on a series of qualitative and quantitative outcome measures, patient outcomes were found to improve noticeably, ranging between 46% and 68% of all coworkers treated. Positive outcomes included improved (self-reported) physical health status, reduced feelings of social isolation, and an increase in overall emotional well-being (Figures 6.23.6 and 6.23.7).[3] One might hope, someday, a large network of horticultural-based mental health treatment centers such as Sydenham Garden will exist. Such a proposition could be structured similar to the Maggie's Centres, a network of alternative community-based health centers (also established as an antihospitalist alternative) for persons, in this case, with a cancer diagnosis who seek non-hospital-based support. For its part, the Maggie's Centre network has grown significantly over the past 20 years and it now includes 13 sites (at this writing) in the United Kingdom and Hong Kong.[4]

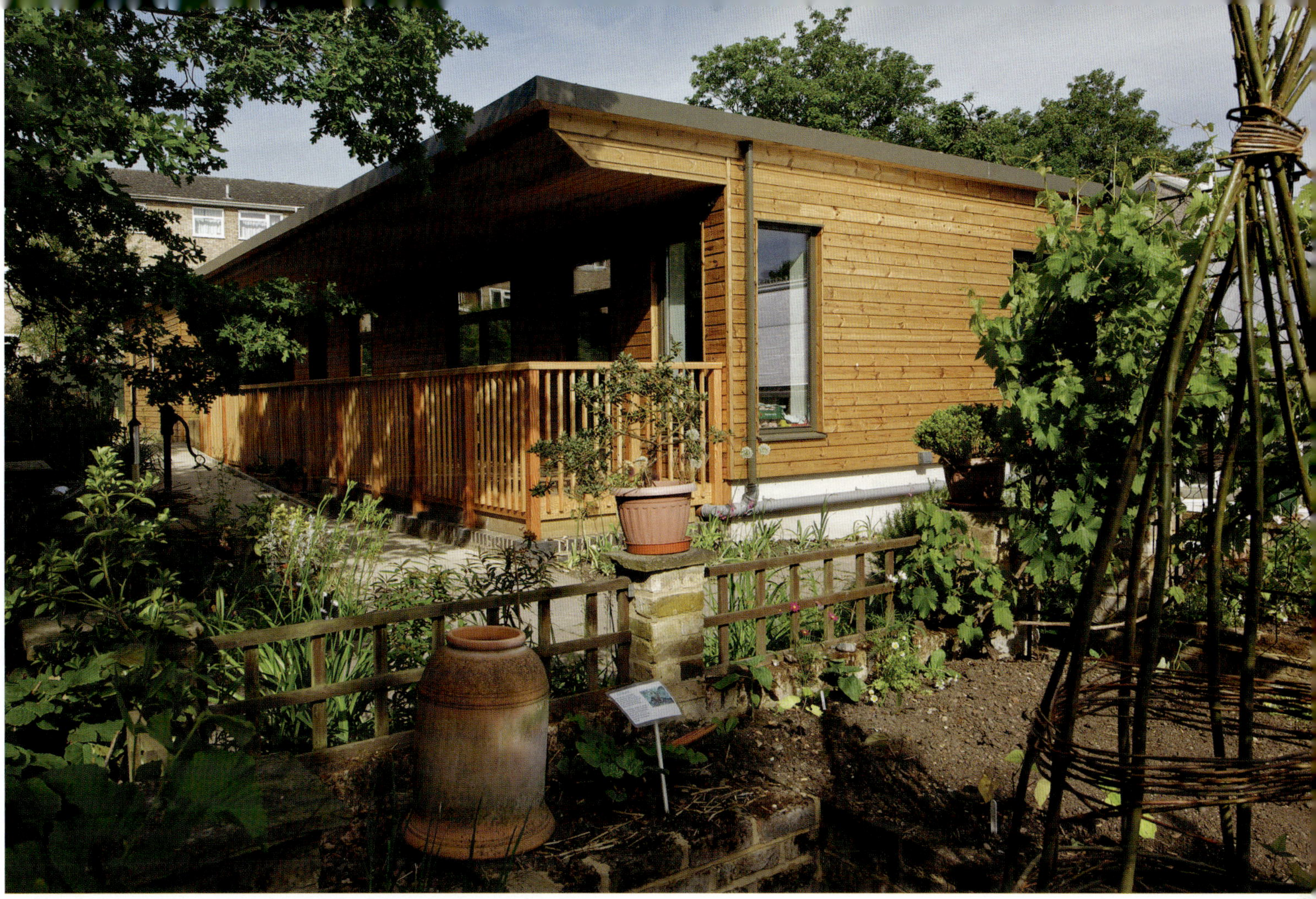

6.23.2 The center is naturalistically woven into a dense urban context in London.

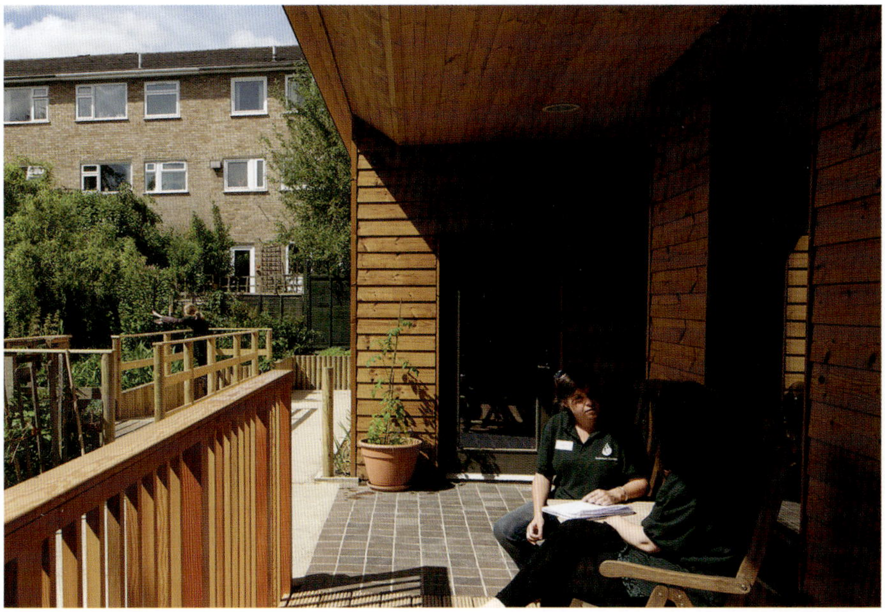

6.23.3 Linear side porches function as consult space and an intermediate zone between exterior and interior realms.

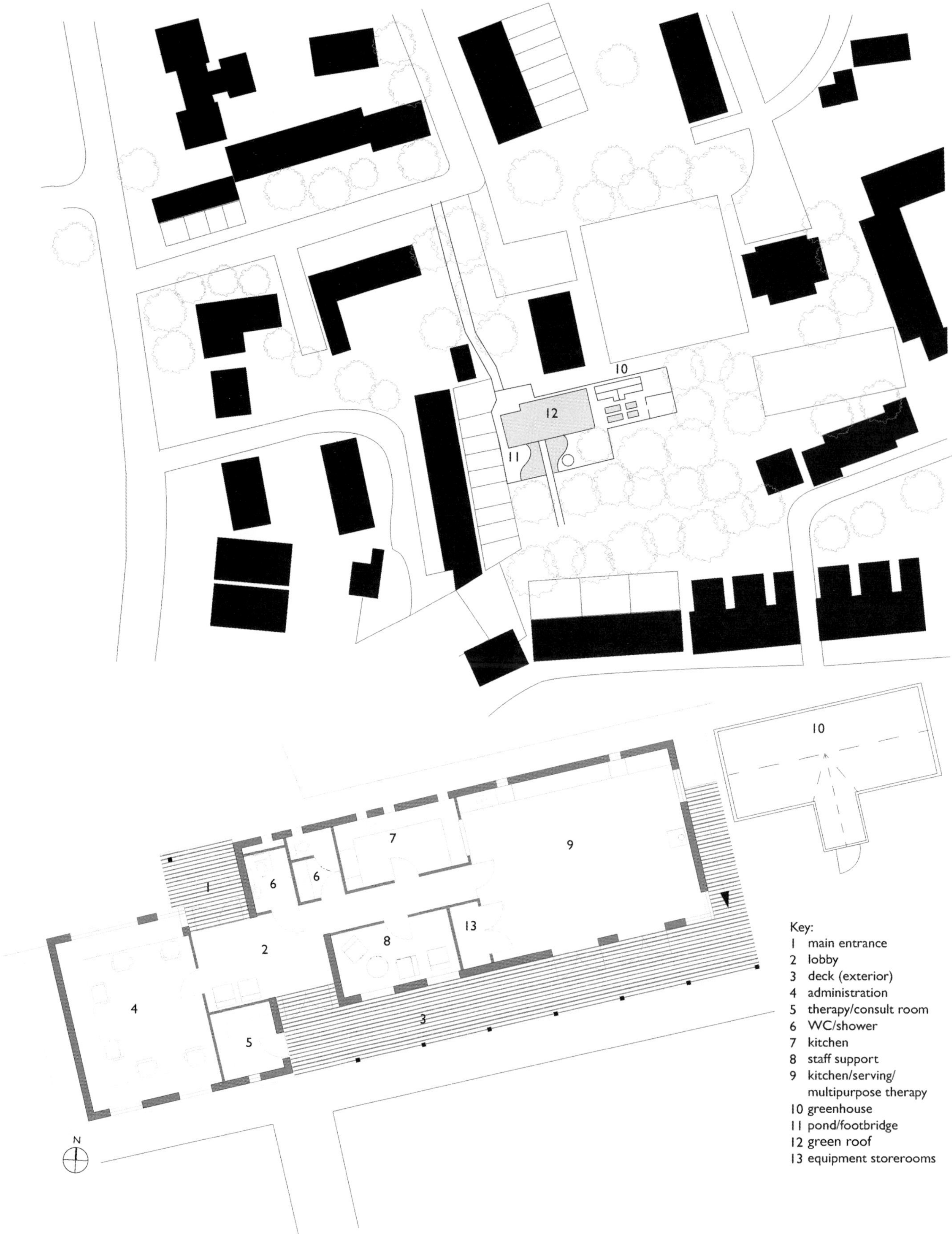

6.23.4a–b The center is in a mixed-use neighborhood and stands apart from the midrise housing blocks in close proximity.

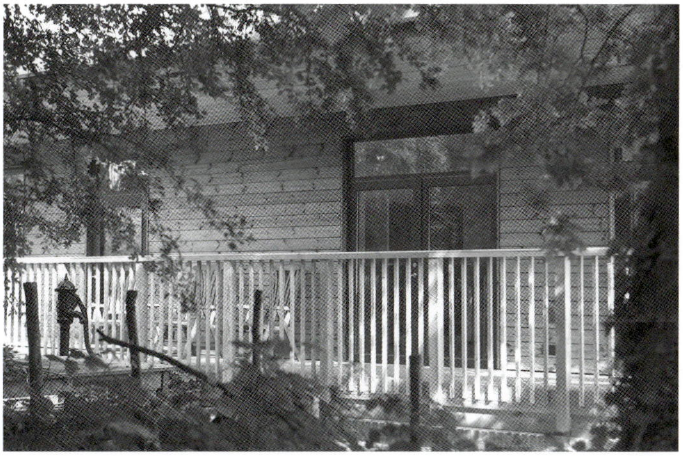

6.23.5 Natural materials and finishes are featured throughout the campus.

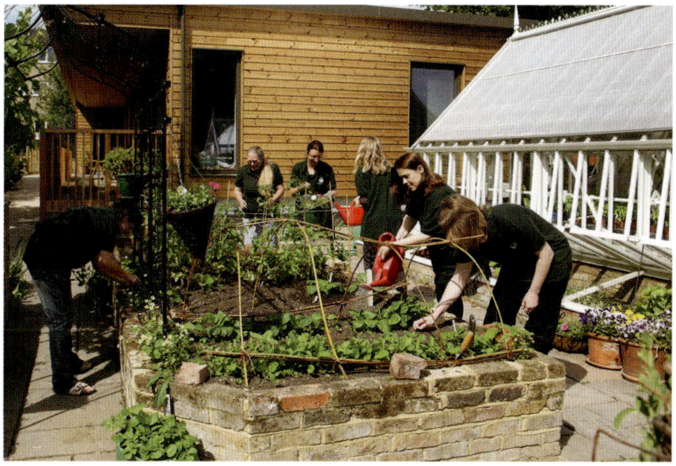

6.23.7 The therapeutic gardening program fosters camaraderie and shared purpose at Sydenham Garden.

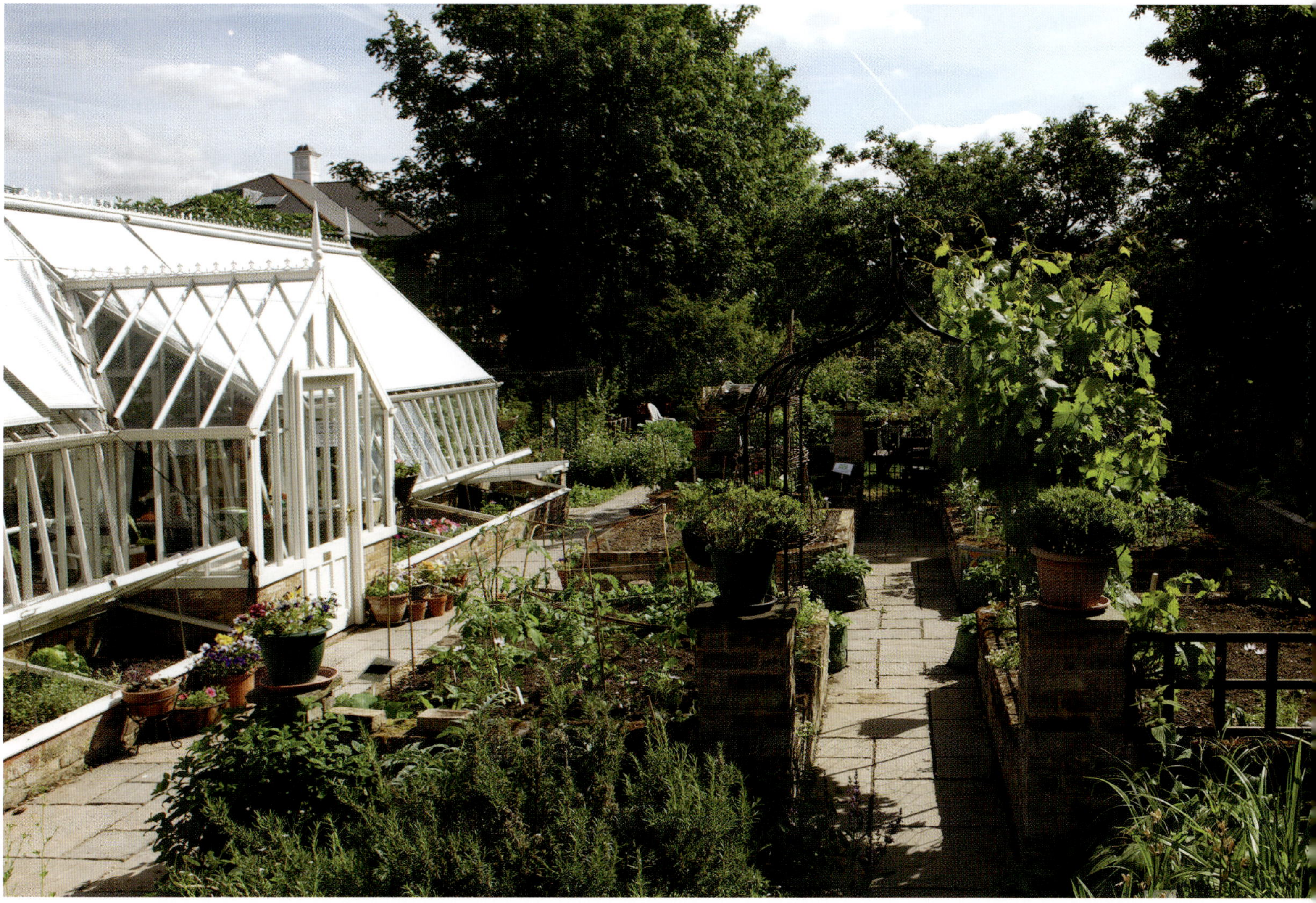

6.23.6 Multiple garden plots and a greenhouse serve as settings for horticultural therapy sessions.

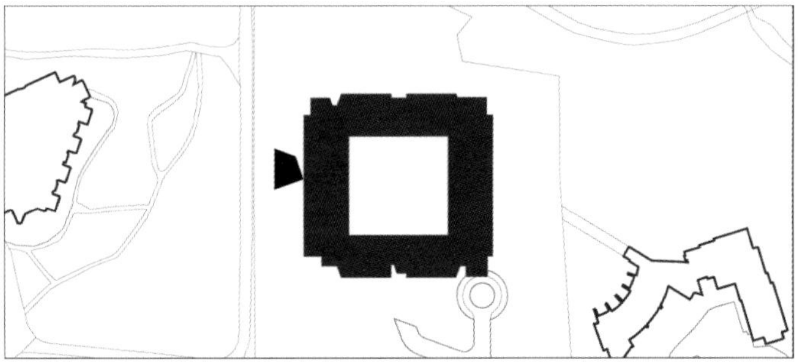

24 Leaside Behavioural Health Centre, Toronto, Ontario, Canada

ARCHITECT: Gabriel Valdivieso, Quito, Ecuador
LANDSCAPE ARCHITECT: Gabriel Valdivieso, Quito, Ecuador
CLIENT: Leaside Behavioural Health Network, Toronto
FEATURED MATERIALS: Glass, steel, masonry, wood interior, exterior sheathing
COMPLETED: 2015 (proposal)
INPATIENT BEDS: 32/outpatient clinic
SITE/PARKING: 12 acres/68 (below) and12 (at grade)
HOSPITAL/TREATMENT CENTER SIZE: 48,000 square feet
NURSES' WORKSTATION: Hybrid

Context/site

This proposed 32-bed mental health treatment center for adults provides inpatient and outpatient services. It was developed in an advanced graduate design studio at the University of Toronto (directed by this author). The site borders a wooded ravine and creek at the edge of a residential district, near Sunnybrook Hospital and next to a 60-bed inpatient rehabilitation hospital operated by the Toronto Rehabilitation Hospital. This facility is to be affiliated with Toronto Rehab's 425-bed main facility in the University Health District downtown. A 75-bed substance abuse treatment facility operated by a for-profit service provider is next door. Leaside is to provide rehabilitation, psychiatric, and substance abuse mental health services in a normative quasi-residential atmosphere. The building treads lightly on its site (currently a surface parking lot), maintaining existing view corridors to an adjoining residential neighborhood, through to a wooded ravine that borders the site to the north. Direct access to this ravine is maintained with access via bike and pedestrian paths. By lifting the main structure up at key intervals, a degree of site openness is attained, further preserving existing views throughout the site (Figure 6.24.1). This two-level hospital was inspired, by Herzog & de Meuron's REHAB Basel, in Basel, Switzerland (2002).[5]

At Rehab Basel, similarly, an undifferentiated box was subjected to a process of addition by subtraction through the elimination of volumes of varying size and proportion. This yielded, here, a large center courtyard cut-out yielding relative transparency – theraserialization – extending from the public arrival zone on the first level into the inpatient residential units on the upper level, to a winter garden in proximity on the site and connected via internal walkway (Figure 6.24.2). The central courtyard destigmatizes the facility and its environs, secures a large common outdoor space, and avoids the presence of intimidating perimeter walls and fences. This allows contact with nature from the major spaces used by patients. Priority is placed on 'site repairing' what once was a residual land parcel. To this end, a 68-car parking garage is located directly beneath the building. The public arrival zone leading to the main entrance provides direct views into the commons/courtyard. It features (saved) mature trees, a therapy garden, outdoor amphitheater, and a canopied terrace. The surrounding landscape features an additional horticultural therapy garden, recreation fields, and a small pond that can double as an ice rink in winter; most outdoor amenities are designed to be used by the immediate neighborhood, without disturbing the center's core functions, nor security requirements.

Building/unit

Four residential wings, equivalent in size, function, and aesthetic, house eight bedrooms and a chill/seclusion room, a space located directly across from the nurses' station (Figure 6.24.3a–b). Circulation and day/activity rooms on this level have full-height windows, providing full views into the commons/courtyard. The nurses' stations are hybrid, consisting of an open-access workstation and a shielded zone nearby, in proximity. A small break room and dining area is provided, as are general staff supports. Circulation on the four residential units is single loaded, with patients' rooms positioned on the outboard side, in plan, surrounding the large open space at the center of the partí. Patient rooms are single occupancy, with a private bath/shower unit positioned on the corridor (inboard) side. Roof overhangs are exaggerated to provide additional protection from the elements. Occupants' spatial orientation and navigation is of high concern, and in response, the single-loaded circulation facilitates views to the center of the complex, as well as

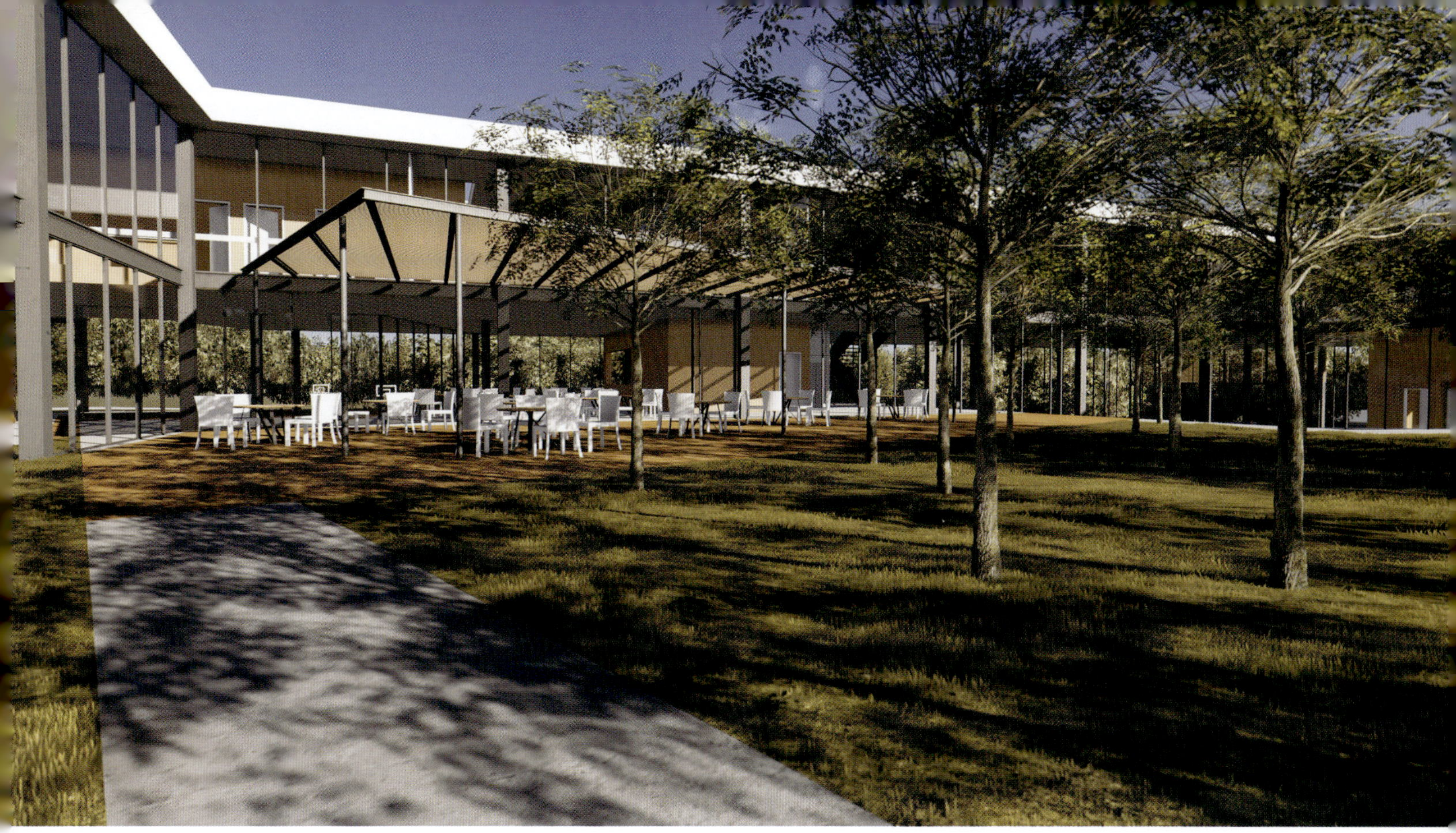

6.24.1 The commons/courtyard at the (proposed) Leaside Behavioural Health Centre in Toronto.

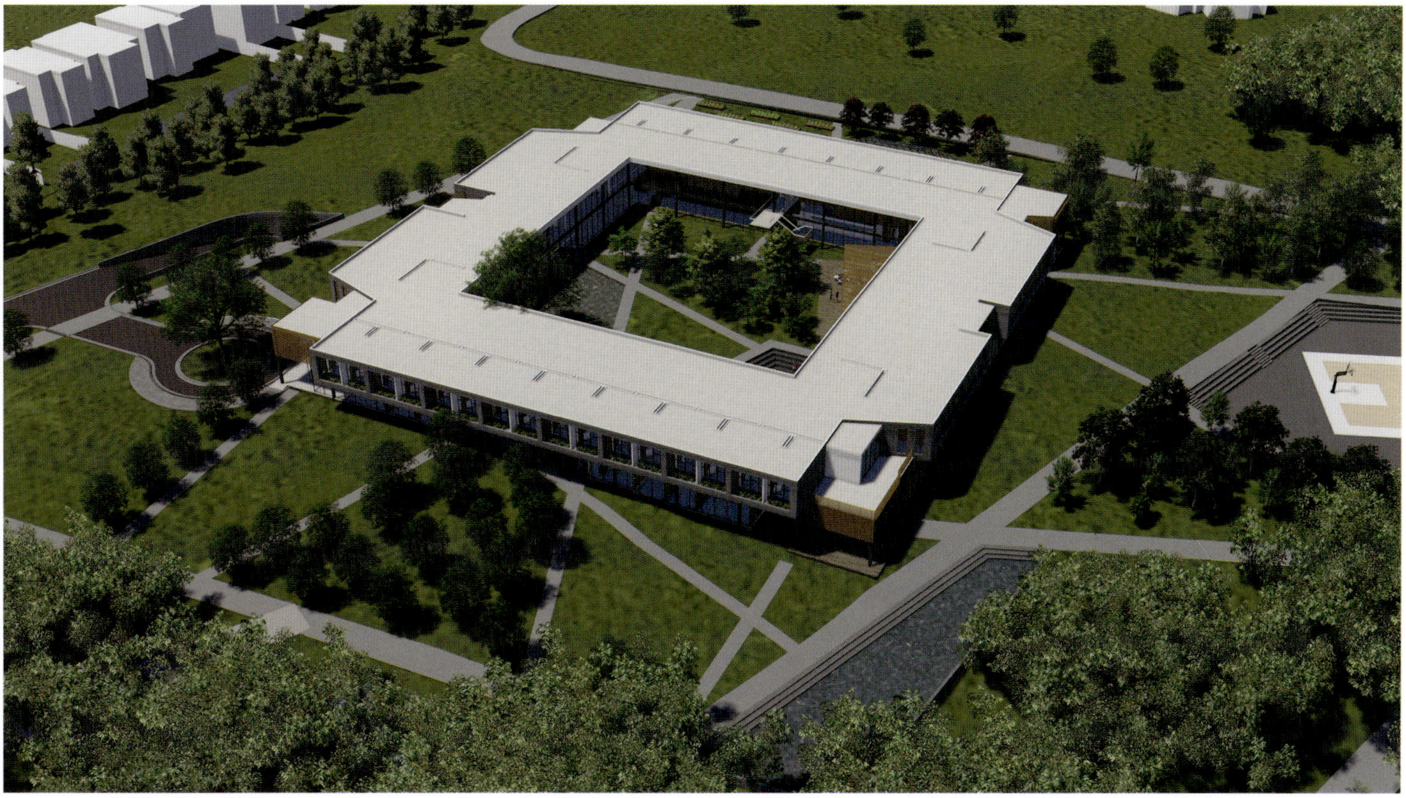

6.24.2 The partí is a large rectangle with a significant volume removed from the center accentuating and drawing it closer to its wooded-ravine site context.

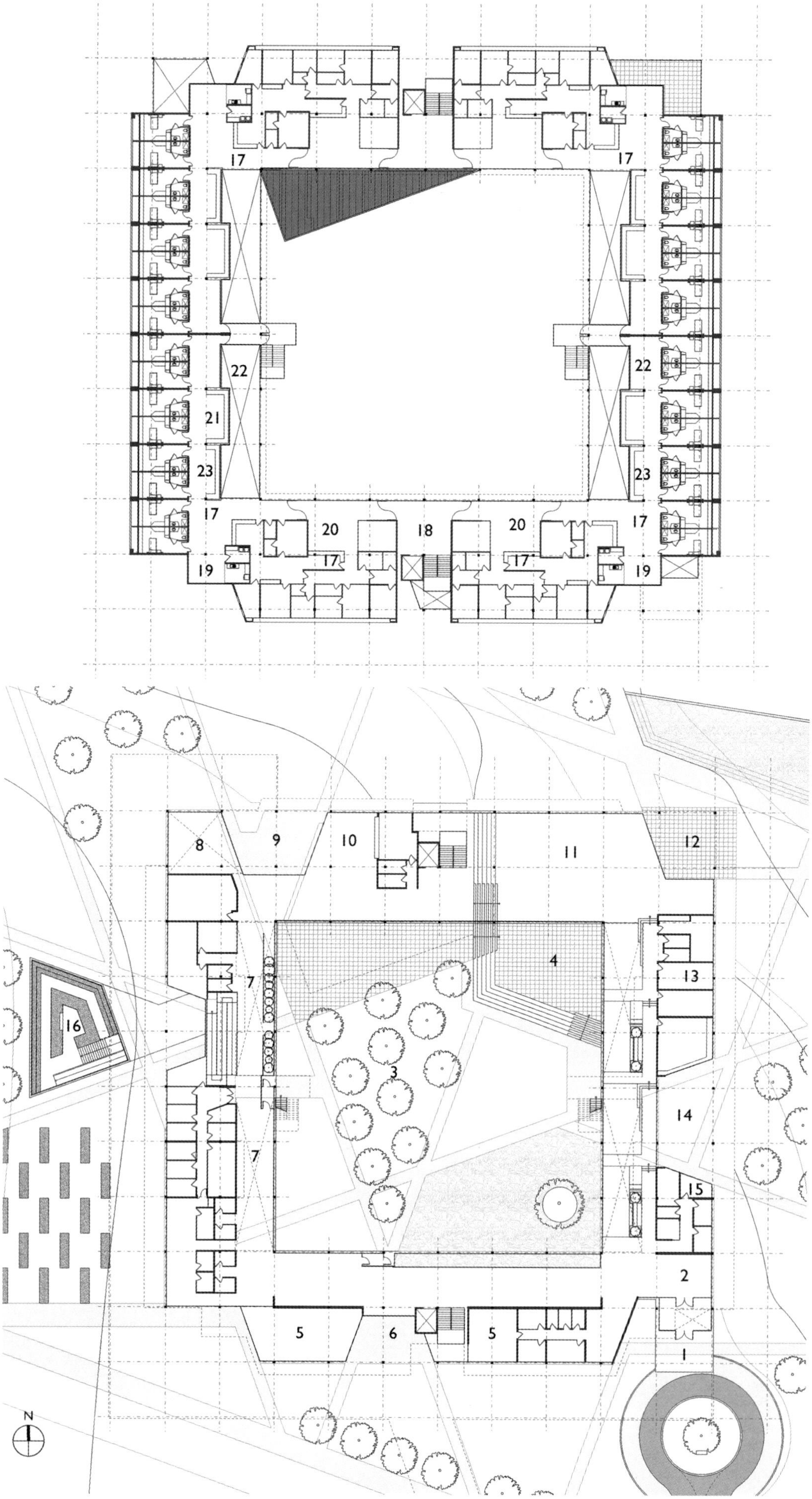

Key:
1 main arrival/entrance
2 reception
3 courtyard
4 terrace (exterior)
5 outpatient clinic
6 therapy room (exterior)
7 administration/staff
8 social space
9 exterior deck
10 dining/kitchen
11 gym/fitness
12 exterior patio
13 therapy rooms/library
14 play area (exerior)
15 admissions
16 winter garden (greenhouse)
17 nurses' station/support
18 residential units 1–4
19 dining/kitchenette
20 living room
21 multimedia pods 1–4
22 art therapy
23 dayroom

6.24.3a–b Arrival and support functions are housed on the main level, with residential units housed above.

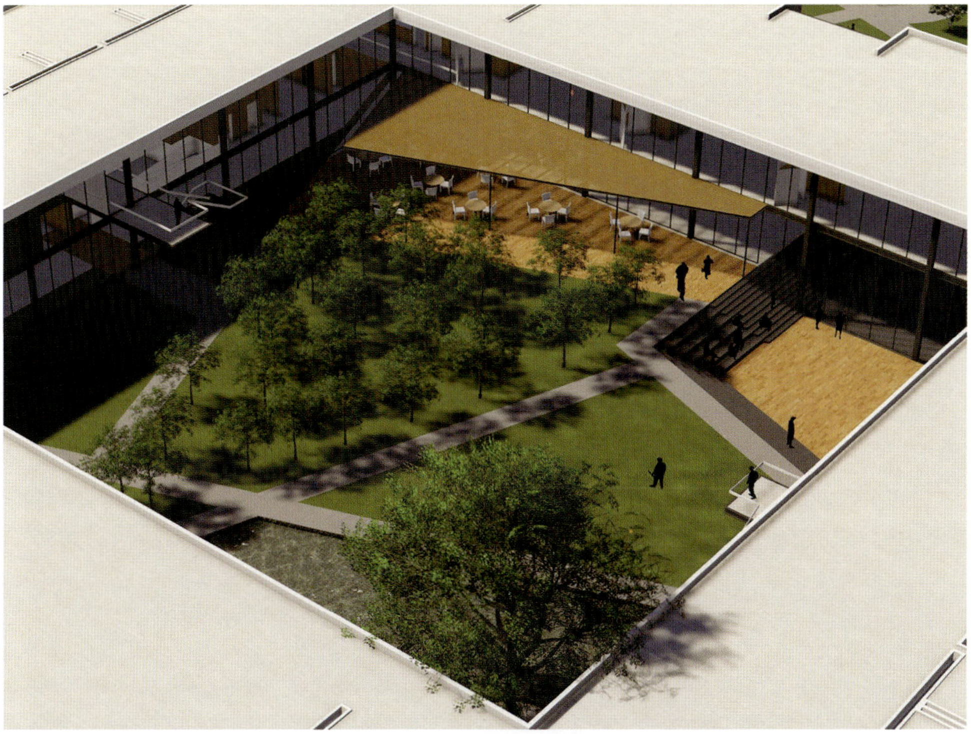

6.24.4 The commons/courtyard houses an exterior sheltered terrace, walking paths, gardens, mini amphitheater, and a stand of trees.

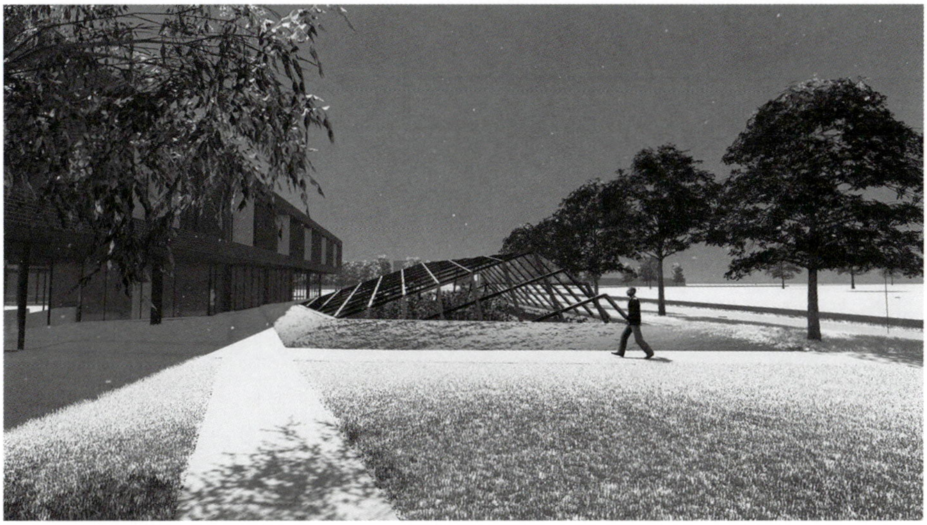

6.24.5 The winter garden is autonomous from the main structure, connected via an underground passageway.

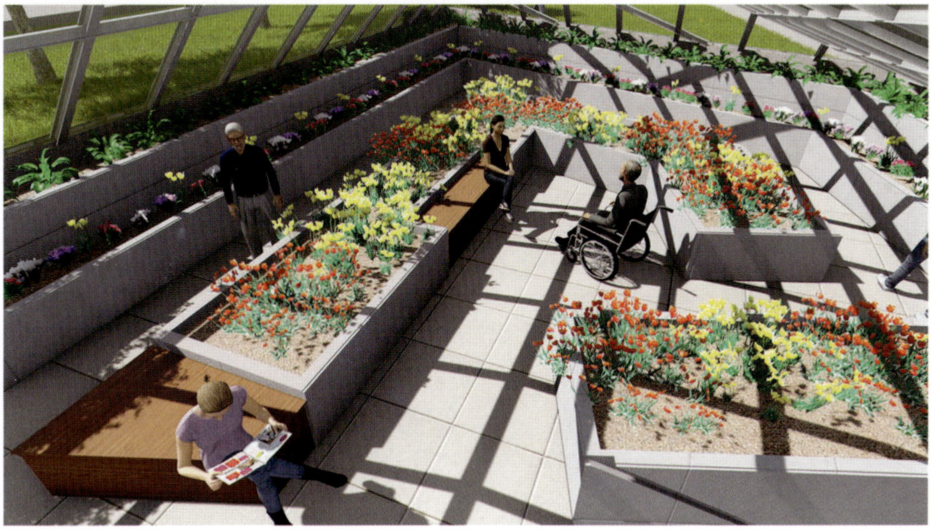

6.24.6 Interior view of the winter garden, illustrating seating areas, the garden, and vegetation.

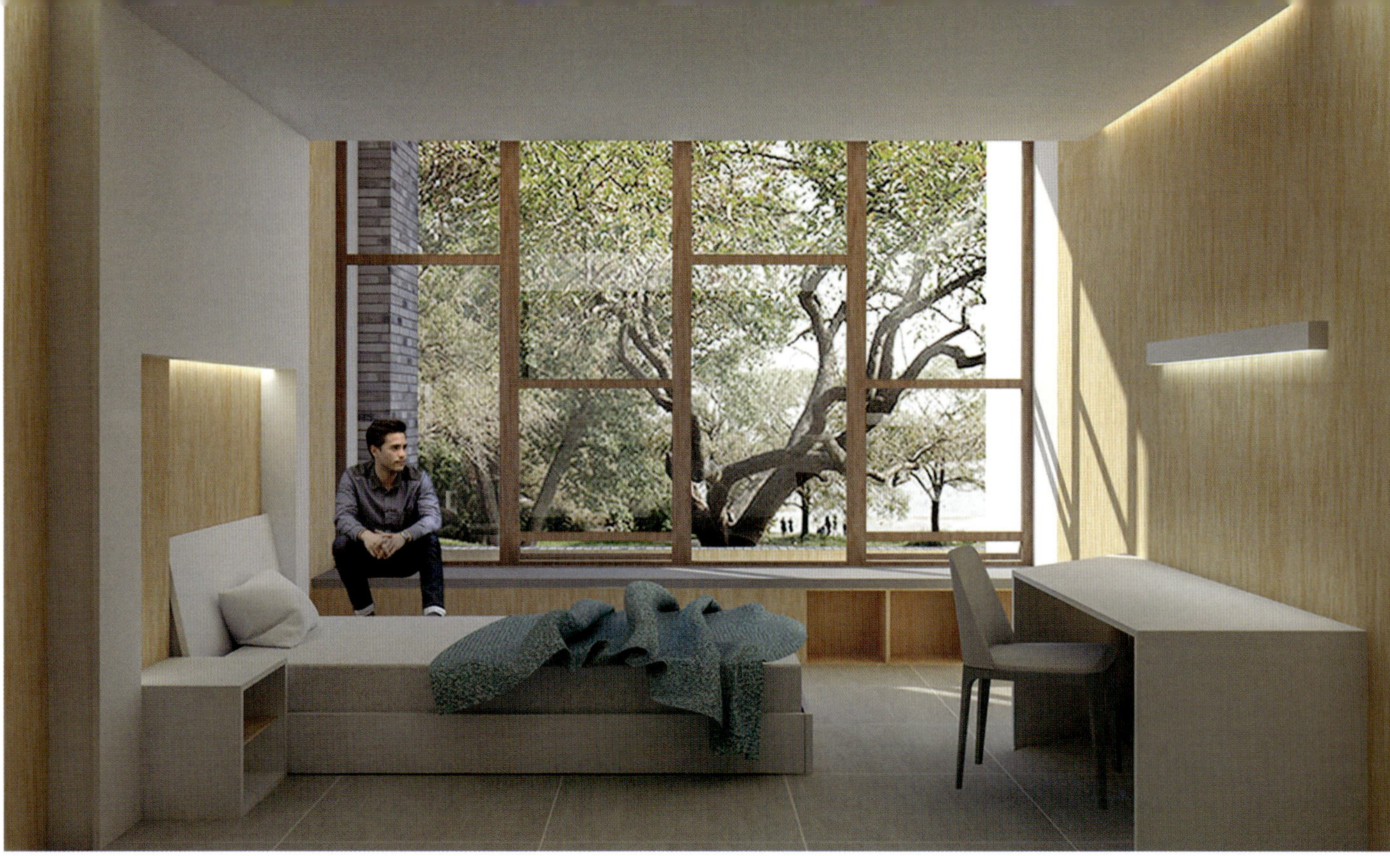

6.24.7 Patient rooms feature operable inset windows, views of the wooded site, and full-length window seat. Windows can be mechanically obscured (in part or completely) in support of privacy and confidentiality.

outward to the surrounding community, adjacent wooded ravine and public park (Figure 6.24.4).

Level 1 houses a gymnasium and recreational therapy unit, the main dining and kitchen supports, a nondenominational chapel, a multipurpose room with bleachers, and a library/resource room organized around the main circulation loop. The continuous main circulation artery surrounding the commons/courtyard is an interior 'street', where informal seating alcoves, plantings, and changes in level afford patients a variety of informal respite and consult spaces – a significant departure from traditional double-loaded institutional corridors The freestanding winter garden pavilion, physically autonomous, yet connected via an interior pathway to the main structure, allows for year-round use and a connection to nature without physically requiring one to leave the building (Figure 6.24.5 and 6.24.6). Patient rooms are furnished with a dormitory bed-headboard, recessed lighting above, side table, desk, chair, and built-in storage units. The room's ceiling is 9 feet in height, allowing natural light to transmit within, and the walls are sheathed in wood panels, which establish a residential ambiance. A window seat spans the length of the outer wall and the windows are operable, with privacy screens and LED-activated obscured panes (Figure 6.24.7). Sustainable design attributes include extended roof overhangs, roof-mounted solar panels, a geothermal system, cisterns for capturing rainwater for irrigating the grounds and for indoor vegetation, greenwalls, automated smart-window louvers to track the sun's incident angle throughout the day, and a narrow building footprint to maximize transmission of natural ventilation and light into the maximum number of interior spaces.

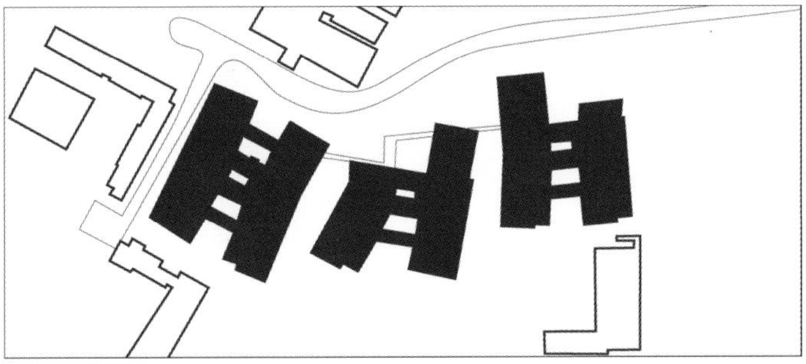

25 New psychiatric hospital, Bispebjerg, Denmark

ARCHITECT: Friis & Moltke Architects, Aarhus, Denmark/PLH Arkitekter, Copenhagen, Denmark
LANDSCAPE ARCHITECT: Moller & Gronborg, Copenhagen, Denmark
CLIENT: Capital Region of Denmark Health Ministry, Copenhagen
FEATURED MATERIALS: Stone, masonry, glass, steel, wood
COMPLETED: 2018–2022 (all phases)
INPATIENT BEDS: 200
SITE/PARKING: 12 acres/100
HOSPITAL/TREATMENT CENTER SIZE: 125,500 square feet
NURSES' WORKSTATION: Shielded

Context/site

This psychiatric hospital in Denmark replaces the historic Bispebjerg Hospital north of Copenhagen. It won a design competition held in 2015–2016, and is built on a portion of the old asylum grounds. Inpatient services were relocated to this new hospital and the heritage facility was renovated for noninpatient services. Its site slopes approximately 20 feet, making possible a series of stepped elements, with the main public arrival zone occupying the lowest level. Above, two floors house central supports and inpatient residential units, with the uppermost floor housing additional residential units and therapy/treatment spaces. A public access road leads to the main entrance, traversing four therapeutic gardens on the grounds. These extend the building into the landscape and simultaneously connect a series of inpatient units. The building's floor plates are shifted and cantilevered, shading outdoor terraces and extending into additional roof gardens. The campus master plan was governed by three core provisos: to achieve maximum openness, maximum accessibility, and maximum freedom of choice for inhabitants – patients, staff, and visitors.

In general, this institution's campus plan is somewhat informal. The articulation of the upper floor plates results in a series of *residences* (in the architects' words). However, in their scale, they are perhaps more aptly described as *pavilions* (Figures 6.25.1 and 6.25.2), and self-referential insofar as they deploy hierarchically as open spaces of varying size and type, some geared to support physical activity, and others for quieter, more contemplative use. The transparency achieved in the three pavilions results from the presence of extensive windows within a deductive compositional strategy – spaces surrounding the open courts 'breathe' as part of a total landscape, as open spaces weave in between various building elements. The is was to maximize natural light transmission, to establish a residential ambiance, and to avoid gloomy, shadowed pockets of outdoor space. The pavilions' formal positioning, together with the aforementioned deployment strategy, contributes to an atmosphere 'of being on a university campus', in the architects' words. The aesthetic of this decentralized replacement campus strongly brakes from the harsh institutionalism of the old psychiatric hospital it replaced (Figure 6.25.3a–b).

Building/unit

The public realms are bright, spacious, and open. Various seating alcoves are positioned along the circulation arteries between and next to the three principal residential units; these compartmentalized spaces have lower ceilings, wood paneling, and flooring to set them apart from the publicness of adjacent main corridors. They serve as semipublic 'rooms' themselves and as extensions of open courtyards (at grade and on the roofs). Adjacent larger spaces, by contrast, are designed for more active socialization in the common areas connected to the pavilions. The overarching goal is to coordinate a network of paths with courtyards to maximize individuals' spatial orientation while reinforcing an alternative, antihospital aesthetic. A subterranean service network connects the entire campus, with vertical connections occurring at four intervals. Each pavilion is configured as an H in plan, as two wings linked by architectural 'connectors'. The first of these is single loaded (on Level 2), the second, at midsection in plan, is double loaded, while a third connector variant is a multipurpose/dining *bridge* suspended above an exterior roof court, with access provided to the roof terrace (Figure 6.25.4 and 6.25.5).

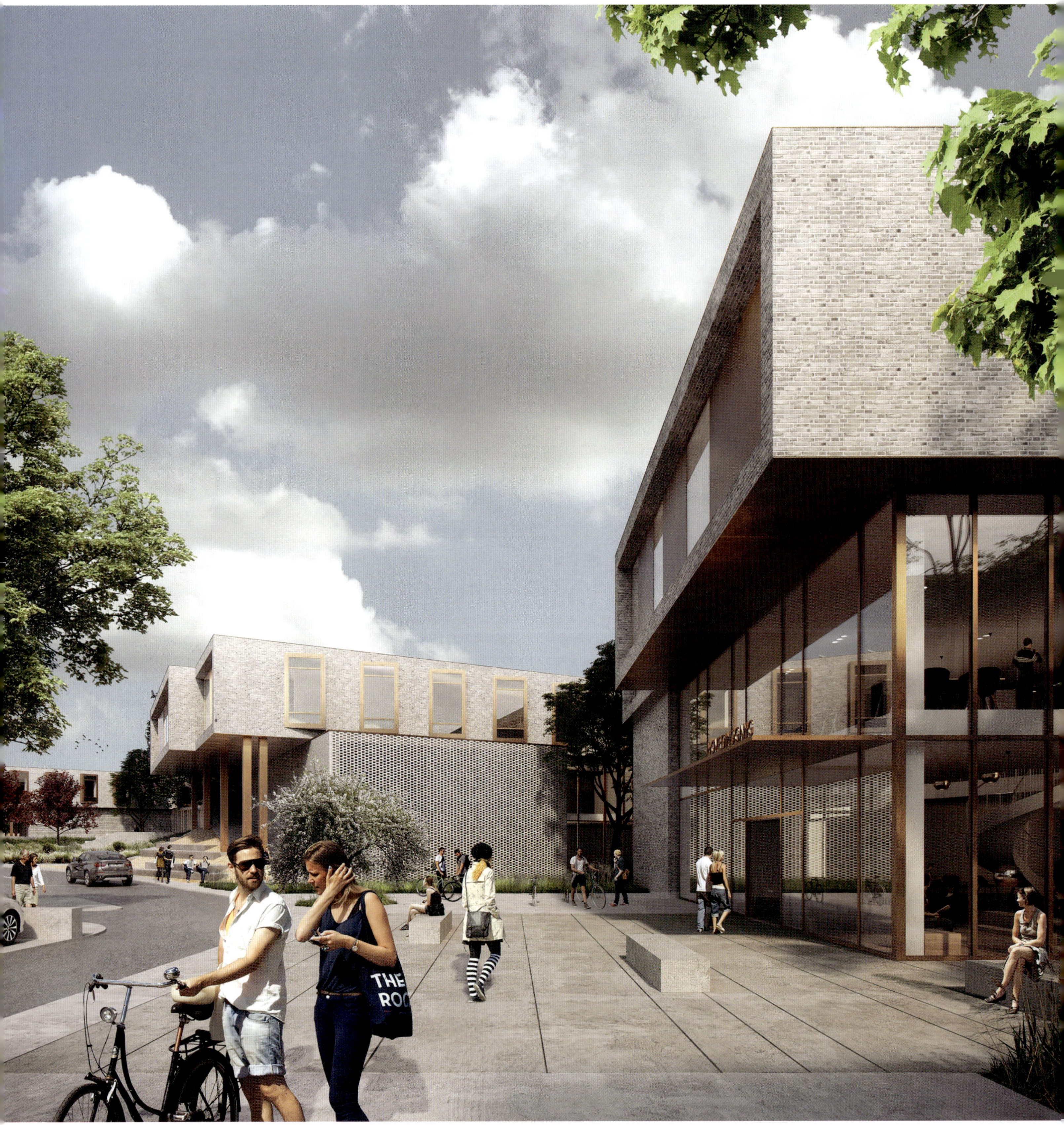

6.25.1 The public vehicular approach to the replacement psychiatric hospital in Bispebjerg, Denmark.

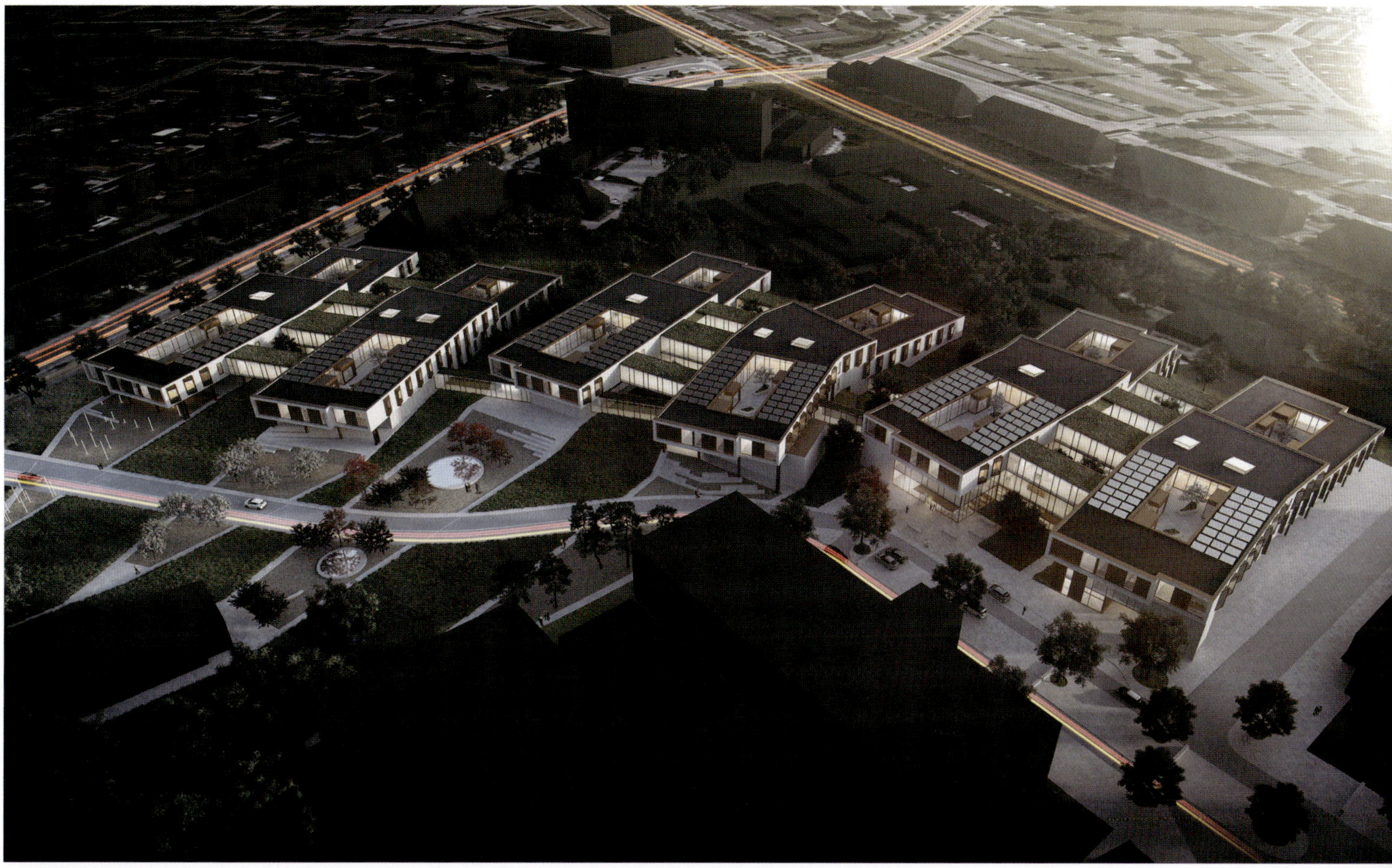

6.25.2 This large complex is decentralized, resulting in six interconnected pavilions and related support functions.

Each residential unit, on the uppermost level, houses a 16-bed residential unit (32 beds total), accessed by means of a dedicated arrival (elevator/stair) vestibule. The unit revolves around the nurse's workstation and associated spaces. These are located on the inboard side, with windows overlooking the roof courts; the nurses' station desk is oriented to face the unit's day/activity room (a tight condition that may result, however, in circulation bottlenecks). In each pavilion, two therapy/counseling rooms and four seating alcoves are provided. Patient rooms are single occupancy; each has a private bath/shower unit on the inboard side along the corridor. Corridors are single loaded, resulting in every occupant's bedroom door being directly across from either a roof terrace or a dayroom, and the various day/activity rooms have skylights (Figures 6.25.6 and 6.25.7). All patient rooms are private and provided with a built-in window seat, with the bed positioned with its headboard opposite the corridor-side wall, with all wall and floor surfaces in the room natural wood finishes. The bed typical is double width (vs. the twin-size bed in mental health facilities). The outer wall of the patient room houses a storage bin and bookcase and a triangular desk that facilitates a direct sight line from the corridor, and in turn, from corridor to the window seat. It is likely this replacement hospital will become a benchmark with regards to the design and construction of residential psychiatric treatment centers in Europe and beyond.[6]

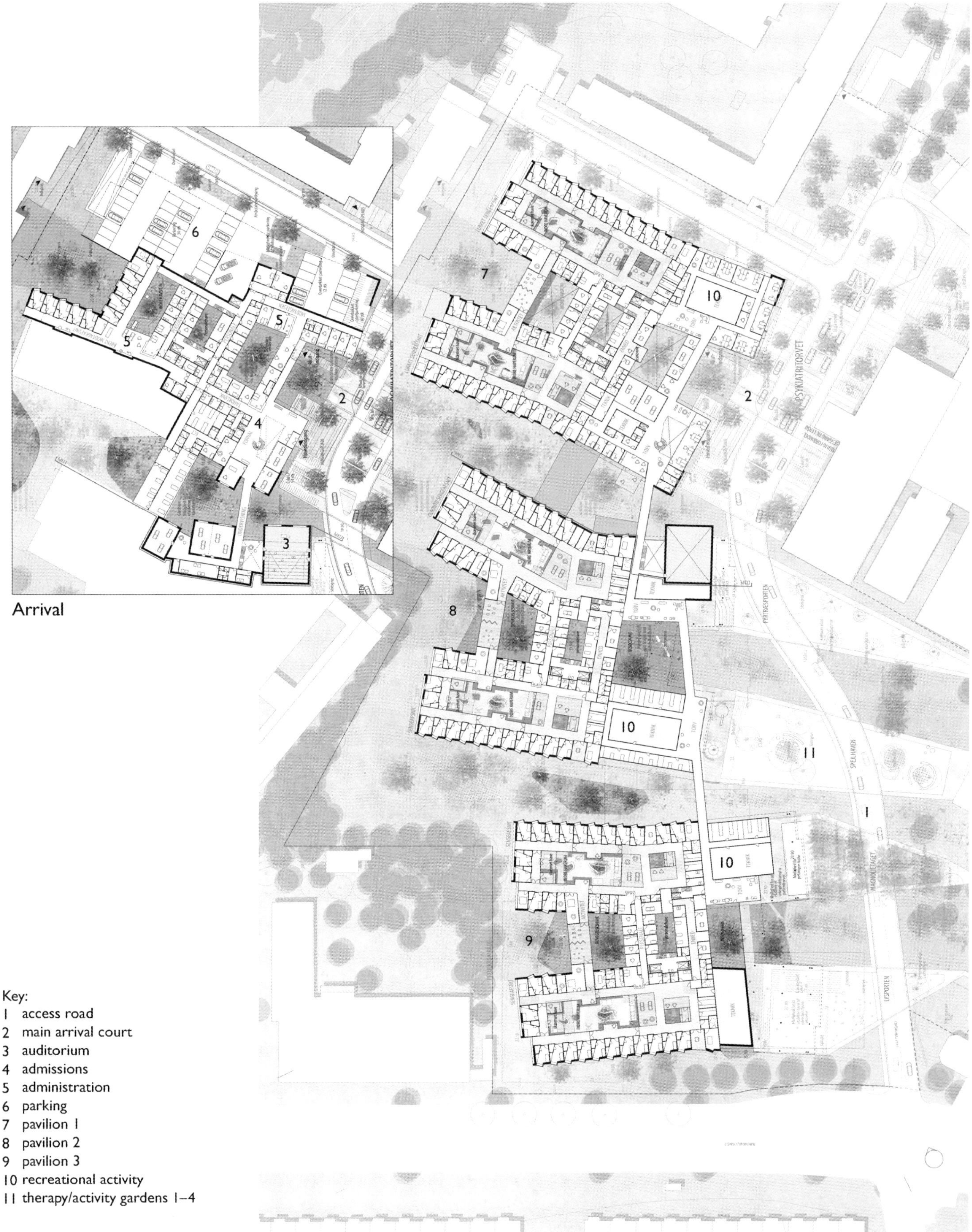

Arrival

Level 1

Key:
1 access road
2 main arrival court
3 auditorium
4 admissions
5 administration
6 parking
7 pavilion 1
8 pavilion 2
9 pavilion 3
10 recreational activity
11 therapy/activity gardens 1–4

6.25.3a–b Three pavilions house inpatient residential units and therapy support functions.

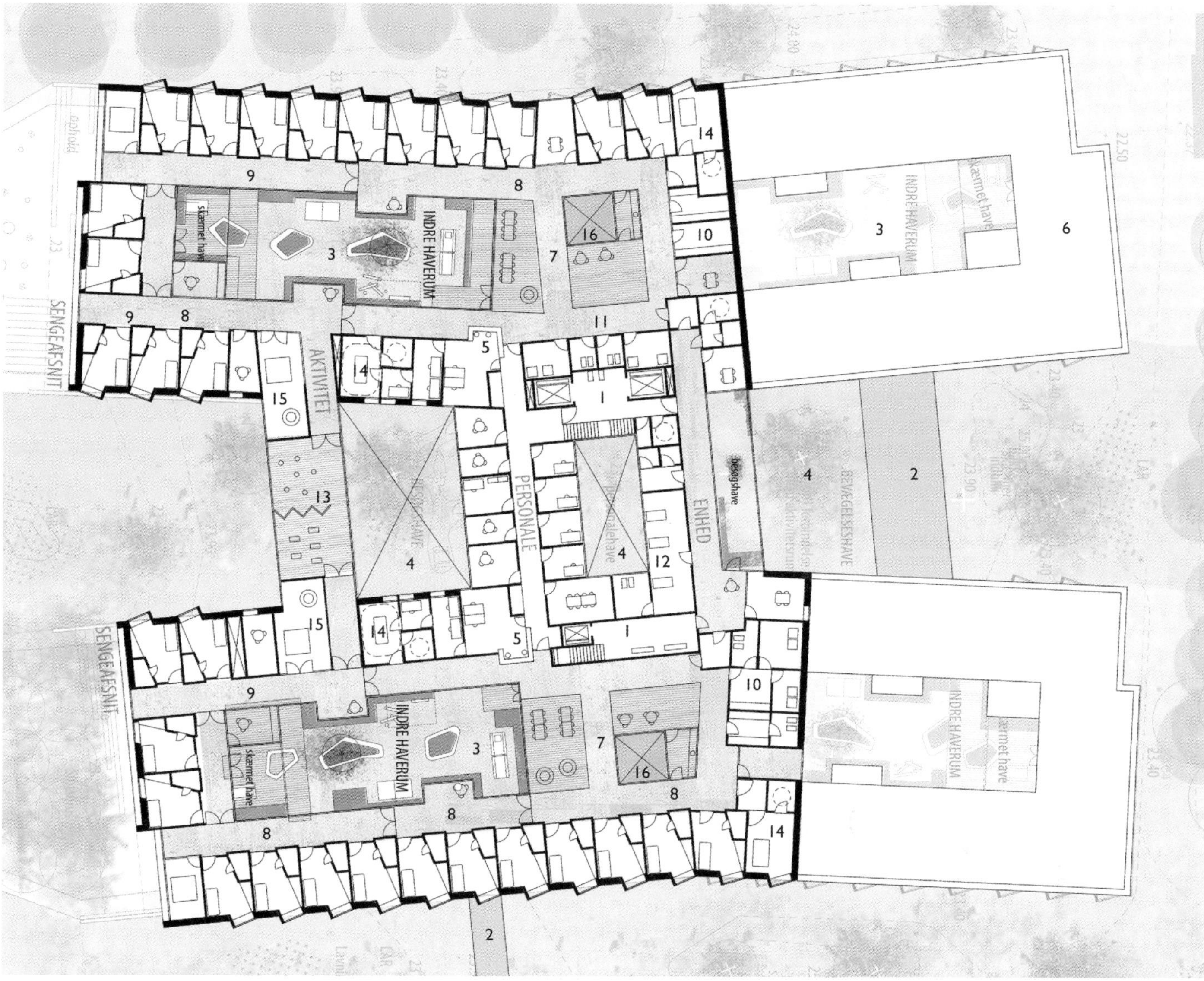

Level 2

Key:

1	arrival lobby/elevator	9	acute observation unit
2	circulation connector	10	supplies/equipment
3	secured courtyard	11	counseling
4	semipublic courtyard	12	staff support
5	nurses' workstation	13	multipurpose/dining
6	Level 1 inpatient unit	14	seclusion
7	dayroom	15	kitchen/staging
8	inpatient unit	16	skylight

6.25.4 Residential pavilions feature a high percentage of single-loaded corridors, affording views of pocket courtyards that support varied therapy treatment and social activities.

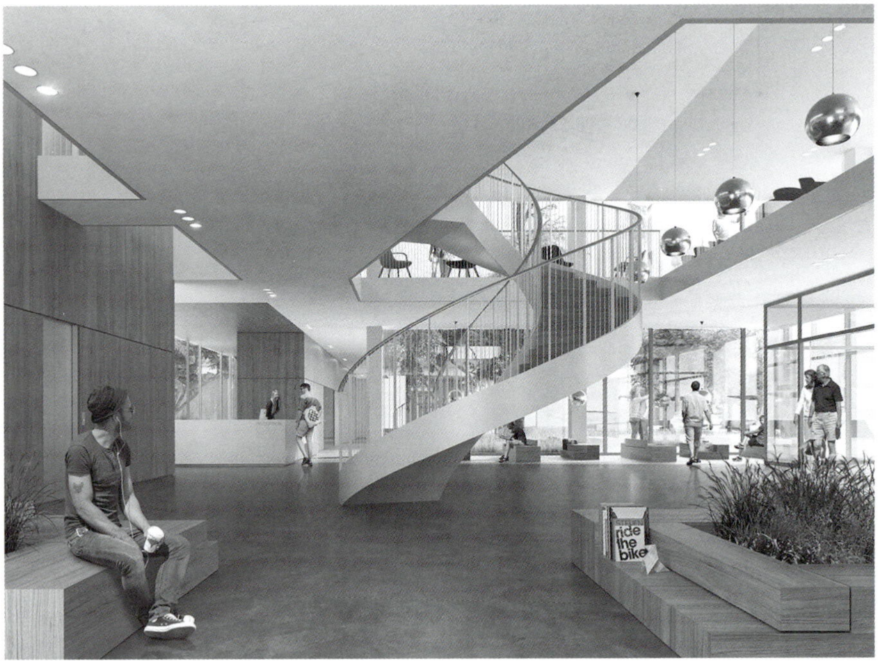

6.25.5 The public realm features elevated walkways, volumes of varied sizes and proportions, and transparency.

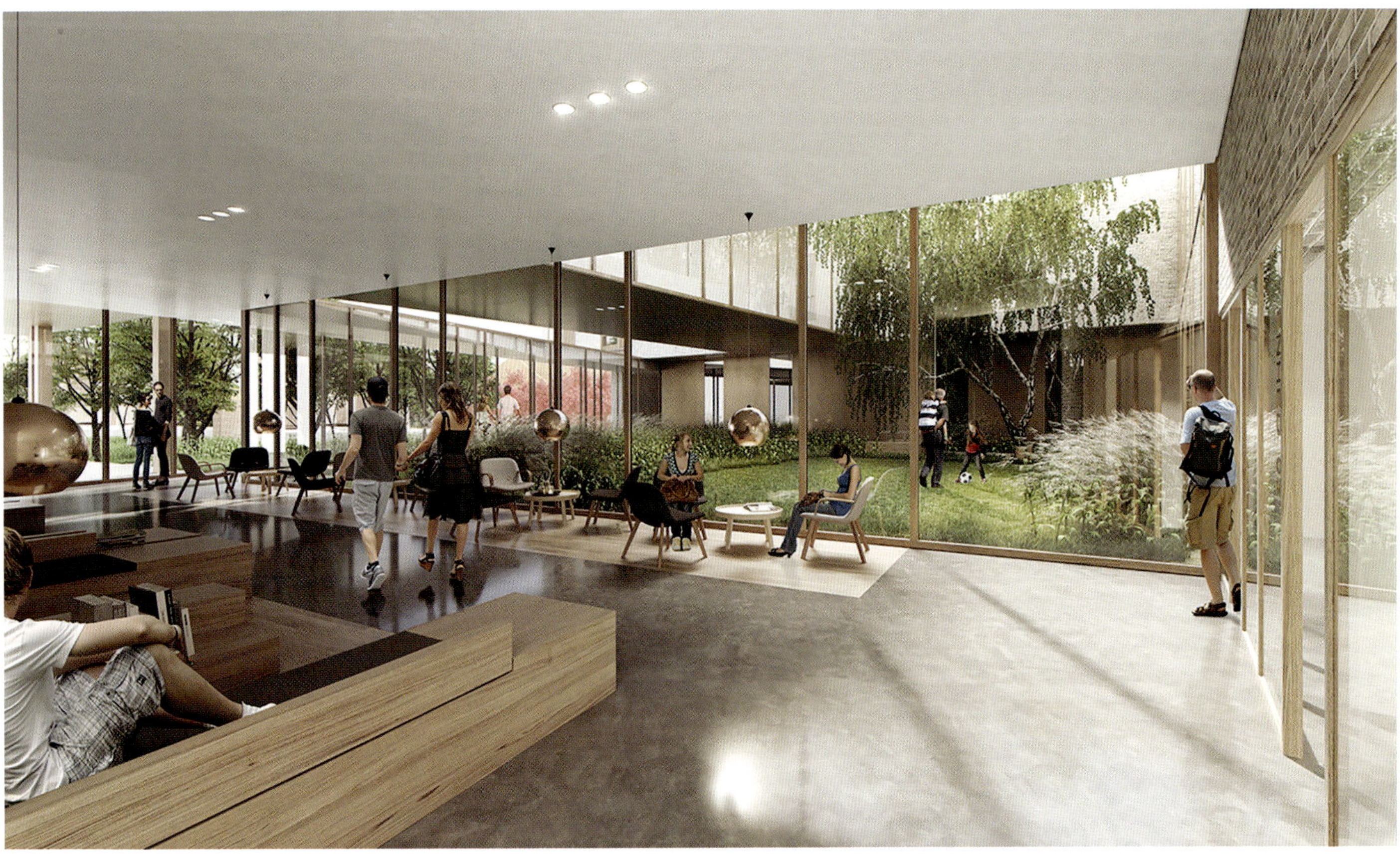

6.25.6 Social activity spaces overlook and directly access exterior courtyards.

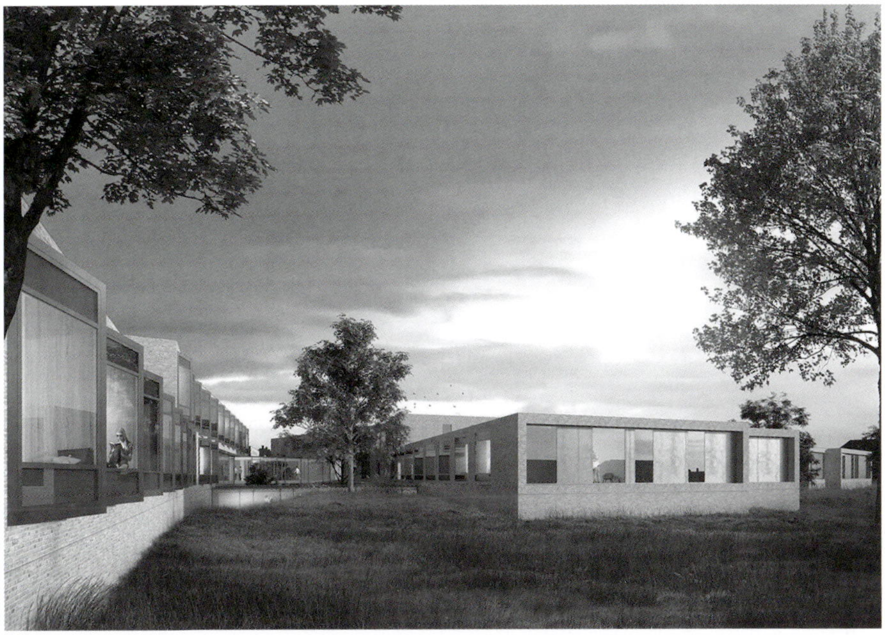

6.25.7 Landscaped exteriors are configured to foster high use by patients.

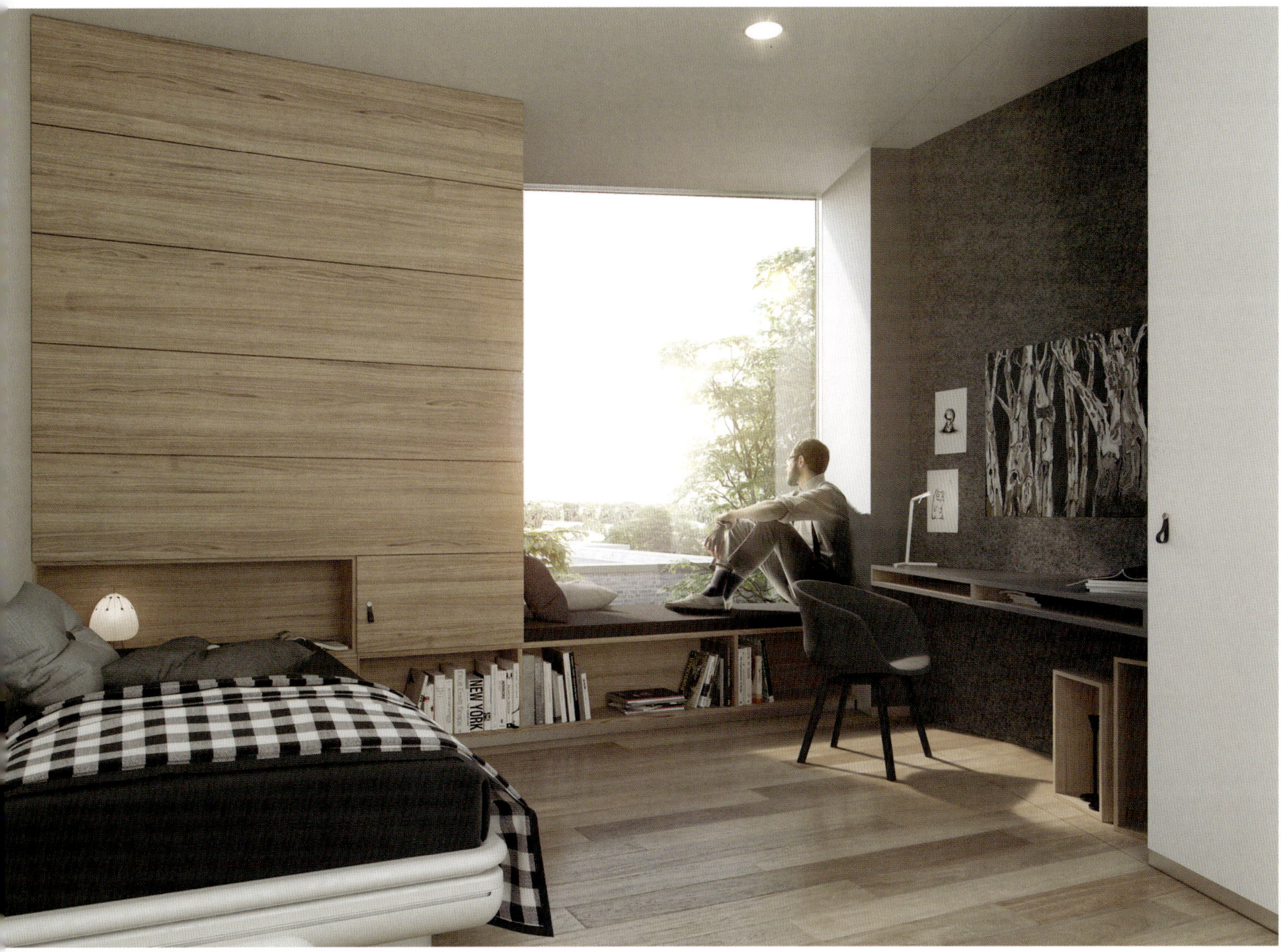

6.25.8 Patient rooms feature a built-in window seat, desk, bed/headwall unit, and views of the surrounding landscape.

Notes and References

Chapter 1

1 Murray, Christopher J.L. and Alan D. Lopez, eds. (1996) *The Global Burden of Disease: A Comprehensive Assessment of Mortality and Disability From Diseases, Injuries, and Risk Factors in 1990 and Projected to 2020*. Cambridge, MA: Harvard School of Public Health, with the World Health Organization and World Bank. Summary Report, Introduction.

2 Anon (2016) 'China, India face huge mental health burden: studies', *The Japan Times*, 18 May. Online. Available at www.japantimes.co.jp/news/2016/05/08/asia-pacific/science-health-asia-pacific/html (accessed 15 May 2017). This finding drew upon years of public health research sponsored by the World Health Organization (WHO) working together with an international coalition.

3 Carey, Benedict (2016) 'China and India burdened by untreated mental disorders', *The New York Times*, 18 May. Online. Available at http://www/nytimes.com/2016/05/19/health/china-andindia-burdened_unit&version=latest&contentPlacement=4&pgtype=sectionfront.html (accessed 20 May 2016).

4 Ibid.: 12.

5 Sugar, J.A., A. Kleinman and L. Eisenberg (1992) 'Psychiatric morbidity in developing countries and American psychiatry's role in international health', *Hospital Community Psychiatry*, 43(4): 355–360.

6 Ibid.: 3.

7 Ibid.: 7. To calculate total DALYs for a given condition in a population, years of life lost (YLLs) and years lived with disability of known severity and duration (YLDs) for that condition must each be estimated, then the total summed. For example, to calculate DALYs incurred through road traffic accidents in India in 2016, add the total years of life lost in fatal road accidents and the total years of life lived with disabilities by the survivors of such accidents.

8 Ibid.: 21.

9 Ibid.: 39.

10 Whiteford, Harvey A., Louisa Degenhardt, Jürgen Rehm, Amando J. Baxter, Alize J. Ferrari, Holly E. Erkstine, Fiona J. Charlson, Rosanna E. Norman, Abraham D. Flaxman, Nicole Johns, Roy Burstein, Christopher J.L. Murray and Theo Vos (2013) 'Global burden of disease attributable to mental and substance abuse disorders: findings from the Global Burden of Disease Study 2010', *The Lancet*, 382(3): 1575–1586. While acute schizophrenia was found to be the most highly weighted disability of all such disorders, it did not rank highly in terms of YLDs because of its low occurrence compared with anxiety, depressive, and substance abuse disorders.

11 United Nations (2016) *World Population Prospects*. New York: United Nations. Online. Available at http://esa.un.org/unpd/wpp/Publications/Files/Key_Findings_WPP_2015.pdf (accessed 12 June 2016).

12 McKenzie, Kwame (2008) 'Urbanization, social capital and mental health', *Global Social Policy*, 8(3): 359–377.

13 World Bank (2000) *World Development Report 1999–2000*. Washington, DC: World Bank. Urbanization is a powerful attractor governed in part by an economic shift in these places away from agriculture to industry, trade, and services.

14 Peen, Jaap and Jack Dekkar (1997) 'Admission rates for schizophrenia in the Netherlands: an urban/rural comparison', *Acta Psychiatry Scandinavia*, 96(4): 301–305.

15 Sundquist, Kirsten and Frank K. Sundquist (2004) 'Urbanization and incidence of psychosis and depression: follow-up study of 4.4 million women and men in Sweden', *British Journal of Psychiatry*, 184(2): 293–298. One recent study in Germany found among a sample of 4,181 individuals, higher levels of urbanization were linked to higher 12-month occurrence rates for almost all major psychiatric disorders (with the exception of substance abuse and psychotic diagnoses), concluded to be attributed to the prevalence of environmental stressors in dense urban settings.

16 Dekkar, Jack, Jaap Peen, Jurrijn Koelen, Filip Smit and Robert Schoevers (2008) 'Psychiatric disorders and urbanization in Germany', *BMC Public Health*, 8(17): 1186–1195. Also Srivastava, Kalpana (2009) 'Urbanization and mental health', *Industrial Psychiatry*, 18(2): 75–77.

17 McKenzie (2008): 361.

18 Ibid.: 362.

19 Harpham, Trudy (1994) 'Urbanization and mental health in developing countries: a research role for social scientists, public health professionals and social psychiatrists', *Social Science and Medicine*, 39(2): 233–245.

20 World Health Organization (1991) *Health Trends and Emerging Issues in the 1990s and the Twenty-First Century: Monitoring, Evaluation and Projection Methodology Unit*. Geneva: World Health Organization.

21 Boydell, James and Kwame McKenzie (2008) 'Society, place and space', in Craig Morgan, Kwame McKenzie and Paul Fearon (eds.) *Society and Psychosis*. London and Philadelphia, PA: Cambridge University Press: 77–95. Also see Halpern, David (1995) *Mental Health and the Built Environment: More Than Bricks and Mortar?* London: Routledge.

22 Krabbendam, Lawrence and James Van Os (2005) 'Schizophrenia and urbanicity: a major environmental influence – conditional on genetic risk', *Schizophrenia Bulletin*, 31(4): 795–799.

23 McKenzie (2008): 364.

24 Putnam, Robert (2001) *Bowling Alone: The Collapse and Revival of American Community*. New York: Simon & Schuster.

25 McKenzie (2008): 366.

26 Ibid.: 372.

27 United Nations Centre for Human Settlement (2001) *Cities in a Globalizing World*. London: Earthscan.

28 McKenzie (2008): 373. Also Barton, H. and C. Tsouroū (2000) *Healthy Urban Planning: A WHO Guide to Planning for People*. London: E&FN Spon. Also see Barton, H., C. Micham and C. Tsourou (2003) *Healthy Urban Planning in Practice: The Experience of European Cities*. London: WHO.

29 IPCC (2014) *Climate Change 2014. Synthesis Report. Continuation of Working Groups I, II and III to the Fifth Assessment Report of the Intergovernmental Panel on Climate Change*. Geneva, Switzerland: IPCC.

30 McMichael, Anthony J. (1993) *Planetary Overload*. Cambridge: Cambridge University Press. Also see McMichael, Anthony J., Claire McMichael, Henry Berry and Kathryn J. Bowen (2009) 'Climate change, displacement and health', in J. McAdam (ed.) *Climate Change and Displacement: Multidisciplinary Perspectives*. Oxford: Hart Publishing.

31 Horton, Robert (2007) 'Launching a new movement for mental health', *The Lancet*, 370(4): 806.

32 Berry, Helen Louise, Kathryn Bowen and Tord Kjellstrom (2010) 'Climate change and mental health: a causal pathways framework', *International Journal of Public Health*, 55(5): 123–132.

33 Foa, Edna B., Daniel J. Stein and Alexander C. McFarlane (2006) 'Symptomatology and psychopathology of mental health problems after disaster', *Journal of Clinical Psychiatry*, 67(3): 15–25.

34 Norris, Fran H., Mathew J. Friedman and Patricia J. Watson (2016) '60,000 disaster victims speak: Part II. Summary and implications of the disaster mental health research', *Psychiatry*, 65(3): 240–260. Adverse impacts on individuals' physical health will occur due to environmental stressors (i.e., extreme heat exposure, heat exhaustion, flooding, sea level rise, coastal subsidence, intense windstorms caused by hurricanes and cyclones, drought, and associated food shortages). Indirect consequences will likely be experienced across communities dislocated due to adverse environmental events (i.e., agricultural dislocation, socioeconomic hardship postdisaster, disrupted or lost interpersonal relationships, and the adverse effects of forced migration and diasporas).

35 Haq, S., S. Kovats, H. Reid and D. Satterwaite (2007) 'Reducing risks to cities from disasters and climate change', *Environmental Urbanism*, 19(2): 3–15.

36 US Department of Commerce (2006) *Gulf Coast Recovery: 7 Months After the Hurricanes*. Washington, DC: Economics and Statistics Administration. Online. Available at www.esa.doc.gov/reports/2008/April2006.pdf (accessed 12 June 2016).

37 Galea, S., C.R. Brewin, M. Gruber, R.T. Jones, D.W. King and L.A. King (2007) 'Exposure to hurricane-related stressors and mental illness after Hurricane Katrina', *Archives of General Psychiatry*, 64(2): 1427–1434. The deleterious aftereffects of catastrophes such as Hurricane Katrina in 2005 can persist for years. New Orleans's recovery was painfully slow, compounded by a freestanding 'mental health disaster' that unfolded in the aftermath. The situation in New Orleans was precarious beforehand, but after Katrina would morph into a full-blown crisis.

38 Verderber, Stephen (2009) *Delirious New Orleans: Manifesto for an Extraordinary American City*. Austin, TX: University of Texas Press. Also Verderber, Stephen (2009) 'The unbuilding of historic neighborhoods in post-Katrina New Orleans', *Journal of Urban Design*, 14(3): 257–277.

39 Kessler, R.C., S. Galea, M.J. Gruber, N.A. Sampson, R.J. Ursano and S. Wessely (2008) 'Trends in mental illness and suicidality after Hurricane Katrina', *Molecular Psychiatry*, 13(4): 374–384.

40 Adeola, Francis O. (2009) 'Katrina cataclysm: does duration of residency and prior experience affect impacts, evacuation, and adaptation behavior among survivors?', *Environment and Behavior*, 41(3): 459–489. Also see DeWeever, A. Jones (2008) *Women in the Wake of the Storm: Examining the Post-Katrina Realities of the Women of New Orleans and the Gulf Coast*. Washington, DC: Institute for Women's Policy Research. The occurrence of serious mental illness virtually doubled, with nearly half of respondents in one study exhibiting symptoms of PTSD. Higher levels of hurricane-related loss and stressors were associated with worse health outcomes, when controlling for baseline sociodemographic and health outcome measures. Conversely, individuals with greater personal resources experienced a lower level of stress, although all respondents, regardless of income level, race, gender, or background, experienced increased stress and grief over sheer physical loss.

41 Rhodes, Jean, Christina Paxson, Cecelia Elena Rouse, Mary Waters and Elizabeth Fussell (2010) 'The impact of Hurricane Katrina on the mental and physical health of low-income parents in New Orleans', *American Journal of Orthopsychiatry*, 80(2): 237–247.

42 UNHCR (2016) *Global Trends/Forced Displacement in 2015*. New York: United Nations. Online. Available at www.unhcr.org/afr/news/latest/2016/6/5763b65a4/global-forced-displacement-hits-record-high.html (accessed 22 December 2016). Also Sengupta, Somini (2016) 'Record 65 million displaced by global conflicts, U.N. says', *The New York Times*, 20 June. Online. Available at www.nyt.com.2016/06/20/world/middleeast/record-65-million-dosplaced.html (accessed 14 January 2017).

43 Zivin, K., M. Paczkowski and S. Galea (2011) 'Economic downturns and population mental health: research findings, gaps, challenges and priorities', *Psychological Medicine*, 41(6): 1343–1348.

44 Goldman-Mellor, Sidra J., Katherine B. Saxton and Ralph C. Catalano (2010) 'Economic contraction and mental health', *International Journal of Mental Health*, 39(2): 6–31.

45 Harvard Medical School (2015) *The World Mental Health Survey Initiative*. Boston, MA: Harvard Medical School. Online. Available at www.hcp.med.harvard.edu/wmh/html (accessed 12 June 2016). Also see WHO (2014) *Mental Health Atlas 2014*. Geneva, Switzerland: World Health Organization. Online. Available at www.apps.who.int/iris/bitstream/10665/178879/1/9789241565011_eng.pdf?ua=1&ua=1.html (accessed 10 June 2016).

46 SAMHSA (2015) *Key Substance Abuse and Mental Health Indicators in the United States: Results From the 2015 National Survey on Drug Use and Health*. Washington, DC: US Department of Health and Human Services. Online. Available at www.samhsa.gov/data/sites/default/files/NSDUH-FFRI-2015/html (accessed 12 January 2017). Also WHO (2010) *Global Strategy to Reduce the Harmful Effects of Alcohol*. Geneva, Switzerland: World Health Organization.

47 Leighton, Alexander H. (1959) *My Name Is Legion: Volume 1 of the Stirling County Study*. New York: Basic Books. This dilemma was rectified in the 1980s with the development of the Diagnostic Interview Schedule (DIS), the first psychiatric interview designed for widespread use by healthcare professionals. Also see Robins, L.N., J.E. Helzer, J.L. Croughan and K.S. Ratcliff (1981) 'National Institute of Mental Health Diagnostic interview schedule: its history, characteristics and validity', *Archives of General Psychiatry*, 38(4): 381–389.

48 Kessler, R.C. et al. (2004) 'Prevalence, severity, and unmet need for treatment of mental disorders in the World Health Organization Mental Health Surveys', *Journal of the American Medical Association*, 291(21): 2581–2590.

49 Kohn, Robert, Shektar Saxena, Itzhak Levav and Benedetto Saraceno (2004) 'The treatment gap in mental health care', *Bulletin of the World Health Organization*, 82(11): 858–866. Median rates of untreated cases of these disorders were calculated across 37 research studies. The median treatment gap for schizophrenia, including related non-affective psychoses, was 32%. For other disorders, the gap was the following: depression, 56%; dysthymia, 56%; bipolar disorder, 50.2%; panic disorder, 55.9%; GAD, 57.5%; and OCD, 57.3%. Alcohol and substance abuse and dependency had the widest treatment gap at 78.1%.

50 Wilson, Claire, Mohammed T. Yasamy, Jodi Morris, Atieh Novin, Khalid Saeed and Sebastiana D. Nkomo (2014) 'Mental health services: the African gap', *Journal of Public Mental Health*, 13(3): 132–141.

51 Kigozi, Fred, Josuha Ssebunnya, Dorothy Kizza, Sara Cooper and Sheila Ndyanabangi (2010) 'An overview of Uganda's mental health care system: results from an assessment using the World Health Organization's Assessment Instrument for Mental Health Systems (WHO-AIMS)', *International Journal of Mental Health Systems*, 4(1): 1–9. Online. Available at www.ijmhs.com/content/4/1/1 (accessed 12 March 2017).

52 Vicente, Benjamin, Sandra Saldivia and Robert Kohn (2012) 'Epidemiology of mental disorders, use of service, and the treatment gap in Chile', *International Journal of Mental Health*, 41(1): 7–20.

53 Docherty, Mary and Graham Thornicroft (2015) 'Specialist mental health services in England in 2014: overview of funding, access and levels of care', *International Journal of Mental Health Systems*, 34(9): 11–18.

54 Pearson, Caryn, Teresa Janz and Jennifer Ali (2013) *Mental and Substance Use Disorders in Canada*. Ottawa: Statistics Canada Health Statistics Division. Online. Available at www.statcan.gc.ca.html (accessed 12 February 2017).

55 Mental Health Network: NHS Confederation (2014) *Key Facts and Trends in Mental Health*. London: NHS Confederation.

56 Corrigan, P.W., F.E. Markowitz and A.C. Watson (2004) 'Structural levels of mental illness stigma and discrimination', *Schizophrenia Bulletin*,

30(3): 481–491. Also see Thornicroft, Graham (2006) *Shunned: Discrimination Against People With Mental Illness*. Oxford: Oxford University Press.

57 Connellan, Kathleen, Mads Gaardboe, Damien Riggs, Clemence Due, Amanda Reinschmidt and Lauren Mustillo (2013) 'Stressed spaces: mental health and architecture', *Health Environments Research & Design Journal*, 6(4): 127–168.

58 Needham, Ian, Christopher Abderhalden, Ruud J.G. Halfens, Joachim E. Fischer and Theo Dassen (2005) 'Non-somatic effects of patient aggression on nurses: a systematic review', *Journal of Advanced Nursing*, 49(3): 283–296.

59 Ibid.: 285.

60 Ulrich, Roger S., Lennart Bogren and Stefan Lundin (2012) 'Toward a design theory for reducing aggression in psychiatric facilities', Paper presented at ARCH12: Architecture/Research/Care/Health Conference, Chalmers University, Gothenburg, Sweden, 12 pp.

61 Ibid. These variables consisted of single-patient rooms with private bathrooms, smaller units with fewer number of beds, moveable seating in spacious dayrooms and lounges, low noise levels with good acoustics, window views overlooking nature, therapeutic gardens accessible to patients, nature-themed art (no abstract art), exposure to natural daylight, staff workstations close to activity areas with direct visibility, and comprehendible facility and campus navigability and wayfinding.

62 Bowers, Len, Teresa Allan, Alan Simpson, Julia Jones, Marie Van Der Merwe and Debra Jeffrey (2009) 'Identifying key factors associated with aggression on acute inpatient psychiatric wards', *Issues in Mental Health Nursing*, 30(3): 260–271. Also Bowers, Len, D. Stewart, C. Papadopoulos, C. Dack, J.H. Ross, H. Khanom, and D. Jeffrey (2011) *Inpatient Violence and Aggression: A Literature Review. Report From the Conflict and Containment Reduction Research Programme*. London: Institute of Psychiatry, Kings College.

63 Chaudhury, Habib (2005) 'Advantages and disadvantages of single versus multiple occupancy rooms in acute care environments', *Environment and Behavior*, 37(6): 760–786. Also Chaudhury, Habib, Atyia Mahood and Maria Valente (2008) 'Characteristics of a successful flexible unit', *Environment and Behavior*, 40(2): 205–232.

64 Papoulias, Constantina (2014) 'The psychiatric ward as a therapeutic space: systematic review', *British Journal of Psychiatry*, 205(3): 171–176.

65 Gross, Ray, Yehuda Sasson, Moshe Zarhy and Joseph Zohar (1998) 'Healing environment in psychiatric hospital design', *General Hospital Psychiatry*, 20(6): 108–114.

66 Verderber, Stephen (2006) *Innovations in Hospice Architecture*. London and New York: Routledge.

67 Verderber, Stephen (2014) 'Residential hospice environments: evidence-based architectural and landscape design considerations', *Journal of Palliative Care*, 30(2): 69–82.

68 *Interval 1: Respondent profiles* – For the caregiver, the experience of working in a mental health treatment environment – and particularly a psychiatric hospital – can be stressful over time. Caregivers are subject to random acts of physical violence and verbal abuse and stigma from colleagues employed in other domains of the health professions and from the general public. They are scrutinized by patient advocacy grassroots organizations and public regulatory agencies. Some caregivers work full time, others part time. Some volunteer, donating their services. For caregiver respondents, it is important to develop a baseline profile that encompasses individual differences and thereby allows for comparative analysis. For patient respondents, the main variable is whether one is admitted to treatment voluntarily or involuntarily.
Interval 2 and Interval 4: Caregiver and patient backgrounds – For the patient, the treatment experience can be highly stressful, characterized by uncertainty and fear: fear of what lies ahead in treatment, uncertainty as to how long one will be hospitalized, and what lies beyond. Importantly, the patient possesses fundamental rights. In Phase I of learning about the patient respondent, this aspect of the investigative model centers on personal attributes. For the *patient respondent*, age, gender, race, and ethnicity are documented. Date of admittance is recorded as is one's medical history and personal occupation (if applicable, for adult patients). The level of family support is rated on a Likert scale (i.e., a five-point scale, indicating low to high) and this or a prevalidated psychometric rating scale can be applied to learn about psycho-emotional status. Location of the treatment facility is documented. In Phase II, composed of background and profile variables of a more probing nature than in Phase I, for the patient, his or her severity of condition, length of residency, and daily activities and range of physical spatial range are assessed. The patient's privacy and desire for social contact are assessed. Morale, personal outlook, and emotional adjustment to the unit or program are assessed, as are acceptance of her or his condition and the desire to recover and leave the institution or outpatient treatment program. Finally, the patient's level of active engagement with nature and the outdoor environs is assessed. For the *caregiver respondent*, age, gender, ethnicity, race, and occupation is ascertained together with department and unit, length of employment at the facility, and total length of work experience in one's current professional role. Distance from home to work, the typical work shift (day, evening, other) one works, and the hours worked per week are recorded. Also, one's place of residence and the geographic location of the facility are documented. Phase II background variables, more probing in nature than Phase I variables, center on caregiver morale, overall attitude, and outlook pertaining to one's career and position. This is augmented with information gathered on satisfaction with one's current job and its attendant responsibilities, the rate of staff turnover, and absenteeism rates. This is followed by a caregiver self-assessment of numerous aspects of his or her work, colleagues, and supervisors, including rapport with patients, patient satisfaction with staff and

administration, quality of the facility and grounds, quality of facility relative to market competitors, degree of visual contact with the outside world while at work, and staff cohesiveness and support provided by the administration.

69 *Interval 3: Built Environment* – These variables are classified within two clusters, *site context/building attributes* and *common area/patient room attributes*. Site context attributes consist of documentation of the facility and adjoining land uses, locational context, landscaping of the immediate grounds, if a greenhouse or garden exists on the site, gardens, topography assessment, facility energy conservation 'quotient' (i.e., total composite annual energy usage), the level of perceived thermal comfort in interior spaces, and occupants' ability to control indoor ambient conditions (i.e., lighting levels, temperature, and humidity levels). The theraserialization quotient (see Chapters 4 and 5) of the facility is documented and rated on perhaps a five-point scale in terms of the level of transparency and connectivity between indoors and outdoors and occupant's proclivity to meaningfully engage the grounds surrounding the facility. Building 'sectional variability' is rated in terms of the facility's ceiling heights and whether they are conventionally shaped or otherwise (i.e., sloping, with skylights, clerestories, or other forms). The number of facility floor levels is also documented, as is the facility and site aesthetic style, and any facility expansion options (if any) are documented. Regarding the common areas and the patient room and bathroom, all furnishings and equipment are documented. Are the furnishings fixed, or moveable? Natural daylight, ventilation, and artificial illumination is documented, as is the level of noise and the nursing staff workstation location within the residential unit. The degree of visual openness on the unit is documented. The number of patient rooms on a unit is documented as are opportunities for occupants to engage in prospect and refuge behaviours: do staff personnel have a place of their own to obtain respite (on-site)? Similarly, for the patient, what privacy affordances exist, as opportunities to be alone, if even briefly? As for evidence-based strategies for ceiling design in healthcare facilities, see Verderber, Stephen, Vicki Barrington and Susan Chester (1984) 'Ceiling design in the hospital rehabilitation environment: the patient's perspective', in Donna Duerk and Donald Campbell (eds.) *The Challenge of Diversity*. Washington, DC: Environmental Design Research Association: 164–172.

70 Verderber, Stephen (1986) 'Dimensions of person-window transactions in the hospital environment', *Environment and Behavior*, 18(4): 450–466.

71 Laursen, J., A. Danielsen and J. Rosenburg (2014) 'Effects of environmental design on patient outcome: a systematic review', *Health Environments Research & Design Journal*, 7(4): 108–119.

72 *Interval 5: Translation* – This phase of the research investigation draws together all prior intervals and steps with the goal of making sense of results, causal effects, and their implications for the patient and the caregiver. This is the point where comparisons become possible. For the patient, the relative stress level is assessed, as is the overall emotional outlook and self-assessment of well-being. For the caregiver, the same occurs, supplemented by a staff composite index that aggregates all independent variables – personal characteristic data and built environment attribute data – into a single index for the purpose of statistical data analysis. A pre- and postoccupancy assessment of the facility is conducted at this point in the research protocol, documenting changes that (may have) occurred in the physical setting during the course of the research.

Interval 6: Behavioural outcomes and design recommendations – This final stage consists of data analyses to ascertain patient health status and the probability of relapse and readmittance and the efficiency of the center's partial hospitalization program (if one exists). Stress-induced aggressions are recorded, as are incidences of violent acts. Similarly, for the caregiver respondent, incidents of stress-induced aggressive acts are recorded. Statistical data analyses then probe if these behaviours are influenced by personal background characteristics, job performance-related attributes, physical setting attributes, or some combination thereof. The results of all research steps are then synthesized into a set of planning and design recommendations.

73 Ulrich, Roger S., Craig Zimring, Xuemei Zhu, Jennifer DuBose, Hyun-Bo Soo, Young-Seon Choi, Xiaobo Quan and Anjali Joseph (2008) 'A review of the research literature on evidence-based healthcare design', *Health Environments Research & Design Journal*, 1(3): 101–165.

74 Bowers et al. (2011).

75 Laursen et al. (2014).

76 Ulrich, Roger S. (2013) 'Designing for calm', *The New York Times*, 11 January: SR12. Online. Available at www.nytimes,com/2013/01/13/opinion/sunday/building-a-space-for-calm.html (accessed 12 March 2017).

77 Ibid. Ulrich writes,

> It should come as no surprise that violence in mental health facilities causes psychological and often physical harm to healthcare workers and patients. What's shocking is how prevalent it is. Globally, a third of all patients admitted for psychiatric care are involved in violent incidents, according to a 2011 analysis by researchers at King's College in London. In Sweden . . . it's estimated that more than half of psychiatric care staff members are exposed to physical violence each year, an experience mirrored in many other countries . . . research suggests, however, that there's an effective solution that has largely been overlooked – to calm emotionally troubled patients through architecture. Currently, questions about design at psychiatric care facilities are viewed through the prism of security. How many

guard and isolation rooms are needed? Where should we put locked doors and alarms? . . . For patients, the stress of mental illness itself can be intensified by the trauma of being confined for weeks in a locked ward . . . Likewise, architectural designs that minimize noise and crowding, enhance patients' coping and sense of control, and offer calming distractions can reduce trauma . . . Providing dayrooms and other shared spaces with moveable seating, for example, gives patients the ability to control their personal space and interactions with others . . . single-patient bedrooms with private toilets increase building costs – but that is arguably offset by the reduced trauma for patients and hospital workers . . . Colleagues from Chalmers University of Technology and Sahlgrenska University Hospital and I recently performed a study using a psychiatric hospital, Östra Hospital in Gothenburg, that opened in 2006. Of the ten architectural features researchers have identified that are likely to diminish stress and aggression, Östra has nine. Data on aggressive incidents were compiled for the hospital and compared with those from two other psychiatric facilities. One was an older facility replaced by Östra, which had only one of the stress-reducing features. A third institution located in the same region also had just one of these architectural elements. Despite the wide differences in design, though, the three hospitals were similar with respect to the number of beds, types of patients, treatment protocols and staffing levels. The drop in the use of patient restraints – a proxy for incidents of aggression – was striking. The number of patient sedations at Östra was 21 percent lower than at the hospital it replaced, and the use of physical restraints fell by more than twice that (44 percent). At the third facility – which operated during the years of both the old and the new hospitals and therefore served as an experimental control – the use of both forms of restraint continued to rise, suggesting that the difference was probably not because of a general improvement in care procedures over the period examined . . . studies like this one have limitations, certainly. It's hard to know for sure that there weren't major differences in patient care and training between the old facility and the new. But evidence from myriad studies and design research strongly supports the notion that architectural design can reduce violence. The principles, moreover, have implications for the wider health care system . . . to reduce the odds of aggression, it's time we put our growing understanding about stress-reducing design into architectural practice.

78 Ulrich, Roger S. (2006) 'Evidence-based health-care architecture', *The Lancet*, 368(6): S38–S39. In this brief essay in the *Lancet* in 2006, Ulrich made a similar broad-brush case for the role of evidence-based health-care design although, here, he presents somewhat more evidence within the essay itself compared to the pilot study-level data he cited in the 2013 *New York Times* op-ed (see above).

79 This led to interesting back-and-forth correspondences published in the *Journal of Health Environments Research & Design* on the relative merits (and limitations) of empirically driven evidence-based methodologies and their appropriateness in architecture. See Hamilton, D. Kirk (2014) 'Intuitive hypothesis and the excitement of discovery', *Health Environments Research & Design Journal*, 7(2): 140–143. Also see Lundin, Stefan (2015) 'In search of the happy balance – Intuition and evidence', *Health Environments Research & Design Journal*, 8(2): 123–126. Based on his award-winning design work at the new Östra Psychiatric Hospital, Lundin was subsequently invited to consult on the design of the Centre for Addiction and Mental Health (CAMH) in Toronto, Canada, in 2014 (see Chapter 4).

80 Editorial (2016) 'Not a solution for mental patients', *The Japan Times*, 7 July. Online. Available at www.japantimes.co.jp/opinion/2014/07/07/editorials/solution-mental-patients/#.V362FYe6Xdk (accessed 12 September 2016). In Japan, in 2014, nearly 65,000 psychiatric inpatients had been hospitalized for more than 10 years, a number considered extremely high by WHO standards. A main reason for Japan's continuing high number of warehoused mentally ill is its culture, which traditionally has labeled these persons 'outcasts'. Similarly, in China, widespread social stigma suppresses public and government support for the construction of a new (and badly needed) generation of treatment facilities, and new policies for successfully mainstreaming large numbers of former inpatients into everyday community life.

81 Meadows, Graham N. and Philip M. Burgess (2007) 'Perceived need for mental health care: findings from the 2007 Australian survey of mental health and well being', *Australian and New Zealand Journal of Psychiatry*, 43(12): 624–634.

82 Seaman, Andrew M. (2014) 'Shrinking psych hospitals may be linked with rising prison populations', *Reuters.com*. Online. Available at www.reuters.com/article/us-psychiatry-prison-population-idUSKBN0JQ26W20141212 (accessed 14 October 2016). Psychiatric hospital data were compared to current prison population data. The reason 1990 was selected was because in that year these six counties all signed a single declaration to reduce the number of psychiatric beds and to correspondingly increase the availability of outpatient mental health services. For example, the number of psychiatric beds in Argentina dropped by about a third between 1990 and 2012 although its prison population swelled by 137%. In Bolivia, the number of psychiatric beds declined by 2%. Meanwhile, its prison population swelled by 16%. This finding echoed that of the English researcher Lionel Sharples

Penrose back in 1939. His main finding then became known as the Penrose hypothesis.

83 Akbar, Jay (2015) 'Startling images of abuse inside Africa's "psychiatric prisons"', *The Daily Mail*, 4 November. Online. Available at www.dailymail.co.uk/news/article-3301484/Startling-images-abuse-inside-Africa-s-psychiatric-prisons.html (accessed 9 March 2017). In Somaliland, in Africa, psychiatric patients are routinely chained up by their ankles in solitary confinement for 23 hours at a time, force-fed tranquilizers, then beaten. Similar mistreatment continues across the continent, including in South Sudan, the Democratic Republic of Congo, Uganda, Kenya, and Nigeria.

84 Torrey, E. Fuller (2016) 'A dearth of psychiatric beds', *Psychiatric Times*, 49(2): 16. Online. Available at www.psychaitrictimes.com/psychiatric-emergencies/dearth-psychiatric-beds.html (accessed 23 March 2017). Also see Karlin, Bradley E. and Robert A. Zeiss (2006) 'Environmental and therapeutic issues in psychiatric hospital design: toward best practices', *Psychiatry*, 47(10): 23. Online. Available at www.psychiatryonline.org/doi/full/10.1176/ps.2006.57.10.1376.html (accessed 12 February 2017). However, this figure is overestimated because in most states existing psychiatric beds are largely occupied by court-ordered long-stay forensic patients and therefore are not readily available for the admission of nonforensic patients.

85 Anon (2015) 'Former Michigan mental asylum finds new life', *Modern Healthcare*, 45(21): 36. This large psychiatric institution in Michigan operated for more than a century a half mile from the center of town on a picturesque site along Lake Michigan. Its centerpiece was the former inpatient ward and administration building, known simply as Building 50. It is a five-level structure designed in the Victorian-Italianate style, with high ceilings, large windows, and red rooftop spires. In the basement level, the 'Mercato' features narrow, twisting passageways where 'incorrigible' patients were once chained to the walls.

86 Hall, Neal (2012) 'Closure of Riverview Hospital marks end of era in mental health treatment', *Vancouver Sun*, 19 July. Online. Available at www.vancouversun.com/health/Closure+Riverview+Hospital+marks+mental+health+treatment/6967310/story.html (accessed 14 March 2017).

Chapter 2

1 Goshen, Charles E., ed. (1959) *Psychiatric Architecture: A Review of Contemporary Developments in the Architecture of Mental Hospitals, Schools for the Mentally Retarded and Related Facilities.* Washington, DC: The American Psychiatric Association. An interdisciplinary team had visited and documented over a 5-year period numerous facilities in North America and in Europe distilling 'guiding' planning and design principles. In the introductory essay, 'A Review of Psychiatric Architecture and the Principles of Design', Charles E. Goshen summarized the state of the art in the late 1950s. He began by recounting the background against which its precepts had been based, summarizing the work of Dr. Thomas Kirkbride, the 'famous psychiatrist' in Philadelphia in the 1850s, and his architect, Samuel Sloane, who first conceptualized 'mental hospital' architecture as a specified field. Kirkbride had advocated two parallel and closely integrated sets of principles applicable to psychiatric care – moral treatment of the insane, and architectural specifications for a new generation of specialized hospitals.

2 Ibid.: 1. Kirkbride believed no asylum should be so large its superintendent would not know every patient individually – 250 was considered the maximum number of patients treatable under this system. The combined effect of isolationism and restrictiveness resulted in no significant further architectural advancements in the 20th century prior to 1960. This was particularly the case in the state-run institutions, although some architectural innovation did take place in the private sector.

3 Ibid.: 2.

4 Ibid.: 3.

5 Goffman, Erving (1961) *Asylums: Essays on the Social Situation of Mental Patients and Other Inmates.* New York: Doubleday Anchor Books.

6 Lammers, Stephen and Allan Vershey (1998) *On Moral Medicine: Theological Perspectives in Medical Ethics.* Grand Rapids, MI: William B. Eerdmans Publishing: 855.

7 Goffman: 6.

8 Ibid.: 7.

9 Ibid.: 16. He wrote,

> In many total institutions the privilege of having visitors or of visiting away from the establishment is completely withheld at first, ensuring a deep initial break with past roles . . . there is a need to obtain initial cooperativeness . . . staff often feel the need to challenge the inmate to balk or to hold his (sic) peace forever. Thus these initial moments of (re) socialization may involve an 'obedience test' and even a will-breaking contest: a (patient) inmate who shows defiance receives immediate visible punishment, which increases until he openly 'cries uncle' and humbles himself (but) once stripped of one's possessions their replacement . . . take the form of standard issue, uniform in character and uniformly distributed.

10 Sedgwick, Peter (1987) *PsychoPolitics*. London: Pluto Press: 5. In the essay 'Notes on the Tinkering Trades', he concluded the medicalization of mental illness and its various treatment modalities are offshoots of the 19th century and the Industrial Revolution and so-called medical models for treating patients were no more than a variation on the way tradespersons and craftsmen of the 19th century had repaired clocks and other mechanized objects: always in the confines of a shop or store, where context and routine remained somewhat of a mystery to the customer. In Sedgwick's view, the book *Asylums* brought Goffman immediate recognition and by the 1970s this work had become required reading in many introductory sociology courses; social scientists and others (including progressive-minded architects) viewed it as powerful and compelling because it provided a rare look into the misery of 'institutional warehouses'.

11 Foucault, Michel (1961) *Folie et Déraison: Historie de la folie à l'âge classique*. Paris: Libraire Pion. An English translation of the complete 1961 edition, titled *History of Madness*, was published in June 2006. Foucault, Michael (2006) *History of Madness* (J. Khalfa, ed./trans.) London and New York: Routledge. He employed phenomenology to narrate the evolving experience of the insane as 'the other' while attributing this evolution to the influence of overarching social structures. This book developed from his earlier writings on psychology, his personal psychological struggles, and his experience working in a psychiatric hospital. He linked the evolutionary decline of widespread leper colonies to the rise of the concept of the relationship between madness and 'unreason' through the Renaissance, the Classical Age of the 17th and 18th centuries, and the modern mid-20th-century experience.

12 Ibid: 24–48. Also see Merquior, J.G. (1985) *Foucault*. Waukegan, IL: Fontana Press. The first asylums were built near the end of the 1700s; these places were built solely for the confinement of the mad under the supervision of medical doctors – justified on the basis the family could no longer afford the level of care required at home. Hence, the community would now be rid of its undesirables, and this was being done as a means to protect the community's quality of life. In time, the insane asylum was seen as the only place where this type of care could be adequately provided, although Foucault viewed treatment in these places as cruel and controlling. He structured a complex, often contradictory narrative in building his thesis, from the contrasting images of leprosy and the 'Ship of Fools' at the beginning and onward, by examining multiple societal conceits and paradoxes, labeling the mad as becoming trapped within an internalized, delirious discourse and within the societal structures erected to confine them to the asylum. Foucault argued that in the Renaissance the insane were portrayed in art as possessing a kind of wisdom and in literature as capable of differentiating what humans are – versus what they pretend (or present themselves) to be. He contended that at the dawn of the Age of Reason, in the mid-1600s, the rational response to the insane, who had until then been relegated to the margins of society, was to isolate them exclusively from society through confinement along with prostitutes, vagrants, and other social undesirables, in newly created institutions across Europe in a process he termed the 'Great Confinement'. Their condition as such warranted extensive systems of punishment and reward aimed at causing the patient/inmate to reverse one's evil/antisocial behaviour. The removal of any and all undesirables from the streets of rapidly growing towns and cities was precipitated by the rise of laws and regulations prescribing strict social conformity. In time, medical doctors viewed insanity as a phenomenon worthy of study and later as a rectifiable condition to be scientifically eradicated.

13 Goshen (1959): 2. These dehumanizing features were (1) the location of the hospital in a remote area with a cordon sanitaire of grounds around it; (2) the construction of large, unadorned brick buildings within extensive grounds, with conspicuous features such as window screens or bars, sun porches heavily grilled, and high fences; (3) the housing of large numbers of patients in single buildings and in large wards; (4) the use of obvious security devices ('This patient must dangerous; he's in a barred room – even the toilets are open to observation'); (5) the use of uniformly drab furniture and colors, and an almost complete absence of accessories commonly recognized as expressions of individuality; (6) widespread use of building materials designed primarily for ease of maintenance, such as tile walls and terrazzo floors; (7) the absence of facilities where patients might store their personal possessions and lack of opportunity for displaying such items as pictures, family photographs, and mementos; (8) the use of uniform clothing for patients, resembling prison garb; (9) mass feeding practices, with no choice of food and the lack of a full set of tableware; (10) mass transportation or 'herding' of patients from one place to another; (11) the lack of privacy for bathing and toilet facilities; (12) the scarcity of orientation devices such as clocks, calendars, newspapers, telephones, and other 'normal' means of keeping in touch with reality; (13) the absence of everyday life activities such as shopping, holidays, and related daily living activities; (14) securely sequestered nursing stations, which tend to limit personnel contact with patients ('How often do you see a nurse hiding herself from patients by busying herself with paperwork in her isolated nursing station?'); (15) the prevalence of accumulated institutional odors; (16) an absence of focal points for patients to take pride in on their unit; and (17) the absence of adequate and commodious social space for patients to receive visitors.

14 Ibid.: 5–6. The remaining sections of the book *Psychiatric Architecture* focus on the presentation of a series of 'progressively designed' case studies of recently built or in-planning facilities embracing the positive attributes called out in the book's introductory essays. After these case studies, an essay on recent progressive European facility design trends is provided, followed by a comprehensive glossary of terminology (a surprising percentage of which remains relevant today).

15 Spiegel, René (1989) *Psychopharmacology: An Introduction.* Chichester and New York: John Wiley & Sons. 'Chapter 2: The history of psychopharmacology': 25–47.

16 Ibid.: 28–29. In the Age of Enlightenment and absolutism, psychiatry developed in different directions across Europe and elsewhere depending on local politics and sociocultural determinants. Spiegel (1989) described the core attributes of this ontology, which occurred in virtually all countries sooner or later as consisting of (1) the spatial segregation of the insane in houses that often lay outside the cities and towns, sometimes in former leper colonies; (2) the gradual rediscovery of the medical model of mental illnesses, premised on pathological anatomical causes; and (3) attempts to return the insane (i.e., social outcasts) to a normalized life by means of work, useful tasks, and regulated daily regimen as a means to support them as contributing members in everyday society. Spiegel notes these three trends were seen as contradictory to an extent, as to how a 'spatially segregated' patient could lead a normalized life in society. In the early Christian Middle Ages, however, a tradition of mercy had arisen. Prayers were said for the possessed and the Church in time saw itself as a haven for the insane and epileptics. Only in the 11th century was the practice of beating the mad in widespread use and by the 14th century there was a change to isolating the insane from the healthy population in lunatic asylums and madhouses. Between the Middle Ages and the modern era were physicians such as Paracelsus (1491–1541), J. Weyer (1515–1588), and F. Platter (1536–1614) who turned against the concept of devil possession, witches, and evil spirits and restored natural causes to center stage in the treatment of mental illness. But they had no new treatments to offer, and prescribed bloodletting and purging to cleanse contaminated bodily fluids, baths and massages for relaxation therapy and to strengthen the body, and soporifics and sedatives to calm the agitated.

17 Spiegel (1989): 31.

18 Spiegel (1989) 'Modern psychopharmaceuticals': 1–47. Psychopharmaceuticals are medications affecting the behaviour and subjective state of humans and are used therapeutically for their psychotropic effects. Other substances with psychotropic effects, such as alcohol, nicotine, cocaine, and heroin, are viewed by society as addictive substances and therefore have no overt therapeutic amenity in Western culture. Analgesic, antiepileptic, and other medications are generally not considered to have psychotic effects. Like other medications, psychopharmaceuticals are classified according to their chemical structure and their applications with patients. Their four general categories are neuroleptics for the symptomatic treatment of schizophrenia and for states of agitation (antipsychotics and major tranquillizers); antidepressants for the treatment of depression (mood equilibrators and mood stimulators) including lithium; tranquillizers for treatment of states of anxiety and tension including sleep-inducing agents (hypnotics); and stimulants used to increase drive and performance, also called psychostimulants and more rarely, analeptics.

19 Casey, J.F., I.F. Bennett, C.J. Lindley, L.E. Hollister, M.H. Gordon and N.N. Springer (1960) 'Drug therapy in schizophrenia: a controlled study of the relative effectiveness of chlorpromazine, promazine, phenobarbital and placebo', *Archives of General Psychiatry*, 2(4): 210–220.

20 Shen, Winston W. (1999) 'A history of antipsychotic drug development', *Comprehensive Psychiatry*, 40(6): 407–414.

21 Spiegel (1989): 37–38. With this trend came a corresponding decline in the traditional role of Freudian psychotherapy. An expanding number of factors – including psychological, interpersonal, sociocultural, and technological determinants – now influenced the efficacy of any given pharmaceutical intervention, thus requiring a new level of regulatory attention. In the 1970s and 1980s, psychodynamic and sociological approaches in psychiatry therefore fell from favor. As psychoanalysis lost its dominance, psychiatrists turned instead to the symptom-based classification system codified in the *Diagnostic and Statistical Manual of Mental Disorders*, 3rd ed., published in 1980.

22 Healy, David (2002) *The Creation of Psychopharmacology*. Cambridge, MA: Harvard University Press.

23 Ban, Thomas A. (2014) 'Psychopharmacology: the beginning of a new discipline', Chapter 23 in Frank Munoz, Charles Gonzalez, Alamo Lopez and Francis Domino (eds.) *History of Psychopharmacology*, Vol. 2. Arlington, MA: NPP Books: 2–3, 2–5.

24 Hall-Flavin, D.K., T.D. Schneekloth and J.D. Allen (2010) 'Translational psychiatry: bringing pharmacogenomic testing into clinical practice', *Psychiatry Weekly*, 5(2): 39–44. The implications of these medications for human genome research are also being explored. They are considered to be at least as effective as typical (i.e., traditional) antipsychotic medications in treating the symptoms of schizophrenia while causing fewer side effects.

25 Shen (1999): 412. In the 2000–2015 period, advancements continued as research identified new, scientifically based treatments for a broadening range of classified mental illnesses. Prozac, for example, has become among the most widely prescribed psychopharmaceuticals of choice for millions across the globe.

26 Ramos, Marco A. (2013) 'Drugs in context: a historical perspective on theories of psychopharmaceutical efficacy', *The Journal of Nervous and Mental Disease*, 201(11): 926–933. This emphasis on exploring and treating the significance of the psychosocial context, by definition, includes the influence of the everyday built environment on mental health and well-being.

27 World Health Organization (2003) *What Are the Arguments for Community Based Mental Health Care?* Geneva: World Health Organization/Health Evidence Network. This new vision for community-based care was premised on providing services closer to where the patient lives, flexible and adaptable to changing conditions in a community, more carefully tailored to each individual's specific needs while

adhering to international conventions of basic human rights, and more closely connected to local community hospitals.

28 Ibid.: 6–7.

29 Haberman, Clyde (2017) 'The quest for a psychiatric cure', *The New York Times*, 16 April. Online. Available at www.nytimes.com/2017/04/16/us/psychiatric-illnesses-lobo.html (accessed 18 April 2017).

30 Foot, John (2015) *The Man Who Closed the Asylums: Franco Basaglia and the Revolution in Mental Health Care*. Rome: Verso.

31 Baker, A., L. Llewelyn Davies and P. Sivadon (1959) *Psychiatric Service and Architecture*. Geneva: World Health Organization. Here, the psychiatric hospital would occupy a central role within a network of hub-and-spoke care providers and facilities. The hospital would shed any resemblances to an asylum or prison and would now symbolize a quasi-domestic 'normalized' environment. A network of proposed associated community-based off-site facilities was to consist of drug dispensaries and 'early treatment centers', alongside day hospitals, protected workshops, and aftercare at home and in the workplace milieu. The emphasis would be on continuity of care.

32 Chrysikou, Evangelia (2014) *Architecture for Psychiatric Environments and Therapeutic Spaces*. Amsterdam: IOS Press: 18–25.

33 Ibid.: 21. The 'day hospital', in this larger equation, was first introduced in the United Kingdom in 1948 with the advent of the NHS, as a place to keep patients closer to their homes while receiving primary care and, in some cases, secondary care.

34 Verderber, Stephen and David J. Fine (2000) *Healthcare Architecture in an Era of Radical Transformation*. New Haven, CT and London: Yale University Press: Chapters 3 and 4.

35 Anon (1965) 'Psychiatric hospitals', *The Architectural Review*, 49(6): 476–478.

36 Anon (1966) 'Hospitals: trends in planning', *Architectural Record*, 49(10): 47–52. In the US, this new building type was created by federal legislation in 1963. This federal agency was officially called the Community Mental Health Facilities Branch of the National Institute of Mental Health. An entirely new agency, the National Institute of Mental Health, would release a series of publications mandating the design attributes of every CMHC.

37 Anon (1967) 'Mental health facilities', *Architectural Record*, 49(2): 141–162.

38 Chrysikou (2014): 22.

39 Ibid.: 24.

40 Anon (1966) 'Improving hospital design: therapeutic environment of new mental hospital', *Progressive Architecture*, 44(8): 164–169. This same issue featured a detailed account of a landmark experiment conducted at the Topeka (Kansas, USA) State Hospital (asylum). See Good, Lawrence and Edith Zeller (1966) 'In-use evaluation of psychiatric facility', *Progressive Architecture*, 44(8): 170–173. There, in 1961, a case study examined the effect of the redesign of one of the existing women's wards, a footprint design conceived in the Kirkbride era. This open ward was subdivided into a series of single-occupancy bedrooms on both sides of a double-loaded corridor. The results of this experiment were mixed, as staff still harbored fears of patients' uncontrolled outbursts, with the reconfigured, more open nurses station seen as providing inadequate security in this regard. The team concluded the hospital could not be converted into a safe and useful facility and recommended building a completely new structure. Advantages would include the opportunity to select a better location and to incorporate the latest 'architectural thinking'. See Anderson, Stephen E., Lawrence Good and Kevin E. Hurtig (1976) 'Designing a mental health center to replace a county hospital', *Hospital and Community Psychiatry*, 27(11): 807–813.

41 Anon (1967) 'Studies show need for psychiatric service in emergency rooms, doctors suggest', *The Modern Hospital*, 108(6): 187.

42 Anon (1968) 'Try to ease crowding in L.A. psychiatric unit', *The Modern Hospital*, 109(8): 47.

43 Dardi, Costantino (1969) 'Concorso Nazionale Ospedale Psichiatrico Salorno-Bolzano', *Lotus*, 29(6): 170–179.

44 Anon (1970) 'News in Italian architecture', *Casabella*, 348(5): 22–25.

45 Editors (1970) 'Health centres', *The Architectural Review*, 57(5): 345–347.

46 Editors (1970) 'Architecture and institutional psychiatry', *Architecture d'Aujourd'hui*, 40(6): 48.

47 Bailey, David R. (1971) 'Hospital's mental health role changed by public funding', *The Modern Hospital*, 44(2): 95–98.

48 Anon (1967) 'Yamanashi prefecture Kita Hospital', *Japan Architect*, 134(8): 43–48.

49 Anon (1973) 'Winnebago children's Neillsville Wisconsin', *Architecture d'Aujourd'hui*, 166(3/4): 38–39.

50 Anon (1974) 'Geha mental hospital', *der baumeister*, 71(4): 291–293.

51 Anderson et al. (1976) *Hospital and Community Psychiatry*.

52 Kuntz, Esther (1979) 'Menninger Foundation plans new 166-bed adult psychiatric hospital', *Modern Healthcare*, 9(10): 50–53.

53 Anon (1975) 'Mental health reform fails', *Modern Healthcare*, 4(6): 45–48.

54 Ibid.: 46.

55 Anon (1978) 'Protest cuts and revisions in Illinois mental health budget', *Modern Healthcare*, 8(1): 40.

56 Anon (1979) 'L'Architecttura è il suo doppio, Unità Ospedaliera Psichiatrica a Girifalco', *Architettura*, 38(4): 24–38.

57 Verderber and Fine (2000): 121.

58 Weeks, Ronald (1980) 'Hospitals', *The Architectural Review*, 48(7): 46–56.

59 Editor (1981) 'Centre de santé mentale', *Architecture d'Aujourd'hui*, 214(2): 66–67.

60 Anon (1981) 'La Salute mentale ala ancora azionalismo, Centro psichiatrico a Tirat Carmel, presso Haifa', *Architettura*, 40(2): 20–34.

61 Emery, Marc (1981) 'Bronx Developmental Centre', *Architecture d'Aujourd'hui*, 213/15(2): 23–24.

62 Verderber and Fine (2000): 137–138.

63 Anon (1982) 'A building adrift', *Progressive Architecture*, 63(5): 152–155.

64 Kuntz, Esther (1981) 'Hospital chains grab psychiatric business from government facilities', *Modern Healthcare*, 11(4): 90–91. Also see Punch, Linda (1982) 'Psychiatric hospitals snapped up', *Modern Healthcare*, 12(5): 106–108. Also Punch, Linda (1983) 'Competition for acquisition of psychiatric hospitals heats up', *Modern Healthcare*, 13(5): 123–124. The Hospital Corporation of America (HCA) alone acquired 25 psychiatric hospitals in 1981. The company sold two hospitals and acquired one for a net gain of 237 beds in 1982. National Medical Enterprises' (NME) psychiatric facility portfolio in 1982 totaled 24 hospitals with 1,977 beds, a 505% increase from 1981. It cost about US$60,000 per bed to construct a psychiatric hospital at this time, compared to double this amount for an acute care community hospital. In time, these investor-owned healthcare systems would dominate the US market and Wall Street would call the shots.

65 Fackelmann, Kathy A. (1985) 'Group contends study proves DRGs won't work in psychiatric hospitals', *Modern Healthcare*, 15(20): 38.

66 White, Elizabeth C. (1985) 'Centers refine their advertising as era of soft-peddling ends', *Modern Healthcare*, 15(10): 74–75.

67 Anderson, Howard J. (1985) 'Hospitals eating disorders units fill empty beds with paying patients', *Modern Healthcare*, 15(22): 62–66.

68 Barkholz, David (1986) 'Systems show strong growth in number of psychiatric beds', *Modern Healthcare*, 16(12): 108–112. Also Wallace, Cynthia (1987) 'Psychiatric hospital industry still growing, but rate of expansion slower than last year', *Modern Healthcare*, 17(12): 92–98. Also Burda, David (1988) 'Investor-owned healthcare systems plan to continue expansion in psychiatric care', *Modern Healthcare*, 18(23): 63–70. Also see Kim, Howard (1989) 'Demand for psychiatric care is expected to maintain the current building boom', *Modern Healthcare*, 19(6): 38–39.

69 Verderber and Fine (2000): 167–169. Also see Valins, Martin (1993) *Primary Health Centers*. London: Butterworth: 68–74.

70 Jencks, Charles (1977) *The Language of Post-Modern Architecture*. Rizzoli: New York: 6–7.

71 Anon (1985) 'Award: Kahi Mohala Psychiatric Hospital, Honolulu', *Modern Healthcare*, 16(22): 66. Also see Anon (1987) 'Award: Kimberly Woods, Columbus, Ohio', *Modern Healthcare*, 17(2): 38. Also Anon (1989) 'Citation: Laurel Ridge Psychiatric Hospital, San Antonio', *Modern Healthcare*, 19(40): 46.

72 Editors (1991) 'Architecture for psychiatric treatment', *Progressive Architecture*, 49(1): 126–127. This author's firm, R-2ARCH, produced a four-volume report, *Architecture for a Changing Psychiatric Treatment Milieu: Research-based Design*, in 1991. The US journal *Progressive Architecture*'s Annual Awards Program recognized this work in evidence-based design, commissioned by HCA. Deliverables included a battery of postoccupancy evaluations conducted at DePaul Hospital's 12-acre campus in New Orleans, 103 campus planning and architectural design considerations, and a schematic design proposal for a new residential pavilion quadrangle sited adjacent to New Orleans's Audubon Park. This project remains unbuilt although the research findings were widely applied in the years since across HCAs nearly 40 self-owned psychiatric facilities nationwide.

73 Crosbie, Michael J. (1993) 'Village, not: the unfulfilled promise of Yale's Psychiatric Institute', *Progressive Architecture*, 48(6): 100–103. Also see Verderber and Fine (2000) for a more detailed description of this psychiatric hospital.

74 Denton, Mark (1995) 'Psychiatric care', *Texas Architect*, 44(1/2): 64–65.

75 Anon (1995) 'Psychiatric center for children, 1995, Leeuwarden', *L'Architettura*, 17(2): 458.

76 Anon (1998) 'Paysage structurant', *Architecture Interieure-Crée*, 12(4): 44–45.

77 Zwoch, di Felix (1987) 'Ganz e Rolfes, Rrigione psichiatrica, Berlin', *Domus*, 687(9): 60–71.

78 Wiser, Stephen A. (1993) 'On the cutting edge: designing Canada's newest psychiatric hospital', *Competitions*, Winter: 6–13.

79 Editor (1992) 'Therapeutic street', *Progressive Architecture*, 48(3): 90.

80 Cooper-Marcus, Clare and Marni Barnes (1999) *Healing Gardens: Therapeutic Benefits and Design Recommendations*. New York: John Wiley & Son: 261–270. Also see McBride, Deborah L. (1998) 'American Sanatoriums: landscaping for health – 1885–1945', *Landscape Journal*, 17(1): 26–36. McBride recounted the history of the Kirkbride asylum movement from the perspective of landscape design and the then-prevailing attitudes toward the therapeutic amenity of nature, from the late 19th century to the end of World War II.

81 Pearson, Clifford A. (1999) 'New York Psychiatric Institute, New York City', *Architectural Record*, 187(7): 138–141.

82 Lutz, Sandy (1995) 'Inpatient stay lengths drop sharply', *Modern Healthcare*, 21 August: 24. Also Lutz, Sandy (1996) 'More upheaval at psych systems', *Modern Healthcare*, 20 May: 76.

83 Editor (1992) 'Federal investigators may get in on the scrutiny of psychiatric facilities', *Modern Healthcare*, 27 April: 52.

84 Japsen, Bruce (1997) 'Psychiatric 'dumping' study: economics often motivates patient transfers', *Modern Healthcare*, 15 December: 22. At the same time, community hospitals were treating many more acutely ill psychiatric patients. Also see Kim, Howard (1990) 'Sicker patients could help hospitals', *Modern Healthcare*, 23 April: 28.

85 Soon, the largest investor-owned for-profit chains began to divest their inventory of 24/7 psychiatric facilities because federal Medicare and private insurance reimbursement rates were now capped, ending the era of (theoretically) unlimited profits.

86 Lutz, Sandy (1992) 'Psych facilities flood the market as chains rush to unload them', *Modern Healthcare*, 12 October: 18. Also see Anon

(1993) 'HCA takes the auction route to unload unwanted psychiatric hospital in Texas', *Modern Healthcare*, 11 January: 40. Also Lutz, Sandy (1993) 'Bad news, falling profits hamper psych providers', *Modern Healthcare*, 24 May: 54. Also Lutz, Sandy (1995) 'Mental healthcare industry suffers another bad year', *Modern Healthcare*, 2 January: 49. Also Saphir, Ann (1999) 'Charter to sell more than half its facilities', *Modern Healthcare*, 15 November: 12.

87 Knapp, M., D. Chisholm, J. Astin, P. Lelliott and B. Audini (1997) 'The cost consequences of changing the hospital-community balance: the mental health residential care study', *Psychological Medicine*, 27(11): 681–692.

88 Smith, C.W. (1958) 'Architectural research and the construction of mental hospitals', *Mental Hospitals*, 9(6): 39–42. Also Baker et al. (1959), and Haun, Paul (1961) 'Architectural considerations', in L. Linn (ed.) *Frontiers in General Hospital Psychiatry*. New York: International University Press: 67–81. Also see Izumi, K. (1968) 'Architectural considerations in the design of places and facilities for the care and treatment of the mentally ill', *Journal of Schizophrenia*, 2(1): 42–52. Also see Moller, C.B. (1968) *Architectural Environment and Our Mental Health*. New York: Horizon Press, for an overview of the shifting societal conditions of the mid-1960s and the architectural profession's prescription for action.

89 Berger, A. and Lawrence R. Good (1963) 'Development of architectural psychology in a psychiatric hospital', *AIA Journal*, 40(12): 76–80. Also see Good, Lawrence R., S.M. Siegel and A.P. Bay (1965) *Therapy by Design: Implications for Architecture and Human Behavior*. Springfield, IL: Charles C. Thomas.

90 Moos, Rudolph and Donald Daniels (1967) 'Differential effects of ward settings on psychiatric staff', *Archives of General Psychiatry*, 17(1): 75–82. Also Moos, Rudolph and Phillip Houts (1968) 'Assessment of the social atmospheres of psychiatric wards', *Journal of Abnormal Psychiatry*, 73(12): 595–604. Also Moos, Rudolph, H. Harris and K. Schonborn (1969) 'Psychiatric patients and staff reaction to their physical environment', *Journal of Clinical Psychology*, 25(4): 322–324.

91 Moos, Rudolph (1989) *The Ward Atmosphere Scale Manual*. Palo Alto: CA: Consulting Psychologists Press.

92 Rice, C., D. Berger, S. Klett, L. Sewall and P. Lemkau (1963) 'The ward evaluation scale', *Journal of Clinical Psychology*, 16: 251–258. Also see Klett, S., D. Berger, L. Sewall and C. Rice (1963) 'Patient evaluation of the psychiatric ward', *Journal of Clinical Psychology*, 19: 347–351. Also DeVries, D.L. (1968) 'Effects of environmental change and of participation on the behavior of mental patients', *Journal of Consulting and Clinical Psychology*, 32: 532–536.

93 Kasmar, J., W. Griffin and J. Mauritzen (1968) 'Effect of environmental surroundings on outpatients' mood and perception of psychiatrics', *Journal of Consulting and Clinical Psychology*, 32(2): 223–226. Also Griffin, W., J. Mauritzen and J. Kasmar (1969) 'The psychological aspects of the architectural environment: a review', *American Journal of Psychiatry*, 125(8): 93–98. Also Zeller, E.V. (1969) *Psychiatric Treatment Environment and Function*. Topeka, KS: The Environmental Research Foundation.

94 Ittelson, William, Harold Proshansky and Leanne G. Rivlin (1970) 'Bedroom size and social interaction of the psychiatric ward', *Environment and Behavior*, 2(3): 255–270. Also Rivlin, Leanne G. and Maxine Wolfe (1972) 'The early history of a psychiatric hospital for children: expectations and reality', *Environment and Behavior*, 4(1): 33–56. Also Holahan, Charles J. and Susan Saegert (1973) 'Behavioral and attitudinal effects of large-scale variation in the physical environment of psychiatric wards', *Journal of Abnormal Psychology*, 82(3): 454–462. Also Willer, B., E. Staslak, P. Pinfold and M. Rogers (1974) 'Activity patterns and the use of space by patients and staff on the psychiatric ward', *Canadian Psychiatric Association Journal*, 14: 561. Also Wolfe, Maxine (1975) 'Room size, group size, and density behavior patterns in a children's psychiatric facility', *Environment and Behavior*, 7(2): 199–224.

95 Davis, C., I. Glick and I. Rosow (1979) 'The architectural design of the psychotherapeutic milieu', *Hospital and Community Psychiatry*, 30(2): 453–460. Also Canter, David and Sandra Canter, eds. (1979) *Designing for Therapeutic Environments: A Review of Research*. New York: John Wiley.

96 Sivadon, P. (1970) 'Principles of psychiatric design', *World Hospitals*, 6(4): 96–101. Also Editors (1971) 'Evaluation: a mental health facility, its users and context', *AIA Journal*, 67(2): 38–41. Also Osmond, Henry and Ken Izumi (1971) 'The mentally ill: the problem of design guidance', in Kenneth Beyes and Sandra Francklin (ed.) *Designing for the Handicapped*. London: George Goodwin, Ltd.

97 Cotton, N. and R. Geraty (1984) 'Therapeutic space design: planning an inpatient children's unit', *Journal of Orthopsychiatry*, 54: 624–636. Also Baldwin, S. (1985) 'Effects of furniture arrangement on the atmosphere of wards in a maximum security hospital', *Hospital and Community Psychiatry*, 36(5): 525–528. Also Main, S., A. McBride and K. Austin (1985) 'Patient and staff perceptions of a psychiatric ward environment', *Issues in Mental Health Nursing*, 12(4): 149–157. Also Jeffers, T. (1991) 'Safety considerations in the psychiatric setting', *The Psychiatric Hospital*, 22(3): 119–122, and Gabb, B., K. Speicher and K. Lodl (1992) 'Environmental design for individuals with schizophrenia: an assessment tool', *Journal of Applied Rehabilitation Counseling*, 23(2): 35–40.

98 Whitehead, C., R. Polsky, C. Crookshand and E. Fik (1984) 'Objective and subjective evaluation of psychiatric ward design', *American Journal of Psychiatry*, 82(6): 454–462. Also Stahler, G., D. Frazer and H. Rappaport (1984) 'The evaluation of an environmental remodeling program on a psychiatric geriatric ward', *Journal of Social Psychology*, 123(2): 101–113. Also Corey, L., M. Wallace, S. Harris and B. Casey (1986) 'Psychiatric ward: a before and after look at how refurbishing affects staff and patient perceptions', *Journal of*

Psychosocial Nursing, 24(10): 10–16, and Gutkowski, S., Y. Ginath and F. Guttmann (1992) 'Improving psychiatric environments through minimal architectural changes', *Hospital and Community Psychiatry*, 43: 920–923.

99 Spivak, Meyer (1984) *Institutional Settings*. New York: Human Sciences Press. Also St. Clair, Ronald (1987) 'Psychiatric hospital design', *The Psychiatric Hospital*, 18(1): 17–22. Also Kiesler, C.A. and A. Sibulkin (1987) *Mental Hospitalization: Myths and Facts About a National Crisis*. Newbury Park, CA: Sage Publications. Also Gulak, M.B. (1991) 'Architectural guidelines for state psychiatric hospitals', *Hospital and Community Psychiatry*, 42(7): 705–707, and American Institute of Architects (1993) *Design Considerations for Mental Health Facilities*. Washington, DC: American Institute of Architects Committee on Architecture for Health.

100 Grosenick, J. and C. Hatmaker (2000) 'Perceptions of the importance of physical setting in substance abuse treatment', *Journal of Substance Abuse Treatment*, 18(4): 29–39. Also Tyson, G., G. Lambert and L. Beattie (2002) 'The impact of ward design on the behavior, occupational satisfaction and well-being of psychiatric nurses', *International Journal of Mental Health Nursing*, 11(6): 94–102. Also Turlington, R. (2004) 'Creating a Planetree inpatient psychiatric unit', *Health Facilities Management*, 17(6): 12–13. Also Kagan, I. and Robert Kigli-Shemesh (2005) 'Relocating into a new building and its effect on uncertainty and anxiety among psychiatric patients', *Journal of Psychiatric and Mental Health Nursing*, 12(11): 603–606, and Cleary, M., G. Hunt and G. Walter (2009) 'A comparison of patient and staff satisfaction with services after relocating to a new purpose-built mental health facility', *Environments and Facilities*, 17(3): 212–217.

101 Middelboe, T., T. Schjødt, K. Byrsting and A. Gjerris (2001) 'Ward atmosphere in acute psychiatric inpatient care: patients' perceptions, ideals and satisfaction', *Acta Psychiatrica Scandinavica*, 103(3): 212–219. Also Müller, M., R. Schlosser, G. Kapp-Steen, B. Schanz and O. Benkert (2002) 'Patients' satisfaction with psychiatric treatment: comparison between open and closed ward', *Psychiatric Quarterly*, 73(2): 93–107. Also Brunt, D. and M. Rask (2005) 'Patient and staff perception of the ward atmosphere in a Swedish maximum-security forensic psychiatry hospital', *The Journal of Forensic Psychiatry & Psychology*, 16(2): 263–276. Also Sorlie, T., A. Parniakov, G. Rezvy and O. Ponomarev (2010) 'Psychometric evaluation of the Ward Atmosphere Scale in a Russian psychiatric hospital', *Nordic Journal of Psychiatry*, 64(6): 377–383, and Beazley, P. and G. Gudjonsson (2011) 'Motivating inpatients to engage with treatment: the role of depression and ward atmosphere', *Nordic Journal of Psychiatry*, 65(2): 95–100.

102 Gaskin, C., S. Elsom and B. Happell (2007) 'Interventions for reducing the use of seclusion in psychiatric facilities', *British Journal of Psychiatry*, 191: 283–303. Also Nanda, U., S. Eisen, R.S. Zadeh and D. Owen (2010) 'Effect of visual art on patient anxiety and agitation in a mental health facility and implications for the business case', *Journal of Psychiatric and Mental Health Nursing*, 185: 386–393.

103 Mahony, J., N. Palyo, G. Napier and J. Giordano (2009) 'The therapeutic milieu reconceptualized for the 21st century', *Archives of Psychiatric Nursing*, 23(6): 423–429. Also Golembiewski, Jan A. (2010) 'Start making sense: applying a salutogenic model to architectural design for psychiatric care', *Facilities*, 28(3/4): 100–117, and Golembiewski, Jan A. (2012) 'Psychiatric design: using a salutogenic model for the development and management of mental health facilities', *World Health Design*, 5(2): 74–79.

104 Saunders, Georgio (2008) 'Studio M10: TBS – Kliniek/Secure Psychiatric Hospital', *Architecture in Nederland*, 49(6): 140–143.

105 Editor (2015) 'William Wake House', *e-architect.co*. Online. Available at www.e-architect.co.uk/england/william-wake-house.html (accessed 10 October 2016).

106 Editors (2010) 'Cleveland Clinic Lou Ruvo Center for Brain Health, Las Vegas, Nevada', *Global Architecture*, 56(3): 43–55.

107 Shekhar, Saxema, Graham Thornicroft, Martin Knapp and Harvey Whiteford (2007) 'Resources for mental health: scarcity, inequity, and inefficiency', *The Lancet*, 370(4): 878–889. Also Knapp, Martin, D. Chisholm, John Astin, P. Lelliott and B. Audini (1997) 'The cost consequences of changing the hospital-community balance: the mental health residential care study', *Psychological Medicine*, 27(6): 681–692. Also Walters, Edgar (2016) 'State spending more on mental health care, but waitlist for beds grows', *The Texas Tribune*, 1 May 2016. Online. Available at www.texasribune.org/2016/05/01/despite-state-spending-dearth-psych-hospital-beds/html (accessed 10 May 2016), and Center for Medicare and Medicaid Services (2014) *The Mental Health Parity and Addiction Equity Act*. Washington, DC: Center for Medicare and Medicaid Services. Online. Available at www.cms.gov/CCIIO/Programs-and-Initiatives/Other-Insurance-Protections/mh-paea_factsheet.html (accessed 12 June 2016).

108 Saphir, Ann (2000) 'Charter restructuring closes 33 hospitals', *Modern Healthcare*, 31 January: 16. Also Saphir, Ann (2000) 'Fiscally challenged: psychiatric industry's hope is in consolidation, focusing services', *Modern Healthcare*, 27 March: 66.

109 Evans, Melanie (2004) 'They're waiting impatiently: despite rising demand, behavioral health services still face lack of hospital capacity, stretched funding sources', *Modern Healthcare*, 4 April: 6. Also Mantone, Joseph (2005) 'Reversal of fortune: after years of scaling back beds because of low occupancy rates, behavioral health facilities are beginning to make a comeback', *Modern Healthcare*, 4 April: 6. By 2002 the situation had further deteriorated, as there were 483 psychiatric hospitals and 1,410 psychiatric units in general acute care hospitals in the United States – 35% and 12% declines, respectively, compared to a mere decade earlier.

110 Lubell, Jennifer (2009) 'No building boom here: many state psych hospitals have given way to community-based care options',

Modern Healthcare, 27 July: 32. Also Zigmond, Jessica (2012) 'Out of the ER: programs aim to redirect psychiatric patients', *Modern Healthcare*, 28 May: 42. Also see Kutscher, Beth (2013) 'Bedding, not boarding: psychiatric patients boarded in hospital EDs create crisis for patient care and hospital finances', *Modern Healthcare*, 18 November: 43.

111 Ross Johnson, Steven (2014) 'Ruling could spur action to address psychiatric boarding crisis', *Modern Healthcare*, 1 September: 44. The United States was now relying upon a new metric that recommended the provision of a mere 50 inpatient psychiatric beds per every 100,000 persons in the general population.

112 Ford, Matt (2015) 'America's largest mental hospital is a jail', *The Atlantic*, 8 June. Online. Available at www.theatlantic.com/politics/archive/2015/06/americas-largest-hospital-is-a-jail.html (accessed 21 May 2017).

Chapter 3

1 Patel, Vikram, Alan J. Fisher, Sarah Hetrick and Patrick McGorry (2007) 'Mental health of young people: a global public-health challenge', *The Lancet*, 369(4): 1302–1313.

2 Williams, Sheila, Jessie Anderson, Rob McGee and Philip A. Silva (1990) 'Risk factors for behavioural and emotional disorder in preadolescent children', *Journal of the American Academy of Child and Adolescent Psychiatry*, 29(3): 413–419. Also see Birmaher, Boris, Neal D. Ryan, Douglas E. Williamson, David A Brent, Joan Kaufman, Ronald E. Dahl, James Perel and Beverly Nelson (1996) 'Childhood and adolescent depression: a review of the past 10 years', *Journal of the American Academy of Child and Adolescent Psychiatry*, 35(4): 1427–1435.

3 Green, H., A. McGinnity, H. Meltzer, T. Ford and R. Goodman (2005) *Mental Health of Children and Young People in Great Britain, 2004*. London: Palgrave Macmillan.

4 Knapp, Martin, Stephen Scott and Julia Davies (1999) 'The cost of antisocial behavior in younger people', *Clinical Child Psychology and Psychiatry*, 4(6): 457–473. Also see Knapp, Michael, Paul McCrone, Eric Fombonne, Jonathan Beecham and Gail Wostear (2002) 'The Maudsley long-term follow-up of child and adolescent depression: 3. Impact of comorbid conduct disorder on service use and costs in adulthood', *British Journal of Psychiatry*, 180(1): 19–23.

5 Birmaher, B., D.E. Williamson, R.E. Dahl, D.A. Axelson, J. Kaufman, L.D. Dorn and N.D. Ryan (2004) 'Clinical presentation and course of depression in youth: does onset in childhood differ from onset in adolescence?' *Journal of the American Academy of Child and Adolescent Psychiatry*, 43(2): 63–70.

6 Rickwood, Debra, Frank P. Deane, Coralie J. Wilson and Joseph V. Ciarocchi (2005) 'Young people's help-seeking for mental health problems', *Australian e-Journal for the Advancement of Mental Health*, 4(2): 1–34.

7 Jukam, Kelsey (2016) 'Report finds Louisiana segregates mental ill', *Courthouse News*, 23 December. Online. Available at www.courthousenews.com/feds-say-louisiana-segregates-mentally-ill-citizens/ (accessed 30 December 2016). Also see Associated Press (2016) 'Louisiana segregates mentally ill in nursing homes instead of giving proper care', *The Times Picayune*, 28 December. Online. Available at www.nola.com/health/index.ssf/2016/12/feds_louisiana_segregates_ment.html (accessed 30 December 2016).

8 Huang, Larke, Beth Stroul, Robert Friedman, Patricia Mrazek, Barbara Friesen, Sheila Pires and Steve Mayberg (2005) 'Transforming mental health care for children and their families', *American Psychologist*, 60(6): 615–627.

9 Ma, Jun, Ky-Van Lee and Randall S. Stafford (2005) 'Depression treatment during outpatient visits by U.S. children and adolescents', *Journal of Adolescent Health*, 37(4): 434–442.

10 Merikangas, Kathleen R., Jian-Ping He, Marcy Burstein, Sonja A. Swanson, Sheli Avenevoli, Lihong Cui, Corina Benjet, Katholiki Georgiades and Joel Swendsen (2010) 'Lifetime prevalence of mental disorders in U.S. adolescents: results from the National Comorbidity Survey Replication – Adolescent Supplement (NCS-A)', *Journal of the American Academy of Child & Adolescent Psychiatry*, 49(10): 980–989.

11 Olfson, Mark, Benjamin G. Druss and Steven C. Marcus (2015) 'Trends in mental health care among children and adolescents', *New England Journal of Medicine*, 372(21): 2029–2038.

12 Klanen, Henrikje and Anne-Claire Crombag (2013) 'What works where? A systematic review of child and adolescent mental health interventions for low and middle income countries', *Social Psychiatry and Psychiatric Epidemiology*, 48(2): 595–611.

13 Gunn, James (2004) 'Foreword', in S. Bailey and M. Dolan (eds.) *Adolescent Forensic Psychiatry*. London: Arnold.

14 Altadottir, H.O., D. Gyllenberg, A. Langridge, S. Sandin, S.N. Hansen, H. Leonard and E.T. Parner (2014) 'The increasing occurrence of reported diagnoses of childhood psychiatric disorders: a descriptive multinational comparison', *European Child & Adolescent Psychiatry*, 24(4): 173–183.

15 Polanczyk, Guilherme V., Giovanni A.A. Salum, Luisa S. Sugaya, Arthur Caye and Luis A. Rohde (2015) 'Annual research review: a meta-analysis of the worldwide prevalence of mental disorders in children and adolescents', *The Journal of Child Psychology and Psychiatry*, 56(3): 345–365.

16 Green, Jonathan, Brian Jacobs, Jennifer Beecham, Graham Dunn, Leo Kroll, Catherine Tobias and Jackie Briskman (2007) 'Inpatient

treatment in child and adolescent psychiatry – a prospective study of health gain and costs', *Journal of Child Psychiatry and Psychiatry*, 48(12): 1259–1267. In England and Wales in 2003, there were 80 units providing a total of only 900 beds for children and adolescents, representing the availability of 7.1 beds per 100,000 population under the age of 18.

17 Kwok, Ka Ho Robin, Sze Ngar Vanesse Yuan and Dennis Ougrin (2016) 'Review: alternatives to inpatient care for children and adolescents with mental health disorders', *Child and Adolescent Mental Health*, 21(1): 3–10.

18 Stephan, Sharon H., Mark West, Sheryl Kataoka, Steven Adelsheim and Carrie Mills (2007) 'Transformation of children's mental health services: the role of school mental health', *Psychiatric Services*, 58(10): 1330–1338.

19 Singh, Swaran P. (2009) 'Transition of care from child to adult mental health services: the great divide', *Current Opinion in Psychiatry*, 22(2): 386–390.

20 Stine, A.G. (2016) 'Watching mental illness from the sidelines', *Tales From the Circus*, 21 June. Online. Available at www.talesfromthecircus.com/watching-mental-illness-from-the-sidelines/ (accessed 14 January 2017).

21 Goldbeck, Lutz and Thomas Ellerkamp (2012) 'A randomized controlled trial of multimodal music therapy for children with anxiety disorders', *Journal of Music Therapy*, 49(4): 395–413.

22 Payman, Vahid (2010) 'An outpatient psychotherapy clinic for the elderly: rationale, establishment and characteristics', *Asia-Pacific Psychiatry*, 2(2): 191–200.

23 Freud, Sigmund (1905) 'On Psychotherapy', in James P. Strachey (ed.) *The Standard Edition of the Complete Psychological Works of Sigmund Freud*, Vol. 7. London: Hogarth Press: 257–268.

24 Abraham, Karl (1919) 'The applicability of psychoanalytic treatment to patients at an advanced age', in Donald Bryan and James P. Strachey (trans., 1957) *Selected Papers of Karl Abraham, M.D.* London: Hogarth Press: 312–317.

25 Jung, Carl (1931) 'The stages of life', in Herbert Read, Martha Fordham and Gregory Adler (eds., 1979) *Collected Works*, Vol. 8. London: Routledge and Kegan Paul: 387–403.

26 Erikson, Erik (1950) *Childhood and Society*. New York: Norton and Company, Inc.

27 Bor, Jonathan S. (2015) 'Among the elderly, many mental illnesses go undiagnosed', *Health Affairs*, 34(5): 727–731. Online. Available at www.content.healthaffairs.org/content/34/5/727.html (accessed 4 January 2017).

28 Institute of Medicine (2012) *The Mental Health and Substance Use Workforce for Older Adults: In Whose Hands?* Washington, DC: Institute of Medicine/National Academies Press. Online. Available at www.iom.edu/reports/2012/The-Mental-Health-and-Substance-Use-Workforce-for-Older-Adults.aspx (accessed 4 January 2017).

29 Bartels, Stephen J., Brent Forester, Kim T. Mueser, Keith M. Miles, Aricca R. Dums, Sarah I. Pratt, Anjana Sengupta, Christine Littlefield, Sheryl O'Hurley, Patricia White and Lois Perkins (2004) 'Enhanced skills training and health care management for older persons with severe mental illness', *Journal of Community Mental Health*, 40(6): 75–90. Also see Hennekens, Charles H., Alissa R. Hennekens, Danielle Hollar and Daniel E. Casey (2005) 'Schizophrenia and increased risks of cardiovascular disease', *Journal of the American Heart Association*, 150(14): 1115–1121.

30 Hendrie, Hugh C., Donald Lindgren, Donald P. Hay, Kathleen A. Lane, Sujuan Gao, Christianna Purnell, Stephanie Munger, Faye Smith, Jeanne Dickens, Malaz A. Boustani and Christopher M. Callahan (2013) 'Comorbidity profile and healthcare utilization in elderly patients with serious mental illnesses', *American Journal of Geriatric Psychiatry*, 21(12): 1267–1276.

31 Byers, Amy L., Kristine Yaffe, Kenneth E. Covinsky, Michael B. Friedman and Martha L. Bruce (2010) 'High occurrence of mood and anxiety disorders among older adults: the National Comorbidity Survey Replication', *Archives of General Psychiatry*, 67(5): 489–496. Also see Reynolds, Kristin, Robert H. Pietrzak, Renée El-Gabalawy, Corey S. Mackenzie and Jitender Sareen (2015) 'Prevalence of psychiatric disorders in U.S. older adults: findings from a nationally representative survey', *World Psychiatry*, 14(1): 74–81.

32 Wuthrich, Viviana M. and Jacqueline Frei (2015) 'Barriers to treatment for older adults seeking psychological therapy', *International Psychogeriatrics*, 27(7): 1227–1236.

33 Lyness, Jeffrey M., Moonseong Heo, Catherine J. Datto, Thomas R. Ten have, Ira R. Katz, Rebecca Drayer, Charles F. Reynolds III, George S. Alexopoulos and Martha L. Bruce (2006) 'Outcomes on minor and subsyndromal depression among elderly patients in primary care settings', *Annals in Internal Medicine*, 144(7): 496–504.

34 Gum, Amber and Patricia A. Areán (2004) 'Current status of psychotherapy for mental disorders in the elderly', *Current Psychiatry Reports*, 6(1): 32–38. Behavioural therapy (BT), cognitive-behavioural therapy (CBT), and problem-solving therapy (PST) are three types of treatment based on the learning theory of personality and focus on teaching the patient new skills to cope with depression and psychosocial problems. Brief dynamic therapy (BDT), interpersonal therapy (IPT), and supportive therapy (ST) focus primarily on the resolution of interpersonal problems and processes through exploration of affect, structured exercise therapy, and bibliotherapy (i.e., the use of reading and recall as a treatment modality). Finally, reminiscence therapy, developed specifically for older adults, is based on Erikson's theory of human psychosocial development and aims to primarily integrate the patient's personal history into how one understands her or his life at this juncture. Of this menu of therapies, CBT and IPT have broad empirical support and are therefore considered to be the most evidence-based therapies in clinical practice.

35 Blake, Holly, Peter Mo, Saul Malik and Stephen Thomas (2009) 'How effective are physical activity interventions for alleviating depressive symptoms in older people? A systematic review', *Clinical Rehabilitation*, 23(3): 873–887.

36 Inventor, Ben R.E., John Henricks, Leslie Rodman, Joel Imel, Lance Holemon and Fernando Hernandez (2005) 'The impact of medical issues in inpatient geriatric psychiatry', *Issues in Mental Health Nursing*, 26(4): 23–46. Acute confusion, or delirium, is a second significant challenge encountered in *geropsychiatric* patients with physical illness comorbidity. Polypharmacy issues represent a third major challenge – inappropriate use or overuse of pharmacological treatments. Institutionalized overmedication is common; too often, a medication is administered prematurely to reduce agitation and unwanted physical behaviours, although treatment *a priori* of depressive symptoms, as well as more active engagement on a daily basis with the built environment of the care setting, has been proven effective.

37 Gerety, Rowan Moore (2013) 'Medicine men', *Slate*, 29 November. Online. Available at www.slate.com/articles/news_and_politics/roads/2013/11/nigeria/psychiatric_care_mentally_ill_nigerians_rely_on_spiritual _healers.html (accessed 12 November 2016). Gerety writes,

> Increase Adeosun, a psychiatrist who manages intake at Nigeria's largest psychiatric hospital, says patients usually only turn up there when their symptoms have reached a 'melting point' when every other option has failed. Most have already put in long stints at churches and mosques – where they are often subjected to fasting and periods of isolation – or in centers run by traditional healers. Flogging and shackling patients is sometimes practiced at all three . . . as a result, psychiatrists typically find themselves treating the 'treatment' as well as the illness, with many patients suffering from symptoms that have been exacerbated by the work of other 'healers' . . . the trick is to convince spiritual healers to modify their treatments and refer cases to professional clinicians.

38 Veerbeek, Marjolein A., Richard C. Oude Voshaar and Anne Margriet Pot (2014) 'Effectiveness and predictors of outcome in routine outpatient mental health care for older adults', *International Psychogeriatrics*, 26(9): 1565–1574.

39 McCaffrey, Ruth (2007) 'The effect of healing gardens and art therapy on older adults with mild to moderate depression', *Holistic Nursing Practice*, 21(2): 79–84. The intent was to determine the effects of two types of garden walks to an art therapy comparison intervention. Three groups were studied. Group 1 walked in a garden alone; Group 2 walked this same garden with a guided imagery leader; and Group 3 participated in an art therapy session. Data were gathered in focus group interviews, a survey instrument known as the Geriatric Depression Scale, and personal stories of sadness and joy preintervention and postintervention. The project was conducted in Florida at a privately administrated botanical park and garden. Sixty participants were recruited and then randomly assigned to one of the three groups. Three 6-week sessions were held with each group and focus group sessions were held afterward where participants were asked numerous preset questions about their experience. Participants in all three groups felt as though the nature interventions they experienced were helpful in relieving their depression and in improving their mood and overall outlook on life.

40 US Census Bureau (2008) *2008 National Population Projections*. Online. Available at www.census.gov/population/www/projections/aummary-tables.html (accessed 12 December 2014). Psychologists, psychiatrists, social workers, art therapists, nurses, physicians, and other frontline care providers have acknowledged the need for more highly trained specialists both capable and passionate about working with the aged. The current number of specialists cannot meet the challenges associated with the demographic shift now underway. The proportion of the US population 65 and older will have increased from 13% in 2010 to 16% by 2020. Before 2023, the proportion of the US population over age 65 will surpass the proportion under 15 years of age.

41 Vogeli, Christine, Alexandria E. Shields, Todd A. Lee, Teresa B. Gibson, William D. Marder, Kevin B. Weiss and David Blumenthal (2007) 'Multiple chronic conditions: prevalence, health consequences, and implications for quality, care management, and costs', *Journal of General Internal Medicine*, 22(Supplement 3): 391–395.

42 Karel, Michele J., Margaret Gatz and Michael A. Smyer (2012) 'Aging and mental health in the decade ahead', *American Psychologist*, 67(3): 184–198. The term *dementia* itself is now used less and in its place the terms *delirium*, *minor neurocognitive disorder*, and *major neurocognitive disorder* are each defined in the latest edition of the DSM.

43 World Vision (2016) 'Syrian refugee crisis: what you need to know', *World Vision*, 22 December. Online. Available at www.worldvision.org/refugees-news-stories/syria-refugee-crisis-faq-war.html (accessed 13 January 2017).

44 Juneau, Gary and Neal S. Rubin (2014) 'A first person account of the refugee experience: identifying psychosocial stressors and formulating psychological responses', *Psychology International*, December. Online. Available at www.apa.org/international/pi/2014/12/global-violence.aspx (accessed 15 January 2017).

45 United Nations High Commissioner for Refugees (UNHCR) (1951) *Convention Relating to the Status of Refugees*. Geneva: United Nations.

46 UNHCR (2015) 'Worldwide displacement hits all-time high as war and persecution increase', *UNHCR*, Geneva. Online. Available at www.unhcr.org/news/latest/2015/6/558193896/worldwide-displacement-

hits-all-time-high-war-persecution-oncrease.html (accessed 12 December 2016).

47 World Health Organization (2007) 'Mental health assistance to the populations affected by the tsunami in Asia', *WHO*, Geneva: World Health Organization. Online. Available at www.who.int/mental.health/resources/tsunami/en/ (accessed 12 November 2016).

48 Inter-Agency Standing Committee (2007) *IASC Guidelines on Mental Health and Psychosocial Support in Emergency Settings*. Geneva: IASC.

49 Murray, Kate E., Graham R. Davidson and Robert D. Schweitzer (2010) 'Review of refugee mental health interventions following resettlement: best practices and recommendation', *American Journal of Orthopsychiatry*, 80(4): 576–585.

50 Fasel, Mina, Jeremy Wheeler and John Danesh (2005) 'Prevalence of serious mental disorder in 7000 refugees resettled in Western countries: a systematic review', *The Lancet*, 365(9467): 1309–1314. Also see Porter, Matthew and Nick Haslam (2005) 'Predisplacement and post-displacement factors associated with mental health of refugees and internally displaced persons: a meta-analysis', *Journal of the American Medical Association*, 294(6): 602–612.

51 Dura-Vila, Gloria, Henrika Klasen, Zethu Makatini, Zohreh Rahimi and Matthew Hodes (2012) 'Mental health problems of young refugees: duration of settlement, risk factors and community-based interventions', *Clinical Child Psychology*, 18(4): 604–623.

52 Bronstein, Israel and Paul Montgomery (2011) 'Psychological distress in refugee children: a systematic review', *Clinical Child and Family Psychological Review*, 14(2): 44–56.

53 UNHCR (2010) 'The Health Information System (HIS) toolkit for use in emergency settings, January 2010. 63. Emergency mental illness report', *United Nations High Commissioner for Refugees*. Geneva: UNHCR. Online. Available at www.unhcr.org/4b7d11dc9.html (accessed 10 June 2013). More recently, however, these figures have been somewhat disputed by external humanitarian aid agencies.

54 World Health Organization (WHO) (2008) 'Integrating Mental Health in Primary Care: A Global Perspective', Geneva: World Health Organization.

55 Rose, Nick, Peter Hughes, Sherese Ali and Lynne Jones (2011) 'Integrating mental health into primary care settings after an emergency: lessons from Haiti', *Intervention*, 9(3): 211–224. A major dilemma encountered was that humanitarian aid organizations were conflicted over whether the best use of their very limited resources was to buttress the two existing hospitals or to invest resources in the construction of new freestanding clinics in outlying rural areas. In retrospect, it was concluded a wiser strategy in the future is to set up referral clinics in existing and newly built portable emergency and fixed-site primary care clinics, triage sites that can serve as referral hubs to the country's two psychiatric hospitals.

56 Rao, Kiran (2006) 'Psychosocial support in disaster-affected communities', *International Review of Psychiatry*, 18(6): 501–505. Also see Silove, Derrick and Z. Steel (2006) 'Understanding community psychosocial needs after disasters: implications for mental health services', *Journal of Postgraduate Medicine*, 52(4): 121–125.

57 Larrance, Ryan, Michael Anastario and Lynn Lawry (2007) 'Health status among internally displaced persons in Louisiana and Mississippi travel trailer parks', *Annals of Emergency Medicine*, 49(5): 590–601.

58 Weisler, Richard H., James G. Barbee and Mark H. Townsend (2006) 'Mental health and recovery in the Gulf Coast after Hurricanes Katrina and Rita', *Journal of the American Medical Association*, 296(5): 585–588. A year later, only 140 of 617 primary care physicians had returned to New Orleans, and only 22 of 196 psychiatrists! Orleans Parish was by then federally designated as a Health Professional Shortage Area.

59 Madrid, Paula A. and Roy Grant (2008) 'Meeting mental health needs following a natural disaster: lessons from Hurricane Katrina', *Professional Psychology: Research and Practice*, 39(1): 86–92.

60 Madrid, Paula A., Heidi Sinclair, Antoinnette Q. Bankston, Sarah Overholt, Arturo Brito, Rita Domnitz and Roy Grant (2008) 'Building integrated mental health and medical programs for vulnerable populations post-disaster: connecting children and families to a medical home', *Prehospital and Disaster Medicine*, 23(4): 314–321.

61 Fritze, Jessica G., Grant A. Blashki, Susie Burke and John Wiseman (2008) 'Hope, despair and transformation: climate change and the promotion of mental health and wellbeing', *International Journal of Mental Health Systems*, 2(13), doi:10 1186/1752-4458-2-13. Online. Available at www.ijmhs.com/content/2/1/13.html (accessed 5 January 2017).

62 Brown, O. (2008) *Migration and Climate Change*. Geneva: International Organization for Migration.

63 Shane III, Leo and Patricia Kime (2016) 'New VA study finds 20 veterans commit suicide each day', *Military Times*, 7 July. Online. Available at www.militarytimes.com/story/veterans/2016/07/07/va-suicide-20-daily-research/8.html (accessed 9 January 2017).

64 Verderber, Stephen (2009) *Delirious New Orleans: Manifesto for an Extraordinary American City*. Austin, TX: University of Texas Press: 167–232.

65 Victorian Health Promotion Foundation (2005) *A Plan for Action 2005–2007: Promoting Mental Health and Wellbeing*. Melbourne: Victorian Health Promotion Foundation.

Chapter 4

1 Yenni, Carla (2007) *The Architecture of Madness: Insane Asylums in the United States*. Minneapolis, MN and London: University of Minnesota Press.

2 Ibid.: 17–18.

3 Stevenson, Christine (2000) *Medicine and Magnificence: British Hospital and Asylum Architecture, 1660–1815*. New Haven, CT: Yale University Press: 34.
4 Yenni (2007): 19.
5 Pugin, Augustus and Thomas Rowlandson (1811) *Microcosm of London*. London: Ackerman.
6 Stevenson (2000): 29–38.
7 Yenni (2007): 21–24.
8 Ibid.: 26.
9 Tuke, Samuel (1813) *Description of the Retreat, an Institution Near York for Insane Persons of Society and Friends*. York: W. Alexander.
10 Yenni (2007): 29.
11 Malin, William G. (1832) *Some Account of the Pennsylvania Hospital, Its Origin, Objects, and Present State*. Philadelphia, PA: Thomas Kite: 14, 17.
12 Waln, Robert (1825) *An Account of the Asylum for the Insane: Established by the Society of Friends Near Frankford in the Vicinity of Philadelphia*. Philadelphia, PA: Benjamin and Thomas Kite. This asylum featured natural ventilation, a more intimate overall scale, and prison-like single rooms. A later institution, the Friends Asylum, built in Frankford (near Philadelphia), was an all-private-room facility built by Quakers and was the first American institution to emphasize moral treatment of the insane. It was linear in plan, symmetrical, with male and female side wings and single-loaded corridors (vs. the double-loaded corridors of the York Retreat).
13 McCandless, Peter (1996) *Moonlight, Magnolia, and Madness: Insanity in South Carolina From the Colonial Period to the Progressive Era*. Chapel Hill, NC: University of North Carolina Press: 56.
14 Yenni (2007): 28.
15 Ibid.: 38.
16 Tomes, Nancy (1994) *The Art of Asylum-Keeping: Thomas Story Kirkbride and the Origins of American Psychiatry*. Philadelphia, PA: University of Pennsylvania Press.
17 Yenni (2007): 41. The Royal Naval Hospital at Plymouth, England (1756–1765), attributed to William Robinson, featured 15 interconnected yet identical (in plan) pavilion structures arranged around a quadrangle. A similar pavilion approach had been adopted by many entrants to the replacement Hotel Dieu design competition held in Paris in the 1780s.
18 Yanni (2007): 42.
19 Yanni (2007): 42. Clarke was one of the commissioners for this new state asylum and it was considered massive for its time. The main structure initially housed 276 beds in its first year of operation, in 1843; its neoclassicism was grand, with a symmetrical Greek Doric main façade portico and flanking three-level wings of identically proportioned windows. In a pattern soon to become common in 19th-century asylum construction, the columniated element housed the superintendent's office and associated administrative functions. On the inner courtyard side, porches overlooked lawns. Patient rooms lined double-loaded corridors in the main structure and in the two connecting wings. A chapel was located on the fourth floor at the center of the main building. Some patients were provided private rooms.
20 Yenni (2007): 43.
21 Bucknill, John Charles (1876) *Notes on Asylums for the Insane in America*. London: J. & A. Churchill: 38.
22 Howard, John G. (1845) 'Letter describing the new Provincial Asylum in Toronto', Toronto: Baldwin Room Archives, Toronto Public Library.
23 Hauch, Valerie (2016) 'How High Park became Toronto's 'Country Sanctuary', *Toronto Star*, 7 April: 44. Online. Available at www.thestar.com.html (accessed 10 April 2016). Howard claimed he had been born illegitimate and was directly descended from the fourth duke of Norfolk, Thomas Howard. However, the Dictionary of Canadian Biography website cites birth records indicating he was the fourth of seven children born to a John and Sarah Corby in England. Howard and his wife did not have children, but apparently he fathered three children with his longstanding mistress, a Mrs. Mary Williams. By 1836, the Howards purchased a 120-acre parcel of wooded land stretching from the shores of Lake Ontario north to Bloor Street West. In 1873 he donated this large parcel to the City of Toronto 'for free use, benefit and enjoyment' of all citizens thereafter. This parcel, since expanded significantly in size, is now known as High Park.
24 Connolly, John (1847) *The Construction & Government of Lunatic Asylums: First Publication*. London: Dawson's of Pall Mall, Reprint, 1968. Nature was to be incorporated as a daily part of every patient's treatment regimen. Patients classified as 'Curable' or 'Recovering' were accorded more time with the attending staff, and provided work activity indoors, as well as outdoors on the grounds.
25 Hudson, Edna (2000) 'Asylum layouts', in Edna Howard (ed.) *The Provincial Asylum in Toronto: Reflections on Social and Architectural History*. Toronto: Toronto Region Architectural Conservancy: 203.
26 Ibid.: 205–209.
27 Hamilton, S.W. and G.A. Kempf (1937) 'A survey of the Ontario Hospitals', New York: Report of the Mental Health Survey Committee, February. Archives for the History of Canadian Psychiatry and Mental Health Services (AHCPMHS), Centre for Addiction and Mental Health, Toronto. This report concluded it was time for the provincial government to rethink its position on the asylum in Toronto. Options included relocating to a new site outside the city or reconstruction in place.
28 AHCPMHS (1950) *Report of the Ontario Health Survey Committee*, Vols. 1–3. Toronto: Ontario Ministry of Health.
29 AHCPMHS (1956); Sneddon, F.W. (1956) *Inspector, Ontario Hospitals, Report of Visit to Ontario Hospital, Toronto, September 7*. As a succession of reports were completed, no mention was made on developing planning or architectural guidelines to renovate or repurpose any existing facility on the Queen Street West campus in Toronto.

30 Court, John (2000) 'From 999 to 1001 Queen Street: A consistently vital resource', in Edna Hudson (ed.) *The Provincial Asylum in Toronto: Reflections on Social and Architectural History*. Toronto: Toronto Region Architectural Conservancy: 185.

31 Ibid.: 187.

32 Ibid.: 189.

33 AHCPMHS. Durost, Henry B. (1972) Interview with Dr. A.L. Swanson in *The Automated Hospital*, 2(1). Toronto: Amsco Canada Ltd. Clinical specialists and administrators believed the need was urgent to destigmatize the mentally ill and this was thought to most likely happen with public relations efforts and by attaining a higher status within the healthcare professions.

34 Jones, Robert F. (1916) 'Hospital for insane, Whitby, Ontario', *Construction*, October: 319–346. The Hospital for the Insane in Whitby, Ontario, opened in summer 1916 and was heralded as state of the art for its cottages and decentralized campus, making full use of its rural location on Lake Ontario, 35 miles east of Toronto. The Whitby psychiatric hospital was antithetical to the aging, 66-year-old asylum in Toronto. A special issue of the Canadian trade magazine *Construction*, in 1916, was devoted its planning, design, and construction.

35 McNeel, B.H. and C.H. Lewis (1960) 'Care of the mentally ill in Ontario: History of treatment, Part I', *Canadian Hospital*, 37(2), February: 102.

36 Henderson, Henry W. (1960) 'Community services', *Canadian Hospital*, 37(2), February: 50.

37 Sussman, Sam (1989) 'Interview with Dr. H.W. Henderson', in Djuwe Joe Blom (ed.) *Pioneers of Mental Health and Social Change, 1930–1989*. London: Ontario Third Eye Publications: 67–70. The decision was made in 1961 by Dr. McNeel in a report stating the old hospital was to be replaced, on the current site, with semiautonomous 'mini-hospitals' and also the construction of the Clarke Institute, on a new site on College Street next to the University of Toronto main campus.

38 AHCPMHS, Henderson Fonds. Urquhart, R.W. Ian (1965) 'A study of the function and operation of the mental health branch and the Ontario hospitals', Toronto: Report to the Ontario Minister of Health, December: 32–33. Also see Henderson, H.W. (1967) 'The changing responsibility of government in the care and treatment of the mentally ill', Presentation at the Annual Meeting, Canadian Psychiatric Association, June.

39 Kahan, F.H. (1965) *Brains and Bricks: The History of the Yorkton Psychiatric Center*. Regina: White Cross Publications.

40 AHCPMHS (1972) *The Automated Hospital*. Toronto: Queen Street Collection.

41 Anon (1975) 'Queen Street Mental Health Centre, Toronto', *Canadian Architect*, 48(9): 32–33.

42 Hudson (2000): 214.

43 Morgan, Gareth (1986) *Images of Organization*. Beverly Hills, CA: Sage Publications.

44 Kelner, Merrijoy J. (1975) 'Spaces and people', *Canadian Architect*, 48(9): 34–40. The team's research methods consisted of focused interviews and behavioural observation. At the outset of a professional journal article describing this study, the research team described the 1850 building as looking like a fortress or prison with its thick walls and small, barred windows. They referred to one of the patient wards, accessible only by thick steel doors with large key locks, as old 'Ward X', and that its corridor, with a floor composed of narrow wooden planks unadorned by rugs or carpets, functioned as an echo chamber. It was remarked how patients socially congregated in the corridors and how at one time this circulation space had served as an overflow dormitory. Old Ward X was characterized as dreary (but clean) and providing no privacy provisions whatsoever for the patient (i.e., no private rooms or private restrooms). The first of the four treatment units was completed in July 1972. This new 'Unit X' was described, by contrast, as a colorful, far more cheerful environment featuring bright, primary shades of blue, red, yellow, and white. The researchers described the bedrooms as small and private with solid wooden doors and modern furnishings. Shatterproof glass windows overlooked the landscaped grounds, and dayrooms featured comfortable colorful sofas and chairs and framed artwork.

45 Ibid.: 36.

46 Ibid.: 36.

47 Ibid.: 37.

48 Ibid.: 39.

49 Ibid.: 40.

50 Hudson (2000): 214. By the late 1980s it was widely held that the province should divest itself from day-to-day operation of its network of psychiatric hospitals. By the mid-1990s this would occur to a large extent, with the support of the province's Services Restructuring Commission (HSRC). It was a clear vote of confidence to 'recast' the former hospital, together with the Clarke Institute, into the new Centre for Addiction and Mental Health (CAMH). The Toronto District Health Council (DHC) recommended realigning the two institutions' catchment areas with Whitby, in order to give Queen Street responsibility for the entire Greater Toronto Area (GTA).

51 Metropolitan Toronto District Health Council (1995) *Directions for Change: Toward a Coordinated Hospital System for Metro Toronto – Final Report of the MTDHC Hospital Restructuring Committee*. September: 142–145. Also see Centre for Addiction and Mental Health (1999) *Annual Report to the Community, 1998–99*. Toronto: Centre for Addiction and Mental Health. Also Anon (1999) 'News from the Centre', *Journal of Addiction and Mental Health*, 2(6), November/December: 2.

52 Author's office visit and interview at Montgomery/Sisam Architects, Toronto, October 2015.

53 In this same year, Phase 1A received an Award for Mental Health Design from the International Academy of Design & Health, and the green space on the northwest edge of the campus is turned over to the City of Toronto for its redesignation as a public park.

54 Institutional light fixtures are specified, as well as heavy-gauge mesh on windows, 'corrections grade' toilets, double-leaf doors that swing in either direction (outward/inward), and an 'anti-barricade' design so patients are unable to seal themselves in during an adverse event. As for gender-related design issues in the patient rooms, women tend to prefer bathtubs more than do men, and elderly patients require age-appropriate visual and sensory cues.

55 Vendeville, Geoffrey (2015) 'Sudden rent hike puts CAMH College St. facility in jeopardy', *Toronto Star*, 7 July. Online. Available at www.thestar.com./news/gta/2015/07/07/sudden-rent-hike-puts-camh-college-st-facility-in-jeopardy.html (accessed 12 August 2015). In 2012, it was decided that the College Street CAMH facility will be retained for the foreseeable future, and its 80 patients would be relocated to Queen Street, with its research unit and the emergency treatment unit to remain at the College Street location until at least 2020. However, CAMH leases the land beneath its structures on College Street and the landlord periodically threatens to forcibly dislocate CAMH so it can erect a condominium complex of four 40-level towers on the site.

56 Verderber, Stephen, Susan Chester and Vicki Barrington (1984), 'Ceiling design in the hospital rehabilitation environment: the patient's perspective', in Donna Duerk and Donald Campbell (eds.) *The Challenge of Diversity. EDRA 15 Proceedings*, San Luis Obispo. Washington, DC: Environment Design Research Association: 164–172.

57 Tse, Mimi M.Y., Jacobus K.F. Ng, Joanne W.Y. Chung and Thomas K.S. Wong (2002) 'The visual effect of visual stimuli on pain threshold and tolerance', *Journal of Clinical Nursing*, 11(4): 462–469. Also see Ulrich, Roger S. (1991) 'Effects of interior design on wellness: theory and recent scientific research', *Journal of Health Care Interior Design*, 3(1): 97–109.

58 Ulrich, Roger S. (1984) 'View through a window may influence recovery from surgery', *Science*, 224: 420–421.

59 Verderber, Stephen (1986) 'Dimensions of person-window transactions in the hospital environment', *Environment and Behavior*, 18(4): 450–466. Also see Verderber, Stephen and David R. Reuman (1987) 'Windows, views and health status in hospital therapeutic environments', *Journal of Architectural and Planning Research*, 4(1): 121–133, and Editor's Errata (1988), *Journal of Architectural and Planning Research*, 5(1): 89–90.

60 Mays, John Bentley (2007) 'Mind over matter', *Canadian Architect*, 75(9): 31–38. Online. Available at www.canadianarchitect.com/freatures/mind-over-matter.html (accessed 10 October 2015).

61 Ibid.: 32.

62 Ibid.: 33.

63 Ibid.: 35.

64 Hudson (2000): 215–216.

65 Sewell, John (2000) 'Epilogue', in Hudson, ed.: 217.

66 Verderber, Stephen (2010) *Innovations in Hospital Architecture*. London: Routledge: 314–319.

67 Gerdin, Karolina (2015) 'Toronto hires Stefan Lundin for the building of a new psychiatric hospital', Toronto: CAMH Public Communications Release.

Chapter 5

1 Karlin, Bradley E. and Robert A. Zeiss (2006) 'Environmental and therapeutic issues in psychiatric hospital design: toward best practices', *Psychiatric Services*, 57(10): 1376–1378.

2 Connellan, Kathleen, Mads Gaardboe, Damien Riggs, Clemence Due, Amanda Reinschmidt and Lauren Mustillo (2013) 'Stressed spaces: mental health and architecture', *Health Environments Research & Design Journal*, 6(4): 127–168. Also see Papoulias, Constantina, Emese Csipke, Diana Rose, Susie McKellar and Til Wykes (2014) 'The psychiatric ward as a therapeutic space: systematic review', *The British Journal of Psychiatry*, 205(3): 171–176.

3 Drahota, Amy, Derek Wad, Heather Mackenzie, Rebecca Stores, Bernie Higgins, Diane Gal and Taraneh P. Dean (2012) *Sensory Environment on Health-Related Outcomes of Hospital Patients* (Review). New York: John Wiley.

4 Hunt, James M. and David M. Simes (2016) *Design Guide for the Built Environment of Behavioral Health Facilities, Edition 7.0*. Chicago: ASHA/AHA/Facilities Guidelines Institute.

5 Hamilton, D. Kirk (2004) 'Four levels of evidence-based practice', *AIA Newsletter*, Washington, DC: American Institute of Architects. Online. Available at www.arch.ttu.edu/courses/2007/fall/5395/392/students/garay/Research/Research.pdf (accessed 6 March 2017).

6 Tachieva, Galina (2010) *Sprawl Repair Manual*. New York: Island Press.

7 From, Lena and Stefan Lundin, eds. (2010) *Architecture as Medicine: The Importance of Architecture for Treatment Outcomes in Psychiatry*. Göteburg, Sweden: ARQ – The Architecture Research Foundation: 262–263.

8 Eris, Evin and Burcin Basyazici Kulac (2014) 'The architect's exam with other spaces: a study on mental asylums', *International Journal of Arts & Science*, 7(1): 83–92.

9 Novotna, Gabriela, Karen A. Urbanoski and Brian R. Rush (2011) 'Client-centered design of residential addiction and mental health care facilities: staff perceptions of their work environment', *Qualitative Health Research*, 21(11): 1527–1538.

10 Chrysikou, Evangelia (2014) *Architecture for Psychiatric Environments and Therapeutic Spaces*. Amsterdam: IOS Press BV: 34–40.

11 Ibid.: 33–70.

12 The Nozoe Psychiatric Hospital, in Kurume, Japan, is an otherwise beautiful facility situated on a gently sloping site. From the exterior, it appears to be a hotel or resort. The majority of inpatients at this psychiatric hospital use communal bath/shower spaces.

13 Shepley, Mardelle M. and Samira Pasha (2013) *Design Research and Behavioural Facilities*. Hawthorne, CA: The Center for Health Design. Online. Available at https://blogs.cornell.edu/healthyfutures/files/2016/01/shepley-pasha-behavior-265fa8a.pdf (accessed 12 August 2015). Also see Shepley, Mardelle M. and Samira Pasha (2017) *Design for Mental and Behavioral Health*. London: Routledge.

14 Antonovsky, Aaron (1979) *Health, Stress and Coping*. San Francisco, CA: Jossey-Bass Publishers.

15 Golembiewski (2010): 100–117.

16 Golembiewski (2012) 'Psychiatric design: using a salutogenic model for the development and management of mental health facilities', *World Health Design*, 5(2): 74–79.

17 Tomes, Nancy (1984) *A Generous Confidence: Thomas Story Kirkbride and the Art of Asylum-Keeping, 1840–1883*. London: Cambridge University Press.

18 Shergill, Sukhwinder S., Gabriele B. Samson, Paul M. Bays, Chris D. Frith and Daniel M. Wolpert (2005) 'Evidence for sensory prediction deficits in schizophrenia', *American Journal of Psychiatry*, 162(1): 2384–2386.

19 Verderber, Stephen (2010) *Innovations in Hospital Architecture*. London: Routledge: 125.

20 Guenther, Robin and Gail Vittori (2013) *Sustainable Healthcare Architecture*. New York: John Wiley.

21 Verderber and Fine (2000): 116–123.

22 Bowden, Kirstie (2012) 'Glimpses through the gates: gentrification and the continuing histories of the Devon County Pauper Lunatic Asylum', *Housing, Theory and Society*, 29(1): 114–139.

23 Verderber (2010): 122.

24 O'Brien, Greg (2014) 'Renovation: construction begins on Buffalo's Richardson Olmstead complex', *Architect*, 10 October. Online. Available at www.architectmagazine.com/design/buildngs/renovation-construction-begins-onrichardson-complex.html (accessed 3 March 2017).

25 Intergovernmental Panel on Climate Change (2014) *Climate Change 2014: Mitigation of Climate Change. IA Models and WGIII: Lessons From IPCC AR5*, College Park, MD, November. Online. Available at www.globalchange.umd.edu/iamc2014/Edenhofer_IAMC_17November.pdf (accessed 2 October 2016).

26 Verderber (2010): 119–120.

27 Musco, Francesco (2016) *Counteracting Urban Heat Island Effects in a Global Climate Change Scenario*. New York: Springer.

28 Watts, Bradley V., Yinong Young-Xu, Peter D. Mills, Joseph M. DeRosier, Jan Kemp, William E. Duncan and Brian Shiner (2012) 'Examination of the effectiveness of the Mental Health Environment of Care Checklist in reducing suicide on inpatient mental health units', *Archives of General Psychiatry*, 69(6): 588–592.

29 Ciancio, Daniela and Christopher Becket, eds. (2015) *Rammed Earth Construction: Cutting-Edge Research on Traditional and Modern Rammed Earth*. Boca Raton, FL: CRC Press. Also see King, Bruce (1996) *Buildings of Earth and Straw: Structural Design for Rammed Earth and Straw-Bale Architecture*. Washington, DC: Island/Ecological Design Press; and Walker, Peter, Rowland Keable, Joseph Marton and Vincent Maniatidis (2010) *Rammed Earth: Design and Construction Guidelines EP62*. Berkshire: IHS BRE Press.

30 Anon (2016) 'Aidlin Darling creates a meditation center at Stanford University with rammed-earth walls', *Dezeen Magazine*, 23 May. Online. Available at www.dezeen.com/2016/05/23/aidlin-darling-design-windhover-spiritual-meditation-centre.html (accessed 3 October 2016).

31 Anon (2015) 'Nkabom House is a prototypical Ghanaian home made from mud and waste plastic', *Dezeen Magazine*, 28 June. Online. Available at www.dezeen.com/2015/06/28/nkabon-house-prototypical-ghana-home-mud-waste.pdf (accessed 3 October 2016).

32 Devin, Ann (1992) 'Psychiatric ward renovation', *Environment and Behavior*, 24(1): 66–84.

33 Bitner, Mary Jo (1992) 'Servicescapes: the impact of physical surroundings on customers and employees', *The Journal of Marketing*, 56(2): 57–71. Also see Fottler, Myron D., Robert C. Ford, Velma Roberts, Eric W. Ford and John D. Spears (2000) 'Creating a healing environment: the importance of the service setting in the new consumer-oriented healthcare system/practitioner application', *Journal of Healthcare Management*, 45(2): 91. Also Passini, Romedi and Paul Arthur (1992) *Wayfinding: People, Signs and Architecture*. New York: McGraw-Hill; and Pangrazio, John R. (2013) 'Planning public spaces for health care facilities', *Health Facilities Management*, 13 January. Online. Available at www.hfmmagazine.com/display/HFM-news-article.dhtml?dcrPath=/templatedata/HF_Common/NewsArticle/data/HFM/magazine (accessed 25 September 2016).

34 Callen, Bonnie L., Jane E. Mahoney, Carey B. Grieves, Thelma J. Wells and Myra Enloe (2004) 'Frequency of hallway ambulation by hospitalized older adults on medical units of an academic hospital', *Geriatric Nursing*, 25(3): 212–217. Also see Carthey, Jane (2008) 'Reinterpreting the hospital corridor: "wasted space" or essential for quality multidisciplinary clinical care?' *Health Environments Research and Design Journal*, 2(4): 17–29.

35 Thompson, John T. and Grace Goldin (1975) *The Hospital: A Social and Architectural History*. New Haven, CT: Yale University Press: 3–4.

36 Jiang, Shan and Stephen Verderber (2016) 'Landscape therapeutics and the design of salutogenic hospitals: recent research', *World Health Design*, 8(1): 40–51.

37 Verderber (2010): 143.

38 Thomson and Goldin (1975): 71. Also see *Microcosm of London*. London: Ackerman, 1808–11; Reprinted 1947.

39 Jiang, Shan and Stephen Verderber (2017) 'On the planning and design of hospital circulation zones: a review of the evidence-based literature', *Health Environments Research & Design Journal*, 10(2): 124–146.

40 Kaplan, Stephen and Marc G. Berman (2010) 'Directed attention as a common resource for executive functioning and self-regulation', *Perspectives on Psychological Science*, 5(1): 43–57.

41 Turner, Kevin (2015) 'Designing for health: challenges and opportunities in psychiatric healthcare design', *Contract Design*, 5 January. Online. Available at www.contractdesign.com/practice/healthcare/designing-for-health-Opportunities-for_Psychiatric-Healthcare-design.html (accessed 7 July 2016).

42 Verderber (2010): 131.

43 Cooper, Randy (2010) *Wayfinding for Healthcare*. Chicago: American Hospital Association Press.

44 Grossman, Ron (2012) 'Debate over Chicago's Prentice Hospital heats up', *Chicago Tribune*, 4 September. Online. Available at www.articles.chicagotribune.com/2012/-09-04/news/ct-met-prentice-20120904_1_landmark.html (accessed 17 October 2016).

45 Verderber, Stephen (1986) 'Dimensions of person-window transactions in the hospital environment', *Environment and Behavior*, 18(4): 450–466.

46 Gemma, Angel (2012) 'A room with a view: asylum art in the 19th century', *University College London*, 6 August. Online. Available at www.blogs.ucl.ac.uk/researchers-in-museums/2012/08/06/a-room-with-a-view.html (accessed 15 October 2016).

47 Lloyd, Chris, Su Ren Wong and Leon Petchkovsky (2007) 'Art and recovery in mental health: a qualitative investigation', *British Journal of Occupational Therapy*, 70(5): 207–214.

48 Sher, Jonathan (2014) 'Special celebration planned Sunday as final salute to 144 years of care', *The London Free Press*, 26 September. Online. Available at www.lfpress.com/2014/09/26/special-celebration-planned sunday-as-final-salute.html (accessed 15 October 2016).

49 Decker, William A. (2007) *Asylum for the Insane: A History of the Kalamazoo State Hospital*. Traverse City, MI: Arbutus Press.

50 Frketich, Joanna (2014) 'New Hamilton hospital campus designed to destigmatize mental illness', *The Hamilton Spectator*, 15 January. Online. Available at www.thespec.com/news-story/4315512-new-hamilton-hospital-campus-designed-to destigmatize-mental-illness.html (accessed 14 October 2016).

51 Turner (2015): 42.

52 Holmberg, Sharon K. and Sharon Coon (1999) 'Ambient sound levels in a state psychiatric hospital', *Archives of Psychiatric Nursing*, 13(3): 117–126.

53 Choiniere, Denise B. (2010) 'The effects of hospital noise', *Nursing Administration Quarterly*, 34(4): 327–333. Also Mazer, Susan E. (2010) 'Music, noise, and the environment of care: history, theory, and practice', *International Journal of Music and Medicine*, 2(3): 182–191.

54 Mazer, Susan E. (2012) 'Creating a culture of safety: reducing hospital noise', *Biomedical Instrumentation & Technology*, September/October: 350–355.

55 Smetzer, James (2002) 'Prescriptions for safety', *American Hospital Association News*, 3 June: 12–16.

56 Mazer, Susan E. (2006) 'Increase patient safety by creating a quitter hospital environment', *Biomedical Instrumentation & Technology*, 40(2): 145–146.

57 Mazer (2012): 353.

58 Nightingale, Florence (1860) *Notes on Nursing: What It Is and What It Is Not*, 1st American ed. New York: D. Appleton & Company: 12–14.

59 Dawson, David L. (2016) 'Feeling threatened at root of hospital attacks, Doctor says design and colors of psychiatric hospital fail to soothe the disturbed', *The Hamilton Spectator*, 16 August. Online. Available at www.pressreader.com (accessed 18 October 2016).

60 Abrahams, Marc (2008) 'Blue is the colour if you have mental illness', *The Guardian*, 24 June. Online. Available at www.tehguardian.com/education/2008/jun/24/highereducation.improbable.html (accessed 18 October 2016).

61 Ajayi, Oo, Kayode Ayinde and Amo Atolagbe (2005) 'An appraisal of the colour of hospital wards on the recovery attitudes of psychiatric patients', *Global Journal of Environmental Sciences*, 4(2): 165–170. Online. Available at www.ajol.info/index.php/gjes/article/view/2441.php (accessed 18 October 2016).

62 Heyden, Tom (2014) 'How patients might design a psychiatric hospital', *BBC News*, 13 May. Online. Available at www.bbc.com/news/blogs-ouch-27206405.html (accessed 17 October 2016).

63 Meyer-Levy, Joan and Rui Zhu (2007) 'The influence of ceiling height: the effect of priming on the type of processing that people use', *Journal of Consumer Research*, 34(8): 125–142.

64 Kaplan and Berman (2010).

65 Thompson and Goldin (1975): 37–40.

66 Bowers, Len, Theresa Allan, Alan Simpson, Julia Jones, Marie Van Der Merwe and Debra Jeffrey (2009) 'Identifying key factors associated with aggression on acute inpatient psychiatric wards', *Issues in Mental Health Nursing*, 30(4): 260–271.

67 Meltzer, Bernard N., John W. Petras and Lawrence T. Reynolds (1975) *Symbolic Interactionism: Genesis, Varieties, and Criticism*. Boston, MA: Routledge and Kegan Paul. Also Herman-Kinney, Nancy J. and Lawrence T. Reynolds (2003) *Handbook of Symbolic Interactionism*. New York: AltaMira.

68 Blumer, Herbert (1969) *Symbolic Interactionism: Perspective and Method*. Englewood Cliffs, NJ: Prentice-Hall. Symbolic interactionism can help to put into perspective why a fortified nurses' station on a postwar modernist psychiatric ward consistently fosters aggressive, hostile outbursts from patients, or why dilapidated and outdated furnishings may become prime targets for vandalism – countertherapeutic messaging is transactionally projected by the physical setting as much as interpersonally between patients.

69 Wood, Victoria J., Sarah E. Curtis, Will Gesler, Ian H. Spencer, Helen J. Close, James Mason and Joe G. Reilly (2013) 'Creating "therapeutic landscapes" for mental health carers in inpatient settings: a dynamic perspective on permeability and inclusivity', *Social Science and Medicine*, 91(10): 122–129.

70 Hunt, Isabelle M., Harriett Bickley, Kirsten Windfuhr, Jenny Shaw, Louis Appelby and Nav Kapur (2013) 'Suicide in recently admitted psychiatric in-patients: a case-control study', *Journal of Affective Disorders*, 144(1–2): 123–128.

71 Andoh, Benjamin (1990) 'The consequences of absconding from mental hospitals', *Mountbatten Journal of Legal Studies*, 44(3): 70–89.

72 CBC News (2012) 'Escape of CAMH patient with violent past probed', *CBC News*, 7 March. Online. Available at www.cbc.ca/news/canada/toronto/escape-of-camh-patient-with-violent-past-probed.html (accessed 2 October 2016).

73 Bentham, Jeremy (1798) 'A proposal for a new and less expensive mode of employing and reforming convicts', in Robin Evans (ed., 1982) *The Fabrication of Virtue: English Prison Architecture: 1750–1840*. Cambridge: Cambridge University Press: 193–235. Also Semple, Janet (1993) *Bentham's Prison: A Study of the Panopticon Penitentiary*. Oxford: Chardon Press.

74 Bowers, Len, Duncan Stewart, Chris Papadopoulos, Charlotte Dack, Jamie Ross, Husnara Khanom and Debra Jeffrey (2011) *Inpatient Violence and Aggression: A Literature Review*. Report from the Conflict and Containment Reduction Research Programme. London: Institute of Psychiatry: Kings College.

75 Mural, Jeffrey R. (2015) 'What's the best nurses' station design for psychiatric hospitals?' *Healthcare Design*, 1 July. Online. Available at www.healthcaredesignmagazine.com/article/what-s-a-best-nurses-station-design-psychiatric-hospitals.html (accessed 7 July 2016).

76 Liu, Wei, Elizabeth Manias and Marie Gerdtz (2014) 'The effects of physical environments in medical wards on medication communication processes affecting patient safety', *Health & Place*, 26(4): 188–198.

77 Doas, Michelle (2016) 'Psychiatric nursing medication administration: is it just a med pass?' *Annals of Psychiatry and Mental Health*, 4(1): 1058–1059.

78 Yeager, Kenneth R., Radu Saveanu, Albert R. Roberts, Gabby Reissland, Dan Mertz, Aavni Cirpili and Ron Makovich (2005) 'Measured response to identified suicide risk and violence: what you need to know about psychiatric patient safety', *Brief Treatment and Crisis Intervention*, 5(2): 121–141.

79 Kho, K., T. Sensky, A. Mortimer and C. Corcos (1998) 'Prospective study into factors associated with aggressive incidents in psychiatric acute admission wards', *British Journal of Psychiatry*, 172(2): 38–43.

80 Moran, Marc (2015) 'Simulation may improve trainee skills with agitated or violent patients', *Psychiatric News*, 31 March. Online. Available at www.psychnews.psychiatryonline.org/doi/full/10.1176/appi.pn.2015.4a8?trendmd-share.html (accessed 15 November 2016).

81 Li, Jie, Mao-Sheng Ran, Yuantao Hao, Zhenhuan Zhao, Yangbo Guo, Jinghua Su and Huixian Lu (2008) 'Inpatient suicide in a Chinese psychiatric hospital', *Suicide and Life Threatening Behavior*, 38(4): 449–455.

82 Janner, Marion and Kathleen R. Delaney (2012) 'Safety issues on British mental health wards', *Journal of the American Psychiatric Nurses Association*, 18(2): 104–111.

83 Chen, Wen-Ching, Chuan-Ju Huang, Jing-Shuang Hwang and Chaio-Chicy Chen (2010) 'The relationship of health-related quality of life to workplace physical violence against nurses by psychiatric patients', *Quality of Life Research Journal*, 191: 1155–1161.

84 Nijman, H., Len Bowers, Kristina Haglund, Elmear Muir-Cochrane, Alan Simpson and M. Ven Der Merwe (2011) 'Door locking and exit security measures on acute psychiatric admission wards', *Journal of Psychiatric and Mental Health Nursing*, 18: 614–621.

85 Trigiani, Tina (2016) 'Nurse beaten by patient over weekend: union accuses CAMH of failing to protect staff', *inews880.com*, 25 October. Online. Available at www.inews880.com/syn/60/177837/camh-nurse-beaten-by-patient-over-weekend.html (accessed 14 November 2016).

86 Anderson, Ashleigh and Sara G. West (2011) 'Violence against mental health professionals: when the treater becomes the victim', *Innovations in Clinical Neuroscience*, 8(3): 34–39. Online. Available at www.ncbi.nlm.nih.gov/pmc/articles/PMC3074201/ (accessed 14 November 2016).

87 Stewart, Duncan, Jamie Ross, Charlotte Watson, Karen James and Len Bowers (2012) 'Patient characteristics and behaviors associated with self-harm and attempted suicide acute psychiatric wards', *Journal of Clinical Nursing*, 21(7–8): 1004–1013.

88 Belanger, Suzanne (2001) 'The S&R challenge: reducing the use of seclusion and restraint in a state psychiatric hospital', *Journal for Healthcare Quality*, 23(1): 19–24. Also Bongar, Bruce M. (1991) *The Suicidal Patient: Clinical and Legal Standards of Care*. Washington, DC: American Psychiatric Association.

89 Vaaler, Arne E., Gunnar Morken and Olav M. Linaker (2005) 'Effects of different interior decorations in the seclusion area of a psychiatric acute ward', *Nordic Journal of Psychiatry*, 59(1): 19–24.

90 Van der Schaaf, R., E. Dusseldorp, W.A. Keuning, W.E. Janssen and E.O. Noorthoorn (2013) 'Impact of the physical environment of psychiatric wards on the use of seclusion', *British Journal of Psychiatry*, 202(10): 142–149.

91 Rogers, Patricia DeProspero and Nancy L. Bocchino (1999) 'Restraint-free care: is it possible?' *American Journal of Nursing*, 99(10): 26–34. Also Perkins, Elizabeth, Helen Prosser, David Riley and Richard Whittington (2012) 'Physical restraint in a therapeutic setting: a necessary evil?' *International Journal of Law and Psychiatry*, 35(1): 43–49.

92 Rakhmatullina, Maryam, Abraham Taub and Theresa Jacob (2013) 'Morbidity and mortality associated with the utilization of restraints', *Psychiatric Quarterly*, 44(7): 1–14. Also Soininen, Paivi, Maritta Valimaki, Toshie Noda, Pauli Puukka, Jyrki Korkeila, Grigori Joffe and

Hanna Putkonen (2013) 'Secluded and restrained patients' perceptions of their treatment', *International Journal of Mental Health Nursing*, 22(1): 47–55.

93 Steinert, Tilman, Peter Lepping, Renate Bernhardsgrütter, Andreas Conca, Trond Hatling, Wim Janssen, Alice Keski-Valkama, Fermin Mayoral and Richard Whittington (2010) 'Incidence of seclusion and restraint in psychiatric hospitals: a literature review and survey of international trends', *Social Psychiatry and Psychiatric Epidemiology*, 45(9): 889–897.

94 Delaney, Kathleen R. and Mary E. Johnson (2012) 'Safety and inpatient psychiatric treatment: moving the science forward', *Journal of the American Psychiatric Nurses Association*, 18(2): 79–80.

95 Needham, Ian, Christopher Abderhalden, Ruud Halfens, Joachim E. Fischer and Theo Dassen (2005) 'Non-somatic effects of patient aggression on nurses: a systematic review', *Journal of Advanced Nursing*, 49(3): 283–296.

96 American Psychiatric Nurses Association (2014) *APNA Position on the Use of Seclusion and Restraint*. Falls Church, VA: American Psychiatric Nurses Association. Online. Available at www.apna.org/i4a/pages/index.cfm?pageid=3728.html (accessed 25 November 2016).

97 Sivak, Kim (2012) 'Implementation of comfort rooms to reduce seclusion, restraint use, and acting out behaviors', *Journal of Psychosocial Nursing and Mental Health Services*, 50(2): 24–34.

98 Appleton, Jay (1975) *The Experience of Landscape*. London and New York: John Wiley.

99 Tuvesson, Hanna, Mona Eklund and Christine Wann-Hansson (2011) 'Perceived stress among nursing staff in psychiatric inpatient care: the influence of perceived atmosphere and the psychosocial work environment', *Issues in Mental Health Nursing*, 32(7): 441–448.

100 Pati, Debajyoti, Tom E. Harvey and Paul Barach (2009) 'Relationships between exterior views and nurse stress: an exploratory examination', *Health Environments Research & Design Journal*, 1(2): 27–38. Also Lottrup, Lene, Patrik Grahn and Ulrika K. Stigsdotter (2013) 'Workplace greenery and perceived level of stress: benefits of access to a green outdoor environment at the workplace', *Landscape and Urban Planning*, 110(2): 5–11.

101 Nejati, Adeleh, Susan Rodiak and Mardelle M. Shepley (2016) 'The implications of high-quality staff break areas for nurses' health, performance, job satisfaction and retention', *Journal of Nursing Management*, 24(2): 512–523.

102 Jiang, Shan and Stephen Verderber (2017) 'On the planning and design of hospital circulation zones: a review of the evidence-based literature', *Health Environments Research & Design Journal*, 8(1): 12–23.

103 Tomes (1984): 48–56.

104 Holahan, Charles J. (1988) *Environmental Psychology*. New York: Random House.

105 Combs, Megan (2014) 'Designing psychiatric units for the geriatric population', *Healthcare Design*, 18 November. Online. Available at www.healthcaredesignmagazine.com/article/designing-psychiatric-units-geriatric-population.html (accessed 28 November 2016).

106 Craig, Jamie-Stewart, Julie Patel, Claire Lee-Jones and Chris Hatton (2000) 'Psychiatric assessment wards for older adults: a qualitative evaluation of two ward models', *International Journal of Geriatric Psychiatry*, 15(8): 721–728.

107 Verderber, Stephen, Shan Jiang, Yanwen Xiao and George Hughes (2014) 'On the evolving role of evidence-based research in healthcare facility design competitions', *Frontiers of Architectural Research*, 3(3): 238–249.

108 Hedaya, Robert J. (2011) 'Light therapy and your mental health', *Psychology Today*, 27 October. Online. Available at www.psychologytoday.com/blog/health-matters/2011/light-therapy-and-mental-health.html (accessed 14 November 2016).

109 Beauchemin, Kathleen M. and Peter Hays (1996) 'Sunny hospital rooms expedite recovery from severe and refractory depressions', *Journal of Effective Disorders*, 40(1-2): 49–51.

110 Facilities Guidelines Institute (2010) *Guidelines for Design and Construction of Healthcare Facilities*. Dallas: TX: Facility Guidelines Institute.

111 Anon (1991) 'Hazard', *Health Devices*, 20(12): 495–496. Online. Available at www.mdsr.ecri.org/summary/detail.aspx?doc_id=8156 (accessed 6 March 2017).

112 *Guidelines for Design and Construction of Healthcare Facilities* (2010): 42.

113 Anon (2015) 'A grand LED marquee: GKD's mediamesh offers a versatile solution for creative and commercial applications', *Architizer*, 15 May. Online. Available at http://architizer.com/blog/gkd-mediamesh-led-marquee/ (accessed 9 March 2017).

114 Verderber, Stephen and Lindsay G. Todd (2012) 'Reconsidering the semi-private inpatient room in U.S. hospitals', *Health Environments Research & Design Journal*, 5(2): 7–23.

115 Perkins, Nathan H. (2013) 'Including patients, staff and visitors in the design of the psychiatric milieu: notes from the field', *Facilities*, 31(9/10): 379–390.

116 Holland Bloorview Rehabilitation Hospital (2017) 'Family accommodation', *Holland Bloorview Rehabilitation Hospital* (Toronto). Online. Available at www.hollandbloorview.ca/clientfamilyresources/visiting-hollandbloorview/familyaccommodation (accessed 9 March 2017).

117 Jenkins, Jimmy (2017) 'After all but disappearing, psychiatric hospitals are coming back', *Marketplace*, 3 March. Online. Available at www.marketplace.org/2017/03/06/health-care/after-all-disappearing-psychiatric-hospitals-are-coming-back.html (accessed 6 March 2017).

118 Serna, Joseph (2016) 'Hospital agrees to pay $450,000 to L.A. to settle homeless patient dumping lawsuit', *The Los Angeles Times*, 25 October. Online. Available at www.latimes.com/local/lanow/la-me-in-homeless-patient-dumping-20161025-snap-story.html (accessed 8 December 2016).

119 Hernandez, Manuel (2014) 'The new psych ED', *Emergency Physicians Journal*, 28(2): 54–58. Online. Available at www.cannondesign.

com/assets/EPI-New-Psych-ED_Spring-2014.pdf (accessed 6 March 2017).

120 Covington, Holly (2001) 'Therapeutic music for patients with psychiatric disorders', *Holistic Nursing Practice*, 15(2): 59–69.

121 Schullian, Dorothy M. and Max Schoen (1948) *Medicine and Music*. North Stratford, NH: Ayer Company Publishers.

122 Nilsson, Ulrica (2008) 'The anxiety and pain-reducing effects of music interventions: a systematic review', *Journal of the Association of Operating Room Nurses*, 87(4): 780–807. Also Nilsson, Ulrica (2009) 'The effect of music intervention in stress response to cardiac surgery in a randomized clinical trial', *Heart Lung*, 38(3): 201–207.

123 Verderber (2010): 132.

124 University of Nottingham (2013) 'Art in the asylum: creativity and the evolution of psychiatry', *Djanogly Gallery at University Park*. Online. Available at www.nottingham.ac.uk/home/events/art-in-the-asylum-creativity-and-the-evolution-of-psychiatry.html (accessed 15 October 2016). Art therapy in mental health treatment is widespread and is defined as art making by individuals who experience mental illness, trauma, and the challenges of everyday living. Through the act of creating art and reflecting on the outcome, self-awareness is increased, and this enhances cognitive abilities and reduces stress and the severity of anxiety disorders.

125 Hogan, Susan (2001) *Healing Arts: The History of Art Therapy*. London: Jessica Kingsley.

126 Riley, Shirley (2001) 'Art therapy with adolescents', *Western Journal of Medicine*, 175(1): 54–57.

127 Teglbjaerg, Hanne Stubbe (2011) 'Art therapy may reduce psychopathology in schizophrenia by strengthening the patients' sense of self: a qualitative extended case report', *Psychopathology*, 44(2): 314–318.

128 Robertson, Terry and Terry Long (2007) *Foundations of Therapeutic Recreation*. Champaign, IL: Human Kinetics.

129 Rodriguez, Tori (2016) 'Animal-assisted therapy linked to psychological benefits', *Psychiatry Advisor*, 10 February. Online. Available at www.psychiatryadvisor.com/therapies/animals-therapy-psychological-mental-health.html (accessed 4 March 2017).

130 Ray, Dee, Sue Bratton, Tammy Rhine and Leslie Jones (2001) 'The effectiveness of play therapy: responding to the critics', *International Journal of Play Therapy*, 10(1): 85–108. Also LeBlanc, Michael and Martin Ritchie (1999) 'Predictors of play therapy outcomes', *International Journal of Play Therapy*, 8(2): 19–34. Also see Timberlake, Elizabeth M. and Marika M. Cutler (2000) *Developmental Play Therapy in Clinical Social Work*. North York, Ontario: Pearson.

131 This condition is relatively the same as at advent of psychotherapy in the late 19th century. In the 70 years when the International Style was predominant, these rooms in psychiatric hospitals were monochromatic, drab, and seemingly interchangeable in function.

132 Miya, Yoshiko and Kazunori Hanyu (2006) 'The effects of interior design on communication and impressions of a counselor in a counseling rom', *Environment and Behavior*, 38(4): 484–502.

133 Kweon, Byoung-Suk, Roger S. Ulrich, Verrick D. Walker and Louis G. Tassinary (2008) 'Anger and stress: the role of landscape posters in an office setting', *Environment and Behavior*, 40(3): 355–381.

134 Ribas, Jose (2012) 'Making therapy offices therapeutic', *PsychotherapySphere.com*, 16 June. Online. Available at www.psychotherapysphere.com/2012/06/16/making-therapy-offices-therapeutic/ (accessed 15 November 2016).

135 Backhaus, Kelly Lynn (2008) 'Client and therapist perspectives on the importance of the physical environment of the therapy room: A mixed methods study', Doctoral dissertation, Denton: TX: Texas Women's University.

136 Freeman, Daniel and Jason Freeman (2016) 'Virtual reality isn't just for gaming – it could transform mental health treatment', *The Guardian*, 5 May. Online. Available at www.theguardian.com/science/blog/2016/may/05/virtual-reality-isnt-just-forgaming.html (accessed 12 October 2016).

137 Moran, Mark (2008) 'Virtual reality is no game in psychiatric treatment', *Psychiatric News*, 16 May. Online. Available at www.psychnews.psychiatryonline.org/doi/full/10.1176/pn.43.10.0012?trendmd-shared=html (accessed 12 October 2016).

138 Senson, Alexander (2016) 'Virtual reality therapy: treating the global mental health crisis', *Techcrunch.com*, 6 January. Online. Available at www.techcrunch.com/2016/01/06/virtual-reality-therapy-treating-the-global-mental-health-crisis.html (accessed 12 October 2016). This technology reaches many populations otherwise unable to travel to a therapist's office, including the homebound, the aged, and persons in remote geographic locales. The need exists for architectural research on identifying optimal typologies for VRET-based treatment.

139 Verderber, Stephen (2005) *Compassion in Architecture: Evidence-Based Design for Health in Louisiana*. Lafayette: Center for Louisiana Studies: Chapter 6.

140 Yenni (2007): 5. After World War II, the rise of the freestanding outpatient mental health clinic coincided with the emergence in the 1960s of a cornucopia of psychotropic drugs for the treatment of mental illnesses – for the first time affording the opportunity to permanently shutter the old asylums together with their less-successful mid-20th-century architectural counterparts.

141 Huynh, Christophe, Joel Tremblay and Marie Josée-Fleury (2016) 'Typologies of individuals attending an addiction rehabilitation center based on diagnosis of mental disorders', *Journal of Substance Abuse Treatment*, 71(4): 68–78.

142 Shepley, Mardelle M. (1995) 'The location of behavioral incidents in a children's psychiatric facility', *Children's Environments*, 12(3): 352–361.

143 Potthoff, Joy K. (1995) 'Adolescent satisfaction with drug/alcohol treatment facilities: design implications', *Journal of Alcohol and Drug Education*, 41(1): 62–73.

144 Wolfe, Maxine (1975) 'Room size, group size, and density behavior patterns in a children's psychiatric facility', *Environment and Behavior*, 7(2): 199–224. Also Lynch, Martin F., Robert W. Plant and Richard M. Ryan (2005) 'Psychological needs and threats to safety: implications for staff and patients in a psychiatric hospital for youth', *Professional Psychology: Research and Practice*, 36(4): 415–425.

145 Madrid, Paula A. and Roy Grant (2008) 'Meeting mental health needs following a natural disaster: lessons from Hurricane Katrina', *Professional Psychology: Research and Practice*, 39(1): 86–92.

146 Kloos, Bret and Greg Townley (2011) 'Investigating the relationship between neighborhood experiences and psychiatric distress for individuals with serious mental illness', *Administration and Policy in Mental Health and Mental Health Services Research*, 38(2): 105–116.

147 Verderber, Stephen (2016) *Innovations in Transportable Healthcare Architecture*. London: Routledge: 111–166.

148 Jiang and Verderber (2015): 15–17.

149 World Wildlife Fund (2016) *Living Planet Report 2016*. Washington, DC: World Wildlife Fund. Online. Available at www.worldwildlife.org.org/pages/living-planet-report-2016.html (accessed 26 October 2016).

150 Erbino, Chantal, Alessandro Toccolini, Ilda Vagge and Paolo S. Ferrario (2015) 'Guidelines for the design of a healing garden for the rehabilitation of psychiatric patients', *Journal of Agricultural Engineering*, 36(4): 43–51.

151 Petros, Anthopoulos and Julia N. Georgi (2011) 'Landscape preference evaluation for hospital environmental design', *Journal of Environmental Protection*, 2(2): 639–647.

152 Jaffe, Eric (2015) 'The (pretty much totally) complete health care case for urban nature', *The Atlantic Citylab*, 20 October. Online. Available at www.citylab.com/weather/2015/10/the-pretty-much-totally-complete-health-case-for-urban-nature/411331/ (accessed 4 March 2017).

153 Dhillon, Sunny and Ian Bailey (2012) 'Life in the shadow of a psychiatric hospital can breed fear that spans generations', *The Globe and Mail*, 1 December. Online. Available at www.theglobeandmail.com/news/british-columbia/life-in-the-shadow-of-a-psychiatric-hospital.html (accessed 31 October 2016).

154 Peters, Terri and Stephen Verderber (2017) 'Territories of engagement in the design of ecohumanist healthcare environments', *Health Environments Research & Design Journal*, 10(2): 104–123.

155 Jiang and Verderber (2015): 15.

156 Ibid.: 16.

157 Slessor, Catherine (2015) 'Alder Hey Children's Hospital by BDP', *The Architects Journal*, 2 October. Online. Available at www.architectsjournal.co.uk/buildings/adrer-hey-childrens-hospital-by-bdp.html (accessed 3 March 2017).

158 Marcus, Claire Cooper and Marni Barnes (1999) *Healing Gardens: Therapeutic Benefits and Design Recommendations*. New York: John Wiley.

159 Schneyer, Joshua and M.B. Pell (2016) 'Unsafe at any level: millions of American children missing early lead tests, Reuters finds', *Reuters Investigates*, 9 June. Online. Available at www.reuters.com/investigates/special-report/lead-poisoning-testing-gaps/pdf (accessed 25 October 2016).

160 Al-Dosky, Ahmed H., Dhia J. Al-Timini and Saddam A. Al-Dabbag (2012) 'Lead exposure among the general population of Duhok governorate, Kurdistan region, Iraq', *Eastern Mediterranean Health Journal*, 18(9): 974–979. Online. Available at www.emro.who.int/emhj-volume-18-2012/issue-9/article-11.html (accessed 25 October 2016).

161 Lowe, Cody (2008) 'Sustainable farming vision takes root at Catawba farm', *The Roanoke Times*, 31 October. Online. Available at www.roanoke.com/webmin/news/sustainable-farming-vision-takes-root-at-catawba-farm.html (accessed 25 October 2016).

162 In 1997, the World Health Organization Consultation on Obesity met in Geneva, Switzerland, declaring that throughout history, weight gain and fat storage were viewed as signs of health and prosperity. Yet today, as standards of living rise, weight gain and obesity pose a major threat to global health. Obesity was cited as a key risk factor in the ontology of numerous noncommunicable diseases (NCDs).

163 Waxman, Amalia (2005) 'Why a global strategy on diet, physical activity and health?', in A.P. Simopoulos (ed.) 'Nutrition and fitness: mental health, aging, and the implementation of a healthy diet and physical activity lifestyle', *World Review of Nutrition and Diet*, 95(2): 162–166.

164 Wadden, Thomas A., Terence G. Wilson, Albert J. Stunkard and Robert I. Berkowitz (2011) *Obesity and Associated Eating Disorders: A Guide for Mental Health Professionals*, The Clinics Series: Internal Medicine. Philadelphia, PA: W.B. Saunders.

165 Chiou, Shu-Ti, Jen-Huai Chiang, Nicole Huang and Li-Yin Chien (2014) 'Health behaviors and participation in health promotion activities among hospital staff: which occupational group performs better?' *BioMed Central Health Services Research*, 14(2): 474–483.

166 Metzl, Jonathan M. and Kenneth MacLeish (2015) 'Mental illness, mass shootings, and the politics of American firearms', *American Journal of Public Health*, 105(2): 240–249. A shopworn adage applies: think globally; act locally. This remains the cornerstone, however, of leadership efforts to confront the current global mental health crisis.

167 Editorial (2007) 'Scale up services for mental disorders: a call for action', *The Lancet*, 6 October, 370: 1241–1252. Online. Available at www.who.int/choice/publications/p_2007_Scaling-up_Mental%20health%20services%mental%health.pdf (accessed 25 October 2016).

168 Levin, Aaron (2007) 'Psychiatric hospital design reflects treatment trends', *Psychiatric News*, 42(2): 9.

169 Bowers, Len, Karen James, Alan Quirk, Alan Simpson, James Sugar, Duncan Stewart and John Hodsoll (2015) 'Reducing conflict and containment rates on acute psychiatric wards: the Safewards cluster randomized controlled trial', *International Journal of Nursing Studies*, 52: 1412–1422. Adverse patient-staff occurrences are always of concern

to administrators. Media coverage documents damage caused by various acts of violence, with a single death of a nurse or physician stigmatizing a psychiatric institution for years, if not decades.

170 Anderson, Sulome (2015) 'How patient suicide affects psychiatrists', *The Atlantic*, 20 January. Online. Available at www.theatlantic.com/health/archive/2015/01/how-patient-suicide-affects-psychiatrists.html (accessed 25 October 2016). An unclean physical environment can cause patient illness, such as nosocomial infection, a leading cause of death in acute care hospitals and in long-term care settings for the aged.

171 Consumer Reports (2016) *Special Report: America's Antibiotic Crisis*. Consumer Reports, Online. Available at www.consumerreports.org/cro/health/hospital-acquired-infections/index.html (accessed 25 October 2016).

172 Fedoriw, Larysa M. and Barbara Meijer (2013) 'Infection prevention strategies in inpatient psychiatric units using patient acuity and motivation', *American Journal of Infection Control*, 41(6): S48. Treatment of both preexisting and newly acquired patient infections during psychiatric hospitalization require time-proven policies.

173 World Health Organization (2008) *Policies and Practices for Mental Health in Europe: Meeting the Challenges*. Copenhagen: WHO Regional Office for Europe. Online. Available at www.euro.who.int/InformationSources/Publications/Catalogue/20081009_1 (accessed 26 October 2016).

174 Bradford City Clinical Commissioning Group (2016) *What You Tell Us About Mental Health Services*. Bradford: National Health Service. Online. Available at www.bradfordcityccg.nhs.uk/about-us/our-performance/our-plans-for-mental-health.html (accessed 26 October 2016).

175 Hohenadel, Kristin (2015) 'This is what a psychiatric ward designed by patients looks like', *Slate.com*, 19 March. Online. Available at www.slate.com/blogs/the_eye/2015/03/19/madlove_a_designer_asylum_from_james_leadbitter_the_vacuum_cleaner_is.html (accessed 4 March 2017).

176 US Environmental Protection Agency (2010) *Defining Life Cycle Assessment*, October. Washington, DC: Environmental Protection Agency. Online. Available at www.gdrc.org/uem/lca-define.hyml (accessed 26 October 2016). The aim is, ideally, to construct mental health care environments that tread as lightly on the earth as possible, achieving carbon neutrality and net-regenerative give-backs.

177 Brownell, Elaine (2016) 'Understanding embodied energy in design', *Architect*, 29 April. Online. Available at www.architectmagazine.com/technology/understanding-embodied-energy-in-design.html (accessed 27 October 2016).

178 Canter, David V. and Sandra Canter, eds. (1979) *Designing for Therapeutic Environments: A Review of Research*. London: John Wiley & Sons.

179 Zimring, Craig, Godfried L. Augenbroe, Eileen B. Malone and Blair L. Sadler (2008) 'Implementing healthcare excellence: the vital role of the CEO in evidence-based design', *Health Environments Research & Design Journal*, 1(3): 7–21. Also Cochran, Brian (1978) 'Design and planning of psychiatric facilities', *Hospital and Community Psychiatry*, 29(8): 533–537.

180 Verderber (2010): 169.

181 Hochman, Michael E. (2013) *50 Studies Every Doctor Should Know: The Key Studies that Form the Basis of Evidence-Based Medicine*. Oxford: Oxford University Press.

182 Sadler, Blair L., Leonard L. Berry, Robin Guenther, D. Kirk Hamilton, Frederick A. Hessler, Clayton Merritt and Derek Parker (2011) 'Fable hospital 2.0: the business case for building better health care facilities', *Hastings Center Report*, January-February, 41(1): 12–23.

183 Hessam, Sadatsafavi and John Walewski (2013) 'Corporate sustainability: the environmental design and human resource management interface in healthcare settings', *Health Environments Research & Design Journal*, 6(2): 98–118.

184 Kaplan and Berman (2010). Also see Kaplan, Stephen (1995) 'The restorative benefits of nature: toward an integrative framework', *Journal of Environmental Psychology*, 15(2): 169–182.

185 Dinesh, Arya (2011) 'So, you want to design an acute mental health inpatient unit: physical issues for consideration', *Australian Psychiatry*, 19(2): 163–167.

186 Curtis, Sarah, Wilbert Gesler, Victoria Wood, Ian Spencer, James Mason, Helen Close and Joseph Reilly (2013) 'Compassionate containment? Balancing technical safety and therapy in the design of psychiatric wards', *Social Science and Medicine*, 97(4): 201–209.

187 Eggert, Jon E., Sean P. Kelly, David T. Margiotta, Donna K. Hegvik, Kairi A. Vaher and Rachel Tamiko Kaya (2014) 'Person-environment interaction in a new secure forensic state psychiatric hospital', *Behavioral Sciences and the Law*, 32(4): 527–538.

188 Blumenthal, David (2009) 'Stimulating the adoption of health information technology', *New England Journal of Medicine*, 360(7): 1477–1479.

189 Behavioral Health IT Coalition (2016) 'About Us', *Behavioral Health IT Coalition*, Online. Available at www.bhitcoalition.org/home.html (accessed 31 October 2016).

190 Medved, James P. (2014) 'Top 10 mental health technology statistics of 2014', *Capterra Medical Software Blog*, 13 March. Online. Available at www.blog.capterra.com/top-10-mental-health-technology-statistics-2014.html (accessed 31 October 2016).

191 Horahan, Kevin, Herman Morchel and Lee Stevens (2014) 'Electronic health records during a disaster', *Online Journal of Public Health Informatics*, 5(3): 232–242.

192 Associated Press (2007) 'Katrina flooding "unimaginable": official at nursing home deaths trial', *CBCNews/World*, 17 August. Online. Available at www.cbc.ca/news/world/katrina-flooding-unimaginable-official-at-nursing-home-deaths.html (accessed 31 October 2016).

193 Robinson, Kelly (2013) 'Eight years after Katrina: St. Rita's owners still feel the stigma', *ABC News*, 29 August. Online. Available at www.

abcnews.go.com/US/years-katrina-st-ritas-owners-feel-stigma/story?id=20110312.html (accessed 31 October 2016).

194 Lurie, Nicole, Karen DeSalvo and Kristen Finne (2015) 'Ten years after: progress and challenges remain for U.S. emergency preparedness', *Health Affairs*, 27 August. Online. Available at www.healthaffairs.org/blog/2015/08/27/ten-years-after-hurricane-katrina-progress-and-challenges-remain-for-us-emergency-preparedness/ (accessed 4 March 2017). Also see Rhodes, Jean, Christina Paxton, Cecilia E. Rouse, Mary Waters and Elizabeth Fussell (2010) 'The impact of Hurricane Katrina on the mental and physical health of low-income parents in New Orleans', *American Journal of Orthopsychiatry*, 80(2): 237–247.

195 Ramsey, Donovan X. (2015) 'Recovering from PTSD after Hurricane Katrina', *The Atlantic*, 1 September. Online. Available at www.the atlantic.com/health/archive/2015/09/ptsd-after-hurricane-katrina/403162/ (accessed 4 March 2017). Also see Carey, Benedict (2007) 'Mood problems prevalent after Katrina, survey finds', *The New York Times*, 4 December. Online. Available at www.nytimes.com/2007/12/04/health/research/04katr.html?_r=0 (accessed 4 March 2017).

196 Peters, Terri and Stephen Verderber (2017) 'Territories of engagement in the design of ecohumanist healthcare environments', *Health Environments Research & Design Journal*, 10(2): 104–123.

197 Grunden, Naida and Charles Hagood (2012) *Lean-Led Hospital Design: Creating the Efficient Hospital of the Future*. Boca Raton: CRC Press/Taylor & Francis.

198 International Facilities Management Association (2017) *Operations and Maintenance Benchmarks Survey for Healthcare Facilities*. IFMA. Online. Available at www.ifma.org/docs/default-source/surveys/hcc_ombenchmarksurvey (accessed 9 March 2017).

199 Schwarz, Ken (2015) 'Can salutogenic outcomes be achieved through public private partnerships?' *World Health Design*, 8(6): 68–77.

Chapter 6

1 Simpson, Veronica (2015) 'Care and craftsmanship in a home for the elderly', *designcurial.com*, 20 January. Online. Available at www.designcurial.com/news/brief-encounters-19012015-4491343 (accessed 12 August 2016).

2 Ring, Wilson (2016) 'After Vermont storm, a mental health rainbow', *Chicago Tribune*, 2 September: 14.

3 Albright, Brian (2014) 'Vermont Psychiatric Care Hospital rebuilds after hurricane', *Behavioral Healthcare*, 22(11/12): 36–38. Online. Available at www.http://behavioral.net.html (accessed 12 June 2016).

4 Guenther, Robin and Gail Vittori (2013) 'Case study 40: Helsingor Psychiatric Clinic', in *Sustainable Healthcare Architecture*. New York: John Wiley: 371–374.

5 Moisse, Katie (2012) 'De Hogeweyk Dutch village doubles as nursing home', *ABC News*, 10 April. Online. Available at www.abcnews.go.com/Health/Community/alzheimers-disease-dutch-village.html (accessed 24 August 2016).

6 Fernandes, Edna (2012) 'Dementiaville: how an experimental new town is taking the elderly back to their happier and healthier pasts with astonishing results', *The Daily Mail*. Dailymail.co.uk. Online. Available at www.dailymail.co.uk/news/article-2109801/Dementiaville-How-experimental-new-town-elderly-back-astonishing-results.html (accessed 24 August 2016).

7 Hans, Barbara (2012) 'Living in the moment: Dutch village offers dignified care for dementia sufferers', *Spiegel*, 29 March. Online. Available at www.spiegel.de/international/europe/dutch-village-for-for-elderly-with-dementia-offers-dignified-care.html (accessed 24 August 2016).

8 Anon (2014) 'Reinventing care: bridging the gap between medical and mental health care', *The Hamilton Spectator*, 30 September: A4.

9 Simpson, Veronica (2015) 'Care and craftsmanship in a home for the elderly', *designcurial.com*, 20 January. Online. Available at www.designcurial.com/news/brief-encounters-19012015-4491343 (accessed 12 August 2016).

10 DiNardo, Anne (2015) 'Seattle children's hospital psychiatry and behavioural medicine unit', *Healthcare Design*, 17 April. Online. Available at www.healthcaredesignmagazine.com/article/photo-tour-seattle-children-s-hospital-psychiatry-and-behavioral-medicine-unit.html (accessed 12 August 2016).

11 Sydenham Gardens Board of Directors (2016) 'Annual evaluation of Sydenham Garden, 2015/2016', *Sydenham Garden*. Online. Available at www.sydenhamgarden.org.uk/wp-content/uploads/Sydenham-Garden-Annual-evaluation.pdf (accessed 9 September 2016).

12 Jencks, Charles and Edwin Heathcote (2010) *The Architecture of Hope: Maggie's Cancer Caring Centres*. London: Frances Lincoln.

13 Jencks, Charles (2017) 'Maggie's architecture: The deep affinities between architecture and health', *Architectural Design*, 246(1): 66–75. Also see Verderber, Stephen (2010) *Innovations in Hospital Architecture*, London: Routledge: 250–257.

14 Chatzi-Chousein, Berrin (2015) 'Henning Larsen Architects wins competition of new mental health building at Bispebjerg Hospital', *worldarchitecture.org*, 28 May. Online. Available at www.worldarchitecture.org/architecture-news/cchgf/henning-larson-wins-competition-of-new-mental-health-building-at-bispebjerg-hospital.html (accessed 17 November 2015). Innovations in Architecture+Health Series

APPENDIX

Urban morphology of CAMH since 1860

Six urban analyses were generated. These representations document a trajectory of change from 1860 to 2020 on the CAMH campus and its immediate neighborhood in Toronto (Figures A.1–A.6).

Figure-ground relationships

The first buildings erected on the Queen Street West campus are the original asylum, the superintendent's residence, and the groundskeeper's workshop. The Provincial Exhibition Hall is shown immediately to the south of the asylum (1860). The two Tully Wings (East and West) are built, with additional outbuildings in time erected along the outer security wall perimeter, and this occurs as surrounding land parcels are soon developed into a working-class residential neighborhood. Development occurs to the north and east of the asylum. The Provincial Exhibition Hall is later demolished, although this parcel, situated between the asylum and the lakefront, continues to be used as open space for special events (1900). Sixty years later, the neighborhood on all sides of the asylum has been extensively developed; the 1956 Administration Building is built immediately in front to the asylum, partially obscuring it from Queen West Street; and a heavy rail line, built along the lakeside edge of the asylum, serves the city's burgeoning industries.

Additional outbuildings are added and the formidable, 12-foot-high brick perimeter wall surrounding the asylum campus is fortified. It has few openings and some sections along the front side of the campus are wrought-iron fencing (1960). More recently, the surrounding neighborhood begins to densify further, with the industrial district to the south of the campus transforming into an upscale residential and mixed-use enclave by 2010. Meanwhile, the 1970s campus redevelopment plan's footprint remains intact as of 2015. The CAMH redevelopment plan, when fully completed as envisioned, will result in the aforementioned nine-square campus completely built out with the exception of one parcel (left as a city-run pocket park), and all remaining available unbuilt parcels in the surrounding neighborhood will experience continued redevelopment pressures; in time, they will altogether disappear as a result of urban densification in the form of condo towers and upscale retail establishments (2020).

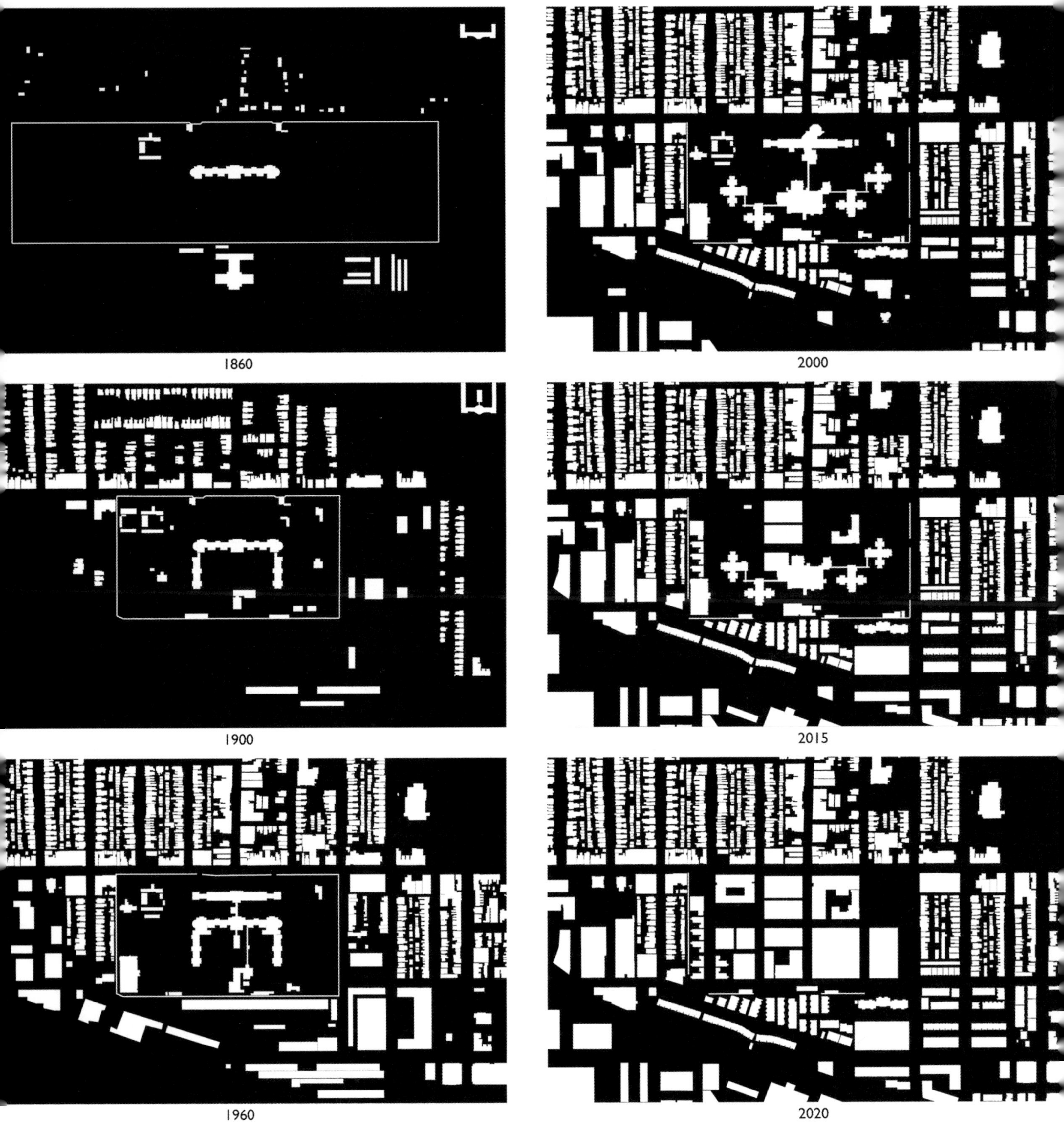

A.1 Figure-ground relationships.

Land use patterns

In the 19th century, the land north of Queen Street West continued to be used as open farmland, miles to the west of the city's growing urban core. To the south of the asylum and the Garrison Military Reserve, the land was originally intended to remain undeveloped. When the heavy rail line was built in the 1850s to the south of the asylum, industry followed, and Toronto's 'Crystal Palace' was soon constructed – that is, the aforementioned Provincial Exhibition Hall immediately south of the asylum (1860). By 1878 when Toronto was awarded the Provincial Fair, the city deemed the site inadequate for handling the increasing size of the crowds, so the hall was demolished and the site sold to the Massey-Harris Manufacturing Company (later Massey-Ferguson), which would later become the largest producer and exporter of agricultural equipment anywhere in the British Empire.

In 1880 the John Abell Engine and Machine Works was built just west of the asylum and north of the rail tracks. In 1894 the Toronto Glass Works was located on the south side of the asylum, and in 1899 it was purchased by the Diamond Glass Company of Montreal. These industries spurred the further construction of working-class neighborhoods so plant workers could live closer to the factories; narrow row houses first appeared soon after the initial asylum building was built. Queen Street West and Ossington Street evolved into vibrant commercial corridors serving new residential enclaves, while the area south of the asylum was transformed into industrial warehouses. The nearby Trinity College is relocated to the University of Toronto campus at this time, and the its former site becomes Trinity/Bellwood Park, a main public open space serving this rapidly growing section of Toronto by 1900. King Street West, directly to the south, becomes lined with underused and abandoned industrial warehouses and car dealerships by the 1960s.

More recently, elementary and middle schools are built nearby. Nonindustrial land uses include numerous artists' lofts and studios. These began to appear in significant numbers along King Street West, and together with the Sudbury Street townhouse enclave a new neighborhood arises by 2000. Queen Street West continues to evolve from a once-blighted low-rise commercial strip into an upscale high-rise residential condo district. This district is now referred to as the Queen West Triangle and designated as an 'Urban Regeneration Zone' by the city. This district encompasses land occupied by the former freight railroad right-of-way, and it extends west to Dovercourt Road. Developers immediately purchased this land, and the city rezoned it to allow ever-denser, taller condo developments.

A similar pattern exists along nearby King Street West, to the south and east of CAMH. Queen Street West, on the north edge of campus, evolves from mom-and-pop groceries, art galleries, small shops, and restaurants into condo towers and upscale retail and restaurants. Meanwhile, the artists who have lived in the neighborhood for decades begin to be displaced due to the relentless forces of urban gentrification. With increasing densification, the need for urban pocket parkland became acute as the city struggled to upgrade its quality-of-life amenities in this regard (2015). Land-redevelopment pressures continued unabated throughout the neighborhoods surrounding CAMH. Densification and gentrification continue to spawn high-rise condo tower developments as most longtime shopkeepers are displaced due to skyrocketing land values. The Centre for Discovery and Knowledge Exchange (CDKE) is to be housed in a Phase 1C building abutting Queen Street West, also housing a storefront art gallery, the Workman Theatre, the Eli Lily Learning Centre, and the CAMH Public Information Centre. As for any remaining open space, by 2020 the sole nearby open green spaces are Shaw Park, Adelaide Common East, and Fennings Park.

Landscape amenities

Queen Street West in the 1850s was little more than an unpaved and muddy farm-to-market road. In time, it becomes the main vehicular approach into the city from the west. Much of the landscape surrounding the asylum is open prairie and agricultural land at this time, and these parcels include thick groves of mature tress (1860). Later, roads in the vicinity of the asylum are paved with brick, and the once-generous tree cover is significantly reduced due to clear-cutting for residential development to the north, west, and east of the asylum. Warehouse construction commences to the south, and very few trees remain in this industrial zone (1900). A significant increase in impervious surfaces occurs in areas surrounding the asylum and particularly to the south during these years, where factories have created large paved staging lots and

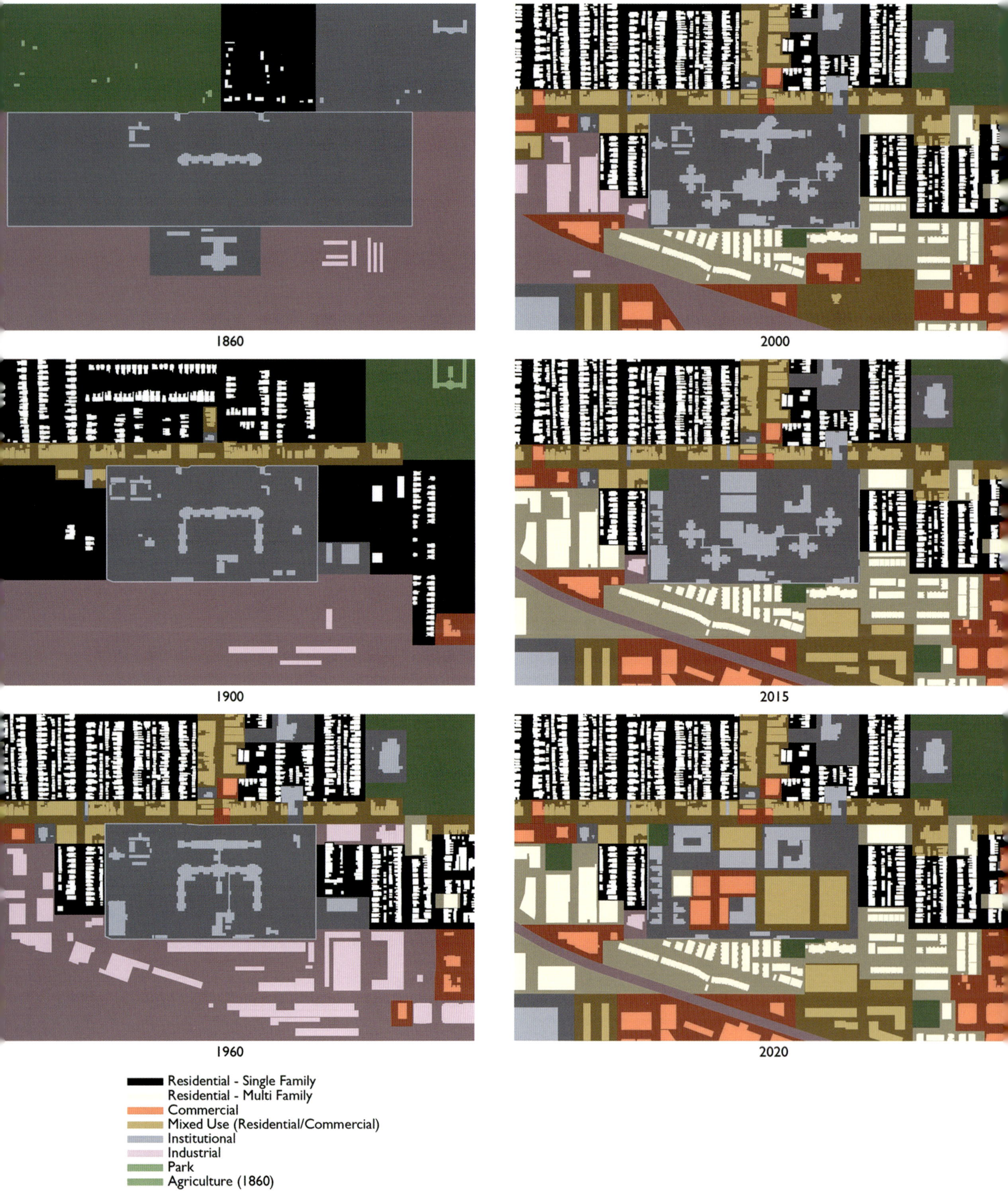
1860
2000
1900
2015
1960
2020
Residential - Single Family
Residential - Multi Family
Commercial
Mixed Use (Residential/Commercial)
Institutional
Industrial
Park
Agriculture (1860)

A.2 Land use.

parking lots for their workers, and the car dealerships located along King Street West are paved over.

As more buildings are constructed on the asylum campus, the amount of tress, open lawns, and ground vegetation becomes noticeably reduced by 1960. A tree-planting program occurs in Trinity Bellwoods Park where Trinity College Circle was once located (upper right in Figure A.3). King Street West is transformed by condo towers to the south. Pocket parks are created: Joseph Workman Park (named after the asylum's first medical superintendent), and the Massey-Harris Park, both south of the CAMH campus, restore somewhat the lost urban tree cover in a district that had suffered from reduced tree cover in the past century. Open green space is eliminated at the heart of the CAMH campus by the construction of the Phase 1A and 1B 'block buildings' that front Queen Street West. Parking is relocated below grade to a recently built deck (2012). Trees and open green space continue to be reduced on the CAMH campus. By 2015, only one undisturbed green space remains. The city commits to constructing a new public park, Lisgar Park, to the west of CAMH on former industrial land. This responds to some extent to the acute need for additional green space and pervious ground surfaces to replace what the CAMH 2020 plan destroyed – although this gesture is of little direct benefit because it is disconnected from the CAMH grounds.

Landmarks and anomalies

The masonry perimeter wall became a formidable landmark soon after its completion in 1850, and it is later expanded in 1889. The asylum is an architectural landmark in the West End section of the city. The Provincial Exhibition Hall, to the south of the asylum, is the second-most iconic building in the immediate area. As for open green space combined with impressive architecture, the Trinity College campus (upper right corner of Figure A.4) would later become a landmark public park. At 16 Ossington Street, Fire Hall No. 9 is completed in 1878. This structure is the oldest intact fire hall (station) in the city of Toronto. This status is attributable to its Italianate Style architecture and an unusual hose tower design. Designed by Stewart and Strickland, prominent architects of the era, the tower is visible from a distance.

Major land parcels of the asylum's once-expansive grounds are sold off to private interests, and the landmark brick wall is rebuilt to reflect this reduced campus footprint (1900). Many warehouses are constructed near to the asylum on and near King Street West and in the blocks directly behind the asylum. The Administration Building, completed in 1956, is an anomaly as it jarringly upstages the old asylum building directly behind it. The Great Hall on Queen Street becomes a citywide landmark. The former Carnegie Library, built in 1909, also on Queen Street West, is now a landmark heritage building, and the postal building (immediately next door) is also granted landmark heritage status by the city by the year 2000. Treatment Units A–D opened in 1972, and the large community building on the CAMH campus emerges as a local landmark. The old asylum structure is demolished in 1976, and later, the bland, modernist Administration Building immediately in front is also demolished (2010). The iconic asylum wall is demolished in some places as new buildings in Phase I of the CAMH redevelopment plan are completed by 2012; these structures are anomalous themselves due to their large scale and contrasting appearance compared to what they replaced (2015).

Other architecturally anomalous buildings are built as part of the anticipated final phase of the CAMH campus redevelopment; multiple city streets are 'pulled into' its once semipastoral grounds. CAMH at this point becomes the so-called *urban village* its architects envisioned, although in reality it is far more akin to an overbuilt mixed-use condo development enclave, with strikingly little open green space remaining. Moreover, the historic asylum wall will have been completely demolished. Sadly, a mere 4.8 acres, or 18% of the campus, will remain as open green space for patients' daily use, while 7.8 acres, or 29% of the campus, will have been given over to newly built, visually intrusive, public street rights-of-way and the aforementioned new 'block buildings'. At this point in time the CAMH campus is completely disconnected from its historic past (2020).

Sound/circulation patterns

In the beginning, asylum patients were encouraged to use the pastoral grounds while accompanied by an attendant, although they were confined within by the imposing brick wall isolating the campus from its semirural surroundings at that time. A raucous, noisy, working-class

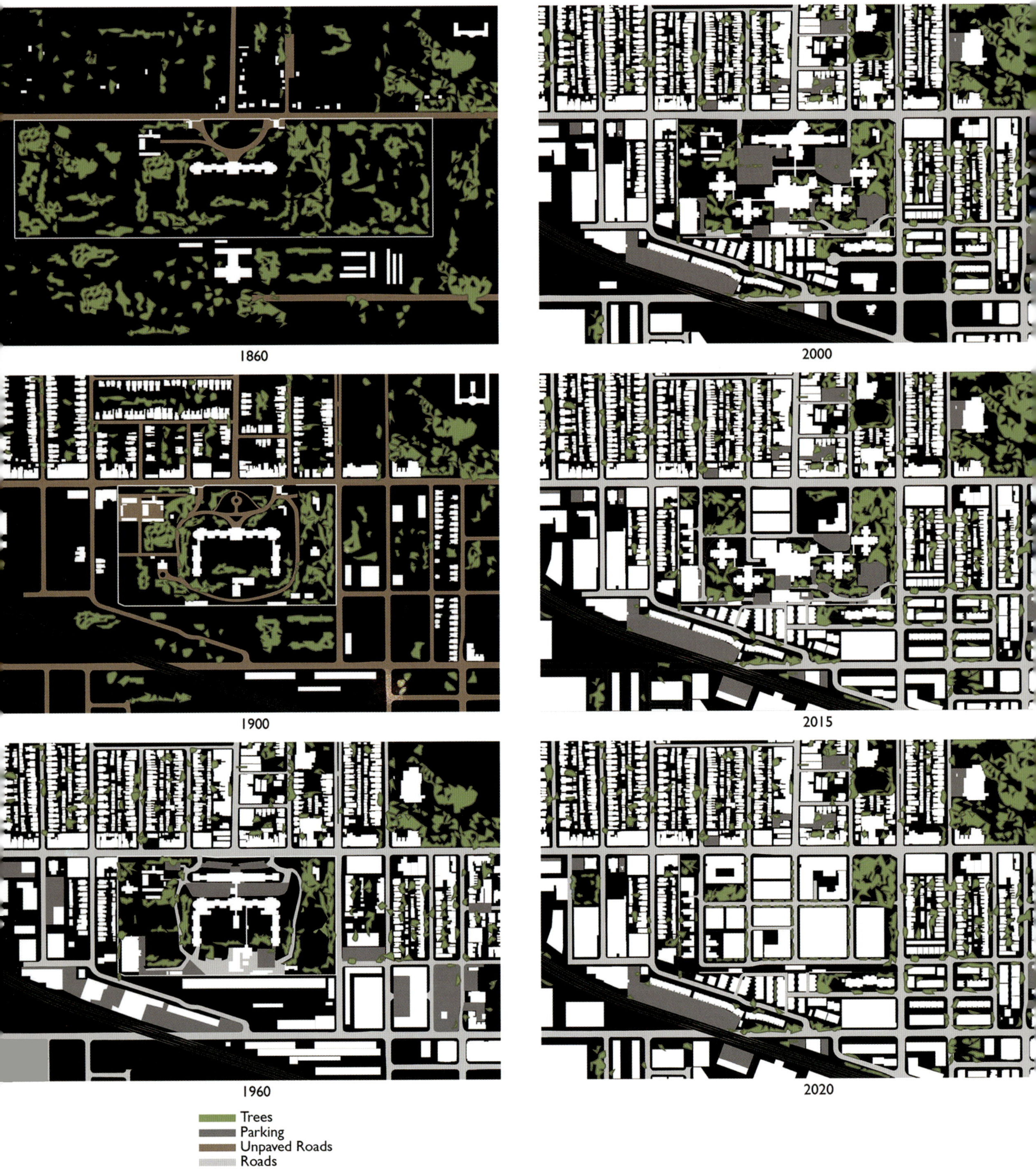

A.3 Landscape.

commercial district would flourish along Queen Street West near the asylum's main entrance. The Provincial Exhibition Hall, directly to the south, stages numerous public events annually, which at times can be heard inside the asylum, particularly during music events with marching bands or circuses that include animal shows (1860). The asylum's grounds are reduced in acreage as the bustling commercial district on Queen Street, combined with the railroad right-of-way to the south, are developed as residential zones to provide more housing in the immediate area for factory workers and others (1900).

Land use intensifies after the streetcar commences operations, and private vehicular traffic further clogs Queen Street West. Noise and traffic generated by the nearby rail yard and industrial district to the south become dominant by 1960. The industrial warehouse zone nearest the asylum begins to decline, as most factories close by 1980, while Queen Street West and Ossington Street evolve into vibrant commercial strips catering to an increasingly upscale clientele. Vehicular traffic volume intensifies further as a result of the construction of many mixed-use condo projects combined with the adaptation of many former industrial buildings by 2000. Unbridled gentrification and urban redevelopment continue throughout the neighborhood in these years and this generates increased traffic volumes, exacerbated by an expanding CAMH where outdoor green space for patient use is greatly diminished by the year 2020.

Transportation amenities

In the 1850s, the main east-west artery in the still largely undeveloped West End is the unpaved Queen Street West. It is one of the only streets that cuts across the entire city at that time and, as mentioned, becomes a major route to downtown (1860). Queen Street West is paved, streetcar service begins in the 1870s, and three additional streets in this rapidly developing district are paved – Ossington, King, and Shaw. Rail lines and the aforementioned freight yard are built to the south of the asylum, although pedestrian amenities such as sidewalks remain very limited in 1900. Sidewalks are soon built along neighboring streets near the asylum, streetcar service is upgraded, the asylum's internal circulation lanes are improved, and the volume of rail yard traffic greatly increases by 1960.

Rail yard traffic soon begins to diminish as a result of rapid deindustrialization of the zone in proximity to the urban waterfront, a waterfront soon repurposed in city master plan documents as public parkland. By contrast, pedestrian and cycling activity increases dramatically due to dozens of mixed-use condo developments being built in the neighborhood. Adjoining commercial corridors emerge as citywide destination points by 2015. By 2020, streetcar and bus service struggles to meet unprecedented ridership volumes due to continued gentrification and densification of the area surrounding CAMH. CAMH contributes to the urban congestion problem in the area as it draws more people to the site than ever before because of the new mixed-use buildings on the campus by 2020. Meanwhile, the public transit infrastructure in the neighborhood remains unchanged from 30 years earlier as urban gentrification and densification growth remain relatively unchecked. Unprecedented pressures are exerted on the straining transit infrastructure as streetcar, auto, bus, and even sidewalk use demand patterns intensify by 2020.

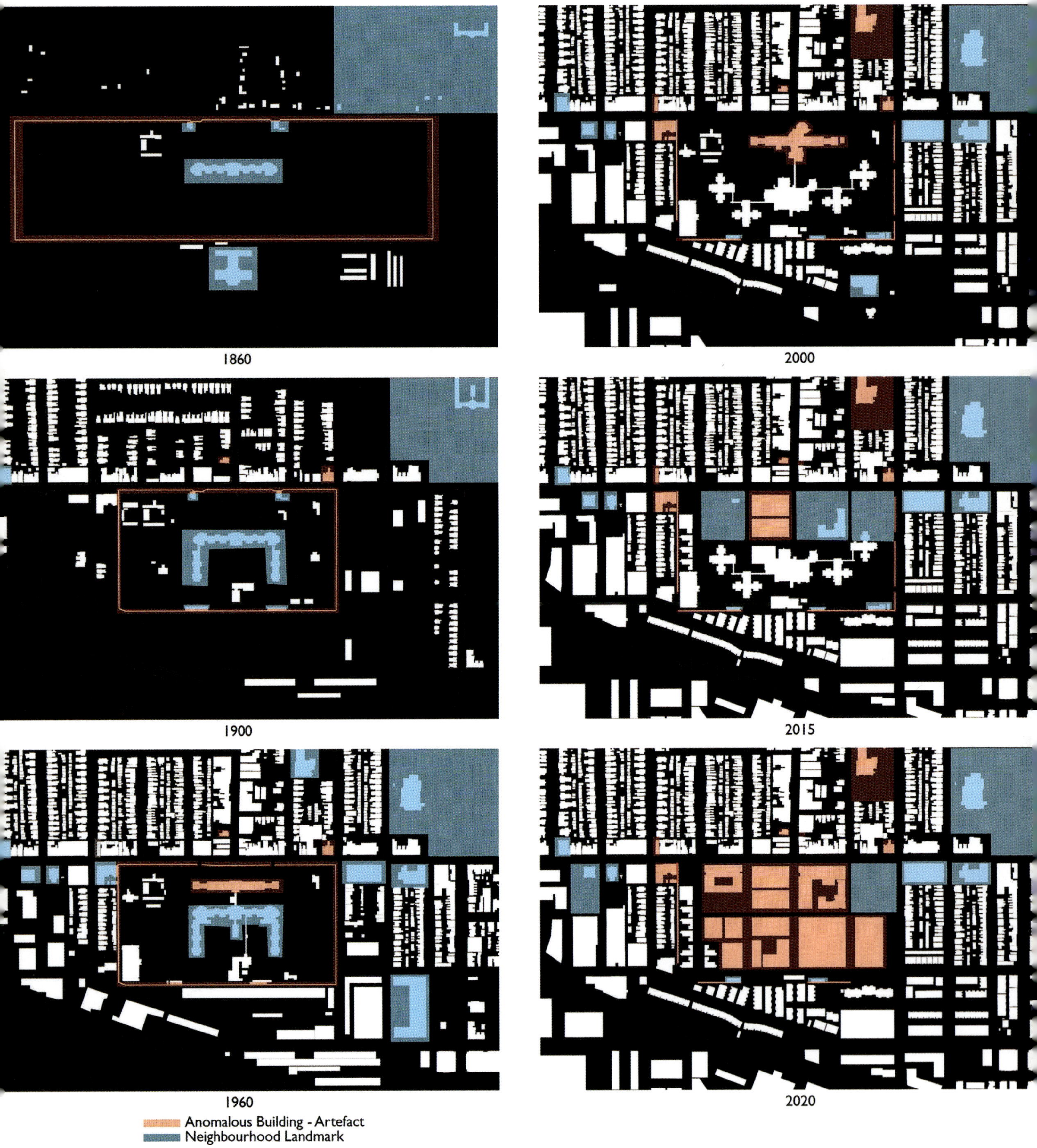

A.4 Landmarks and anomalies.

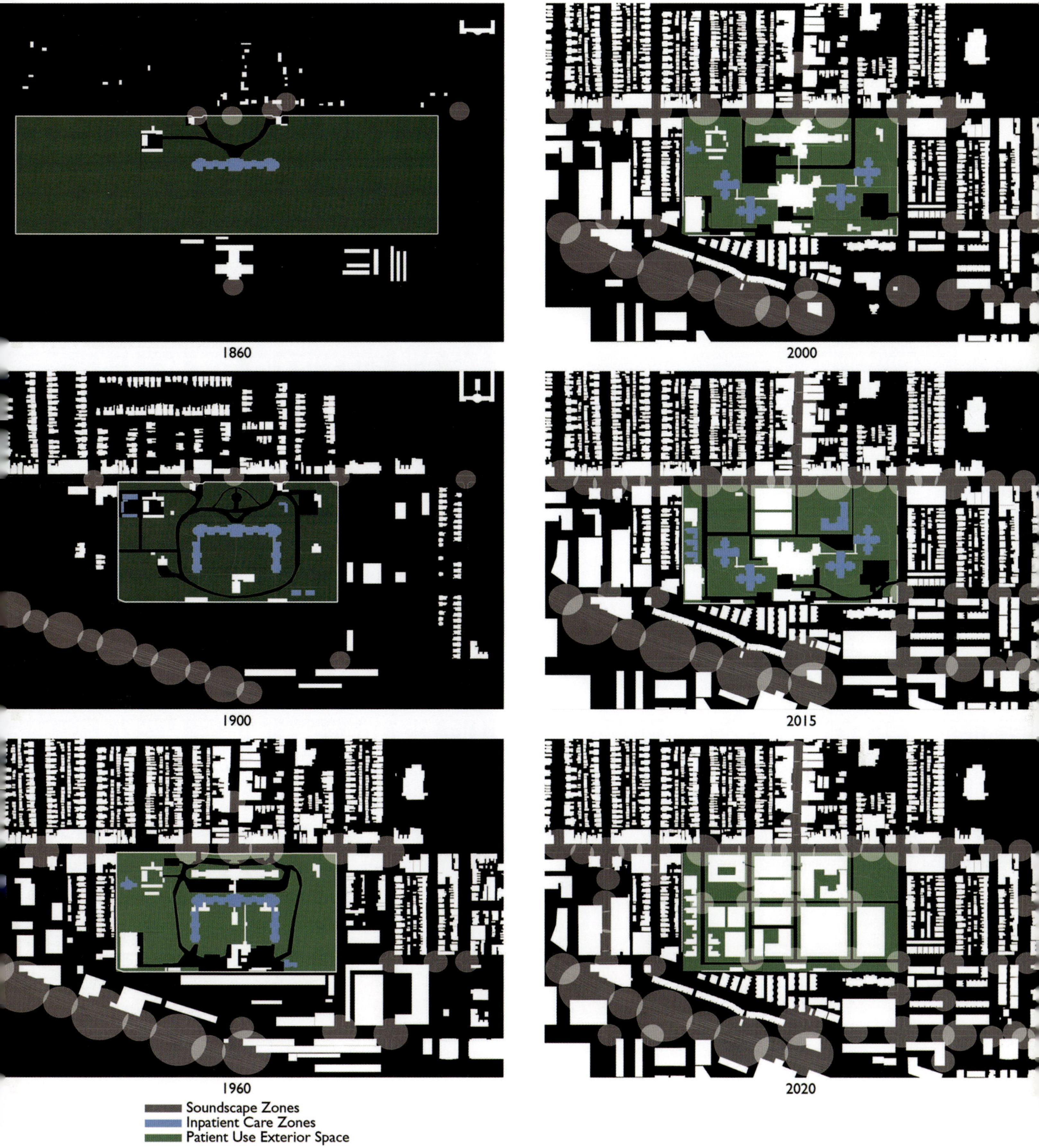

A.5 Sound/circulation patterns.

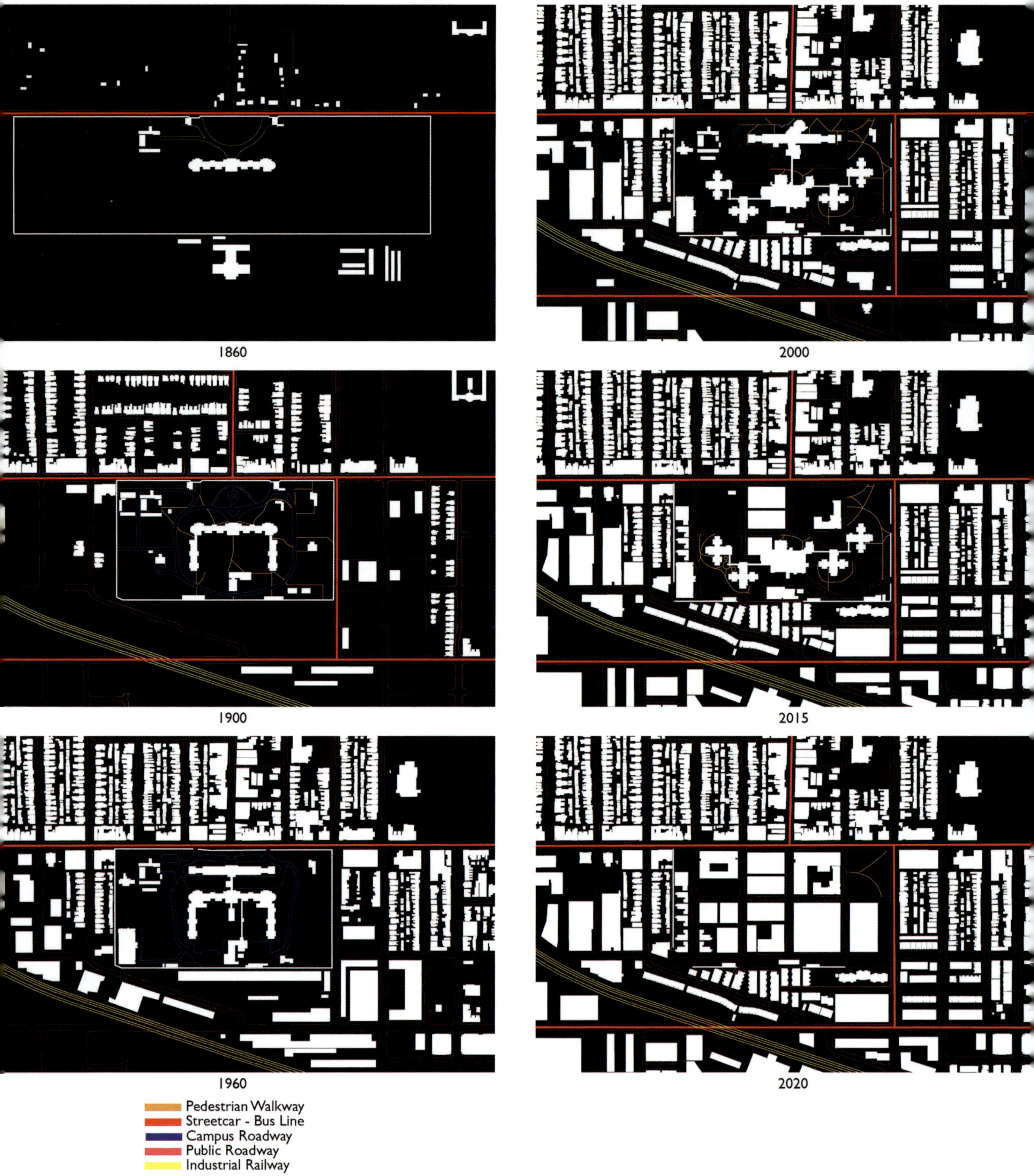

A.6 Transportation.

Postscript

The 25 case studies express diverse locational contexts, user constituencies, programmatic issues, architectural and site-planning concerns, and philosophical positions on the role of the built environment in mental illness and substance abuse treatment. Collectively, patterns become discernible, and 14 design concerns are distilled here. These are grounded in site and landscape, arrival sequences, views and daylighting, prospect-refuge amenities, theraserialization, circulation innovations, inpatient unit design and configuration, inpatient room amenities, community outreach amenities, the presence (or absence) of green roof terraces, gardens and landscaping, sustainable and regenerative energy systems, ecological habitat conservation, and transit and cycling amenities. These concerns are examined, comparatively, across the case studies. It proved interesting to compare and contrast in this regard. and the results of this assessment are presented in Figure 6.26.

Of universal priority across the case studies is a signature arrival sequence to the campus and the facility's main public entrance, high-quality views overlooking nature to varying degrees, the provision of daylighting in internal spaces to maximize therapeutic affordances, user-oriented directional graphics systems, semi-autonomous inpatient residential units and associated therapy/treatment zones, private patient rooms and bathrooms, varied landscape amenities including therapeutic gardens and terraces, and in some instances, green roofs, and contemplative (passive) outdoor spaces together with spaces for recreational (active) therapy activity (to promote prospect-refuge behaviours among patients, care providers, and visitors), and the importance of staff lounges and break rooms. An additional concern of relative high priority was the incorporation of facility energy systems minimally reliant on conventional fossil fuels, the use of low-e glazing and passive design strategies, on-site rainwater management retention systems, microgardens, and landscape design and materials to minimize total campus energy consumption.

Amenities of moderate to high concern across the case studies included a theraserialization concept yet to be embraced widely in psychiatric and substance abuse inpatient/outpatient environments. Many case studies did successfully express this concept to establish interconnectivity between building and landscape, together with other concepts associated with salutogenic healthcare design. In some case studies, high connectivity to the site environs was precluded due to a tight, restrictive urban site. In these cases, the facility, by default, often was turned inward and instead made use of green roof terraces, such as at the Marie Bashir Centre in Sydney, Australia.

Of lessor concern were efforts to promote local habit conservation, including the conservation of plant and animal species on-site. Also, relatively low priority was ascribed to the establishment of direct, sustainable connections to local transit and the cycling routes, including campus/facility connections to mass transit and whether or not this was of priority in the initial campus site selection process. Rural facilities face the greatest challenge in achieving sustainable linkages of this type. Two additional concerns of rather low priority was few case studies featured microfarming plots, public green spaces available for use by the local community, and provided mixed-use amenities within the facility and on the grounds – for example, a neighborhood grocery, branch bank, or coffeeshop housed on the ground level of a multilevel facility, or a daycare center, pharmacy, or a community-use meeting space. In light of Churchill's famous statement on the value of architecture, 'We shape our buildings; thereafter they shape us', we stand at this moment at the precipice of unprecedented opportunity. Architecture and landscape design hold the power to profoundly impact, positively, the lives of individuals who suffer from mental illnesses and substance abuse addictions, globally. Let us not squander this rare opportunity.

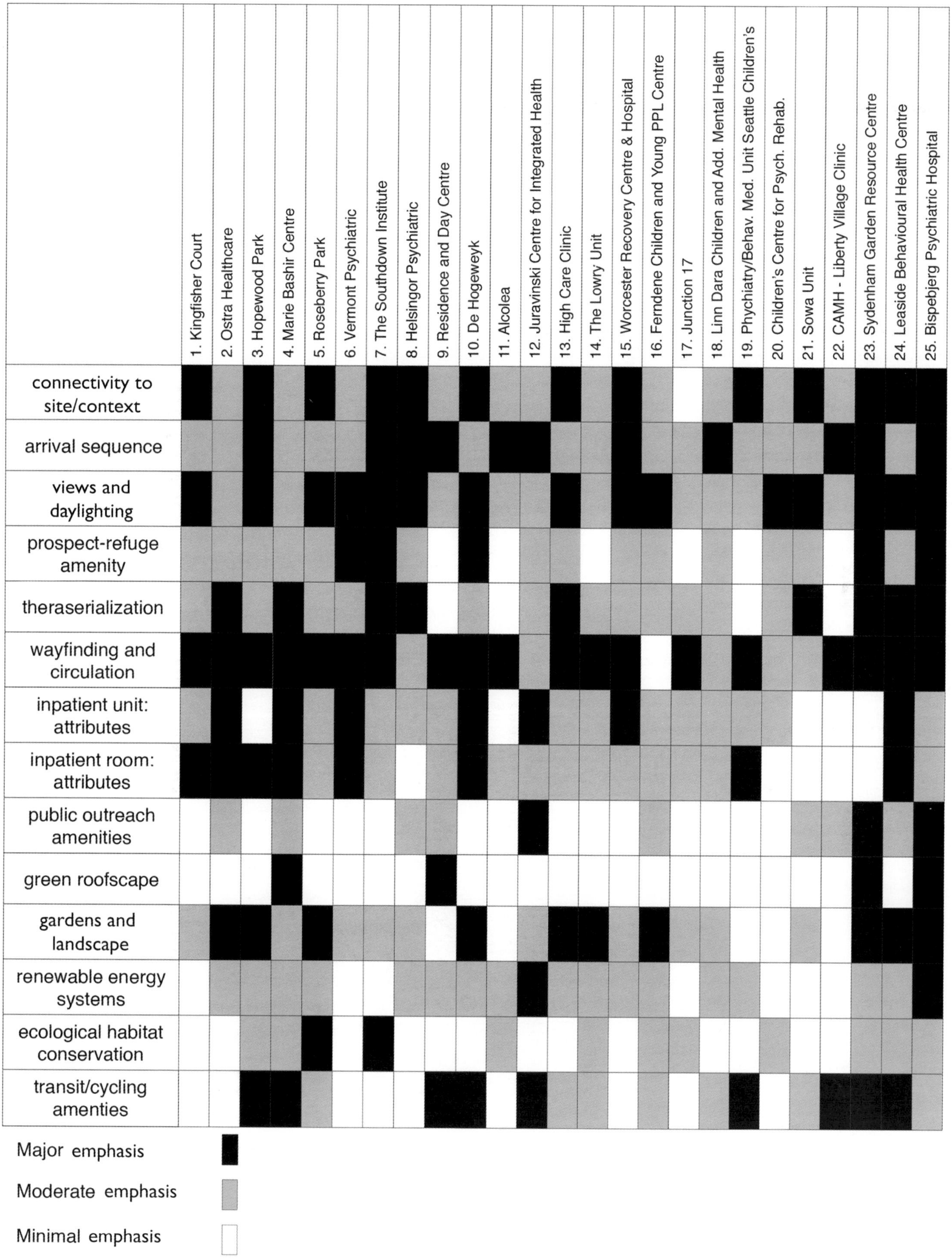

PS.1 Featured landscape and architectural attributes in case studies 1–25.

Index

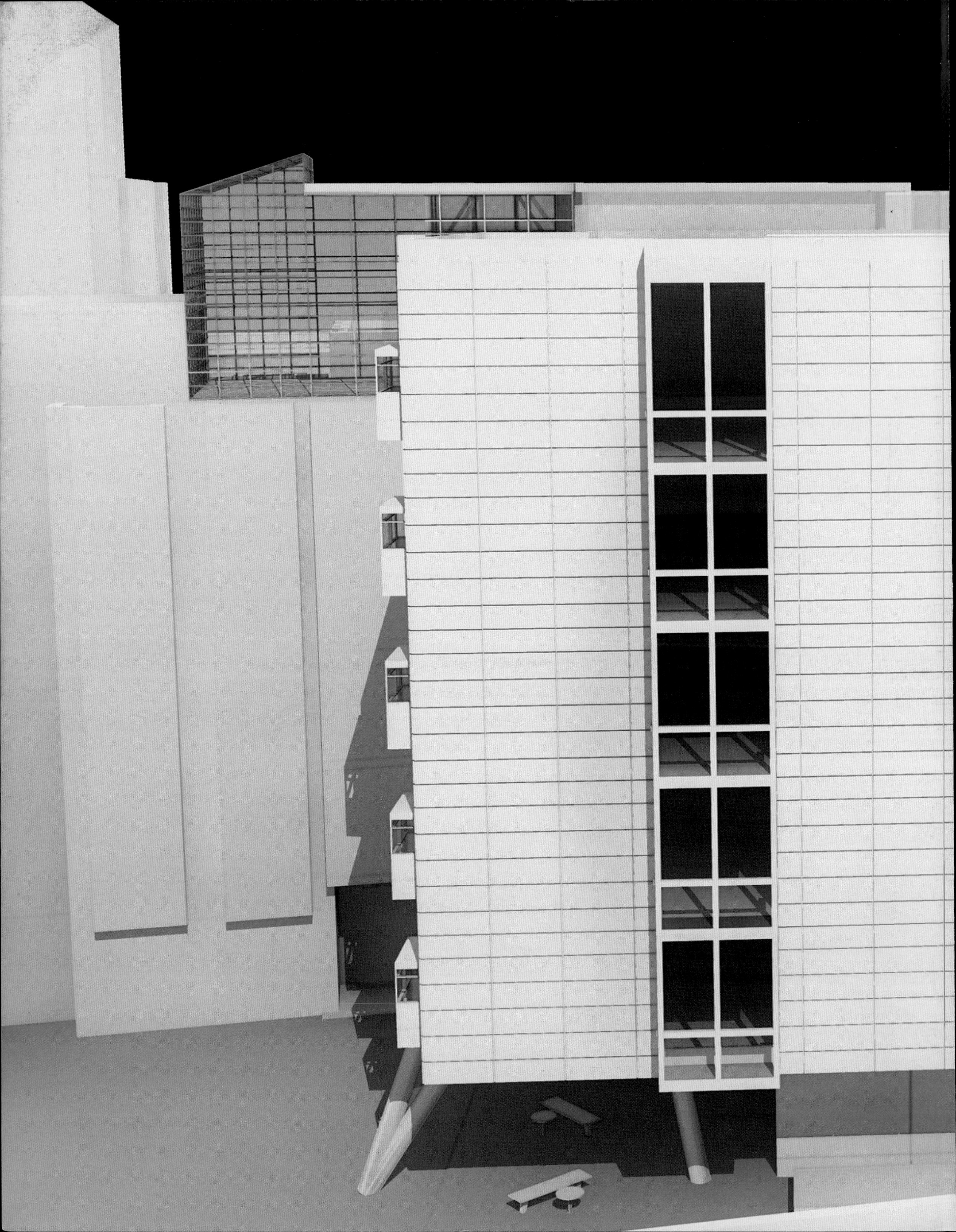

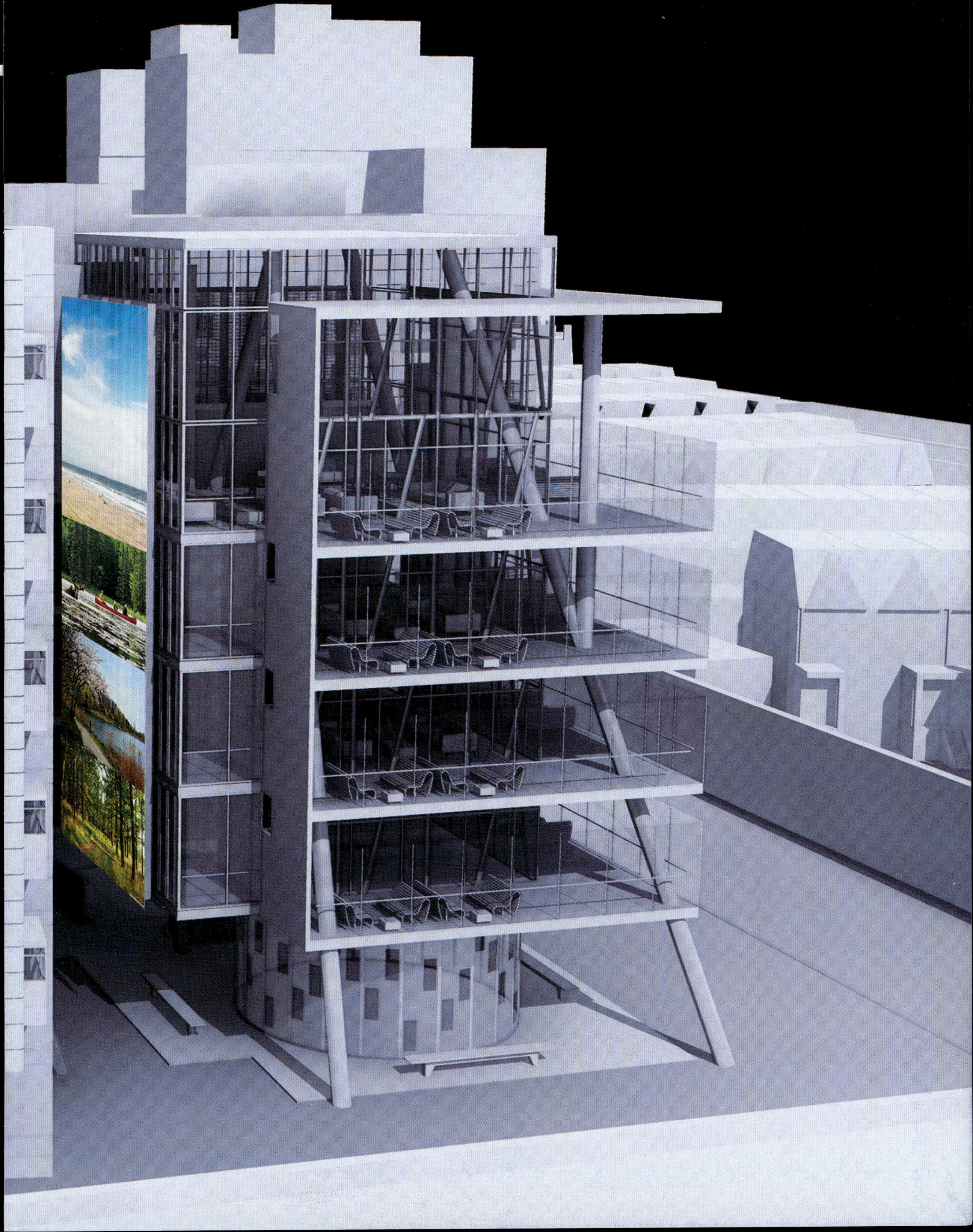

INNOVATIONS IN ARCHITECTURE+HEALTH SERIES

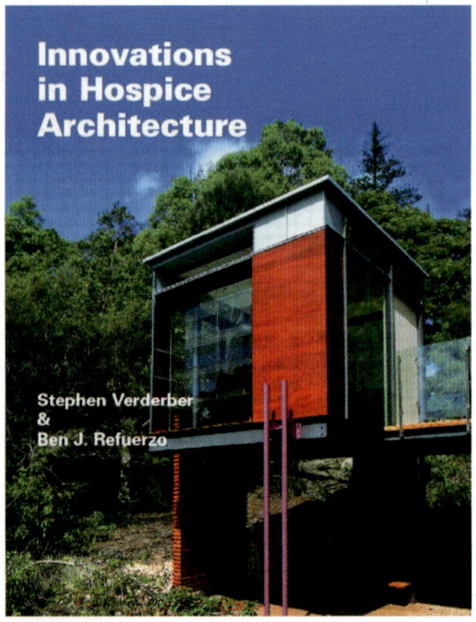

INNOVATIONS IN HOSPICE ARCHITECTURE
BY STEPHEN VERDERBER AND BEN J. REFUERZO

Providing much-needed focus on hospice projects in the context of unprecedented rates of societal ageing, this reference book presents an overview of major recent developments in this rapidly evolving building type. The authors examine the historical origins of the contemporary hospice and the diverse contemporary variations on the basic premise of hospice care, and offer a series of eighteen international case studies of exemplary hospices.

The most innovative work in this area over the past decade has been in Japan, the US, Canada and the UK, and the authors describe and analyze examples both as individual projects and as comparable yet differing approaches. A case study designed by the authors for Hospice Hawaii is presented as a vehicle to explore and test the 74 design considerations presented in Chapter 4. *Hospice Architecture* is essential reading for anyone involved in the planning, design and construction of hospices.

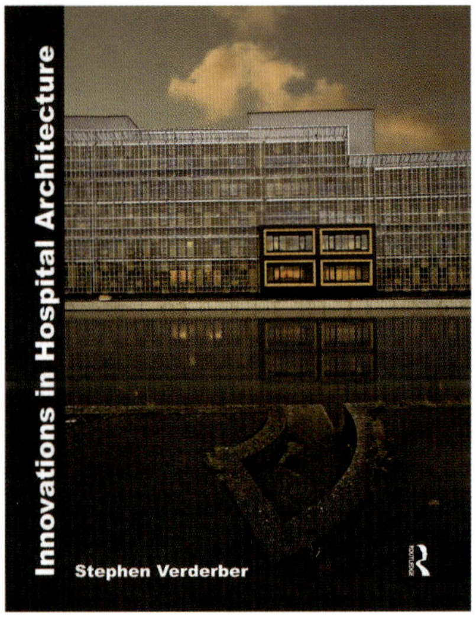

INNOVATIONS IN HOSPITAL ARCHITECTURE
BY STEPHEN VERDERBER

This groundbreaking book captures key recent developments in the rapidly evolving field of sustainable hospital architecture. Today's architects must provide hospitals which enable high-quality care for diverse patient populations in carbon neutral care settings, and this book succinctly considers what needs to be done in order to meet that challenge. The contemporary hospital is viewed in the context of global climate change, the planet's diminishing natural resources and the spiralling cost of operating healthcare facilities.

The future of the hospital is examined, and the author supplies a compendium of 100 planning and design considerations for the building type. The research includes twenty-eight case studies of built and unbuilt hospitals from around the world. These are grouped into five types – autonomous community-based hospitals, children's hospitals, rehabilitation and elderly care centres and hospitals, regional medical centre campuses, and visionary (unbuilt) projects.

Extensively illustrated with photographs, diagrams and floor plans, this is essential reading for architects, planners, engineers, product manufacturers, clients, healthcare providers and government agencies involved in the present and future of sustainable healthcare environments.

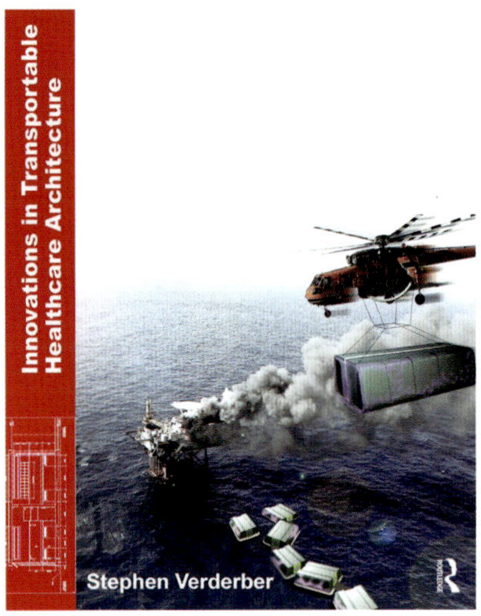

INNOVATIONS IN TRANSPORTABLE HEALTHCARE ARCHITECTURE
BY STEPHEN VERDERBER

Innovations in Transportable Healthcare Architecture is the first book to examine how healthcare architecture can provide far more proactive and effective support in disaster-stricken communities globally. Created for architects and allied professions working across the disaster mitigation spectrum, it provides:

- Global case studies which demonstrate real examples;
- Historical perspectives on redeployables used in past military and civilian contexts;
- Analysis of the advantages, challenges, and opportunities associated with offsite, premanufactured healthcare facilities and their component systems, for permanent installations or reuse on multiple sites;
- Planning and design considerations for transportable offsite-built healthcare architecture;
- State-of-the-art research on pop-up clinics, truck-based configurations, ISO container-based outpatient clinical and trauma care centres, and modularized facilities for contemporary military and civilian contexts.